AF360709

Sensors for Gait, Posture, and Health Monitoring

Sensors for Gait, Posture, and Health Monitoring

Volume 2

Special Issue Editor

Thurmon Lockhart

MDPI • Basel • Beijing • Wuhan • Barcelona • Belgrade

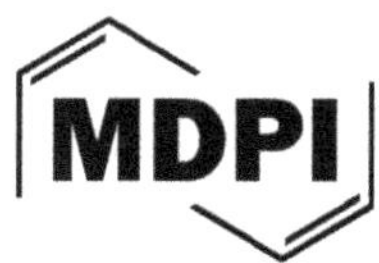

Special Issue Editor
Thurmon Lockhart
Arizona State University
USA

Editorial Office
MDPI
St. Alban-Anlage 66
4052 Basel, Switzerland

This is a reprint of articles from the Special Issue published online in the open access journal *Sensors* (ISSN 1424-8220) from 2017 to 2019 (available at: https://www.mdpi.com/journal/sensors/special_issues/Gait_Recognition).

For citation purposes, cite each article independently as indicated on the article page online and as indicated below:

LastName, A.A.; LastName, B.B.; LastName, C.C. Article Title. *Journal Name* **Year**, *Article Number*, Page Range.

Volume 2
ISBN 978-3-03936-344-5 (Pbk)
ISBN 978-3-03936-345-2 (PDF)

Volume 1-3
ISBN 978-3-03936-348-3 (Pbk)
ISBN 978-3-03936-349-0 (PDF)

© 2019 by the authors. Articles in this book are Open Access and distributed under the Creative Commons Attribution (CC BY) license, which allows users to download, copy and build upon published articles, as long as the author and publisher are properly credited, which ensures maximum dissemination and a wider impact of our publications.

The book as a whole is distributed by MDPI under the terms and conditions of the Creative Commons license CC BY-NC-ND.

Contents

About the Special Issue Editor

Thurmon Lockhart is Professor in the Biomedical Engineering and Biological Design program in the School of Biological Health and Systems Engineering at Arizona State University, Tempe, AZ. He is also Adjunct Professor at the Barrow Neurological Institute, Research Affiliate at the Mayo Clinic College of Medicine, Division of Endocrinology, and Guest Professor at Ghent University in Belgium. His research focuses on the identification of injury mechanisms and the quantification of sensorimotor deficits and movement disorders associated with aging and neurological disorders on fall accidents. His academic grounding in biomechanical modeling, nonlinear dynamics, human postural control, gait mechanics, and wearable biosensor design underscore a fundamental capacity to provide unique clinical solutions to injury prevention utilizing both engineering and biomedical principles. He has translated research findings into practice by reaching a significant number of external organizations and individuals. His outreach efforts have impacted several organizations, including UPS, the US Navy, Los Alamos National Security, the DOE, GE, and BP. In recognition of these scientific achievements, Prof. Lockhart and co-workers were awarded the Alexander C. Williams, Jr., Design Award from the Human Factors and Ergonomics Society in 2008. His research was recently featured on the PBS NOVA ScienceNow and Good Morning America programs and in the Fortune, AgingWell, Men's Health, and Discover magazines.

Preface to "Sensors for Gait, Posture, and Health Monitoring"

The acquisition of gait and postural characteristics during active and passive movements provides important information about limb propulsion and postural control strategies and provides insight into performance and risk of injury. These measures were traditionally assessed by utilizing motion capture systems and force plates. Although modern motion capture laboratories collect precise gait and posture data, they are expensive and immobile and require serial (single person at-a-time data capture) and clustered data collection, limiting the use of motion capture in the field to obtain more realistic motion profiles that may be applicable to various interventions.

As such, in recent years, many technologies for gait and posture assessments have emerged. Wearable sensors, active and passive in-house monitors, and many combinations thereof all promise to provide accurate measures of gait and posture parameters. The objective of this Special Issue is to address and disseminate the latest gait and posture monitoring systems as well as various mathematical models/methods that characterize mobility functions.

This Special Issue explores the core scientific issues associated with the use of custom-designed, wearable, wireless sensor nodes for continuous, non-invasive gait–posture–activity monitoring and analysis in order to accurately study the relationship between these monitoring variables and physical and psychological health conditions to predict adverse medical events in a variety of populations. This type of assessment will dramatically expand the clinical usefulness of these analyses and pave the way for identifying potential adverse health conditions and appropriate interventions for those most at risk.

Thurmon Lockhart
Special Issue Editor

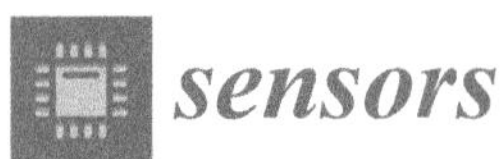 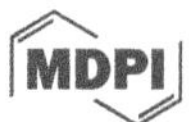

Article

Gait Shear and Plantar Pressure Monitoring: A Non-Invasive OFS Based Solution for e-Health Architectures

Cátia Tavares [1,2,*], M. Fátima Domingues [1,3], Anselmo Frizera-Neto [4], Tiago Leite [2], Cátia Leitão [1,2], Nélia Alberto [1], Carlos Marques [1], Ayman Radwan [1], Eduardo Rocon [3], Paulo André [5] and Paulo Antunes [1,2]

[1] Instituto de Telecomunicações, Campus Universitário de Santiago, Aveiro 3810-193, Portugal; fatima.domingues@ua.pt (M.F.D.); catia.leitao@ua.pt (C.L.); nelia@ua.pt (N.A.); carlos.marques@ua.pt (C.M.); aradwan@av.it.pt (A.R.); pantunes@ua.pt (P.A.)

[2] Department of Physics & I3N, University of Aveiro, Campus Universitário de Santiago, Aveiro 3810-193, Portugal; tmpl@ua.pt

[3] CSIC-UPM, Ctra. Campo Real, Arganda del Rey 28500, Madrid, Spain; e.rocon@csic.es

[4] Telecommunications Laboratory, Electrical Engineering Department, Federal University of Espírito Santo, Espírito Santo 29075-910, Brazil; frizera@ieee.org

[5] Department of Electrical and Computer Engineering and Instituto de Telecomunicações, Instituto Superior Técnico, University of Lisbon, Lisbon 1049-001, Portugal; paulo.andre@lx.it.pt

* Correspondence: catia.tavares@ua.pt; Tel.: +351-234-377-900

Received: 26 March 2018; Accepted: 20 April 2018; Published: 25 April 2018

Abstract: In an era of unprecedented progress in sensing technology and communication, health services are now able to closely monitor patients and elderly citizens without jeopardizing their daily routines through health applications on their mobile devices in what is known as e-Health. Within this field, we propose an optical fiber sensor (OFS) based system for the simultaneous monitoring of shear and plantar pressure during gait movement. These parameters are considered to be two key factors in gait analysis that can help in the early diagnosis of multiple anomalies, such as diabetic foot ulcerations or in physical rehabilitation scenarios. The proposed solution is a biaxial OFS based on two in-line fiber Bragg gratings (FBGs), which were inscribed in the same optical fiber and placed individually in two adjacent cavities, forming a small sensing cell. Such design presents a more compact and resilient solution with higher accuracy when compared to the existing electronic systems. The implementation of the proposed elements into an insole is also described, showcasing the compactness of the sensing cells, which can easily be integrated into a non-invasive mobile e-Health solution for continuous remote gait monitoring of patients and elder citizens. The reported results show that the proposed system outperforms existing solutions, in the sense that it is able to dynamically discriminate shear and plantar pressure during gait.

Keywords: gait analysis; e-Health application; physical rehabilitation; shear and plantar pressure sensor; biaxial optical fiber sensor; multiplexed fiber Bragg gratings

---

1. Introduction

Between 2015 and 2050, the world's population aged over 60 years is expected to double from about 12% up to 22% (up to about 2 billion), with the group aged 80 years and over growing most rapidly (predictably will quadruple from approximately 100 million to 434 million people) [1]. Many elderly and patient groups experience varying degrees of mobility impairments, which require closer monitoring. Assistive devices play a pivotal role in their lives and have a great impact on their ability to live independently and perform basic daily tasks. The assistive products market is set to expand significantly in response to the ageing population and disability trends, with a global market for home medical equipment expected to grow from $27.8 billion in 2015 to nearly $44.3 billion by 2020 [2]. This growing demand for e-Health solutions will improve healthcare services and quality of life by providing autonomy and mobility during daily activities.

Non-invasive continuous monitoring of an individual's health conditions, rehabilitation status, or assistance appears as a natural evolution of current healthcare services by providing patients with continuous remote support when required while guaranteeing autonomy and free mobility. Following this direction and towards improving the quality of life of physically impaired citizens by increasing their mobility, our team has been working on different practical solutions for the continuous remote monitoring of patients [3–5].

The monitoring and analysis of the shear and plantar pressure involved in gait is crucial for the evaluation of patients under physical rehabilitation processes, as well as for the control of rehabilitation exoskeletons in order to correct abnormal plantar pressures due to the uneven load distribution resulting from poor foot sensitivity [6,7]. Moreover, shear in particular, plays a major role in the diagnosis of foot ulceration in diabetic patients. The existence of shear forces presupposes friction between the skin-foot and the shoe. An abnormal increase of shear forces in a given plantar area can cause callosities or the so-called pressure ulcers. This health condition can occur when the tissue is compressed under pressure during gait/walk. Diabetic patients tend to lose sensitivity in the extremities of the body and the feet are one of the most affected areas. By losing sensitivity in the foot plantar areas, the patient involuntarily begins to modify the gait pattern and to adopt less correct postures that lead to the appearance of wounds, which due to their insensitivity in most cases are discovered late. An early discovery of irregularities in the gait pattern of individuals at risk is the first step in reducing the occurrence of ulceration and its treatment. Although shear stress has been identified as a pathogenic factor in the development of plantar ulcers, due to a lack of validated shear stress sensing devices, only studies related to plantar pressures are widely reported [6]. During the last few decades some methods have been proposed for the measurement of plantar shear stress [6], nonetheless, there is a lack of systems able to accurately monitor shear and plantar pressure simultaneously during gait. The work reported in this paper intends to fill such a gap while providing an ambulatory solution based on state-of-the-art optical fiber sensing technology able to be integrated as an enabler in e-Health architectures.

As a first step, we have developed a non-invasive solution for the continuous remote monitoring of foot plantar pressure during gait (walking). Our previous efforts have concentrated on pressure distribution through a strategically placed network of optical fiber sensors (OFSs) [3–5]. In the present work, we take a step forward by presenting the design and implementation of a fiber Bragg grating (FBG)-based platform for the simultaneous measurement of shear force (F_S) and vertical force (F_V), which can be useful in various applications in addition to e-Health. The proposed architecture comprises a compact and accurate biaxial OFS-based on two in-line FBGs (FBG1 and FBG2) placed individually in two adjacent cavities. For the demodulation of the optical signal registered by the designed optical sensing cell, a system of two equations was used, correlating the sensitivities of both FBGs with the F_V and F_S forces [8]. Moreover, we also present the design and integration of the sensing architecture in an insole for continuous monitoring of F_S and F_V (from which is calculated the plantar pressure), during the gait movement of patients.

The rest of this paper is organized as follows. Section 2 provides a survey of the state-of-the-art technology in monitoring shear and vertical forces, highlighting the advantages of the proposed solution. Section 3 introduces the design and calibration of the sensors and the implemented experimental protocols. Section 4 showcases the implantation of five sensing cells in an insole for gait analysis purposes. Section 5 discusses a potential e-Health architecture based on optical fiber sensors for gait analysis. The conclusion is drawn in Section 6.

2. Related Work

Vertical force sensors are nowadays required for a wide number of applications in diverse areas such as industrial production and structural health monitoring, artificial intelligence, robotic exoskeletons, and other health applications [3–5,9–16]. There are several types of F_V sensors, which are characterized essentially by the transduction mechanisms and technology used for converting forces into electrical signals, such as piezo resistivity and capacitance [11,14–16]. In addition to these electronic mechanisms, other transduction methods, such as OFSs are frequently used for the measurement of these type of forces [3–5,17].

Apart from the F_V sensors, devices with additional sensing properties, such as temperature and shear, are highly desired in equipment for medical applications. Specifically, sensors capable of simultaneously measuring F_V and F_S are highly required for the haptic perception of robotic hands, prosthetic skin, and to monitor the stress under the foot to prevent its ulceration [3–6,18–23].

Several studies have been published, using different technologies for the simultaneous sensing of F_V and F_S, namely strain gauge technology [21,24], piezoelectric materials [22,25], capacitive sensors [26], micro strip antennas, and coils [27] to name a few. All these types of sensors have the great disadvantage of using electricity at the point of contact with the user of the equipment, non-immunity to electromagnetic radiation, and thus require the use of several electric cables, usually one for each sensor cell, when multiple points are monitored simultaneously. As an example of the drawbacks presented by electronic devices, the sensor developed by Chen et al. can only be used as a static equipment because, despite having a small detection area of 1.9 cm × 1.9 cm, the overall structure of the sensor is very large [24]. In the work presented by Heywood et al., problems with the electrical insulation of the four layers that constitute the sensor to avoid the short circuits were reported [26]. Also, the work developed by Moahmmad et al. has limitations on the maximum pressure that it can withstand, which is about 0.25 psi [27]. In this context, OFSs appear as an alternative technology to sense these variables, with several advantages over their electronic counterparts. Such advantages include their immunity to electromagnetic interference, remote operation and sensing capability, small dimensions, lightweight, and geometrical versatility, making the technology increasingly used as sensing devices in several areas, with special significance in the biomedical engineering and biomechanics areas [3–5,9,28,29].

Although few, there are already some works reporting the development of optical fiber based F_V and F_S sensors. In 2000, Koulaxouzidis et al. demonstrated that three optical fibers with one FBG each (one on the horizontal and the other two on the diagonals), embedded in a block of solid elastomer, could be used for the measurement of in-shoe shear stress [30]. The Bragg wavelength shift was found to be almost linear under shear stress, in the range between −120 kPa and 120 kPa, yielding to a sensitivity of 4.35 pm/kPa. In 2013, Zhang et al. used a similar method to produce a sensor for the measurement of the same parameters. However, in this case only two optical fibers with FBGs were used (one on the horizontal and the other on the diagonal directions), embedded in a soft polydimethylsiloxane matrix [8]. The sensitivities achieved were 0.82 pm/Pa for vertical pressure and 1.33 pm/Pa for shear. Moreover, in 2005, Wang et al. used a different sensing mechanism, consisting of an array of optical fibers, lying in perpendicular rows and columns separated by elastomeric pads [31]. In their design, the measurements of plantar and shear pressures are based on intensity attenuation in the fibers due to physical deformation. The pressure measurement relies on the force induced light loss from the two affected crossing fibers, while the shear measurement depends on relative position changes in these pressure points between the two fiber mesh layers. This method was later used by other researchers [32–34], where they tried to improve the quality of the obtained data, but still with the disadvantage of a high number of fibers for each measuring point, hence its high complexity and large sensor size.

Although some previous efforts reported the use of OFSs, all those works have used complex designs with more than one optical fiber, which increases their fragility and lowers their application feasibility.

With the aim of reducing the complexity of the sensing device without compromising its performance, we present the design and implementation of an FBG-based sensor for simultaneous measurement of F_V and F_S. Our proposed solution stands out from previously reported ones because of the minimalism of the sensor structure and its accurate feedback. In an insole with several points of analysis it is important to use the least invasive technology possible, to reduce the amount of fiber inside the insole (with a limited size and thickness), and decrease the number of fracture and possible rupture points along the fiber. As this detection method has the ability to multiplex several sensors in the same fiber, it was possible to design an insole with several points of analysis using only one optical fiber.

3. Sensing Cell Design and Implementation

3.1. Sensing Cell Design

In the designed architecture, we used a sensing system comprising two multiplexed FBGs with a 2 mm-length, FBG1 and FBG2, spaced by 9 mm, inscribed in a photosensitive optical fiber (GF1, Thorlabs® Newton, NJ, USA), using the phase mask method with a UV KrF pulsed excimer laser (Bragg StarTM Industrial-LN, Coherent, Dieburg, Germany) operating at 248 nm. A 5 mJ pulse energy was applied with a repetition rate of 500 Hz. The central Bragg wavelength of the FBGs is 1560.9 nm and 1557.6 nm, for FBG1 and FBG2, respectively.

The optical fiber containing the multiplexed FBGs was incorporated in a small cell (9.0 mm × 16.0 mm × 5.5 mm) composed by two cavities, as shown in Figure 1. The cavity in which the FBG1 was placed (cavity 1) was mechanically isolated with a cork wall with a thickness of 2 mm, while the cavity containing the FBG2 (cavity 2) was designed and 3D printed with a hard polymer (polylactic acid, PLA) with a 1.2 mm thick wall. To protect the optical fiber and provide the necessary robustness to the sensing cell, both cavities were then filled with a thermosetting epoxy resin [17], which becomes a semi-rigid structure bounded to the optical fiber, after the curing process. Despite the epoxy resin stiffness, the applied F_V and F_S still induce deformation in the cell area and consequently in the optical fiber sensors without compromising their feedback. It should be noted that no bonding points were added in the cross section between the optical fiber and the cavities' boundaries. In that way, a vertical force applied in the cell top area will compress the epoxy resin vertically, inducing the stretching of the fiber embedded in its interior. On the other hand, a horizontal force, applied along the longitudinal axis of the fiber (left to right on the image), will compress the resin and the fiber containing the sensors against the PLA hard wall.

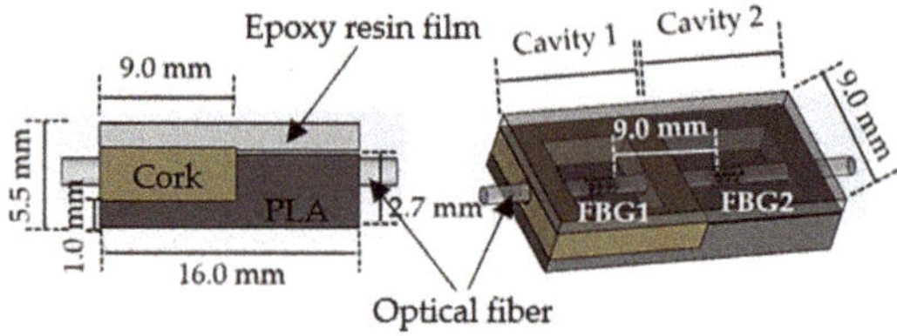

Figure 1. Schematic illustration of the designed sensing cell for simultaneous vertical forces (F_V) and shear forces (F_S) measurement.

Due to its near zero Poisson coefficient [35], the cork walls in cavity 1 provide the necessary mechanical isolation from lateral forces (applied out of the sensing cell area), while, simultaneously, offering the necessary elasticity for the FBG1 to be actuated under vertical forces and longitudinal shear stresses.

Additionally, in order to induce different sensitivities in the FBGs, the walls of cavity 1 were designed to be slightly higher than the walls of cavity 2 (gap of 0.8 mm), and in that way, the response obtained from FBG1 can be enhanced when compared with the FBG2, since the latter is more concealed due to the hard polymer wall. To make the contact area uniform, a 2 mm thick layer of epoxy resin was placed on the top of the sensing cell, as shown in Figure 1.

3.2. Calibration and Performance Testing Methodology

The optical sensing cell feedback is processed in terms of the Bragg wavelength shift ($\Delta\lambda$). The dependence of this parameter with the strain variations ($\Delta\varepsilon$) can be translated by Equation (1) [4]:

$$\Delta\lambda = K_\varepsilon . \Delta\varepsilon \tag{1}$$

where K_ε is the sensor sensitivity to strain variations.

For the demodulation of the reflected optical signal, it was necessary to calibrate each FBG, independently, to F_V and F_S. To do so, a 3-axial electronic force sensor, composed of one biaxial (MBA400, Futek, Irvine, CA, USA) and one uniaxial (TPP-3/75, Transdutec, Barcelona, Spain) unit was used. The designed optical fiber based sensing cell (designated hereinafter as FBGs cell) was firmly attached to the three-axial sensing unit in order to guarantee that any perturbation induced in the FBGs cell would be also registered by the electronic sensing mechanism. Figure 2 is a schematic representation of the experimental setup implemented.

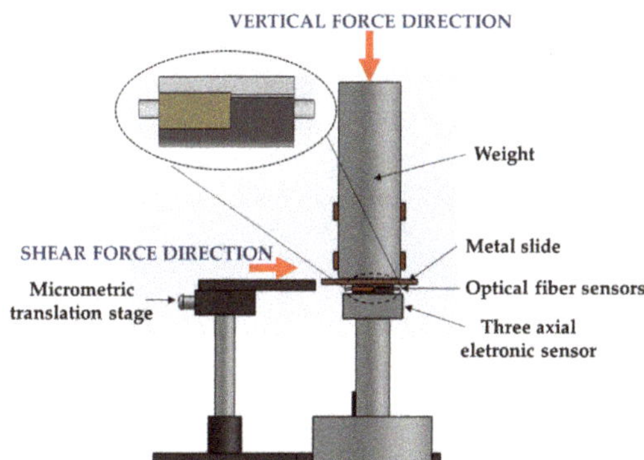

Figure 2. Representation of the experimental setup for the calibration and testing of the fiber Bragg grating (FBGs) cell.

The data retrieved from the electronic sensor was acquired through an analog-to-digital converter (USB-6008, National Instruments, Austin, TX, USA), while the optical signal given by the FBGs cell was acquired by an interrogation system (I-MON 512 USB, Ibsen, Farum, Denmark).

For the calibration of the FBGs cell to F_S, a metal slide placed between the sensing units and a metal cylinder bar (3 kg) was horizontally dragged with the help of a translation stage [8], as shown in Figure 2. The translation stage pushed the metal slide parallel to the sensors' top area, inducing an F_S in both sensing units (electronic and optical). During this test, the F_V was maintained constant ($\Delta F_V \approx 0$ N). For the calibration to F_V, a variable force was applied on the cylindrical bar, while the F_S was kept constant ($\Delta F_S \approx 0$ N). During these procedures (F_S and F_V calibration), the values registered by both sensing systems were simultaneously acquired for further comparison/calibration.

After the calibration, in order to evaluate the FBGs performance under the simultaneous application of F_V and F_S, the procedures described previously were performed simultaneously: the metal slide was propelled horizontally while an F_V was applied in the cylindrical bar, as seen in Figure 2. During the implementation of this protocol, both sensors (electronic and optical) were simultaneously acquiring the data modulated in the sensing units. The obtained results are presented and discussed in the next subsections.

Also, the system hysteresis was tested, by inducing increasing and decreasing vertical forces in the sensing cell.

3.3. Calibration Results

Figure 3 shows the data simultaneously acquired by the electronic and optical systems, for the F_V (a) and F_S (b) characterization procedures. The F_V characterization, Figure 3a, clearly shows the increase of the registered pressure with the load applied over time. In the case of the optical sensor, this increase is translated by a continuous wavelength shift towards higher wavelengths in both FBGs. Such a shift is caused by the longitudinal distension (stretching) of the resin under vertical compression, which will induce the elongation of the embedded optical fiber and consequently the positive Bragg wavelength shift. In the representation of the shear calibration data (see Figure 3b), the periodic variations induced by the translation stage movements are visible in both sensors.

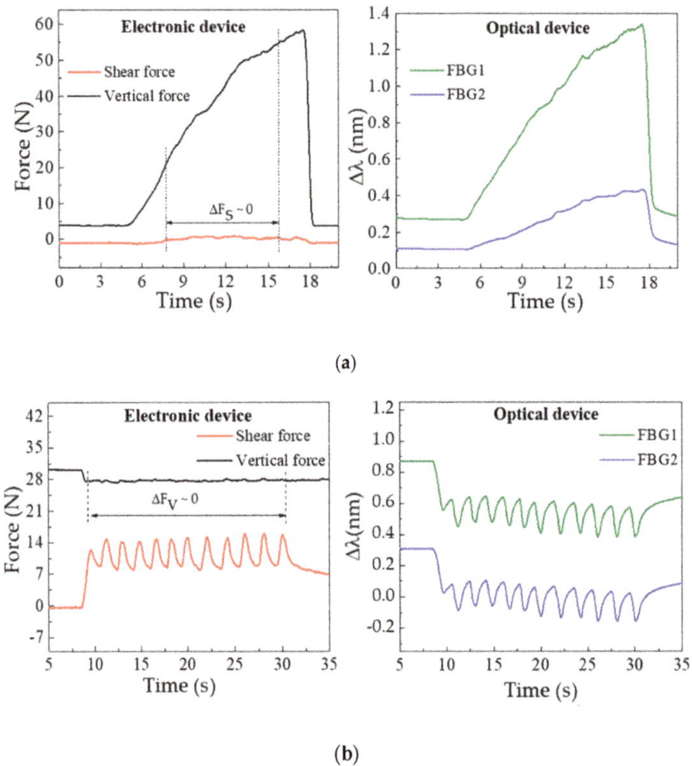

Figure 3. Data acquired by the three-axial electronic (left) and optical fiber (right) based systems, for the (**a**) vertical and (**b**) shear forces characterization.

In the electronic device, the increasing force corresponds to the movement of the translation stage given by one complete turn of the micrometric screw (360°). Once that turn is complete there is a relaxing moment till the new turn is started, which corresponds to the decrease (return to initial state) of the applied force. In the represented characterization process, there is a total of 12 turns. In the optical sensor response, this data is inverted, hence the shear applied in the cell will longitudinally compress the resin and the embedded optical fiber, resulting in a negative Bragg wavelength shift.

From the characterization procedures, the sensitivities of FBG1 and FBG2 were calculated for both the F_V and F_S applied. Towards that, for each value registered by the three-axial electronic sensor, the correspondent Bragg wavelength shift (given by the optical sensor) was correlated, as presented in Figure 4.

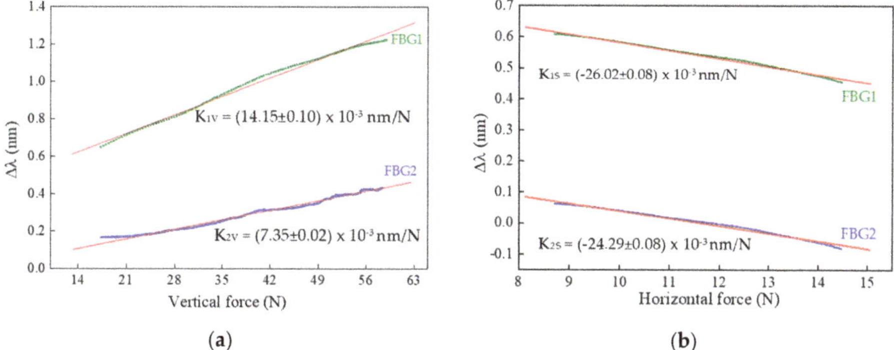

Figure 4. Calibration data obtained for FBG1 and FBG2 during the variation of the applied forces: (**a**) vertical (with $\Delta F_S \approx 0$ N) and (**b**) shear (with $\Delta F_V \approx 0$ N). Symbols are the acquired data and the red line corresponds to the linear fit ($R^2 > 0.99$).

From the calibration representation, a linear dependence of the Bragg wavelength shift with the applied force is verified. The sensitivities obtained for FBG1 and FBG2 as a function of the vertical (K_{1V} and K_{2V}) and shear forces (K_{1S} and K_{2S}) were:

$$K_{1V} = (14.15 \pm 0.10) \times 10^{-3} \text{ nm/N}, \quad K_{1S} = -26.02 \pm 0.08) \times 10^{-3} \text{ nm/N},$$
$$K_{2V} = (7.35 \pm 0.02) \times 10^{-3} \text{ nm/N}, \quad K_{2S} = (-24.29 \pm 0.08) \times 10^{-3} \text{ nm/N}.$$

The substantial discrepancy in the vertical force sensitivity values obtained for the two FBGs is due to the height difference between the walls of cavity 1 and 2, since there is a gap of 0.8 mm between the wall of cavity 2 and the top of the cell. However, once the fiber is not fixed in any point of the cell, its longitudinal movements are similarly transmitted to FBG1 and FBG2, and therefore their sensitivities to shear forces are not as different as that of the vertical forces.

The results obtained for the hysteresis tests are presented in Figure 5. The maximum values found were 0.07 nm for FBG1 and 0.05 nm for FBG2.

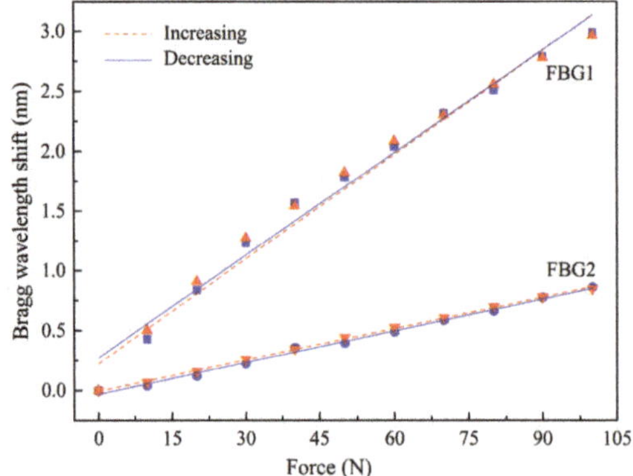

Figure 5. Bragg wavelength shifts as function of increasing and decreasing loadings.

3.4. Implementation: Simultaneous F_V and F_S Loadings

After the calibration, and using the same experimental setup as depicted in Figure 2, the sensor was tested for simultaneous F_S and F_V loadings. The Bragg wavelength shifts, modulated in the optical fiber sensors under simultaneous shear and vertical loadings, can be related to the applied forces by a two-equation system [8]:

$$\begin{bmatrix} F_V \\ F_S \end{bmatrix} = \begin{bmatrix} K_{1V} & K_{1S} \\ K_{2V} & K_{2S} \end{bmatrix}^{-1} \begin{bmatrix} \Delta\lambda_{FBG1} \\ \Delta\lambda_{FBG2} \end{bmatrix} \quad \begin{bmatrix} F_V \\ F_S \end{bmatrix} = \begin{bmatrix} 14.15 \times 10^{-3} & -26.02 \times 10^{-3} \\ 7.35 \times 10^{-3} & -24.29 \times 10^{-3} \end{bmatrix}^{-1} \begin{bmatrix} \Delta\lambda_{FBG1} \\ \Delta\lambda_{FBG2} \end{bmatrix} \tag{2}$$

where $\Delta\lambda_{FBG1}$ and $\Delta\lambda_{FBG2}$ are the Bragg wavelength shift of FBG1 and FBG2, respectively.

In Figure 6, the values acquired for the electronic and optical sensing units during this test are presented, as well as the data acquired after the application of Equation (2). The plot in Figure 6a corresponds to the values registered by the 3-axial electronic force sensor, while the data depicted in Figure 6b are the corresponding Bragg wavelength shift values acquired through the optical sensing cell.

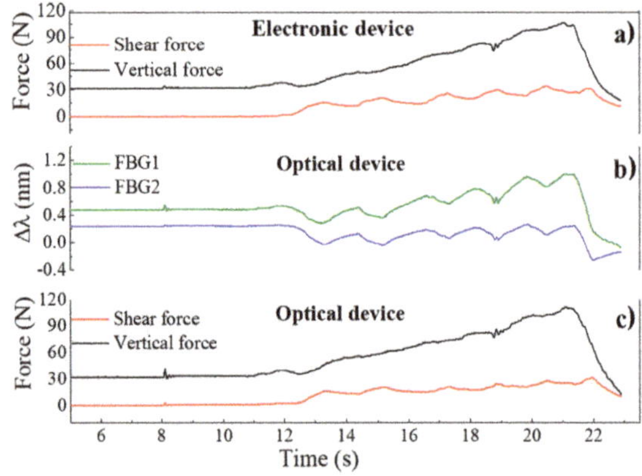

Figure 6. Response to the applied forces as a function of time for the: (**a**) electronic sensor; (**b**) FBGs cell, with the response as Bragg wavelength shift; (**c**) FBGs cell, the forces are calculated by applying Equation (2) to the registered wavelength shifts.

After applying Equation (2) to the $\Delta\lambda$ values obtained from the optical sensing unit, it is possible to obtain the correspondent force values, as presented in Figure 6c, which match the values acquired by the electronic sensors. Moreover, when comparing both sensors' responses, the differences between the curves obtained by the optical and the electronic sensor have a normalized root mean square error value of $RMSE_V = 0.025$ for F_V and $RMSE_S = 0.053$ for F_S, as presented in Figure 7, indicating the reliable performance of the optical sensor and its suitability to monitor F_V and F_S, simultaneously.

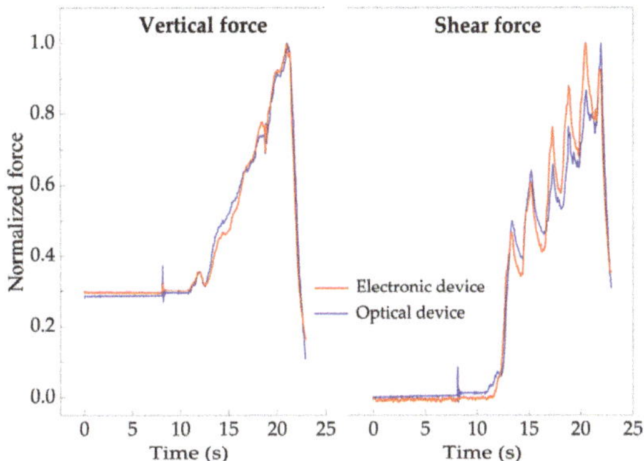

Figure 7. Comparison between the normalized values acquired with the three-axial sensor and the FBGs cell ($RMSE_V = 0.025$ and $RMSE_S = 0.053$).

The compactness, accuracy and reliability of the presented solution is demonstrated in shoe insoles for non-invasive gait pattern analysis (Section 4), however, its application in rehabilitation exoskeleton robots has great potential and will also be considered in our future work.

4. Gait Simultaneous Shear and Plantar Pressure Monitoring

In this section, we present the integration of the sensing architecture described before in an insole for the continuous and simultaneous monitoring of shear and plantar pressure during gait. This proposed solution is compact in size, non-invasive and could be used continuously during a daily routine, without jeopardizing the mobility of patients nor their autonomy while providing an early assessment of the gait pattern abnormalities of individuals at risk.

4.1. Insole Design and Implementation

Considering the foot plantar anatomy, the most at risk areas to develop neuropathic ulcers are the regions covering the bony prominences, where the load is heavily applied. Such areas are located under the metatarsal heads. Nonetheless, the shear stress measured in the great toe and heel are also reported as key points of analysis [6].

During gait, the value of vertical reaction forces and anterior-posterior (AP) forces (shear) are related to the body weight. As for vertical forces, a typical maximum (over the plantar area) is obtained with a force corresponding to 120% of the body weight at the early stance and toe-off moments [36,37]. For the anterior posterior forces, they are considerably smaller and can reach up to 25% of the body weight [36,37]. Locally wise, the area in which the vertical force will have a higher amplitude is the heel area, with a force that can reach up to 80% of the body weight [37].

Bearing in mind such key areas and gait pattern features, we have designed and produced an insole incorporating a total of five sensing cells, similar to the one described in Section 3. A single optical fiber, containing a total of 10 FBGs, was incorporated in the insole, as depicted in Figure 8.

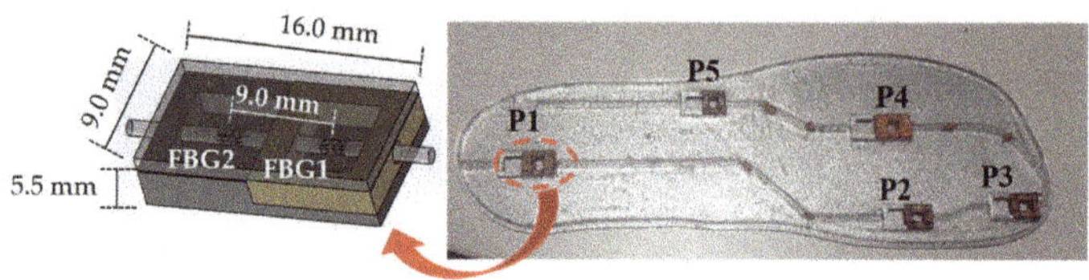

Figure 8. Photograph of the insole used for shear and plantar pressure monitor, incorporating five FBGs cells (as also schemed).

The FBGs cells were placed in the key points of analysis for the foot plantar pressure and shear stress monitor, namely, heel (P1), midfoot (P5), metatarsal (P2 and P4) and toe (P3). The Bragg wavelength and grating periodicity for each FBG are presented in Table 1.

Table 1. Bragg wavelength and grating periodicity for each FBG.

		Bragg Wavelength (nm)	**Grating Period (nm)**
P1	FBG1	1535.1	522.1
	FBG2	1547.1	526.2
P2	FBG1	1540.4	524.0
	FBG2	1543.8	525.1
P3	FBG1	1549.2	527.0
	FBG2	1555.7	529.1
P4	FBG1	1537.1	522.8
	FBG2	1552.8	528.2
P5	FBG1	1557.9	529.9
	FBG2	1561.4	531.1

4.2. Shear and Plantar Pressure Results

With the developed system, by monitoring the wavelength shift experienced by the FBGs in each cell, it is possible to simultaneously monitor the patient's gait pattern, as well as the plantar pressure (corresponding to the vertical force mention in previous sections, for unit of area) and shear stress distribution. Nonetheless, prior to its dynamic application, it is necessary to calibrate each sensing cell to pressure and shear. In that way, the procedure described in Section 3.2 was performed individually for each sensing cell, from which the sensitivities values K_{1V}, K_{2V} (to vertical forces) and K_{1S}, K_{2S} (to shear) were obtained for each FBGs cell.

Figure 9 displays the optical spectra obtained for the developed insole during the vertical force calibration of the FBGs cell "P5". Since the whole system is placed in one optical fiber with 10 multiplexed FBGs, the Bragg wavelength corresponding to each FBG is also visible. However, during the calibration process, only the FBGs corresponding to the sensing cell inserted in P5 responds to the local applied loads. Such a characteristic confirms the good isolation of the designed sensing cell to forces applied in its surroundings, and its suitability for a precise local analysis. Additionally, the presented design (size, number and location of the sensing cells) can be customized according to a doctor prescription and each patient/situation's specific needs.

After calibration, the insole was placed in a shoe for a dynamic monitoring test. During the test, the interrogation system was continuously acquiring the Bragg wavelength shift registered in each point, while the subject (female with 45 kg) was walking.

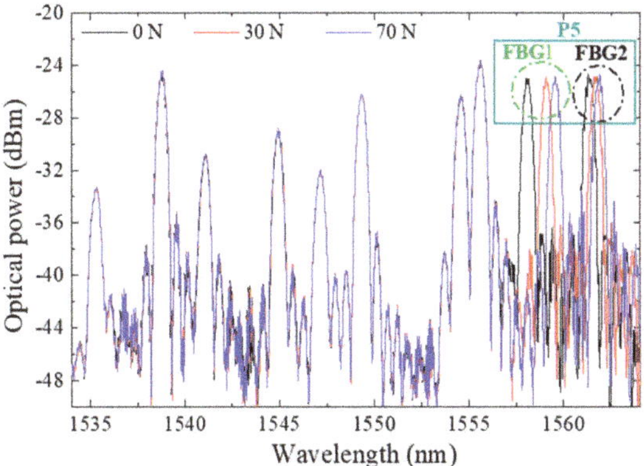

Figure 9. Optical spectra obtained during the pressure calibration of FBGs cell "P5".

Figure 10 represents the registered Bragg wavelength shift for each FBG, in the 5 points, during a 3 s gait. Due to a malfunction in the interrogation system, the Bragg wavelength acquired for FBG1 in P1 had extensive value gaps along time (Bragg wavelength returned as zero) and therefore its values were ignored.

For the global set of the remaining sensing cells, it is clear that each point is activated according to the pressure pattern expected during gait. The stance phase (foot in contact with the floor) and swing phase (foot without contact with the floor) are also clear in this representation [3].

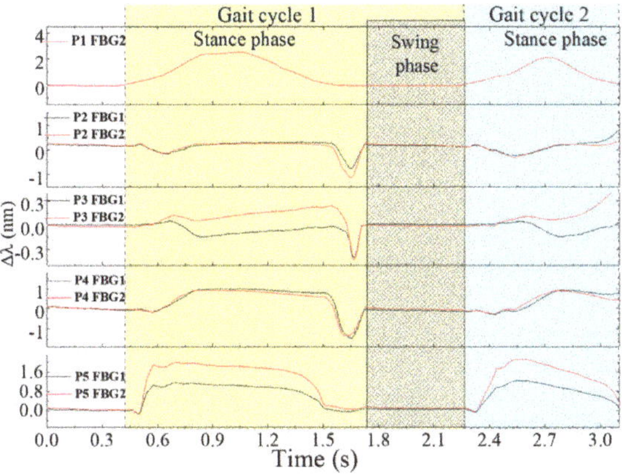

Figure 10. Bragg wavelength shifts in time, registered for each FBG in the 5 points of analysis.

Moreover, the instant in which the shear is a dominant force in the gait cycle is clearly visible (end of the stance phase), as well as the areas in which it is more predominant, namely, the metatarsal (P2 and P4) and the toe (P3) areas.

In order to retrieve the values of plantar vertical and shear forces from the raw data plotted in Figure 10, we apply Equation (2) to each point. The resultant curve, obtained for point 2, located at one of the metatarsal heads (critical point for shear analysis), is depicted in Figure 11.

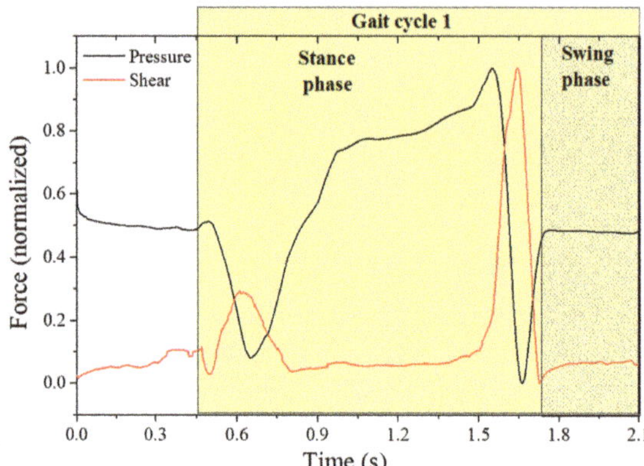

Figure 11. Plantar pressure and shear stress retrieved from the sensing cells in the insole during gait.

As it can be seen, it is possible to differentiate the plantar vertical force and the AP shear stress curve, as reported previously [3,6]. From the obtained curves, it is also observed that the maximum shear stress occurs first in the beginning of the foot-flat phase and again, with higher intensity, at the rising of the heel and the toe-off phase, which corresponds to the backward acceleration force under the metatarsal areas [6].

It is worth noting here that the shear stress evaluated with the referred system is the AP longitudinal shear, and to evaluate the medial-lateral stress, a different sensing cell configuration should be designed. However, and as stated before (and shown in Figure 9), lateral forces do not affect the proposed sensing cells performances for AP shear stress and plantar pressure. Also, it should be noticed that the estimated dynamic range can reach up to at least ~350 N (considering the sensor at heel area, where a typical vertical force of 80% of the body weight is applied).

So, the designed system presented in this paper is a reliable solution for the simultaneous monitoring of plantar pressure and shear stress during gait. Although the developed insole is composed of resin, which is a semi-rigid material, due to its flexibility and the small thickness used for this application, it is possible to be integrated inside the orthopedic insoles, for more comfortable wear. Its application as e-Health tool can provide a clear advantage to patients prone to develop neuropathic ulcers, by early alerting them to correct their posture and walking pattern [4,38]. Also, the incorporation of such devices in rehabilitation exoskeletons will allow the mitigation of the existing gap regarding the monitoring of shear forces.

5. Suitable Non-Invasive e-Health Solution

It has been emphasized throughout this paper the importance of the compact size of the sensing architecture, in addition to its resilience. These two properties render the architecture suitable for integration within a non-invasive e-Health system for the continuous monitoring of patients and elderly citizens. The proposed insole design, described in Section 4, would comprise one part of the whole mobile e-Health solution, used to continuously monitor patients for irregularities in their gait movement. The envisioned overall non-invasive monitoring solution is shown in Figure 12. The system comprises three components: the sensing element, the interrogator system, and the mobile app on a smartphone. The first part, which is the optical fiber sensing architecture, has been extensively explained throughout the paper. It is basically represented by the insole integrated with the optical FBGs cells, as explained in previous section.

The second part is the interrogator system, required to acquire the signal modulated in the sensing points. This can be translated into shear and vertical pressure, based on the proposed system of two equations, as explained in Section 3.

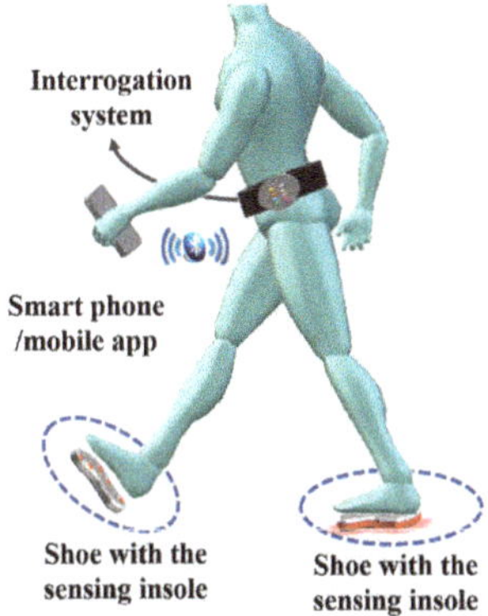

Figure 12. Non-invasive e-Health optical fiber sensing architecture for shear and plantar pressure gait analysis.

The last component is a mobile app installed on a smartphone. The mobile app has multiple roles. First, it is used as a data processing tool to analyze the acquired measurements from the sensing system. Second, the app uses the smartphone as a gateway for transmitting the measured data to the cloud, as shown in our previous work [3]. Additionally, the app can be used to display the results, when required by the patient. The user (patient or his/her doctor) is able to use the app to view the statistics from the measured data over a period of time. Although the system is continuously measuring the pressures, the main requirement is not the instantaneous display of measured values, but the average overall performance of monitored patients/elders during their actual daily routines. Hence the results are continuously transmitted to the cloud for a more elaborate analysis by medical personnel (i.e., the doctor, nurse or physical therapist), eliminating the requirement for high computational and energy capabilities at the mobile device [38]. It is worth mentioning here that the overall e-Health solution is still under development and results obtained from the system will be presented in future work.

6. Conclusions

In this work, a novel compact and efficient optical fiber based solution for the simultaneous sensing of vertical and shear forces is presented. The proposed architecture is accurate and resilient compared to existing solutions. The results obtained from the developed sensing cell show similar behavior to the three-axial electronic force sensor used for comparison, with a $RMSE_V = 0.025$ and $RMSE_S = 0.053$ between them. These values show that the developed device achieved the necessary accuracy while offering all the optical fiber sensor technology advantages, like immunity to electromagnetic interference and humid environments. Moreover, the proposed one-dimensional configuration is a reliable solution, which facilitates the production and incorporation of the sensing cell elements in other devices. Additionally, the presented sensing element, being able to infer and discriminate shear from vertical forces, has a great potential for incorporation into insoles for the measurement of plantar pressure (vertical force) and shear force. This measurement has high potential in different contexts/scenarios, including the prevention and study of pressure ulcers or in monitoring the performance of athletes during training; in electronic skin (e-skin) technologies; intelligent and rehabilitation robotic exoskeletons; human-machine interaction devices or even biomimetic prosthesis.

As for future work, it is our intention to optimize the cell to be able to retrieve both shear forces, anteroposterior and medial lateral, and validate its functionality within several individuals of both genders and of different age groups. Furthermore, its integration in an overall non-invasive e-Health architecture is being assembled, which will allow us to evaluate the forces during gait remotely and in a real time, enabling the monitoring of patients and elder citizens during their active lifestyle routines, without jeopardizing their mobility or freedom.

Author Contributions: Cátia Tavares, M. Fátima Domingues and Tiago Leite designed, implemented, tested the optical device and wrote the manuscript. Anselmo Frizera-Neto and Paulo Antunes contributed for the optical device production, its optimization and for the experimental setup design. Cátia Leitão, Nélia Alberto and Carlos Marques worked on the optical device optimization and testing. Ayman Radwan implemented the algorithm for data analysis and contributed for device optimization. Eduardo Rocon, Paulo André and Paulo Antunes guided the research and supervised the overall work. All the authors contributed to the discussions, data analysis and the revision of the manuscript.

Acknowledgments: This work is funded by FCT/MEC through national funds and when applicable co-funded by FEDER–PT2020 partnership agreement under the projects UID/EEA/50008/2013, within the WeHope (Cátia Tavares) and PREDICT (FCT-IT-LA) (Nélia Alberto) scientific actions, and 5G-AHEAD IF/FCT- IF/01393/2015/CP1310/CT0002 (Ayman Radwan). The financial support from FCT through the fellowships SFRH/BPD/101372/2014 (M. Fátima Domingues) and SFRH/BPD/109458/2015 (Carlos Marques) is also acknowledged. Anselmo Frizera-Neto acknowledges CAPES PGPTA (88887.095626/2015-01), CNPq (304192/2016-3) and FAPES (72982608, 80599230). Eduardo Rocon acknowledges the financial support from the XoSoft project at CSIC-UPM, Madrid-Spain, contract H2020-ICT24-2016-688175.

Conflicts of Interest: The authors declare no conflict of interest. The founding sponsors had no role in the design of the study; in the collection, analyses, or interpretation of data; in the writing of the manuscript, and in the decision to publish the results.

References

1. World Health Organization. Aging and Health. Available online: http://www.who.int/mediacentre/factsheets/fs404/en/ (accessed on 13 February 2018).

2. McWilliams, A. Global Markets and Technologies for Home Medical Equipment. Available online: https://www.bccresearch.com/market-research/healthcare/home-medical-equipment-technologies-market-report-hlc054d.html (accessed on 20 April 2018).

3. Domingues, F.; Tavares, C.; Leitão, C.; Frizera-Neto, A.; Alberto, N.; Marques, C.; Radwan, A.; Rodriguez, J.; Postolache, O.; Racon, E.; et al. Insole optical fiber Bragg grating sensors network for dynamic vertical force monitoring. *J. Biomed. Opt.* **2017**, *22*. [CrossRef] [PubMed]

4. Domingues, F.; Alberto, N.; Leitão, C.; Tavares, C.; Lima, E.; Radwan, A.; Sucasas, V.; Rodriguez, J.; André, P.; Antunes, P. Insole optical fiber sensor architecture for remote gait analysis-an eHealth Solution. *IEEE Internet Thing J.* **2017**. [CrossRef]

5. Domingues, M.F; Tavares, C.; Alberto, N.; Leitão, C.; Antunes, P.; André, P.; Rocon, E.; Sucasas, V.; Radwan, A.; Rodriguez, J. Non-invasive insole optical fiber sensor architecture for monitoring foot anomalies. In Proceedings of the IEEE Global Communications Conference, Singapore, 4–8 December 2017.

6. Rajala, S.; Lekkala, J. Plantar shear stress measurements—A Review. *Clin. Biomech.* **2014**, *29*, 475–483. [CrossRef] [PubMed]

7. Bayón, C.; Lerma, S.; Ramírez, O.; Serrano, J.I.; Del Castillo, M.D.; Raya, R.; Belda-Lois, J.M.; Martínez, I.; Rocon, E. Locomotor training through a novel robotic platform for gait rehabilitation in pediatric population. *J. Neuroeng. Rehabil.* **2016**, *13*, 98. [CrossRef] [PubMed]

8. Mohammad, I.; Huang, H. Pressure and shear sensing based on microstrip antennas. *Proc. SPIE* **2012**, *8345*. [CrossRef]

9. Leitão, C.; Antunes, P.; Pinto, J.; Bastos, J.; André, P. Carotid distension waves acquired with a fiber sensor as an alternative to tonometry for central arterial systolic pressure assessment in young subjects. *Measurement* **2017**, *95*, 45–49. [CrossRef]

10. Hammock, M.; Chortos, A.; Tee, B.; Tok, J.; Bao, Z. 25th Anniversary Article: The Evolution of Electronic Skin (E-Skin): A Brief History, Design Considerations, and Recent Progress. *Adv. Mater.* **2013**, *25*, 5997. [CrossRef] [PubMed]

11. Luo, N.; Dai, W.; Li, C.; Zhou, Z.; Lu, L.; Poon, C.; Chen, S.-C.; Zhang, Y.; Zhao, N. Flexible piezoresistive sensor patch enabling ultralow power cuffless blood pressure measurement. *Adv. Funct. Mater.* **2016**, *26*, 1178–1187. [CrossRef]
12. Jung, S.; Kim, J.; Kim, J.; Choi, S.; Lee, J.; Park, I.; Hyeon, T.; Kim, D. Reverse-micelle-induced porous pressure-sensitive rubber for wearable human-machine interfaces. *Adv. Mater.* **2014**, *26*, 4825–4830. [CrossRef] [PubMed]
13. Mesquita, E.; Arede, A.; Silva, R.; Rocha, P.; Gomes, A.; Pinto, N.; Varum, H.; Antunes, P. Structural health monitoring of the retrofitting process, characterization and reliability analysis of a masonry heritage construction. *J. Civ. Struct. Health Monit.* **2017**, *7*, 405–428. [CrossRef]
14. Minami, K.; Kokubo, Y.; Maeda, I.; Hibino, S. Analysis of actual pressure point using the power flexible capacitive sensor during chest compression. *J. Anesth.* **2017**, *31*, 152–155. [CrossRef] [PubMed]
15. Voinea, J.; Butnariu, S.; Mogan, G. Measurement and geometric modelling of human spine posture for medical rehabilitation purposes using a wearable monitoring system based on inertial sensors. *Sensors* **2016**, *17*, 3. [CrossRef] [PubMed]
16. Choi, S.; Cho, H.; Lissenden, C. Selection of shear horizontal wave transducers for robotic nondestructive inspection in harsh environments. *Sensors* **2016**, *17*, 5. [CrossRef] [PubMed]
17. Ferreira, L.; Antunes, P.; Domingues, F.; Silva, P.; André, P. Monitoring of sea bed level changes in nearshore regions using fiber optic sensors. *Measurement* **2012**, *45*, 1527–1533. [CrossRef]
18. Zang, Y.; Zhang, F.; Di, C.; Zhu, D. Advances of flexible pressure sensors toward artificial intelligence and health care applications. *Mater. Horiz.* **2015**, *2*, 140–156. [CrossRef]
19. Tiwana, M.; Shashank, A.; Redmond, S.; Lovell, N. Characterization of a capacitive tactile shear sensor for application in robotic and upper limb prostheses. *Sens. Actuators A Phys.* **2011**, *165*, 164–172. [CrossRef]
20. Puangmali, P.; Althoefer, K.; Seneviratne, L.; Murphy, D.; Dasgupta, P. State-of-the-art in force and tactile sensing for minimally invasive surgery. *IEEE Sens. J.* **2008**, *8*, 371–381. [CrossRef]
21. Chen, W.; Lee, P.; Park, S.; Lee, S.; Shim, V.; Lee, T. A novel gait platform to measure isolated plantar metatarsal forces during walking. *J. Biomech.* **2010**, *43*, 2017–2021. [CrossRef] [PubMed]
22. Kärki, S.; Lekkala, J.; Kuokkanen, H.; Halttunen, J. Development of a piezoelectric polymer film sensor for plantar normal and shear stress measurements. *Sens. Actuators A Phys.* **2009**, *154*, 57–64. [CrossRef]
23. Hamatani, M.; Mori, T.; Oe, M.; Noguchi, H.; Takehara, K.; Amemiya, A.; Ohashi, Y.; Ueki, K.; Kadowaki, T.; Sanada, H. Factors associated with callus in patients with diabetes, focused on plantar shear stress during gait. *J. Diabetes Sci. Technol.* **2016**, *10*, 1–7. [CrossRef] [PubMed]
24. Yavuz, M.; Erdemir, A.; Botek, G.; Hirschman, G.; Bardsley, L.; Davis, B. Peak plantar pressure and shear locations—Relevance to diabetic patients. *Diabetes Care* **2007**, *30*, 2643–2645. [CrossRef] [PubMed]
25. Razian, M.; Pepper, M. Design, development, and characteristics of an in-shoe triaxial pressure measurement transducer utilizing a single element of piezoelectric copolymer film. *IEEE Trans. Neural Syst. Rehabil. Eng.* **2003**, *11*, 288–293. [CrossRef] [PubMed]
26. Heywood, E.J.; Jeutter, D.C.; Harris, G.F. Tri-axial plantar pressure sensor: Design, calibration and characterization. In Proceedings of the 26th Annual International Conference of the IEEE Engineering in Medicine and Biology Society, San Francisco, CA, USA, 1–5 September 2004.
27. Alberto, N.; Bilro, L.; Antunes, P.; Leitão, C.; Lima, H.; André, P.; Nogueira, R.; Pinto, J.L. Optical fiber technology for e-Healthcare. In *Handbook of Research on ICTs and Management Systems for Improving Efficiency in Healthcare and Social Care*; IGI Global: Hershey PA, USA, 2013; pp. 180–200.
28. Domingues, F.; Radwan, A. Optical fiber sensors in IoT. In *Optical Fiber Sensors for IoT and Smart Devices*; Springer: Cham, Switzerland, 2017; pp. 73–86.
29. Koulaxouzidis, A.; Holmes, M.; Roberts, C.; Handerek, V. A shear and vertical stress sensor for physiological measurements using fibre Bragg gratings. In Proceedings of the 22nd Annual International Conference of the IEEE Engineering in Medicine and Biology Society, Chicago, IL, USA, 23–28 July 2000.
30. Zhang, Z.; Tao, X. Soft fiber optic sensors for precision measurement of shear stress and pressure. *IEEE Sens. J.* **2013**, *13*, 1478–1482. [CrossRef]
31. Wang, W.; Ledoux, W.; Sangeorzan, B.; Reinhall, P. A shear and plantar pressure sensor based on fibre-optic bend loss. *J. Rehabil. Res. Dev.* **2005**, *42*, 315–326. [CrossRef] [PubMed]
32. Liu, C.; Chou, G.; Liang, X.; Reinhall, P.; Wang, W. Design of a multi-layered optical bend loss sensor for pressure and shear sensing. *Proc. SPIE* **2007**, *6532*. [CrossRef]

33. Soetanto, W.; Nguyen, N.; Wang, W. Fiber optic plantar pressure/shear sensor. *Proc. SPIE* **2011**, *7984*. [CrossRef]
34. Chang, C.; Liu, C.; Soetanto, W.; Wang, W. A platform-based foot pressure/shear sensor. *Proc. SPIE* **2012**, *8348*. [CrossRef]
35. Silva, S.; Sabino, M.; Fernandes, E.; Correlo, V.; Boesel, L.; Reis, R. Cork: Properties, capabilities and applications. *Int. Mater. Rev.* **2005**, *50*, 345–365. [CrossRef]
36. Perry, J.; Davids, J.R. Gait analysis: normal and pathological function. *J. Pediatr. Orthop.* **1992**, *12*, 815. [CrossRef]
37. Wearing, S.C.; Urry, S.R.; Smeathers, J.E. Ground reaction forces at discrete sites of the foot derived from pressure plate measurements. *Foot Ankle Int.* **2001**, *22*, 653–661. [CrossRef] [PubMed]
38. Radwan, A.; Domingues, M.F.; Rodriguez, J. Mobile caching-enabled small-cells for delay-tolerant e-Health apps. In Proceedings of the 2017 IEEE International Conference on Communications Workshops, Paris, France, 21–25 May 2017; pp. 103–108.

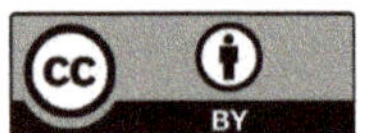 © 2018 by the authors. Licensee MDPI, Basel, Switzerland. This article is an open access article distributed under the terms and conditions of the Creative Commons Attribution (CC BY) license (http://creativecommons.org/licenses/by/4.0/).

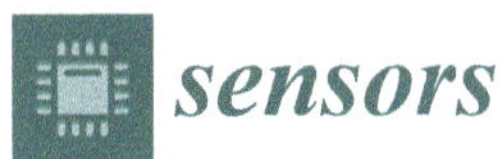 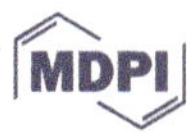

Article

Wearable Sensors and the Assessment of Frailty among Vulnerable Older Adults: An Observational Cohort Study

Javad Razjouyan [1,2], Aanand D. Naik [1,3,4], Molly J. Horstman [1,3], Mark E. Kunik [1,3,4], Mona Amirmazaheri [2], He Zhou [2], Amir Sharafkhaneh [3] and Bijan Najafi [2,3,*]

[1] VA HSR&D, Center for Innovations in Quality, Effectiveness and Safety,
     Michael E. DeBakey VA Medical Center, Houston, TX 77030, USA; javad.razjouyan@va.gov (J.R.);
     anaik@bcm.edu (A.D.N.); mhorstma@bcm.edu (M.J.H.); mkunik@bcm.edu (M.E.K.)
[2] Interdisciplinary Consortium on Advanced Motion Performance (iCAMP), Division of Vascular Surgery and
     Endovascular Therapy, Michael E. DeBakey Department of Surgery, Baylor College of Medicine,
     One Baylor Plaza, MS: BCM390, Houston, TX 77030, USA; Mona Amirmazaheri@bcm.edu (M.A.);
     he.zhou2@bcm.edu (H.Z.)
[3] Department of Medicine, Baylor College of Medicine, Houston, TX 77030, USA; amirs@bcm.edu
[4] South Central Mental Illness Research, Education and Clinical Center (MIRECC), Houston, TX 77030, USA
*   Correspondence: najafi.bijan@gmail.com or Bijan.najafi@bcm.edu; Tel.: +1-713-798-7536;
     Fax: +1-713-798-1158

Received: 12 March 2018; Accepted: 24 April 2018; Published: 26 April 2018

Abstract: *Background:* The geriatric syndrome of frailty is one of the greatest challenges facing the U.S. aging population. Frailty in older adults is associated with higher adverse outcomes, such as mortality and hospitalization. Identifying precise early indicators of pre-frailty and measures of specific frailty components are of key importance to enable targeted interventions and remediation. We hypothesize that sensor-derived parameters, measured by a pendant accelerometer device in the home setting, are sensitive to identifying pre-frailty. *Methods:* Using the Fried frailty phenotype criteria, 153 community-dwelling, ambulatory older adults were classified as pre-frail (51%), frail (22%), or non-frail (27%). A pendant sensor was used to monitor the at home physical activity, using a chest acceleration over 48 h. An algorithm was developed to quantify physical activity pattern (PAP), physical activity behavior (PAB), and sleep quality parameters. Statistically significant parameters were selected to discriminate the pre-frail from frail and non-frail adults. *Results:* The stepping parameters, walking parameters, PAB parameters (sedentary and moderate-to-vigorous activity), and the combined parameters reached and area under the curve of 0.87, 0.85, 0.85, and 0.88, respectively, for identifying pre-frail adults. No sleep parameters discriminated the pre-frail from the rest of the adults. *Conclusions:* This study demonstrates that a pendant sensor can identify pre-frailty via daily home monitoring. These findings may open new opportunities in order to remotely measure and track frailty via telehealth technologies.

Keywords: frailty; pre-frail; wearable sensor; physical activity; sedentary behavior; moderate-to-vigorous activity; steps

---

1. Introduction

According to a 2014 United States Census Bureau report, the population aged 65 and over has been projected to grow from 43.1 million in 2012 to 83.7 million in 2050 [1]. One of the distinctive health states related to the aging process is frailty [2]. The prevalence of frailty in the ambulatory population is about 15% and the prevalence of pre-frailty is about 45% [3]. Frailty places older adults at risk for dramatic changes in physical and mental well-being following challenges to their health, such as an infection, injury, or medication interactions [4]. Frailty is an independent predictor of adverse outcomes, including falls, delirium, hospitalization, and mortality [5]. Identifying patients at risk for frailty (pre-frail adults) would enable healthcare providers to intervene from an early stage so as to mitigate some of the potential adverse sequelae [6].

Although there is no consensus on the definition of frailty, recent efforts have focused on a standardization of the definition so as to enhance its application in clinical care [7]. Geriatricians used to say, "I know it when I see it, but what I see may not be the same as what everyone else sees" [8]. The definition of frailty has evolved from the stereotypical description of a "thin, stooped, slow octogenarian" person [9]. Approaches introduced by Fried [10] and Rockwood [11] have had the strongest empirical and conceptual support.

Fried and colleagues developed a frailty phenotype theory based on mutually exacerbating cycles of negative energy balance, sarcopenia, and diminished strength and tolerance for exertion in the community dwelling geriatric population [7]. In this theory, the frailty phenotype is associated with declining energy and reserve [10]. Fried proposed five core clinical criteria for the impairment that is underlying frailty, namely, shrinking, exhaustion, inactivity, slowness, and weakness [10]. Older adults are classified as frail, pre-frail, or robust. An individual meeting the threshold of impairment for three of these criteria are classified as frail. The individual meeting criteria for one or two components is classified as pre-frail. Those meeting none of the impairment criteria are classified as non-frail or robust. Individuals meeting the pre-frail criteria can potentially benefit more from clinical intervention [12] compared with those meeting the frail and non-frail (robust) criteria [13]. Furthermore, a greater variety of interventions are potentially available to pre-frail older adults, who require less supervision than frail older adults [14].

The Fried frailty phenotype has several diagnostic limitations. The Fried approach has been described as impractical in a busy clinic settings [15], not designed for inpatient or bed-bound older patients [16], not sensitive to subtle physiological changes [17], and as failing to account for the important domain of cognition function [18]. Additionally, the approach's reliance on questionnaires to identify weight loss, exhaustion, and energy expenditure suffers from participant bias [19–22].

To overcome limitations of the Fried frailty phenotype, researchers have proposed wearable sensors as an alternative to assessing the frailty phenotype [15,23–25]. These wearable sensors can address the challenges in measuring frailty, such as feasibility, practicality, ease of use, accessibility, reproducibility, and reliability, without hindering daily activity in the outpatient or inpatient settings [15,23,24]. Previous studies using a wrist sensor, by Lee et al., have demonstrated that a 20-s upper extremity test is capable of predicting frailty in the outpatient setting [26] and in community dwelling settings [27]. Schwenk et al. have shown that multiple sensor-based physical activity monitors, which measure posture (walking, standing, sitting, lying, and postural transition from sit-to-stand and stand-to-sit) and gait parameters (stride length, gait speed, gait velocity, and cadence), are capable of discriminating between non-frail, pre-frail, and frail patients [24]. Other studies have shown that sensor-derived activity levels (sedentary behaviors, light and moderate-to-vigorous activity) have a high correlation with frailty status [28] and are capable of discriminating between different frailty statuses [29–32]. They found that an increase in the sedentary behavior and a decrease in the high intensity activity, such as moderate-to-vigorous activity, is a strong predictor of frailty progression. Interestingly, Theou et al. showed that a single parameter, the number of steps, which is derived from a wearable sensor is significantly correlated with the progression of frailty [31]. Furthermore, studies of sensor-based in-home sleep monitors have found an association between sleep disruptions and [33] the existence of frailty [34].

While few studies proposed daily step measurement for in-place monitoring frailty status, to our knowledge, no prior studies have examined fine-grain characteristics of daily physical activities, such as activity behavior (e.g., sedentary), activity postures (e.g., sitting, standing, lying, and walking), and walking characteristics (e.g., number of taken steps), which are measured by a single senor into a cohesive model. Such models are potentially valuable because they would provide a clinical and technical validation of these sensor-derived parameters, and serve as a basis for future studies developing predictive models of change between frailty categories. In particular, there are very few studies that are enabled to identify pre-frailty using wearable-based activity monitoring. Pre-frailty is considered as the early stage of frailty [35–37]. While several studies have suggested that frailty is not an irreversible process, it has been hypothesized that the early detection of a pre-frail status may provide a window of opportunity for timely preventive or therapeutic interventions, which may delay the progression of frailty and even reverse it [35–37]. Thus, the early detection of pre-frailty may provide a unique opportunity to provide a timely intervention and is desperately needed. Therefore, the purpose of this study is to examine the ability of a practical wearable platform (a pendant accelerometer), to remotely monitor the frailty stages using daily activity monitoring, with an emphasis on distinguishing pre-frailty. Specifically, our first aim was to determine which sensor-derived parameters—including walking characteristics (e.g., daily number of taken steps); activity patterns, including postures (i.e., sitting, standing, and lying) and walking durations; activity patterns, including sedentary, light, and moderate-to-vigorous activities; and sleep parameters, including total sleep time and sleep efficiency—are capable of discriminating between the three frailty categories. The second aim was to identify the most significant independent parameters in order to discriminate the pre-frail from other groups. Finally, our third aim was to build a composite model that would have a promising performance so as to discriminate the pre-frail stage from non-frail and frail stages.

2. Materials and Methods

2.1. Participants and Assessment

2.1.1. Participants Recruitment

We recruited ambulatory older adults that were $\geq$60 years of age, who were able to walk 15 feet (~4.5 m) independently, with or without aid. Participants were enrolled from outpatient clinics or community dwelling settings. Exclusion criteria were severe cognitive impairment (a Mini-Mental State Examination [MMSE] score $\leq$16) [38] and those unable/unwilling to consent. Participants who met the eligibility criteria signed written consent form. This study was approved by the local institutional review boards.

2.1.2. Demographic and Clinical Characteristics

Trained clinical coordinators collected patient demographic and clinical characteristics. The measures were history of falls, height, weight, and fear of falling, which was assessed by the Fall Efficacy Scale-International (FES-I) [39]. Participants' depression scale was measured using the Center for Epidemiologic Studies Depression Scale (CES-D) [40].

2.1.3. Frailty Assessment

We used the Fried frailty phenotype assessment to stratify the participants into three groups, namely, non-frail, pre-frail, and frail [10]. The Fried frailty assessment consisted of five phenotypes, namely, shrinking (losing more than 10 lb. in prior year unintentionally), exhaustion (self-reported questionnaire), inactivity (self-reported questionnaire), slowness (prolonged performance during 15-feet walk test), and weakness (decreased grip strength) [10]. If the participants' performance placed them in the lowest quartile for a phenotype, they received one point for that phenotype. For the final score, the sum of all of the one points (*SUM*) was calculated and the subject was classified into one of three groups:

$$Frailty\ Status = \begin{cases} nonFrail/Robust: & SUM = 0 \\ preFrail: & 0 < SUM \leq 2 \\ Frail: & SUM \geq 3 \end{cases}$$

2.2. Sensor Based Assessment

We used a pendant sensor (PAMSys™, BioSensics LLC, Watertown, MA, USA), which was placed at the sternum (Figure 1). The participants were instructed to keep the sensor on for 48 h and then return it to the center, through either a paid envelope or collection by the study coordinators. The PAMSys had three dimensional accelerations that recorded the gravity and inertial accelerations, with a sampling frequency of 50 Hz. The sensor had a built-in memory that allowed for the saving of data and also downloading it to the computer via the company software that was provided. We used PAMWare™ software (BioSensics, Watertown, MA, USA) to download, calibrate, and normalize (to gravity or g) the data. All of the physical activity and sleep parameters were extracted from the pendant sensor. However, two different validated algorithms were used to extract the physical activities and sleep parameters using chest acceleration, as described in our previous studies [41–44].

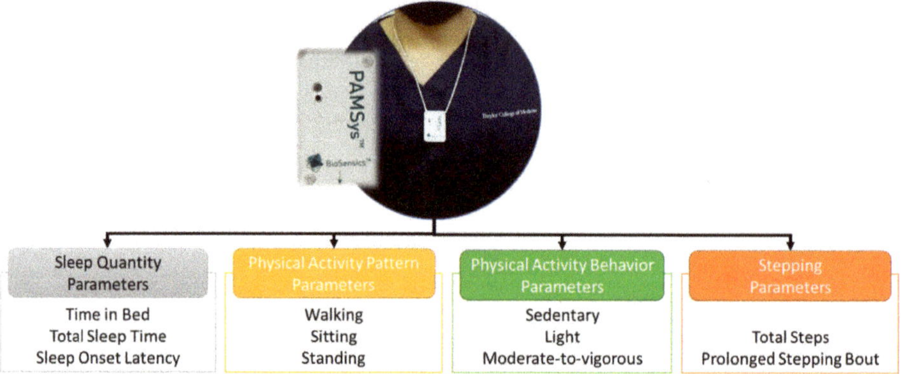

Figure 1. The sensor placement (above) and the common parameters (below) that were extracted, based on validated algorithm, namely: sleep quantity, physical activity patterns, physical activity behaviors, and stepping count.

2.2.1. Physical Activity Behavior Parameters

For the purpose of this study, the physical activity behavior parameters that were considered were sedentary behavior (Sed), light activity (Lgt), and moderate-to-vigorous activity (MtV). Sedentary behavior was defined as an activity with less than 1.5 metabolic equivalent (MET), such as sitting or lying [45,46]. Light activity was defined as an activity between ≥1.5 MET and MET <3.0, such as hanging out the washing, ironing and dusting, and working at a standing workstation [46]. Moderate-to-vigorous activity referred to an activity demanding ≥3.0 MET, such as brisk walking, recreational activities, climbing stairs, etc. [46].

To measure the physical activity levels in each category, we calculated the mean amplitude deviation (MAD) [47]. Before we calculated the MAD, several steps were taken. Firstly, we preprocessed the data in order to remove the high frequency activities that had not originated from human body [41]. We used a wavelet filter bank (Daubechies [48]) with a cut-off at 12.5 Hz. The wavelet filter was used, as it has been shown to keep the morphology of signal better than the other filters [49]. Then, we calculated the following:

$$r_i = \sqrt{x_i^2 + y_i^2 + z_i^2} \tag{1}$$

Here, r_i is the norm acceleration containing the static and dynamic component of the body accelerations for each sample (i). The (x_i, y_i, z_i) are the three-dimensional accelerations. For each 6-s epoch, the average r_i (R_{ave}) of the 300 samples (=6 s $\times$ 50 Hz) was calculated as follows:

$$R_{ave} = \frac{1}{N} \sum_{i=1}^{N=6\,s} r_i \tag{2}$$

The MAD value for each epoch was calculated as the absolute sum of distance from R_{ave} as follows:

$$MAD = \frac{1}{N} \sum_{i=1}^{N=300} |r_i - R_{ave}| \tag{3}$$

The MADs for all of the possible epochs were calculated. The unit of MAD is in the milligravity, where 1 g is equal to 1000 mg. We used three cut-points to classify activity level into sedentary (MAD < 20), light (20 $\leq$ MAD < 90) and moderate-to-vigorous (MtV: MAD $\geq$ 90). This method had, on average, a very high sensitivity and specificity of 98% and 96%, respectively, in order to detect the physical activity levels [47].

2.2.2. Non-Wear Time and Valid Day of Monitoring

We excluded the intervals when participants did not wear the sensors. These non-wear periods occurred during aquatic activities, such as bathing, or because the participant forgot to wear the sensor. We used a method that was validated in older adults [50], which defined non-wear periods as $\geq$90 min with no MAD (allowing for 2 interrupted minutes with MAD of <20).

A valid day of monitoring was defined as $\geq$8 hours of wear [45,50]. We used the valid day with the wear time annotation to report the physical activity parameters. The average of the activity parameters over the 2 days were reported to have reached the highest inter-class correlation (ICC) [51].

For each valid day of monitoring, we calculated the following parameters:

- Total activity: the sum of the all of the specific activity (Sed, Lgt, and MtV).
- Percentage activity: the total activity duration of a specific activity, divided by the total duration of wear time, excluding the nocturnal time in bed.
- Median activity: the 50th percentile of the bout of the specific activity.
- Health and Human Services (HHS) guideline, %: The percentage of participants who met the U.S. Department of HSS recommendations that an adult should have at least 300 min of moderate-to-vigorous activity per week [52]. To calculate this parameter, we estimated those who had at least 42 min (300 min/7 days = ~42 min) of moderate-to-vigorous physical activities per day.

The bout of activity was the consecutive, continuous interval of an activity without any interruption, such as Sed, Lgt, or MtV.

2.2.3. Physical Activity Pattern and Stepping Parameters

The postural parameters that were calculated from the PAMSys sensor's raw data included lying, sitting, standing, walking, and the number of steps. The algorithm first detected the episodes of walking, which was three consecutive steps with less than specific time intervals [42–44,53]. The steps were determined by the peaks in vertical acceleration, where the signal passed through a wavelet-based band pass filter, with absolute values greater than a certain threshold. Standing, sitting, and lying were considered non-walking intervals. Lying intervals were identified when the vertical acceleration was close to zero gravity. In the other words, during the lying intervals, the vertical vector was at a right angle with the frontal plain. Sitting and standing were identified through the pattern changes in frontal-vertical vectors. The sensitivity (87% to 99%) and specificity (87% to 99%) of the algorithm was reported previously [43].

The postural data was reported for each 24 h period and the average was calculated for the final outcomes, as follows:

- Posture, %: the duration of each posture (lying, sitting, standing, walking) in 24 h.
- Total steps: the total number of steps per day.
- Longest unbroken posture, s: the maximum duration of an unbroken bout for each posture.
- Median posture, s: the median duration of a bout for each posture.
- Longest unbroken stepping bout: the number of steps during the longest bout of stepping without interruption.
- Median stepping bout: the number of steps in the median bout of stepping without interruption.

2.2.4. Sleep Quantity Parameters

Using the physical activity algorithm [41,44], the start and end of sleep during night time were recorded in order to estimate the time spent in the bed and out of the bed. The sleep algorithm was applied only during the time in the bed. The method for extracting sleep parameters of interest, using a chest accelerometer, was described in detail in our previous study [41]. In summary, firstly, the acceleration data passed through a band pass filter, then a vector magnitude/norm of acceleration was built and a minute wise signal was calculated. Next, a feature vector, which consisted of an activity intensity in the moment and a standard deviation of the activities as well as any sleep position changes, was built for each minute and fed to a model. Finally, the model estimated the sleep/wake conditions. From the sleep/wake signal, the sleep quantity parameters were extracted as follows:

- Time in bed (TiB), hours: the total duration of a participant's time in bed.
- Total sleep time (TST), hours: the total duration of nocturnal sleep.
- Sleep onset latency (SOL), min: the total interval of the time to fall asleep, from the beginning of TiB.
- Wake after sleep onset (WASO), min: the total duration of the time awake, after sleep onset until sleep offset.
- Sleep efficiency (SE), %: the percentage of TST to onset of sleep to last offset of sleep.
- Supine, %: the total duration of supine during TiB.
- Prone, %: the total duration of prone during TiB.
- Sides, %: the total duration of side lying (left or right) during TiB.

2.3. Statistical Analysis

We used the Fisher exact test to evaluate the differences between the categorical variables (demographic or clinical characteristics). We used the ANCOVA with the Tukey LSD post hoc test, which was performed on the SPSS (IBM, V24.0.0), in order to test the significance level between the three groups of non-frail, pre-frail, and frail. We also estimated the Cohen's d effect size (d), where $d \approx 0.2, 0.5$, and 0.8 were considered as small, medium, and large, respectively.

We selected independent variables in two of the steps [54]. In the first step (filter method [54]), we chose parameters from the sensor-derived parameters that had a p-value less than 0.05 and a $d \geq 0.4$. In the second step (embedded method [54]), these independent predictors were fed to a model in order to discriminate the pre-frail from the two other groups (non-frail and frail). The Receiver Operating Characteristic (ROC) curve, performance (sensitivity, specificity, and accuracy), and area under the curve (AUC), were calculated based on the one-vs-rest method [55]. Of the independent predictors, those with an AUC greater than 0.7 were used to develop discrimination models. To select the independent predictors, the whole dataset was used [56,57].

We developed four models as follows: (1) the step model: using step parameters, such as the total number of steps; (2) the physical activity pattern (PAP) model: PAP parameters such as the total walking and postures duration; (3) the physical activity behavior (PAB) model: PAB parameters, such as sedentary; and (4) the combined model: all of the parameters such as total number of steps, total walking, and sedentary. To train and test the model, we used a k-fold cross validation (k = 5). In this method, the dataset was randomly partitioned into five subsamples [58,59]. Four partitions were used to train each model and one partition, which was not used for training, was used for validating each model. This step performed for five times. The average and standard deviation of the performance parameters for the validation phase were reported. The performance parameters that were measured for each model were sensitivity, specificity, accuracy, and the AUC [59].

3. Results

3.1. Demographic and Clinical Characteristics

Originally, 163 participants had consented to participant in this study. Data from 10 participants was excluded because of low wear-time (*n* = 3), less than two days of recording (*n* = 5), and forgetting to put on the sensor (*n* = 2). The remaining 153 participants (75 ± 10 years and 79% female) were included in the study, where 42 (27%) were considered as non-frail, 78 (51%) pre-frail, and 33 (22%) frail (Table 1). In the progression of the frailty status among the participants, we observed a trend in several demographic characteristics, such as BMI, depression, fear of falling, cognitive dysfunction, number of the prescribed medication, and number of comorbidities. The pre-frail group had a significantly higher BMI than the non-frail group (*p*-value ≤ 0.001). Depression in the frail group was significantly higher than in the pre-frail group (*p*-value = 0.002). A fear of falling in the pre-frail group was lower than that in the frail group (*p*-value = 0.006) (Table 2).

Table 1. Demographic and clinical characteristics reported by mean ± standard deviation.

Parameter	Non-Frail (N)	Pre-Frail (P)	Frail (F)	N vs. P (*p*-Value)	P vs. F (*p*-Value)
Number of participants	42	78	33		
Age, years	74.02 ± 7.37	75.25 ± 11.53	78.03 ± 11.20	0.527	0.191
BMI, kg/m^2	25.21 ± 5.64	29.76 ± 6.88	31.18 ± 7.01	0.000	0.289
Depression (CES-D)	6.62 ± 5.64	8.75 ± 7.14	12.89 ± 6.33	0.083	0.002
Concern for fall (SFES-I)	20.69 ± 4.22	23.43 ± 11.14	29.69 ± 15.89	0.182	0.006
Gender (female), %	82%	54%	51%	0.001	0.247
Number of prescribed medication, N	2.5 ± 1.8	4.1 ± 3.8	6.0 ± 3.4	0.530	0.520
Number of over the counter medication, N	3.0 ± 2.5	2.7 ± 2.2	2.5 ± 2.5	0.150	0.080
Number of comorbidities, N	2.3 ± 1.8	3.7 ± 2.2	4.7 ± 1.7	0.710	0.490
Fall history:					
0 falls	71%	69%	69%	0.177	0.425
1–3 falls	24%	30%	23%	0.090	0.800
>3 falls	4%	1%	9%	0.368	0.020

BMI—body mass index; CES-D—Center for Epidemiologic Studies Depression; FES-I—Fall Efficacy Scale-International.

Table 2. Results of sensor derived parameters assessment, stratified by frailty status.

Parameters	Non-Frail (N) †	Pre-Frail (P) †	Frail (F) †	*p*-Value (Effect Size ‡)	
				N vs. P	P vs. F
Sleep Quantity					
Time in bed, min	494.3 ± 114.4	434.7 ± 125.3	402.4 ± 127.6	0.010 (0.50)	0.209 (0.26)
Sleep onset latency, min	16.9 ± 7.5	18.5 ± 7.9	20.0 ± 8.4	0.290 (0.20)	0.369 (0.18)
Total sleep time, min	367.5 ± 86.2	321.9 ± 116.5	300.9 ± 119.4	0.027 (0.45)	0.360 (0.18)
Wake after sleep onset, min	103.7 ± 48.0	89.4 ± 41.7	75.5 ± 43.0	0.081 (0.32)	0.129 (0.33)
Sleep efficiency, %	78.4 ± 9.3	77.5 ± 10.9	79.6 ± 11.6	0.650 (0.09)	0.333 (0.19)
Sleep supine position, %	43.6 ± 21.0	41.2 ± 23.2	47.5 ± 31.4	0.594 (0.11)	0.222 (0.23)
Sleep prone position, %	14.7 ± 17.5	12.3 ± 16.7	18.8 ± 23.3	0.484 (0.14)	0.091 (0.32)
Sleep side position, %	34.6 ± 17.1	34.6 ± 24.2	19.7 ± 21.1	0.994 (0.00)	0.001 (0.65)

Table 2. *Cont.*

Parameters	Non-Frail (N) †	Pre-Frail (P) †	Frail (F) †	*p*-Value (Effect Size ‡)	
				N vs. P	P vs. F
Physical Activity Pattern					
Total sit, %	43.3 ± 15.6	46.9 ± 17.1	45.7 ± 17.1	0.253 (0.22)	0.734 (0.07)
Total stand, %	16.9 ± 5.8	13.6 ± 5.8	11.3 ± 5.7	0.003 (0.57)	0.060 (0.40)
Total walk, % *	8.7 ± 3.9	5.1 ± 3.3	3.2 ± 3.2	0.000 (1.02)	0.012 (0.57)
Total Lye, %	30.9 ± 15.6	34.3 ± 20.4	39.7 ± 20.9	0.348 (0.19)	0.188 (0.26)
Longest unbroken sitting bout, s	5356.7 ± 3499.1	5351.3 ± 3042.0	5576.5 ± 3927.4	0.993 (0.00)	0.749 (0.06)
Median sitting bout, s	96.2 ± 72.9	89.6 ± 105.2	81.1 ± 92.0	0.712 (0.07)	0.666 (0.09)
Longest unbroken standing bout, s	385.3 ± 387.3	550.6 ± 723.8	553.2 ± 360.5	0.132 (0.28)	0.983 (0.00)
Median standing bout, s	15.0 ± 3.2	13.3 ± 7.5	13.3 ± 11.7	0.247 (0.29)	0.983 (0.00)
Longest unbroken walking bout, s *	351.3 ± 347.9	187.9 ± 223.9	110.3 ± 132.4	0.001 (0.56)	0.002 (0.42)
Median walking bout, s *	9.7 ± 1.0	9.0 ± 1.5	8.3 ± 1.9	0.020 (0.51)	0.018 (0.43)
Stepping Parameters					
Total step, N/1000 *	12.2 ± 6.1	6.7 ± 4.2	4.3 ± 4.3	0.000 (1.04)	0.018 (0.57)
Longest unbroken stepping bout, N *	694.3 ± 743.0	322.9 ± 411.0	162.5 ± 184.2	0.000 (0.62)	0.006 (0.57)
Median stepping bout, N	13.5 ± 2.2	10.8 ± 4.7	8.8 ± 5.2	0.001 (0.75)	0.113 (0.38)
Physical Activity Behavior					
Median Sedentary bout, s	323.8 ± 2044.6	491.1 ± 4243.4	29.7 ± 16.7	0.783 (0.05)	0.497 (0.15)
Total sedentary, h *	9.6 ± 2.6	11.7 ± 3.2	13.2 ± 4.2	0.001 (0.73)	0.029 (0.40)
Total sedentary, %	70.4 ± 12.7	81.1 ± 8.9	84.9 ± 7.0	0.000 (0.98)	0.066 (0.47)
Median light bout, s *	10.8 ± 2.2	9.6 ± 2.8	8.3 ± 2.5	0.011 (0.50)	0.013 (0.51)
Total light, h	3.2 ± 1.3	2.4 ± 1.2	2.1 ± 0.9	0.001 (0.62)	0.206 (0.29)
Total light, prc	23.7 ± 9.9	16.7 ± 7.7	13.9 ± 6.2	0.000 (0.79)	0.105 (0.39)
Median MtV, s	6.8 ± 1.9	6.8 ± 2.4	6.3 ± 1.8	0.990 (0.00)	0.267 (0.24)
Total MtV, min *	47.7 ± 30.7	19.6.3 ± 20.5	11.2 ± 14.6	0.000 (1.08)	0.047 (0.47)
Total MtV, % *	6.0 ± 4.0	2.2 ± 2.4	1.2 ± 1.5	0.000 (1.13)	0.066 (0.50)
HHS guideline, % (N)	50.0	16.0	3.1	0.000 (-)	0.109 (-)

†—average ± standard deviation; ‡—effect size calculated based on Cohen's *d* effect size for normal distribution (*d*) or for those who reject the normality (*r*), *—parameters that *p*-value < 0.05 and *d/r* ≥ 0.4; MtV—moderate-to-vigorous activity; bout—consecutive interval of a physical activity behavior without interrupt; HHS guideline—U.S. Department of Health and Human Services recommended guideline for the MtV duration.

3.2. Sleep Quantity Parameters

In the sleep parameters, we observed a trend of reduction in TiB and TST, and a trend of increase in SOL in the progression of frailty. Specifically, TiB (*p*-value = 0.010, *d* = 0.50) and TST (*p*-value = 0.027, *d* = 0.45) differed significantly in non-frail and pre-frail groups (Table 2). Interestingly, the sleep side position (*p*-value = 0.001, *d* = 0.65) was significantly different in the pre-frail and frail group. No sleep quantity parameters were capable of discriminating between the three groups of frailty statuses.

3.3. Physical Activity Pattern Parameters

In the physical activity pattern parameters, we observed a trend of reduction in standing and walking, and a trend of increase in the lying duration (Table 2). Specifically, the standing duration was significantly different between the pre-frail and non-frail (*p*-value = 0.003, *d* = 0.57). The total duration of walking, longest unbroken walking bout, and the median walking bout were capable of discriminating between the comparisons group of groups. When each parameter was fed into the model in order to identify the pre-frail group, only the total walking duration and longest unbroken walking bout had an AUC of >0.7, while the median walking bout showed an AUC of <0.7, and specificity, less than 50% (Table 3).

3.4. Stepping Parameters

All of the stepping parameters showed a trend of decline by frailty progression (Table 2). The total number of steps and the longest unbroken stepping bout were significantly different between the non-frail vs. pre-frail, and the pre-frail vs. frail groups, and they showed a significant independent predictor with an AUC > 0.7 for pre-frail status (Table 3). The median stepping bout was not significant between the groups and was also rejected when it was independently fed to the model, for an AUC < 0.7 (Table 3).

Table 3. The performance of each parameter to discriminate the pre-frail group from the non-frail and frail groups.

	Sensitivity †, %	Specificity †, %	Accuracy †, %	AUC
Physical activity behaviors				
Total sedentary, h *	91.9 ± 3.8	66.7 ± 4.4	76.3 ± 1.9	0.91 ± 0.03
Median light bout, s	100.0 ± 0.0	0.0 ± 0.0	51.9 ± 0.2	0.50 ± 0.00
Total MtV, min *	85.4 ± 3.3	77.8 ± 4.9	78.8 ± 1.7	0.92 ± 0.02
physical activity patterns				
Total walk, % *	86.1 ± 4.5	73.7 ± 6.7	78.0 ± 1.9	0.90 ± 0.02
Longest unbroken walking bout, s *	84.2 ± 5.6	67.9 ± 6.8	73.0 ± 1.6	0.87 ± 0.02
Median walking bout, s	85.3 ± 8.1	32.4 ± 13.2	59.0 ± 2.2	0.64 ± 0.02
stepping parameters				
Total step, N/1000 *	88.9 ± 3.0	74.0 ± 3.4	78.7 ± 1.2	0.89 ± 0.02
Longest unbroken stepping bout, N *	85.0 ± 5.7	75.8 ± 4.3	75.3 ± 1.9	0.88 ± 0.03

†—average ± standard deviation; AUC—area under the curve; *—parameters with asterisks were used later to develop the model.

3.5. Physical Activity Behavior Parameters

In the overall physical activity behavior parameters, we observed a reduction trend (from non-frail to frail) in the duration of light activity and moderate-to-vigorous activity, and a trend of increase in sedentary behavior (Table 2). Specifically, the percentage of sedentary behavior (p-value < 0.001, $d = 0.98$), duration of light activity (p-value = 0.001, $d = 0.62$), percentage of light activity (p-value < 0.001, $d = 0.79$), and percentage of MtV activity (p-value < 0.001, $d = 1.13$), differed significantly between the non-frail and pre-frail groups. Among the parameters, the total duration of sedentary behavior, median light activity, and total duration of MtV, differed significantly between the groups. The median light activity had a very low specificity and AUC; therefore, it was not considered for building the model so as to discriminate the pre-frail from other groups. However, the total sedentary and MtV was used in building this model. Also, we observed a trend of reduction in the percentage of participants in each group who met the physical activity recommendation from the HHS. The odds of meeting the HHS guidelines in the non-frail and pre-frail groups varied significantly (p-value < 0.001)

3.6. Performance of Models for Discriminating Pre-Frail Status

Among the non-combined models, the stepping model and the physical activity pattern (PAP) model had the same level of high sensitivity (88.6%), while the specificity of physical activity behavior (PAB) was the highest (77.9%). The accuracy of PAB and PAP were slightly (less than 2%) higher than the stepping model (Table 4). Overall, the four models showed a large AUC of ≥0.8 (Table 4). The combined model was a composite of all of the sensory parameters that were independently predictive of pre-frail status (see Table 3). This combined model had the highest sensitivity, specificity, accuracy, and AUC (91.8%, 81.4%, 84.7%, and 0.88, respectively) for identifying the pre-frail status (Table 4).

Table 4. The performance of models to separate the pre-frail group from the rest of the groups (non-frail and frail).

Models	Sensitivity †, %	Specificity †, %	Accuracy †, %	AUC †
Step Model	88.6 ± 3.8	77.5 ± 1.3	79.7 ± 0.5	0.87 ± 0.02
Physical Activity Pattern Model	88.6 ± 3.3	74.2 ± 1.7	80.6 ± 0.4	0.85 ± 0.02
Physical Activity Behavior Model	87.1 ± 6.1	77.9 ± 2.0	80.4 ± 0.6	0.85 ± 0.03
Combined Model	91.8 ± 4.2	81.4 ± 2.2	84.7 ± 0.4	0.88 ± 0.03

AUC—area under the curve; †—the mean ± standard deviation reported for the validation datasets based on a 5-fold cross validation; Step Model—the total number of steps and longest unbroken stepping bout; Physical Activity Pattern Model—the total walk and longest unbroken walking bout; Physical Activity Behavior Model—the total steps and longest unbroken stepping bout; Combined Model—all of the mentioned parameters.

4. Discussion

This study examined the association between the measurable physical activities, from a pendant accelerometer-based sensor, and the different frailty stages. Prior frailty studies, which had used sensor-derived parameters, were often based on the supervised assessment of motor performances (e.g., gait assessment, balance, Timed Up & Go, etc. [24,60–62]), which were unsuitable for the remote monitoring of the frailty stages. There were few studies that attempted to determine the frailty stages based on activity monitoring [32]. However, to our knowledge, none of the prior studies took into account both the daytime and nighttime (e.g., sleep) activities in order to distinguish the pre-frailty stage. The current study used and determined the most sensitive and independent metrics that were measurable from a single pendant sensor, including the physical activity pattern/stepping, physical activity behaviors, and sleep parameters, in order to discriminate among the frailty categories in community-dwelling older adults. Furthermore, we examined which activity-derived parameters were the most sensitive in order to distinguish pre-frailty, which was known as a potentially reversible frailty stage [35–37]. From a model construction standpoint, we not only used uni-variate, multi-variable analysis, and embedded feature selections, but we also applied a decision trees model, which had been shown to be a more robust model than conventional multi-variable models (e.g., the linear regression of logistic regression model) [62,63]. Together, the proposed approach allowed for distinguishing the pre-frailty stage from the other stages during activities of daily living, via a simple and practical wearable platform. More specifically, the results suggested that the most sensitive descriptors of the pre-frailty stage were total sedentary duration, total moderate-to-vigorous activity duration, total walking duration as a percentage of 24 h activities, longest unbroken walking bout, total daily steps, and longest unbroken steps.

While several instruments were proposed for assessing frailty (e.g., the frailty index, proposed by Rockwood et al. [11], and the frailty phenotypes, proposed by Fried et al. [10]), they were unsuitable for in-place and remote monitoring of the frailty stages, because they often required a supervised administration of the test, relied on subjective or semi-objective data obtained from self-reported inactivity and/or availability of patient health records, and were often insensitive to change over time [26,64]. The proposed model/platform and its practical form factor (using a pendant instead of securing a sensor to the chest) might have addressed these limitations and thus could have facilitated the development of a telehealth platform, based on wearables and activity monitoring. Most importantly, the results of this study suggested that a single pendant sensor could distinguish the pre-frail stage from other frailty stages. In addition, we previously demonstrated that two days of activity monitoring would be enough to determine the frailty stages [51]. This in turn, might have allowed for the tracking of changes in the frailty stages, with a relatively high time resolution (48 h), which would have provided a window of opportunity for timely preventive or therapeutic interventions that might have delayed the progression of frailty and identifying modifiable factors. This might have contributed to the deteriorating resilience (e.g., medication adverse effect, depression, immobility, etc.).

Our results were in agreement with previous studies, which suggested that total number of steps, amount of sedentary behaviors, and moderate-to-vigorous activity were associated with the progression of the frailty stages [31,32,60,61]. However, to our knowledge, this was the first study that integrated a greater variety of sensor-based measurable physical activity metrics, including steps, sleep, activity pattern, and activity behavior, into a cohesive model in order to determine the independent descriptors of the frailty stages. In addition, our study was able to demonstrate which activity related parameters, which were measurable by a pendant sensor, allowed for determining the pre-frailty stage. Our results suggested that in order to more accurately discriminate between the pre-frail and non-frail stages, a more comprehensive set of measurable physical activity categories, including sleep, activity pattern, stepping parameters, and activity patterns, could enable a significant discrimination, with effect sizes ranging from medium to large. The largest effect sizes were observed for the total walk duration, as a percentage of 24 h activities; total daily number of steps; and MtV behavior (Cohen's effect, size $d > 1.00$). The discrimination between the pre-frail and frail was, however, more challenging. Nevertheless, the moderate effect sizes were observed when the total walk, total step, longest unbroken steps number, median light bout activity, or total MtV activities were considered ($d > 0.50$). Using the univariate analysis, none of the sleep parameters were enabled to simultaneously distinguish the pre-frail from other groups, and thus were excluded from the model design. Among the remaining parameters, the most sensitive parameters were the total sedentary duration, total MtV duration, and total walk duration, which were able to identify the pre-frail from the other groups with an AUC of greater than 0.90.

Overall, we found that the frail group had the highest sedentary behaviors, which was an indicator of functional disability, as was reported in previous studies [65]. Furthermore, as previous literature had mentioned, we observed that the frail group had the highest sedentary duration, which might have led to a higher comorbidity [66]. The HSS guidelines emphasized the importance of meeting the physical activity requirements, namely, having more than 300 min per week of moderate-to-vigorous activity. We observed that the odds of meeting the guideline recommendation were significantly lower in the frail group, which might have increased the risk of adverse health outcomes [67,68].

Further investigation would be needed into the association between frailty status and light activity, which included domestic chores like instrumented activity of daily living (e.g., cooking, household tasks, etc.). In our study, light activity was unable to discriminate between the frail and pre-frail, but it did enable the distinguishing of the pre-frail from non-frail stage. A study on older females with Parkinson's disease reported an association between light activity duration and cognitive dysfunction [69]. Thus, light activity might have been representative of instrumental activities of daily living or cognitive function. On the other hand, recent studies suggested that the combination of frailty and cognitive impairment (cognitive frailty) could have better determined the prospective decline in motor and cognitive performance [70–73]. Our study did not incorporate cognitive function into the model, because it was based on the Fried frailty phenotypes, which did not include cognitive performance. Thus, further exploration would be warranted to better understand the association between light activity and frailty phenotype progression, mediated by measures of cognitive function and changes in cognitive function. Indeed, future studies investigating sensory-derived data as measures for cognitive function that integrate physical performance-based models (as presented in the current study) could provide a more holistic understanding of the progression of the frailty stages in older adults.

We observed a reduction in nocturnal sleep parameters, such as total sleep time and time in bed, and an increase in sleep onset latency in the advancing frailty stages. The same observation was reported in a previous cohort of older community-dwelling men ($n = 3133$), where the odds of sleep disturbances had increased by the risk of frailty [34]. In our study, the non-frail group had significantly lower sleep disturbances, but group comparison between the pre-frail and frail did not achieve a statistically significant level in our sample.

Finally, in order to examine the robustness of a predictive multiple variables model, so as to identify the pre-frail group among other groups, we used k-fold cross validation (k = 5) method, in which a 20% randomly selected dataset were used for the validation of the model. Using this approach, namely, stepping; the physical activity pattern; and physical activity behavior models were able to distinguish between the pre-frail from the others groups, with an AUC of 0.87, 0.85, and 0.85, respectively. The combination model improved on the discriminative power, with an AUC of 0.88.

To improve the level of comfort and mimic the telehealth platforms, which often incorporated a pendant sensor (e.g., personal emergency response system [PERS], such as pendant automatic fall detectors), we used a pendant accelerometer to monitor sleep and activities instead of securing the sensor on the chest, which had been used in previous studies [41,43]. This approach might have affected the accuracy of the activity detection, as well as the estimation of the sleep parameters of interest. Despite this potential limitation, the measured parameters achieved a statistically significant level so as to distinguish the pre-frailty stages, thus creating a more realistic sensor-based method in order to monitor the frailty stages and their fluctuation over time, without hindering the everyday activities of daily living. In addition, the proposed study design could have facilitated the integration of the designed model in the currently available pendant PERS platforms.

5. Limitations

This study had several limitations. The sample size (n = 163) was relatively small and may be insufficient to represent the general older adults population. In addition, the feature selection was done based on the entire sample, and the sample size might have been insufficient for the purpose of the k-fold cross validation model. However, as recommended by the prior literature, this approach was shown to be more robust than the conventional approaches for relatively small sample size studies [56,57]. To better examine the validity and reliability of the proposed model, another study was needed to confirm that the results remained the same when using an independent and larger dataset. Therefore, the results needed to be confirmed in a larger sample, in order to be generalized. As this was a cross-sectional study, the sensitivity to change over time for the proposed model was unclear and needed to be verified in another study. In addition, the ability of the proposed model to predict the prospective adverse health outcomes, including mortality or loss of independency, should have been examined in another study. We used the Fried physical phenotypes criteria to determine the frailty stages, which carried some limitations, including a lack of consideration for cognitive function and using the categorical stages (non-frail, pre-frail, and frail) instead of a continuous scale. Fine tuning the model outputs in comparison with other well-established frailty assessment tools, such as the frailty index (an alternative frailty conceptual model that measures accumulation of deficits and provides a continuous scale instead of categorical), might have been useful for designing a more sensitive to change metric for the purpose of longitudinal studies. Two days of continuous monitoring (48 h) might not have been sufficient in order to represent the overall in-place activities of older adults. However, as suggested in our previous study [51], two days of continuous monitoring yielded a reliable representation of daily physical activities in a geriatric population, in particular among those with the frailty status, because of the reduction in the activities complexities or day-to-day variation, as suggested by previous studies [74–76]. On the other hand, in order to determine the causal factors that might have led to physical frailty, for instance in response to medication, a high time resolution, to determine frailty phenotypes, might have been considered as an advantage of the proposed approach. However, future studies were needed that would examine whether the proposed frailty model was sensitive to change and could track changes in the frailty stages over time.

6. Conclusions

We demonstrated that a single pendant accelerometer enables determining the frailty stages, including pre-frailty, via an in-place monitoring of the spontaneous daily physical activity, including the day time and night time. Among the measurable parameters, using a single pendant accelerometer-based device, a combination of step parameters (e.g., number of daily taken steps, longest unbroken steps), activity behavior (e.g., moderate-to-vigorous and sedentary activities), and postures (e.g., duration of standing, walking, and longest unbroken walking bout duration) enables the distinguishing of the pre-frailty stage among non-frail and frail stages, with AUC of 0.88. The proposed model and the form factor of the sensor that was used (pendant instead of securing sensor to the skin) provide advantages, compared with the conventional frailty assessment tools, for the purpose of in-place and prolonged screening (over days and months). In addition, it doesn't require a supervised administration of testing (unsupervised monitoring of frailty stages); it is objective; and does not need patient health records, demographics, or self-report, which makes it easy and cost-effective for deployment for in-place monitoring platforms. It can also facilitate in the development of a telehealth platform, based on wearable technology, to determine the modifiable factors that are significant for the advancing frailty stages (e.g., use of medication, which may negatively impact subject resilient; sleep deprivation; depression; cognitive decline; etc.). These potential applications, however, need to be validated in future studies.

Author Contributions: B.N., A.D.N., M.E.K., A.S. and J.R. helped with the study design and interpretation of the data. J.R., H.Z. and M.A. helped on data collection and analyzing. All of the authors read the manuscript and participated in writing the manuscript.

Funding: This research was partly funded by the National Institute of Health/National Institute of Aging (Award number: 2R42AG032748-04) and the U.S. Department of Veterans Affairs, Veterans Health Administration, Health Services Research and Development Service. J.R. was also funded by receives support from the Big Data-Scientist Training Enhancement Program (BD-STEP).

Acknowledgments: J.R. is the Post-doctoral research fellow at the Center for Innovations in Quality, Effectiveness and Safety (CIN 13-413), Michael E. DeBakey VA Medical Center, Houston, TX, USA and he receives support from the Big Data-Scientist Training Enhancement Program (BD-STEP). The content is solely the responsibility of the authors and does not necessarily represent the official views of the sponsors. The authors would like to thank Kimberly Macellaro, a member of the Baylor College of Medicine Michael E. DeBakey Department of Surgery Research Core Team, for her editorial assistance during the preparation of this manuscript.

Conflicts of Interest: While the overlap with this study is minimal, using activity monitoring to determine frailty is protected by a patent pending (US20150272511 A1). The patent is owned by University of Arizona, and B.N. is listed as a co-inventor on this patent pending. Other author(s) declared no potential conflicts of interest with respect to the research, authorship, and/or publication of this article.

References

1. Ortman, J.M.; Velkoff, V.A.; Hogan, H. An Aging Nation: The Older Population in the United States. Available online: http://bowchair.com/uploads/9/8/4/9/98495722/agingcensus.pdf (accessed on 25 April 2018).
2. Papanikitas, A.; Spicer, J. *Handbook of Primary Care Ethics*; CRC Press: Boca Raton, FL, USA, 2017.
3. Bandeen-Roche, K.; Seplaki, C.L.; Huang, J.; Buta, B.; Kalyani, R.R.; Varadhan, R.; Xue, Q.-L.; Walston, J.D.; Kasper, J.D. Frailty in older adults: A nationally representative profile in the United States. *J. Gerontol. Ser. A* **2015**, *70*, 1427–1434. [CrossRef] [PubMed]
4. British Geriatrics Society. *Fit for Frailty: Consensus Best Practice Guidance for the Care of Older People Living with Frailty in Community and Outpatient Settings*; British Geriatrics Society: London, UK, 2015.
5. Ensrud, K.E.; Ewing, S.K.; Cawthon, P.M.; Fink, H.A.; Taylor, B.C.; Cauley, J.A.; Dam, T.T.; Marshall, L.M.; Orwoll, E.S.; Cummings, S.R. A comparison of frailty indexes for the prediction of falls, disability, fractures, and mortality in older men. *J. Am. Geriatr. Soc.* **2009**, *57*, 492–498. [CrossRef] [PubMed]
6. Rodriguez-Mañas, L.; Fried, L.P. Frailty in the clinical scenario. *Lancet* **2015**, *385*, e7–e9. [CrossRef]
7. Xue, Q.-L. The frailty syndrome: Definition and natural history. *Clin. Geriatr. Med.* **2011**, *27*, 1–15. [CrossRef] [PubMed]
8. Chen, X.; Mao, G.; Leng, S.X. Frailty syndrome: An overview. *Clin. Interv. Aging* **2014**, *9*, 433–441. [PubMed]
9. Cohen, M.S.; Paul, E.; Nuschke, J.D.; Tolentino, J.C.; Mendez, A.V.C.; Mira, A.-E.A.; Baxter, R.A.; Stawicki, S.P. Patient Frailty: Key Considerations, Definitions and Practical Implications. In *Challenges in Elder Care*; InTech: Princeton, NJ, USA, 2016.

10. Fried, L.P.; Tangen, C.M.; Walston, J.; Newman, A.B.; Hirsch, C.; Gottdiener, J.; Seeman, T.; Tracy, R.; Kop, W.J.; Burke, G. Frailty in older adults: Evidence for a phenotype. *J. Gerontol. Ser. A* **2001**, *56*, M146–M157. [CrossRef]

11. Mitnitski, A.B.; Mogilner, A.J.; Rockwood, K. Accumulation of deficits as a proxy measure of aging. *Sci. World J.* **2001**, *1*, 323–336. [CrossRef] [PubMed]

12. Dedeyne, L.; Deschodt, M.; Verschueren, S.; Tournoy, J.; Gielen, E. Effects of multi-domain interventions in (pre) frail elderly on frailty, functional, and cognitive status: A systematic review. *Clin. Interv. Aging* **2017**, *12*, 873–896. [CrossRef] [PubMed]

13. Makizako, H.; Shimada, H.; Doi, T.; Tsutsumimoto, K.; Suzuki, T. Impact of physical frailty on disability in community-dwelling older adults: A prospective cohort study. *BMJ Open* **2015**, *5*, e008462. [CrossRef] [PubMed]

14. Cameron, I.D.; Fairhall, N.; Gill, L.; Lockwood, K.; Langron, C.; Aggar, C.; Monaghan, N.; Kurrle, S. Developing interventions for frailty. *Adv. Geriatr.* **2015**, *2015*, 1–7. [CrossRef]

15. Toosizadeh, N.; Joseph, B.; Heusser, M.R.; Jokar, T.O.; Mohler, J.; Phelan, H.A.; Najafi, B. Assessing upper-extremity motion: An innovative, objective method to identify frailty in older bed-bound trauma patients. *J. Am. Coll. Surg.* **2016**, *223*, 240–248. [CrossRef] [PubMed]

16. Juma, S.; Taabazuing, M.-M.; Montero-Odasso, M. Clinical frailty scale in an acute medicine unit: A simple tool that predicts length of stay. *Can. Geriatr. J.* **2016**, *19*, 34–39. [CrossRef] [PubMed]

17. Buchman, A.; Wilson, R.; Bienias, J.; Bennett, D. Change in frailty and risk of death in older persons. *Exp. Aging Res.* **2009**, *35*, 61–82. [CrossRef] [PubMed]

18. Khezrian, M.; Myint, P.K.; McNeil, C.; Murray, A.D. A Review of Frailty Syndrome and Its Physical, Cognitive and Emotional Domains in the Elderly. *Geriatrics* **2017**, *2*, 36. [CrossRef]

19. Da Câmara, S.M.A.; Alvarado, B.E.; Guralnik, J.M.; Guerra, R.O.; Maciel, Á.C.C. Using the Short Physical Performance Battery to screen for frailty in young-old adults with distinct socioeconomic conditions. *Geriatr. Gerontol. Int.* **2013**, *13*, 421–428. [CrossRef] [PubMed]

20. Kiely, D.K.; Cupples, L.A.; Lipsitz, L.A. Validation and comparison of two frailty indexes: The MOBILIZE Boston Study. *J. Am. Geriatr. Soc.* **2009**, *57*, 1532–1539. [CrossRef] [PubMed]

21. Melzer, D.; Lan, T.-Y.; Tom, B.D.; Deeg, D.J.; Guralnik, J.M. Variation in thresholds for reporting mobility disability between national population subgroups and studies. *J. Gerontol. Ser. A* **2004**, *59*, 1295–1303. [CrossRef]

22. Tudor-Locke, C.E.; Myers, A.M. Challenges and opportunities for measuring physical activity in sedentary adults. *Sports Med.* **2001**, *31*, 91–100. [CrossRef] [PubMed]

23. Joseph, B.; Toosizadeh, N.; Jokar, T.O.; Heusser, M.R.; Mohler, J.; Najafi, B. Upper-extremity function predicts adverse health outcomes among older adults hospitalized for ground-level falls. *Gerontology* **2017**, *63*, 299–307. [CrossRef] [PubMed]

24. Schwenk, M.; Mohler, J.; Wendel, C.; Fain, M.; Taylor-Piliae, R.; Najafi, B. Wearable sensor-based in-home assessment of gait, balance, and physical activity for discrimination of frailty status: Baseline results of the Arizona frailty cohort study. *Gerontology* **2015**, *61*, 258–267. [CrossRef] [PubMed]

25. Zhou, H.; Sabbagh, M.; Wyman, R.; Liebsack, C.; Kunik, M.E.; Najafi, B. Instrumented trail-making task to differentiate persons with no cognitive impairment, amnestic mild cognitive impairment, and Alzheimer disease: A proof of concept study. *Gerontology* **2017**, *63*, 189–200. [CrossRef] [PubMed]

26. Lee, H.; Joseph, B.; Enriquez, A.; Najafi, B. Toward Using a Smartwatch to Monitor Frailty in a Hospital Setting: Using a Single Wrist-Wearable Sensor to Assess Frailty in Bedbound Inpatients. *Gerontology* **2017**. [CrossRef] [PubMed]

27. Toosizadeh, N.; Mohler, J.; Najafi, B. Assessing upper extremity motion: An innovative method to identify frailty. *J. Am. Geriatr. Soc.* **2015**, *63*, 1181–1186. [CrossRef] [PubMed]

28. Del Pozo-Cruz, B.; Mañas, A.; Martín-García, M.; Marín-Puyalto, J.; García-García, F.J.; Rodriguez-Mañas, L.; Guadalupe-Grau, A.; Ara, I. Frailty is associated with objectively assessed sedentary behaviour patterns in older adults: Evidence from the Toledo Study for Healthy Aging (TSHA). *PLoS ONE* **2017**, *12*, e0183911. [CrossRef] [PubMed]

29. Galan-Mercant, A.; Cuesta-Vargas, A. Clinical frailty syndrome assessment using inertial sensors embedded in smartphones. *Physiol. Meas.* **2015**, *36*, 1929–1944. [CrossRef] [PubMed]

30. Haider, S.; Luger, E.; Kapan, A.; Titze, S.; Lackinger, C.; Schindler, K.E.; Dorner, T.E. Associations between daily physical activity, handgrip strength, muscle mass, physical performance and quality of life in prefrail and frail community-dwelling older adults. *Qual. Life Res.* **2016**, *25*, 3129–3138. [CrossRef] [PubMed]
31. Theou, O.; Jakobi, J.M.; Vandervoort, A.A.; Jones, G.R. A comparison of physical activity (PA) assessment tools across levels of frailty. *Arch. Gerontol. Geriatr.* **2012**, *54*, e307–e314. [CrossRef] [PubMed]
32. Blodgett, J.; Theou, O.; Kirkland, S.; Andreou, P.; Rockwood, K. The association between sedentary behaviour, moderate–vigorous physical activity and frailty in NHANES cohorts. *Maturitas* **2015**, *80*, 187–191. [CrossRef] [PubMed]
33. Ensrud, K.E.; Blackwell, T.L.; Ancoli-Israel, S.; Redline, S.; Cawthon, P.M.; Paudel, M.L.; Dam, T.-T.L.; Stone, K.L. Sleep disturbances and risk of frailty and mortality in older men. *Sleep Med.* **2012**, *13*, 1217–1225. [CrossRef] [PubMed]
34. Ensrud, K.E.; Blackwell, T.L.; Redline, S.; Ancoli-Israel, S.; Paudel, M.L.; Cawthon, P.M.; Dam, T.T.L.; Barrett-Connor, E.; Leung, P.C.; Stone, K.L. Sleep Disturbances and Frailty Status in Older Community-Dwelling Men. *J. Am. Geriatr. Soc.* **2009**, *57*, 2085–2093. [CrossRef] [PubMed]
35. Lang, P.O.; Michel, J.P.; Zekry, D. Frailty syndrome: A transitional state in a dynamic process. *Gerontology* **2009**, *55*, 539–549. [CrossRef] [PubMed]
36. Mohler, M.J.; Fain, M.J.; Wertheimer, A.M.; Najafi, B.; Nikolich-Zugich, J. The Frailty syndrome: Clinical measurements and basic underpinnings in humans and animals. *Exp. Gerontol.* **2014**, *54*, 6–13. [CrossRef] [PubMed]
37. Mohler, J.; Najafi, B.; Fain, M.; Ramos, K.S. Precision Medicine: A Wider Definition. *J. Am. Geriatr. Soc.* **2015**, *63*, 1971–1972. [CrossRef] [PubMed]
38. Tombaugh, T.N.; McIntyre, N.J. The mini-mental state examination: A comprehensive review. *J. Am. Geriatr. Soc.* **1992**, *40*, 922–935. [CrossRef] [PubMed]
39. Yardley, L.; Beyer, N.; Hauer, K.; Kempen, G.; Piot-Ziegler, C.; Todd, C. Development and initial validation of the Falls Efficacy Scale-International (FES-I). *Age Ageing* **2005**, *34*, 614–619. [CrossRef] [PubMed]
40. Lewinsohn, P.M.; Seeley, J.R.; Roberts, R.E.; Allen, N.B. Center for Epidemiologic Studies Depression Scale (CES-D) as a screening instrument for depression among community-residing older adults. *Psychol. Aging* **1997**, *12*, 277–287. [CrossRef] [PubMed]
41. Razjouyan, J.; Lee, H.; Parthasarathy, S.; Mohler, J.; Sharafkhaneh, A.; Najafi, B. Improving Sleep Quality Assessment Using Wearable Sensors by Including Information From Postural/Sleep Position Changes and Body Acceleration: A Comparison of Chest-Worn Sensors, Wrist Actigraphy, and Polysomnography. *J. Clin. Sleep Med.* **2017**, *13*, 1301–1310. [CrossRef] [PubMed]
42. Aminian, K.; Najafi, B.; Büla, C.; Leyvraz, P.-F.; Robert, P. Spatio-temporal parameters of gait measured by an ambulatory system using miniature gyroscopes. *J. Biomech.* **2002**, *35*, 689–699. [CrossRef]
43. Aminian, K.; Najafi, B. Capturing human motion using body-fixed sensors: Outdoor measurement and clinical applications. *Comput. Anim. Virtual Worlds* **2004**, *15*, 79–94. [CrossRef]
44. Najafi, B.; Armstrong, D.G.; Mohler, J. Novel wearable technology for assessing spontaneous daily physical activity and risk of falling in older adults with diabetes. *J. Diabetes Sci. Technol.* **2013**, *7*, 1147–1160. [CrossRef] [PubMed]
45. Troiano, R.P.; Berrigan, D.; Dodd, K.W.; Masse, L.C.; Tilert, T.; McDowell, M. Physical activity in the United States measured by accelerometer. *Med. Sci.Sports Exerc.* **2008**, *40*, 181–188. [CrossRef] [PubMed]
46. US Department of Health and Human Services. Physical Activity Guideline. Available online: http://www.health.gov/paguidelines (accessed on 25 April 2018).
47. Vähä-Ypyä, H.; Vasankari, T.; Husu, P.; Mänttäri, A.; Vuorimaa, T.; Suni, J.; Sievänen, H. Validation of cut-points for evaluating the intensity of physical activity with accelerometry-based mean amplitude deviation (MAD). *PLoS ONE* **2015**, *10*, e0134813. [CrossRef] [PubMed]
48. Rioul, O.; Vetterli, M. Wavelets and signal processing. *IEEE Signal Process. Mag.* **1991**, *8*, 14–38. [CrossRef]
49. Ogden, T. *Essential Wavelets for Statistical Applications and Data Analysis*; Springer: Berlin, Germany, 2012.
50. Dunlop, D.D.; Song, J.; Semanik, P.A.; Chang, R.W.; Sharma, L.; Bathon, J.M.; Eaton, C.B.; Hochberg, M.C.; Jackson, R.D.; Kwoh, C.K. Objective physical activity measurement in the osteoarthritis initiative: Are guidelines being met? *Arthrit. Rheumatol.* **2011**, *63*, 3372–3382. [CrossRef] [PubMed]
51. De Bruin, E.D.; Najafi, B.; Murer, K.; Uebelhart, D.; Aminian, K. Quantification of everyday motor function in a geriatric population. *J. Rehabil. Res. Dev.* **2007**, *44*, 417–428. [CrossRef] [PubMed]

52. Pate, R.R.; Pratt, M.; Blair, S.N.; Haskell, W.L.; Macera, C.A.; Bouchard, C.; Buchner, D.; Ettinger, W.; Heath, G.W.; King, A.C. Physical activity and public health: A recommendation from the Centers for Disease Control and Prevention and the American College of Sports Medicine. *JAMA* **1995**, *273*, 402–407. [CrossRef] [PubMed]

53. Najafi, B.; Aminian, K.; Paraschiv-Ionescu, A.; Loew, F.; Bula, C.J.; Robert, P. Ambulatory system for human motion analysis using a kinematic sensor: Monitoring of daily physical activity in the elderly. *IEEE Trans. Biomed. Eng.* **2003**, *50*, 711–723. [CrossRef] [PubMed]

54. Jović, A.; Brkić, K.; Bogunović, N. A review of feature selection methods with applications. In Proceedings of the 2015 38th International Convention on Information and Communication Technology, Electronics and Microelectronics (MIPRO), Opatija, Croatia, 25–29 May 2015; pp. 1200–1205.

55. Chatfield, K.; Simonyan, K.; Vedaldi, A.; Zisserman, A. Return of the devil in the details: Delving deep into convolutional nets. *arXiv*, 2014.

56. Singhi, S.K.; Liu, H. Feature subset selection bias for classification learning. In Proceedings of the 23rd International Conference on Machine Learning, Haifa, Israel, 27–29 June 2010; pp. 849–856.

57. Guyon, I.; Elisseeff, A. An introduction to variable and feature selection. *J. Mach. Learn. Res.* **2003**, *3*, 1157–1182.

58. Refaeilzadeh, P.; Tang, L.; Liu, H. Cross-validation. In *Encyclopedia of Database Systems*; Springer: Berlin, Germany, 2009; pp. 532–538.

59. Arlot, S.; Celisse, A. A survey of cross-validation procedures for model selection. *Stat. Surv.* **2010**, *4*, 40–79. [CrossRef]

60. Parvaneh, S.; Mohler, J.; Toosizadeh, N.; Grewal, G.S.; Najafi, B. Postural Transitions during Activities of Daily Living Could Identify Frailty Status: Application of Wearable Technology to Identify Frailty during Unsupervised Condition. *Gerontology* **2017**, *63*, 479–487. [CrossRef] [PubMed]

61. Schwenk, M.; Howe, C.; Saleh, A.; Mohler, J.; Grewal, G.; Armstrong, D.; Najafi, B. Frailty and technology: A systematic review of gait analysis in those with frailty. *Gerontology* **2014**, *60*, 79–89. [CrossRef] [PubMed]

62. Shumway-Cook, A.; Brauer, S.; Woollacott, M. Predicting the probability for falls in community-dwelling older adults using the Timed Up & Go Test. *Phys. Ther.* **2000**, *80*, 896–903. [PubMed]

63. Rudolfer, S.M.; Paliouras, G.; Peers, I.S. A comparison of logistic regression to decision tree induction in the diagnosis of carpal tunnel syndrome. *Comput. Biomed. Res.* **1999**, *32*, 391–414. [CrossRef] [PubMed]

64. Lee, H.; Joseph, B.; Najafi, B. Optimized Upper Extremity Frailty Parameters for Assessing Frailty in Trauma Patients. *Innov. Aging* **2017**, *1*, 618. [CrossRef]

65. Tremblay, M.S.; Kho, M.E.; Tricco, A.C.; Duggan, M. Process description and evaluation of Canadian Physical Activity Guidelines development. *Int. J. Behav. Nutr. Phys. Act.* **2010**, *7*, 42. [CrossRef] [PubMed]

66. Hassapidou, M.; Papadopoulou, S.K.; Vlahavas, G.; Kapantais, E.; Kaklamanou, D.; Pagkalos, I.; Kaklamanou, M.; Tzotzas, T. Association of physical activity and sedentary lifestyle patterns with obesity and cardiometabolic comorbidities in Greek adults: Data from the National Epidemiological Survey. *Hormones* **2013**, *12*, 265–274. [CrossRef] [PubMed]

67. Thorp, A.A.; Healy, G.N.; Winkler, E.; Clark, B.K.; Gardiner, P.A.; Owen, N.; Dunstan, D.W. Prolonged sedentary time and physical activity in workplace and non-work contexts: A cross-sectional study of office, customer service and call centre employees. *Int. J. Behav. Nutr. Phys. Act.* **2012**, *9*, 128. [CrossRef] [PubMed]

68. Peterson, M.J.; Giuliani, C.; Morey, M.C.; Pieper, C.F.; Evenson, K.R.; Mercer, V.; Cohen, H.J.; Visser, M.; Brach, J.S.; Kritchevsky, S.B. Physical activity as a preventative factor for frailty: The health, aging, and body composition study. *J. Gerontol.* **2009**, *64*, 61–68. [CrossRef] [PubMed]

69. Roland, K.P.; MD Cornett, K.; Theou, O.; Jakobi, J.M.; Jones, G.R. Physical activity across frailty phenotypes in females with Parkinson's disease. *J. Aging Res.* **2012**, *2012*, 1–8. [CrossRef] [PubMed]

70. Ruan, Q.; Yu, Z.; Chen, M.; Bao, Z.; Li, J.; He, W. Cognitive frailty, a novel target for the prevention of elderly dependency. *Ageing Res. Rev.* **2015**, *20*, 1–10. [CrossRef] [PubMed]

71. Kelaiditi, E.; Canevelli, M.; Andrieu, S.; Del Campo, N.; Soto, M.E.; Vellas, B.; Cesari, M. Impact of Cholinergic Treatment Use Study, D.S.A.G. Frailty Index and Cognitive Decline in Alzheimer's Disease: Data from the Impact of Cholinergic Treatment USe Study. *J. Am. Geriatr. Soc.* **2016**, *64*, 1165–1170. [CrossRef] [PubMed]

72. Kelaiditi, E.; Cesari, M.; Canevelli, M.; van Kan, G.A.; Ousset, P.J.; Gillette-Guyonnet, S.; Ritz, P.; Duveau, F.; Soto, M.E.; Provencher, V.; et al. Cognitive frailty: Rational and definition from an (I.A.N.A./I.A.G.G.) international consensus group. *J. Nutr. Health Aging* **2013**, *17*, 726–734. [CrossRef] [PubMed]

73. Zhou, H.; Lee, H.; Lee, J.; Schwenk, M.; Najafi, B. Motor Planning Error: Toward Measuring Cognitive Frailty in Older Adults Using Wearables. *Sensors* **2018**, *18*, 926. [CrossRef] [PubMed]
74. Bussmann, J.B.; van den Berg-Emons, R.J. To total amount of activity and beyond: Perspectives on measuring physical behavior. *Front. Psychol.* **2013**, *4*, 463. [CrossRef] [PubMed]
75. Moufawad El Achkar, C.; Lenoble-Hoskovec, C.; Paraschiv-Ionescu, A.; Major, K.; Bula, C.; Aminian, K. Physical Behavior in Older Persons during Daily Life: Insights from Instrumented Shoes. *Sensors* **2016**, *16*, 1225. [CrossRef] [PubMed]
76. Paraschiv-Ionescu, A.; Perruchoud, C.; Buchser, E.; Aminian, K. Barcoding human physical activity to assess chronic pain conditions. *PLoS ONE* **2012**, *7*, e32239. [CrossRef] [PubMed]

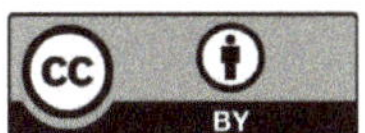

© 2018 by the authors. Licensee MDPI, Basel, Switzerland. This article is an open access article distributed under the terms and conditions of the Creative Commons Attribution (CC BY) license (http://creativecommons.org/licenses/by/4.0/).

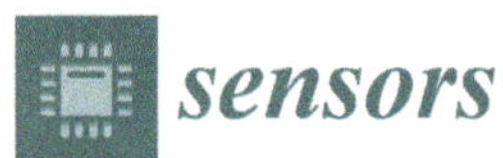 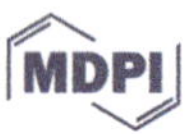

Article

Improving Fall Detection Using an On-Wrist Wearable Accelerometer

Samad Barri Khojasteh [1,†], José R. Villar [2,*,†,‡], Camelia Chira [3,†], Víctor M. González [2,†] and Enrique de la Cal [2,†]

1   Sakarya University, 54050 Sakarya, Turkey; samad.khojasteh@ogr.sakarya.edu.tr
2   Electric, Electronic, Computers and Systems Engineering Department, University of Oviedo, 33003 Oviedo, Spain; vmsuarez@uniovi.es (V.M.G.); delacal@uniovi.es (E.d.l.C.)
3   Computer Science Department, Babes-Bolyai University, 400084 Cluj-Napoca, Romania; cchira@cs.ubbcluj.ro
*   Correspondence: villarjose@uniovi.es; Tel.: +34-985-182-597
†   These authors contributed equally to this work.
‡   Current address: Computer Science Department, University of Oviedo, EIMEM, c/Independencia 13, 33004 Oviedo, Spain.

Received: 12 March 2018; Accepted: 23 April 2018; Published: 26 April 2018

Abstract: Fall detection is a very important challenge that affects both elderly people and the carers. Improvements in fall detection would reduce the aid response time. This research focuses on a method for fall detection with a sensor placed on the wrist. Falls are detected using a published threshold-based solution, although a study on threshold tuning has been carried out. The feature extraction is extended in order to balance the dataset for the minority class. Alternative models have been analyzed to reduce the computational constraints so the solution can be embedded in smart-phones or smart wristbands. Several published datasets have been used in the Materials and Methods section. Although these datasets do not include data from real falls of elderly people, a complete comparison study of fall-related datasets shows statistical differences between the simulated falls and real falls from participants suffering from impairment diseases. Given the obtained results, the rule-based systems represent a promising research line as they perform similarly to neural networks, but with a reduced computational cost. Furthermore, support vector machines performed with a high specificity. However, further research to validate the proposal in real on-line scenarios is needed. Furthermore, a slight improvement should be made to reduce the number of false alarms.

Keywords: fall detection; wearable sensors; elderly people monitoring

1. Introduction

Fall Detection (FD) is a very active research area, with many applications in health care, work safety, etc. [1]. Even though there are plenty of commercial products, the best rated products only reach an 80% success rate [2,3]. There are basically two types of FD systems: context-aware systems and wearable devices [4,5]. FD has been widely studied using context-aware systems, i.e., video systems [6]; nevertheless, the use of wearable devices is crucial because of the high percentage of elderly people and their desire to live autonomously in their own house [7].

Wearable-based solutions may combine different sensors, such as a barometer and inertial sensors [8], 3DACC combined with other devices, like a gyroscope [9], intelligent tiles [10] or a barometer in a necklace [11]. By far, 3DACC is the most used option within the literature [12–16]. Different solutions have been proposed to perform the FD; for instance, a feature extraction stage and SVM have been applied directly in [12,14], using some transformations and thresholds with very simple rules for classifying an event as a fall [15–17]. A comparison of classifiers has been presented in [13].

The common characteristic in all these solutions is that the wearable devices are placed on the waist or on the chest. The reason for this location is that it is by far much easier to detect a fall using the sensory system in this placement [18]. Clearly, each location is the best option for some cases, while for other problems, it may not be the best one. For instance, placing the sensor on the waist is valid for patients with severe impairment; however, the requirement to use a belt with some dressing might not be valid in the case of healthy participants. Furthermore, this type of device lacks usability, and people might find it easy to forget them on the bedside table [4,19]. Thus, this research limits itself to use a single sensor, a commercial smart wristband, placed on the wrist.

Furthermore, these previous studies do not focus on the specific dynamics of a falling event: although some of the proposals report good performances, they are just machine learning applied to the FD problem. There are studies concerned with the dynamics in a fall event with sensors located on the waist [20–23], establishing the taxonomy and the time periods for each sequence. Interestingly, it has been found that the vast majority of the solutions have been obtained using data gathered from simulated falls [3,24]; these studies have found that analyzing the solutions with data gathered from real falls produce a high error rate and rather poor performances. As far as we know, FARSEEING (FAll Repository for the design of Smart and sElf-adaptive Environments prolonging Independent livinG) is the first dataset including data from real elderly persons' falls [3]. The data have been gathered from patients suffering an impairment illness while using a 3DACC placed either on the thigh or on the lower back. It seems the data must come from the same population in order to record the inherent behavior of the subjects when falling, which may vary with age [25].

Focusing on FD using a wrist-worn bracelet, there are several works published in the literature. Ngu et al. proposed using a BLE link with a smartphone that has access to intelligent web services [26]. Basically, the agent running on the smartphone gathers the 3DACC data stream, analyzing each sliding window with a one step sample. For each sliding window, up to four features are computed and fed to an SVM, which classifies the window as FALLor NOT_FALL. For training the SVM, the authors proposed a training stage for each user, sending the data stream to an intelligent web service to learn the model. Furthermore, the authors proposed a set of ADL to be performed by the user to gather data, including the fall simulation.

In [27], a smartwatch sends the data to a smartphone, where the detection takes place in the smartphone using Kalman filters and the CUMSUMalgorithm [28] using adaptive thresholds. Similarly, a commercial wrist-worn 3DACC wearable was used together with a smartphone to detect falls and inactivity in [29]. In this case, the wearable delivers the processed data to the BLE-linked smartphone, which includes an implementation of WEKA. With the gathered data, an NN model was trained to discriminate between fall and several ADL; also, a threshold-based inactivity detection is continuously updated. As the authors stated, one of the problems is the energy efficiency of the wearable: the data stream, even with BLE, penalizes the battery life. Furthermore, an important problem refers to computing the models in the wearable, which also reduces the autonomy. Moreover, the authors stated the problem of the "heavy dependence on the availability of a smartphone which should therefore always be within a few meters of the user" [29].

A threshold-based solution was analyzed in [30], where up to four different features were computed for each sliding window with one sample shift. Up to 11 thresholds were defined; their values were found experimentally. The authors reported very good results when the alternative ADLs were walking, sitting and other. When the threshold algorithms ran both on the smartphone and on the wrist worn wearable device, the performance was enhanced between 5 and 15%. Although thresholds have been widely used in the literature, having only this type of discrimination might not apply to the general population. Additionally, depending on the availability of the smartphone, this represents a big challenge as the whole FD is computed in this device. A similar solution is proposed in [31], using threshold-based algorithms in both the smartwatch and in the smartphone.

An alternative solution was proposed in [32], where a smartwatch works autonomously to detect falls and send notifications. Threshold-based solutions were proposed assuming that only those falls for which the user faints are the ones to be detected: in the rest of the cases, the user is in charge of calling the ehealth service. Similarly, [27] made use of an Android smartphone to run threshold-based FD. In these latter studies, the authors proposed a continuous analysis of the acceleration magnitude in order to classify the current motion as FALL or NOT_FALL. As the authors stated in these papers, performing more complex models continuously would drain the battery, severely reducing the autonomy of the solution.

In one of the published solutions, Abbate et al. [33] proposed the use of the inherent dynamics of a fall as the basis of the FD algorithm with the sensor placed on the waist. A fall event detection is run continuously based on peak detection; once a peak is detected, a feature extraction is performed, and a feed forward NN classifies the event as FALL or NOT_FALL. A very interesting point of this approach is that the computational constraints for the first two stages are kept moderate so as to be deployed in a wearable device, although this solution includes a high number of thresholds to tune.

The aim of this study is to develop a wrist wearable solution for FD focused on the elderly. A wrist-worn 3DACC on a smart wristband is proposed to enhance the ergonomic skills of the solution. Based on [33], the solution has been implemented and enhanced with (i) an intelligent optimization stage to improve the peak detection, (ii) a dataset balancing stage to avoid biasing the models towards the majority class, (iii) alternative machine learning methods compared to the one originally proposed in order to reduce the computational complexity and promote a longer battery life. Finally, this study makes use of several published datasets, including real falls [3], simulated falls and ADL [34], ADL only [35] and from ADL and simulated epileptic seizures [36]; all of them are using 3DACC, the former with the sensor on the lower back or on the thigh, the three latter with the sensor placed on a wrist. A comparison between real falls suffered by elderly people and falls from young participants in ideal conditions is included to analyze the validity of the results using the simulated falls. Moreover, a complex cross-validation stage, including training, testing and validation, is performed. To our knowledge, this is the first study considering so many different published datasets and a complex scheme of comparison to analyze different FD solutions.

The remainder of this study is organized as follows. Next, the description of the solution proposed in this research is outlined. Section 3 details the experimentation that has been carried out, while Section 4 shows the experiment results and the discussion on them. The study ends with the conclusions drawn from this research.

2. Fall Detection with a Wrist-Worn Sensor

The block diagram depicted in Figure 1 is defined in this research, which basically is the proposal in [33]. The data gathered from a 3DACC located on the wrist are processed using a sliding window. A peak detection is performed, and if a peak is found, the data within the sliding window are analyzed to extract several features, which are ultimately classified as FALL or NOT_FALL. The FD block is performed with an AI classifier.

The next subsection describes the method for detecting a peak, as well as the feature extraction, while the method for training the FD block is detailed in Section 2.2. For each case, the proposed modifications are included. A discussion on the most suitable models to be used in this approach is held in Section 2.3. Finally, a new stage is included in the process devoted to the tuning of the peak detection threshold; this stage is explained in Section 2.4.

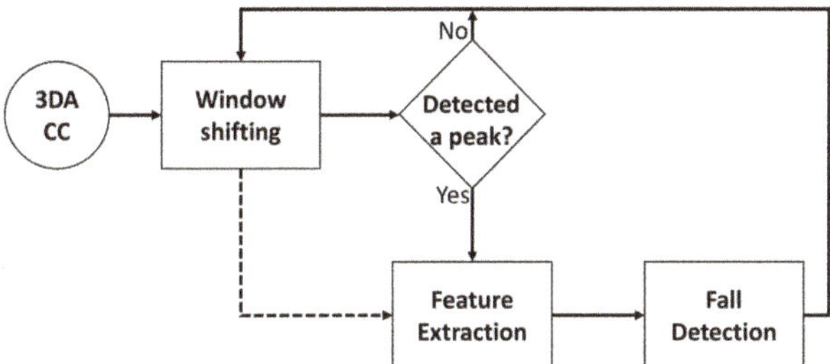

Figure 1. Block diagram of the solution.

2.1. Feature Extraction Based on the Dynamics of a Fall

Abate et al. [33] proposed the following scheme to represent the dynamics within a fall, so a possible fall event could be detected (refer to Figure 2). Let us assume that gravity is $g = 9.8$ m/s. Given the current times tamp t, we find a peak at **peak time** $pt = t - 2500$ ms (Point 1) if at time pt the magnitude of the acceleration a is higher than $th_1 = 3\times g$ and there is no other peak in the period $(t - 2500$ ms$, t)$ (no other a value higher than th_1). If this condition holds, then it is stated that a peak occurred at pt.

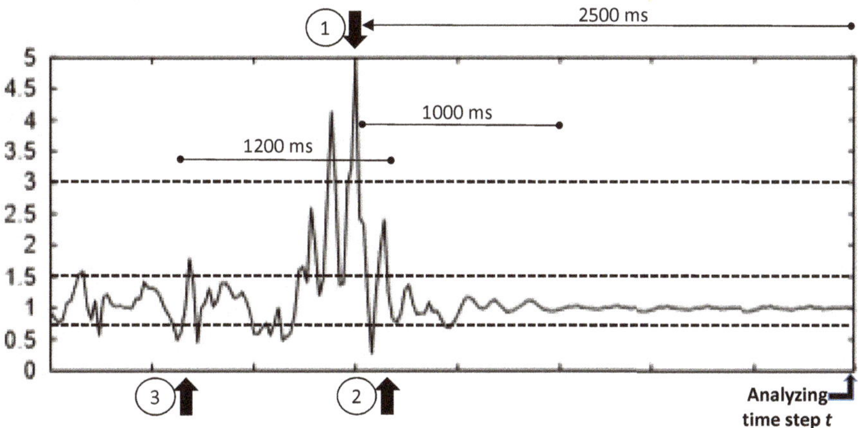

Figure 2. Graph elaborated from [33], showing the evolution of the magnitude of the acceleration in multiples of g. Analyzing the signal at time stamp t, the peak condition described in the text must be found in order to detect a fall. The X-axis represents the time, and each mark corresponds to 500 ms.

When a peak is detected, the feature extraction is performed, computing for this peak time several parameters and features. The **impact end** (*ie*) (Point 2) denotes the end of the fall event; it is the last time for which the a value is higher than $th_2 = 1.5\times g$. Finally, the **impact start** (*is*) (Point 3) denotes the starting time of the fall event, computed as the time of the first sequence of an $a <= th_3$ ($th_3 = 0.8\times g$) followed by a value of $a >= th_2$. The impact start must belong to the interval $[ie - 1200$ ms$, pt]$. If no impact end is found, then it is fixed to $pt + 1000$ ms. If no impact start is found, it is fixed to pt.

With these three times—*is*, *pt* and *ie*—calculated, the following transformations should be computed:

- Average Absolute Acceleration Magnitude Variation, $AAMV = \sum_{t=is}^{ie} \frac{|a_{t+1} - a_t|}{N}$, with N the number of samples in the interval.
- Impact Duration Index, $IDI = ie - is$.

- Maximum Peak Index, $MPI = max_{t \in [is,ie]}(a_t)$.
- Minimum Valley Index, $MVI = min_{t \in [is-500,ie]}(a_t)$.
- Peak Duration Index, $PDI = pe - ps$, with ps the peak start defined as the time of the last magnitude sample below $th_{PDI} = 1.8 \times g$ occurring before pt and pe the peak end defined as the time of the first magnitude sample below $th_{PDI} = 1.8 \times g$ occurring after pt.
- Activity Ratio Index, ARI, calculated as the ratio between the number of samples not in $[th_{ARIlow}0.85 \times g, th_{ARIIhigh} = 1.3 \times g]$ and the total number of samples in the 700-ms interval centered in $(is + ie)/2$.
- Free Fall Index, FFI, the average magnitude in the interval $[t_{FFI}, pt]$. The value of t_{FFI} is the time between the first acceleration magnitude below $th_{FFI} = 0.8 \times g$ occurring up to 200 ms before pt; if not found, it is set to $pt - 200$ ms.
- Step Count Index, SCI, measured as the number of peaks in the interval $[pt - 2200, pt]$.

According to the block diagram, each sample of these eight features is classified as a fall event or not using the predefined model. Therefore, this model has to be trained; this topic is covered in the next subsection.

2.2. Training the FD Model

Provided there exists a collection of TS with data gathered from real falls or from ADL, a training phase can be proposed to train the FD model. Let us consider a dataset containing $\{TS_i^L\}$, with $i = 1 \cdots N$, n the number of TS samples and L the assigned label; that is, a sample of this dataset is a TS_i^L with the data gathered from a participant using a 3DACC on the chosen location, i.e., on a wrist. Let us assume we know a priori whether this TS_i^L includes or not the signal gathered when a fall occurred; therefore, each TS is labeled as $L = FALL$ or $L = NOT\_FALL$.

Now, let us evaluate the peak detection and the feature extraction blocks for each TS. Whenever a TS_i^L has no peak, the TS_i^L is discarded. When a peak is detected for TS_i^L, then the eight features are computed, and label L can be assigned to this new sample. Therefore, a new dataset is created with M being eight features' labeled samples, with $M \leq N$. This dataset was used in [33] to train the feed-forward NN.

Nevertheless, it has been found that this solution (i) might generate more than a sample for a single TS_i^L, which is not a problem, and (ii) certainly will generate a very biased dataset, with the majority of the samples belonging to the class FALL. From their study [33], it can be easily seen that the main reason for a 100% detection is this biased dataset.

Consequently, in this research, we propose to include a dataset balancing stage using SMOTE [37], so at least a 40/60 ratio is obtained for the minority class.

2.3. Model Complexity and the Battery Life

In [33], Abbate et al. made use of a feed-forward NN. Although the number of hidden neurons was set to seven, using a balanced training dataset as stated in the previous section raises this NN parameter up to 20. Basically, the use of any type of NN is a well-known solution that works quite well in computerized environments [12,14]. Nevertheless, it is known that the higher the number of operations with real numbers the higher the effort a computer has to perform; in the context of wearable and mobile devices, this extra cost matters [38].

In previous research, a comparison between models and their suitability to each possible scenario was presented [36,39]. As it has been shown, those models that include high computation seem to perform better. Actually, K-nearest neighbor outperformed many other solutions; however, its implementation in battery feed devices could drain the battery in a relatively short period of time [40].

Therefore, this research proposes to constrain the models to those that include a low computational impact, reducing complex calculations as much as possible. Actually, in this research, only decision trees and rule-based systems are proposed. These models are based on comparison operations, which are much simpler; the hypothesis is that the obtained results are not going to significantly differ from those of an NN. Finally, to obtain a comparison with state-of-the-art modeling [12,14], we also include the SVM as an alternative.

2.4. Tuning the Peak Threshold

As stated in the Introduction of this study, several solutions in the literature are based on thresholds (for instance, [15,20–22], among others). In all of these studies, the thresholds were set up based on the data analysis, either by experts or by data engineers through data visualization.

The solution proposed in [33] is not different. Furthermore, several thresholds are used in that study, not only to detect a peak, but also to compute the extracted features. All of them have been fixed by analyzing the gathered data, establishing some typical values for the features for the class FALL.

However, this can be improved by means of computational intelligence and optimization. In this research, we propose to use well-known techniques (genetic algorithms and simulated annealing) to find the most suitable values for these thresholds. This study, in any case, requires not only optimization, but also some design decisions to modify the features. Therefore, for the purpose of this study, we constrain ourselves to focus on the optimization of the peak threshold, which is the most important threshold as it is the one responsible for finding fall event candidates.

3. Materials and Methods

3.1. Public Datasets

A common way of studying FD is by developing a dataset of simulated falls plus extra sessions of different ADL; all of these TS are labeled and become the test bed for the corresponding study. In this context, a simulated fall is performed by a set of healthy young participants wearing the sensory system, each of them letting him/herself fall towards a mattress from a standing still position.

The vast majority of these datasets were gathered with the sensor attached to the main body, either on the chest, waist, lumbar area or thigh. Interestingly, the UMAFall [34] dataset includes data gathered from 3DACC sensors placed on different parts of the body—ankle, waist, wrist and head—while performing simulated falls; this is the type of data needed in this research as long as the main hypothesis of this study is to perform FD with a sensor worn on a wrist. Furthermore, there is no pattern in the number of repetitions of each activity or fall simulation. Some participants did not simulate any fall; some performed 6 or 9; and one participant simulated 60 falls.

Besides, this research also includes more publicly available datasets. On the one hand, the ADL and simulated epileptic seizure datasets published in [36] are considered because they include a high movement activity, the simulated partial tonic-clonic seizures, followed by a relatively calm period plus some other ADL, all of them measured using 3DACC placed on the dominant wrist. Although this dataset includes neither simulated, nor real falls, it includes activities that share similar dynamics with that proposed for a fall.

Additionally, the DaLiac [35] dataset is also considered in this study. This dataset includes several sensors, one on the wrist and one on the waist, among others. Up to 19 young healthy participants and up to 13 different ADLs are considered, from sitting to cycling.

On the other hand, the FARSEEING dataset [3] is also used for studying the validity of the simulated falls compared with real falls. As stated on the web page, "the FARSEEING real-world fall repository: a large-scale collaborative database to collect and share sensor signals from real-world falls". Data from 15 participants have been gathered for a total of 22 TS; each TS corresponds to a fall: 7 participants (producing 7 TS) have the 3DACC placed on a thigh, while 8 participants (producing 15 TS) have the 3DACC sensor placed on the lower back. Therefore, this dataset is used to validate the simulated falls, so the extent of the conclusions using the available datasets can be determined. Table 1 summarizes the datasets used in this study.

Table 1. Descriptions of the different datasets used in this research. Columns NP, NF and NR stand for the Number of Participants, the Number of Falls in the dataset and the Number of goes for each ADL, respectively. A question mark (?) means that it is not a regular value. The sampling frequency used in gathering the dataset is stated in Hz in the frequency column (Fqcy).

Dataset	NP	NR	NF	Fqcy	Description
UMAFall [34]	17	?	208	20	Includes forward, backward and lateral falls, running, hopping, walking and sitting. Neither do all the participants have every type of activity, nor the same number of goes. Sensors on the wrist, waist, ankle, chest and trouser pocket.
DaLiac [35]	19	1	0	204.8	Sitting, standing, lying, vacuuming, washing dishes, sweeping, walking, up and down stairs, using a treadmill, cycling and rope jumping. Sensors on the wrist, waist, ankle and chest.
Epilepsy [36]	6	10	0	16	Walking at different paces, running, sawing and simulating epileptic partial tonic-clonic seizures. Sensor on the dominant wrist.
FARSEEING [3]	15	?	22	100	22 real falls recorded from 15 elderly people; each of the files might include a description: context of the fall event, where the sensor was located, etc. Sensor located either on the lower back or on the thigh.

3.2. Dataset Comparison

As mentioned before, the published studies on FD use to base their experimentation on simulated falls with healthy participants, the UMA Fall among them, with an age out of the range of the population on which we focus in this research. In this context, it can be argued that the extrapolation of the conclusions could not be straightforward.

Therefore, a comparison of the signals recorded from the waist from UMA Fall and lower back from FARSEEING is performed, so a conclusion about the similarity of the simulated and the real falls can be drawn. This comparison will consider an exhaustive visual comparison of the signals. To do so, signals of falls from the UMA Fall dataset with the same direction—forward, backward or lateral—will be compared with each of the fall signals coming from a sensor placed on the lower back. The idea is to evaluate whether the dynamics from those TS are similar and if they are similar to that mentioned in [20,33].

3.3. A Complete Cross-Validation Scheme

In this research, a complete cross-validation (cv) scheme is performed, that is including training, testing and validation. Each of these stages includes all the TS from the same individual. In other words, once a participant is chosen to become part of the dataset partition, either validation or training and testing, all of his/her TS are included in that partition (refer to Figure 3). Therefore, none of the TS from a participant included in the validation dataset are used in the training and testing: these two partitions—on one side, the validation, and on the other side, the training and testing—are absolutely unrelated.

The first thing that has been done is choosing the participants from the UMA Fall and the simulated epileptic seizures datasets that are preserved for the validation. Fifteen percent of the participants from each dataset have been chosen to be included in the validation dataset. The remaining participants are assigned to the training and testing dataset.

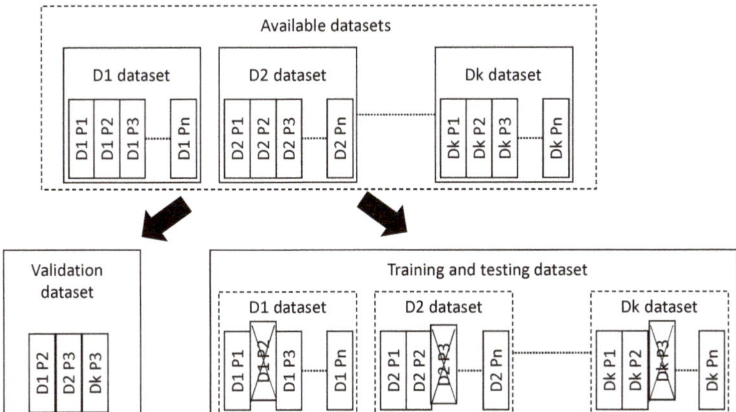

Figure 3. Cross-validation scheme. From the available datasets (D_x), some participants (P_y) (and all of their TS) are preserved for validation purposes. The remaining participants and their TS are all conforming to the training and validation dataset.

On this training and testing dataset, cross-validation is performed. Both 10-fold cv and 5×2 cv based on participants are performed on a participant's basis, as well. This means that for each fold, the participants are grouped for training or for testing. Once a participant is grouped for either training or testing, then all of his/her TS are used in the corresponding process. Again, for each fold, the training and testing partitions do not share any participant's TS; they are completely unrelated.

This scheme is outlined in Figure 3. The advantage of this cv scheme is that it will allow one to evaluate the performance of the solution with unseen participants, those preserved for validation, like would be the case in real life. Furthermore, this scheme allows one to perform training and testing on independent participants. This means that a model is trained with data from a set of participants and then it is tested with data from a different and independent set of participants. Therefore, the training models are tested against data from participants that are totally unseen by them. For sure, this will reduce the performance of the methods, but will allow one to evaluate the robustness of the solutions.

The general process is depicted in Figure 4. The training and testing dataset is used for tuning the threshold to perform the peak detection, this optimization process is detailed in Section 3.4. Once the threshold is obtained, then the peak detection takes place. Each TS included in the training and testing dataset is analyzed to find out whether there exists a peak or not. Those detected peaks are analyzed in depth, extracting the eight features and assigning a label: FALL or NOT_FALL.

This new intermediate dataset, called the model training dataset, might be highly imbalanced; therefore SMOTE is applied to obtain a more suitable dataset to use in the learning process. The learning process is detailed in Section 3.5 and includes up to four types of models: feed forward NN, SVM, DT and RBS. The SMOTE configuration will be to obtain a 40–60% representation of the minority class at least. This balanced dataset and the best model configuration found using a grid scheme are used in the training of the model.

Finally, the validation dataset is considered. It goes through the peak detection block, using the optimized threshold, and whenever a peak is found, the feature extraction stage is executed. Finally, the eight features are classified using the best model found in the previous stage. A TS from the validation dataset will be classified as FALL if a peak is detected and the subsequent classifier outputs the FALL label; otherwise, the TS will be assigned the label NO_FALL.

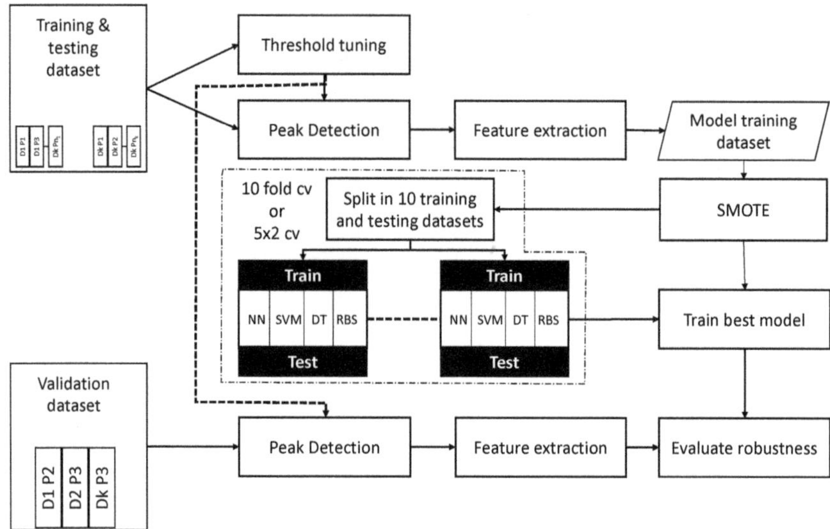

Figure 4. The machine learning process within the cross-validation scheme. The training and testing dataset is used for (i) threshold optimization and (ii) peak detection and feature extraction. The labeled dataset is then used for the machine learning process to find the best modeling option. The best option is then evaluated with the validation dataset once processed so the real performance of the system can be obtained.

To evaluate this validation stage, and every classification result in this study, the standard measurements accuracy, Kappa factor, precision, sensitivity, specificity and the geometric mean of these two latter will be computed. In order to compute the TP, TN, FP and FN, each TS is labeled with FALL if it includes a fall event; otherwise, it is labeled as NOT_FALL. Each TS is evaluated using each of the classifiers; a label FALL is assigned to the TS whenever a peak is detected and the corresponding output of the classifier is FALL; otherwise, the TS is labeled as NOT_FALL. Then, the following formulas hold.

$$Acc = \frac{TP + TN}{TP + TN + FP + FN} \tag{1}$$

$$P_0 = TP + TN \tag{2}$$

$$P_e = (TP + FN) \times (TP + FP) + (TN + FP) \times (TN + FN) \tag{3}$$

$$K = \frac{P_0 - P_e}{1 - P_e} \tag{4}$$

$$Se = \frac{TP}{TP + FN} \tag{5}$$

$$Sp = \frac{TN}{TN + FP} \tag{6}$$

$$Pr = \frac{TP}{TP + FP} \tag{7}$$

$$G = \sqrt{\frac{TP}{TP + FN} \times \frac{TN}{TN + FP}} \tag{8}$$

3.4. Tuning the Peak Detection Threshold

A peak is detected whenever the acceleration magnitude is higher than $3\times g$ as defined in [33] when the sensor is located on the waist. However, is this a valid value when the sensor is located on a wrist? This question will be answered using two metaheuristics: Genetic Algorithms (GA) and Simulated Annealing (SA).

The peak threshold is encoded as a real value ranging from 2.0 to 3.5. As explained in the dataset comparison experiments, these values were collected from the analysis of the TS from the UMA Fall gathered with the sensor on the wrist; for the sake of brevity, these TS are not plotted. The encoded real value represents a possible solution for both GA and SA approaches. The quality of the solution is evaluated using a fitness function based on the sensitivity and specificity obtained by the classification measurements generated using the current peak threshold. The fitness function used to guide the search process of the metaheuristics is the geometric mean of the specificity and the sensitivity, that is $f(x) = G(x)$; see Equation (8).

The GA starts with a population of randomly-generated individuals. Each generation, convex crossover is applied with a certain probability between each individual and a mate selected using a binary tournament. The resulting offspring replaces the first parent if it has a better fitness value. Gaussian mutation is then applied to the current individual with a fixed probability. Mutation perturbs the peak threshold using a zero-mean Gaussian distribution, and the new obtained value is allowed to replace the current individual. This unconditioned replacement enhances the diversity of the population and benefits the search process. The parameter setting is performed with the aim to keep the number of fitness evaluations as low as possible in order to avoid high computational cost. To this end, the peak threshold optimization using GA is based on a population size and generation number of 10, crossover probability of 0.8 and mutation probability of 0.2.

The SA algorithm is based on a single solution initialized with a random value in the considered range $[2.0, 3.5]$. The neighborhood of a solution is defined based on the Gaussian mutation. A new solution y selected from the neighborhood of a current solution x is accepted as the new current solution if it has better fitness or with a probability defined according to the SA approach (as given below).

$$p^{accept} = e^{\frac{f(y) - f(x)}{T}} \tag{9}$$

The probability of accepting a new solution from the neighborhood that does not improve the current fitness value depends on the difference between the fitnesses of the two solutions and on an SA parameter called temperature (denoted by T above). The cooling scheme for the temperature is based on a simple iterative function that returns the current T multiplied by a constant value α. For each value of T starting from the initial temperature to the minimum temperature, several iterations are allowed to select a new neighboring solution. In the current parameter setting, the value of T starts at 1.0, the minimum temperature is 0.1, the value of α is 0.9 and the number of iterations is set to 5. Parameter values for both GA and SA have been selected based on some preliminary experiments according to the results obtained and the computational cost.

3.5. Model Learning

The original solution proposed in [33] made use of a feed-forward NN with 7 hidden neurons. However, in that original paper, the authors did not balance the model training dataset. In our experience, the feature extraction domain was clearly unbalanced toward the FALL label, so obtaining good results for the FALL label does not guarantee a good performance as the specificity might be really poor. Further, if this approach were to be deployed on a smart wristband or similar device, it would be advisable to use low computational models.

Therefore, in this study, several different models are proposed: the feed-forward NN, support vector machines (SVM), C5.0 decision trees (DT) and C5.0 rule-based systems (RBS). The former is the one proposed in the original work, and the two latter are simpler models based on C4.5. Alternatively, SVM is proposed as an alternative state-of-the-art modeling technique that has been applied in FD [12,14]. All of them are implementations included in the caret package for R [41,42].

For each model technique, a grid search for the most interesting parameters will be performed after the balancing stage, even for the NN as long as the model training dataset has changed from that originally published.

4. Results and Discussion

4.1. Dataset Comparison

The FARSEEEING dataset includes up to 15 falls from elderly people using a 3DACC placed on the lower back; for each of them, there might be a break in the circumstances of the fall event. This context information is included in Table 2 with the corresponding ID within this research and within the FARSEEING dataset. Furthermore, in Figure 5, the evolution of the acceleration magnitude is plotted for F1to F8. Although for the majority of the subjects, the $3\times g$ threshold remains valid, some subjects perform with lower peak values; i.e, F3 in the figure. Furthermore, F9 has a peak value below the Abbate et al. threshold, though it has not been included for the sake of space.

Table 2. FARSEEING dataset: Context information of each fall event for subjects wearing a 3DACC placed on the lower back. ID and FRSIDare the Identification within this study and that given in the dataset, respectively. The context is extracted from the FARSEEING documentation [3].

ID	FRSID	Context
F1	17744725-01	Female. After walking with a wheeled walker, stood behind a chair, then fell backwards on the floor. Standing, backward fall.
F2	38243026-05	Female. Fell forward while bending down to fix a shoelace. Bending down, forward fall.
F3	42990421-01	Male. Wanted to pick up an object from the ground. Bending down, forward fall.
F4	42990421-02	Male. Got up from the chair and wanted to walk. Transferring from sitting to standing, forward fall.
F5	42990421-03a	Male. When trying to move to the side, the wheeled walker fell forward. Freezing of movement. Walking, side-forward fall.
F6	72858619-01	Female. Went to the table in the dining room. Fell down backwards on the buttocks. Standing, backward fall.
F7	72858619-02	Female. Person held on the wall, then fell down backwards on the buttocks. Standing, backward fall.
F8	72858619-02	Male. Fell during walking. Walking, unknown fall direction.
F9	74827807-07	Male. Walking, then fell down in front of the entrance of the house. Walking, unknown fall direction.
F10	79761947-03	Female. Changing the hip protector, fell backwards on the ground and hit the toilet. Standing, backward fall.
F11	91943076-01	Female. Changing the hip protector, fell backwards on the ground and Walking, unknown fall direction.
F12	91943076-02	Female. Walking, then fell down opening the door in the entrance hall. Walking, unknown fall direction.
F13	96201346-01	Female. Walking to the bathroom, stopped with freezing and fell from standing position. Walking, left-backward fall.
F14	96201346-02	Female. Standing at the wardrobe, wanted to walk backwards and then fell on buttocks. Standing, backward fall.
F15	96201346-05	Female. Walking backwards from the wash basin, then fell backwards. Standing, backward fall.

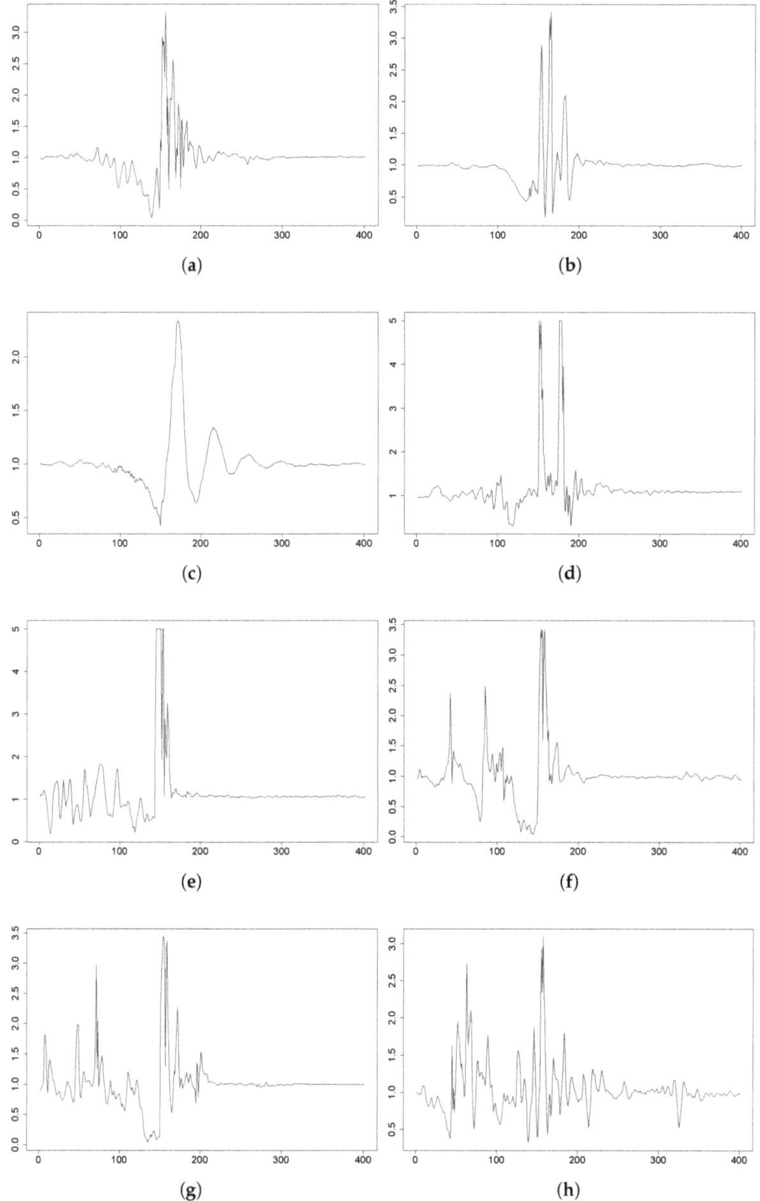

Figure 5. FARSEEING plots of some falls depicting the magnitude of the acceleration during a fall; 400 samples in 4 s. From left to right and top to bottom: F1, F2, F3, F4, F5, F6, F7 and F8. F3 shows a peak below $3\times g$. In all the cases, the sensor is located on the lower back. (**a**) F1: backward fall, 3DACC $\in [0.0, 3.5] \times g$. (**b**) F2: forward fall, 3DACC $\in [0.0, 3.5] \times g$. (**c**) F3: forward fall, 3DACC $\in [0.0, 3.0] \times g$. (**d**) F4: forward fall, 3DACC $\in [0.0, 5.2] \times g$. (**e**) F5: forward fall, 3DACC $\in [0.0, 5.2] \times g$. (**f**) F6: backward fall, 3DACC $\in [0.0, 3.6] \times g$. (**g**) F7: backward fall, 3DACC $\in [0.0, 3.6] \times g$. (**h**) F8: unknown direction, 3DACC $\in [0.0, 3.3] \times g$.

Besides, Figures 6 and 7 depict several fall events from the participants in the UMA Fall dataset. In these figures, P_x refers to the corresponding participant in that dataset, and the plots include the 3DACC magnitude (see Equation (10)) data from the sensor on the waist. Most of the participants did fairly similar to the hypothesis of dynamics and also the thresholds in [33]. Nevertheless, there were also several exceptions; see Figure 6. For instance, Participants 1, 2 and 15 seem to have been falling with fear: their movements were clearly slower. For these participants, some tests were fair, even with a remarkable magnitude value higher than the $3 \times g$ threshold; for some other tests, they performed gently. In some tests, the participant behaved really differently, with the evolution of the magnitude of the acceleration having a totally different shape: Participant 12, the backward fall included in the figure.

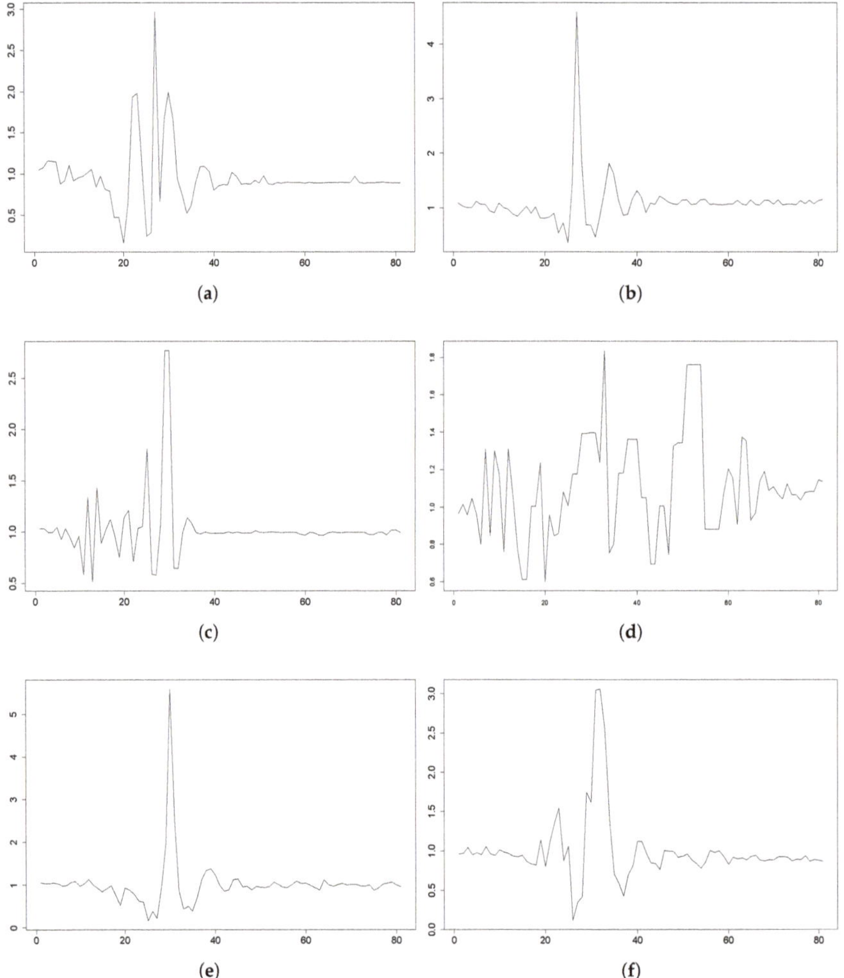

Figure 6. *Cont.*

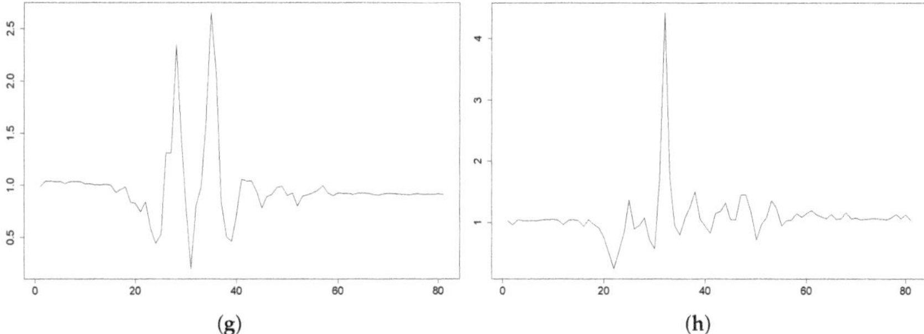

(g) (h)

Figure 6. UMA Fall plots for some falls that behave differently from what was expected. The plots depict the magnitude of the acceleration during a fall in a period of 4 s (80 samples). The data come from the 3DACC sensor on the waist. (**a**) P1: forward fall, 3DACC $\in [0.0, 3.2] \times g$. (**b**) P1: backward fall, 3DACC $\in [0.0, 5.0] \times g$. (**c**) P12: lateral fall, 3DACC $\in [0.0, 2.8] \times g$. (**d**) P12: backward fall, 3DACC $\in [0.0, 2.0] \times g$. (**e**) P9: lateral fall, 3DACC $\in [0.0, 6.0] \times g$. (**f**) P9: forward fall, 3DACC $\in [0.0, 3.2] \times g$. (**g**) P15: forward fall, 3DACC $\in [0.0, 2.8] \times g$. (**h**) P15: backward fall, 3DACC $\in [0.0, 4.5] \times g$.

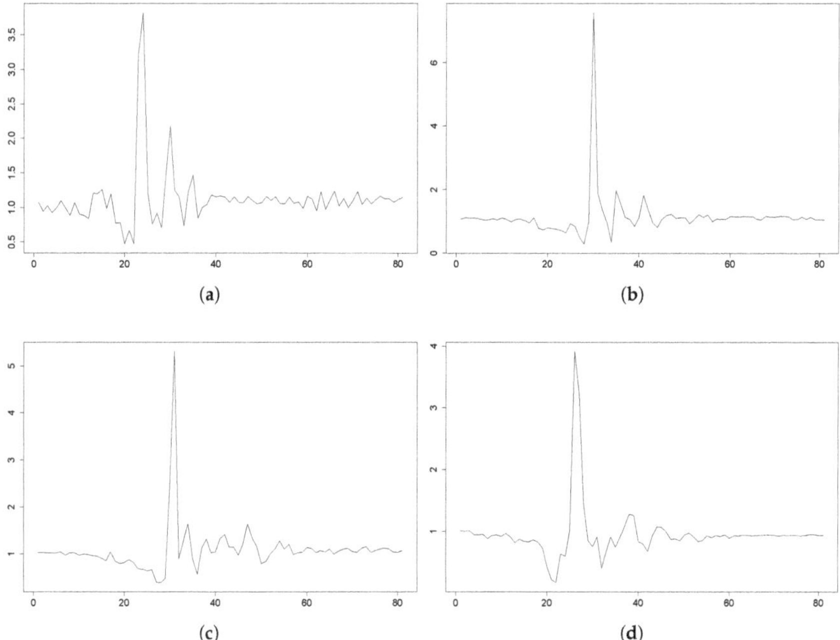

(a) (b)

(c) (d)

Figure 7. *Cont.*

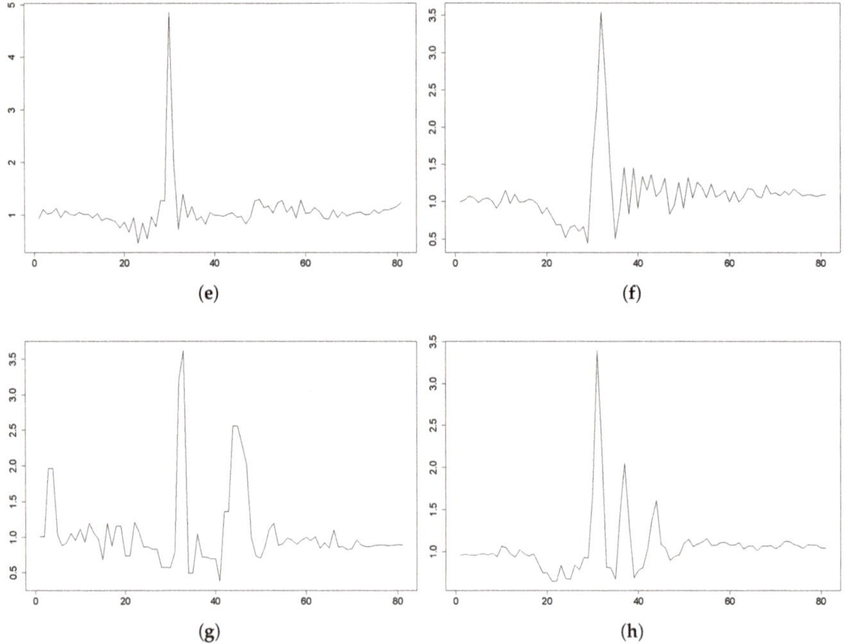

Figure 7. UMA Fall plots for some fall events from participants behaving as expected. The plots depict the magnitude of the acceleration during a fall in a period of 4 s (80 samples). The data come from the 3DACC sensor on the waist. (**a**) P1: backward fall, 3DACC $\in [0.0, 4.0] \times g$. (**b**) P1: backward fall, 3DACC $\in [0.0, 8.0] \times g$. (**c**) P2: lateral fall, 3DACC $\in [0.0, 5.5] \times g$. (**d**) P2: forward fall, 3DACC $\in [0.0, 4.1] \times g$. (**e**) P5: backward fall, 3DACC $\in [0.0, 5.0] \times g$. (**f**) P5: backward fall, 3DACC $\in [0.0, 3.5] \times g$. (**g**) P12: forward fall, 3DACC $\in [0.0, 3.8] \times g$. (**h**) P15: lateral fall, 3DACC $\in [0.0, 3.5] \times g$.

$$\hat{a} = \sqrt[2]{a_x^2 + a_y^2 + a_z^2} \tag{10}$$

However, the majority of the simulations behaved as expected (refer to Figure 7). As seen in these plots, with the independence of the fluctuation of the signal due to the different sampling frequencies, the dynamics can be considered similar to those shown in FARSEEEING, accomplished to some degree with the dynamics proposed in [33]. Still, some differences in this issue can be observed.

On the one hand, the peak threshold is valid for the majority of the cases, but some of the TS behaved under that limit. This will produce a false negative, that is there will be undetected falls. This is the reason why in this research an optimization stage is included in order to tune the peak threshold. The range of possible candidates is defined with the smallest peak threshold found for all the TS from the UMA Fall dataset for the sensor on the wrist: this value has been found to be $2.5 \times g$; therefore, the lower limit was set to $2.0 \times g$. The upper limit of the range is defined as a relatively large threshold, which was estimated as $3.5 \times g$.

On the other hand, the FARSEEING includes some TS that cover walking and a sudden fall; the TS obtained for these cases may change the time periods mentioned in [33]. Moreover, each subject and participant has a different reaction speed. These two ideas must be reconsidered in future work to revisit the definition of the extracted features.

Due to the fact that there were visual differences in the behavior of the different datasets, and also because it would allow a better comprehension of the similarities between the simulated and real falls, a comparison between the TS from the FARSEEING and from the UMA Fall datasets is performed using the algorithm and thresholds proposed in [33]. Table 3 shows the mean and the standard deviation of the values of the extracted features for the TS that include a fall event. Using the Shapiro normality test, it was found that not all features follow a normal distribution; thus, a Mann–Whitney–Wilcoxon test was used to evaluate whether the features from each dataset belonged to the same distribution or not. These results are included in Table 3, as well.

Table 3. Comparison between FARSEEING (sensor on the lower back) and UMA Fall (sensor on the waist) datasets: the mean and standard deviation (Std) of the features computed for all the TS that correspond to a fall. The last row shows the *p*-values from the Mann-Whitney-Wilcoxon test (MWW test), showing that the features from FARSEEING and UMA Fall do not follow the same probability distribution.

Mean	AAMV	IDI	MPI	MVI	PDI	ARI	FFI	SCI
FARSEEING	0.1592	1.2225	4.2345	0.6363	1.2160	0.5933	1.5660	4.7170
UMA Mob	0.5155	1.4619	5.9534	0.4943	1.5911	0.3475	1.3607	2.3730
Std	**AAMV**	**IDI**	**MPI**	**MVI**	**PDI**	**ARI**	**FFI**	**SCI**
FARSEEING	0.1701	2.5817	2.6419	0.3002	2.5817	0.3376	0.8590	3.8098
UMA Mob	0.3889	2.002	2.928	0.2358	1.4173	0.3142	0.8768	1.5238
MWW test	**AAMV**	**IDI**	**MPI**	**MVI**	**PDI**	**ARI**	**FFI**	**SCI**
p-value	2.20×10^{-16}	1.68×10^{-6}	1.54×10^{-7}	0.0009	1.04×10^{-10}	4.53×10^{-6}	0.0022	4.70×10^{-5}

As can be seen, the results clearly show the differences between the simulated and the real falls. This is a very relevant finding as it is normal in the literature to use simulated falls in the evaluation of FD algorithms: now, it is found that there is evidence to not accept simulated falls as valid. Although these differences might be explained because the participants in the FARSEEING datasets suffer from impairment illnesses, it is clear from the obtained results that what is found out in the next subsections needs to be validated in real scenarios, with participants from the population in focus living independently, but keeping a log of any possible fall that might happen so real data could be gathered.

Notwithstanding the differences between the simulated and the real fall datasets found so far, we have no other option than to use the simulated fall dataset because, to the best of our knowledge, there are no publicly available real fall datasets using a 3DACC sensor placed on a wrist. Nevertheless, further research will be needed, as explained before.

Moreover, there are some issues in the UMA Fall dataset that need further addressing. When people fall, they use their arms to protect themselves and to try to grab something to avoid falling. Therefore, there will be much more movement variability, from those who fall without moving the arms to those that frantically try not to fall. Research with sensors worn on the wrist and in real scenarios will be needed.

4.2. Threshold Optimization

The GA and SA algorithms have been run 10 times based on the parameter setting given in Section 3.4. The results obtained have been analyzed according to the fitness function defined to guide the search process. The dataset used in this threshold optimization, following the experiment scheme shown in Figure 4, was the training and testing dataset.

The best fitness value generated by the GA is 0.870 for the peak threshold values 3.09629, 3.09632 and 3.0971. The average fitness over 10 runs is 0.8695, which only slightly deviates from the best run. The best thresholds detected by GA are mostly in the fitness range from 3.093 to 3.109 with a median value of 3.09590.

The SA algorithm obtains similar results to the GA. The best fitness value is 0.869 obtained for the peak threshold values 3.0936, 3.0921, 3.0940 and 3.0984. The average fitness for the 10 SA runs considered is 0.868, which is, as in the case of GA, near the best value obtained. This indicates a stable performance for both algorithms over the independent runs. Most peak values detected by SA range from 3.078 to 3.093 with a median value of 3.09290. As already emphasized, these are fitness values obtained based on the training and testing data. As can be noticed, GA and SA trigger similar results both in terms of the best and average fitness values, as well as the median peak threshold values.

After these optimization stages, and also by the visualization stage performed in the previous subsection, the following thresholds will be compared:

- $th25 = 2.5 \times g$: as the minimum value to detect any peak in the datasets.
- $th3 = 3.0 \times g$: the original proposal from [33].
- $th309 = 3.09290 \times g$: the median of the values obtained from the SA optimization. The median value obtained from the GA runs was $3.09590 \times g$, which is quite a similar value; for the sake of the length, only the SA optimized value will be analyzed.

4.3. Model Training and Cross-Validation Results

Recall that the experimentation design included several published datasets; these datasets were split into training, testing and validation. When splitting, the participants (and all of the TS gathered from them) were assigned either to the training and testing or to the validation datasets. Furthermore, the majority of the available datasets gathered using a wrist-worn 3DACC do not include fall events but ADL, including jumping, simulated seizures or running, among others; this results in a more balanced feature extraction dataset than if only a single dataset were used. Nevertheless, a SMOTE stage was performed to guarantee 40% minority samples in the training and testing dataset.

The best parameter subset was obtained for each pair of threshold and model type using a grid search. The obtained parameter subsets are shown in Table 4 for the feed forward NN, in Table 5 for SVM and in Table 6 for both the decision tree and the rule-based system based on C5.0.

Table 4. Best parameter set found for the feed forward NN and for each threshold.

Threshold	Size	Decay	Max. Iter.	Abs. Tol.	Rel. Tol.
2.5	20	1×10^{-6}	500	4×10^{-6}	1×10^{-10}
3.0	20	1×10^{-4}	1000	4×10^{-6}	1×10^{-9}
3.09290	20	1×10^{-3}	1000	4×10^{-6}	1×10^{-9}

Table 5. Best parameter set found for the SVM and for each threshold.

Threshold	Sigma	C
2.5	0.2	4.5
3.0	0.2	0.7
3.09290	0.20	1.0

Table 6. Best parameter set found for the Decision Tree (DT) and Rule-Based System (RBS) based on C5.0, for each threshold.

Threshold	Model	Winnow	Trials	CF	Bands	Fuzzy Threshold
2.5	DT	FALSE	15	0.5	0	FALSE
2.5	RBS	FALSE	20	0.5	0	FALSE
3.0	DT	FALSE	20	0.05	0	FALSE
3.0	RBS	FALSE	15	0.20	0	FALSE
3.09290	DT	TRUE	10	0.5	0	FALSE
3.09290	RBS	TRUE	5	0.05	0	TRUE

Both 10-fold cv and 5×2 cv were performed, and the obtained results are depicted and shown in Figure 8 and Tables 7 and 8 for threshold $th25$. For both thresholds $th3$ and $th309$, only the 5×2 cv results are included for the sake of both readability and space; Table 9 shows the 5 × 2 cv for threshold *th*3, and Table 10 shows the 5 × 2 cv results for threshold *th*309. Finally, Figure 9 depicts the boxplots for 5 × 2 cv for both *th*3 and *th*309.

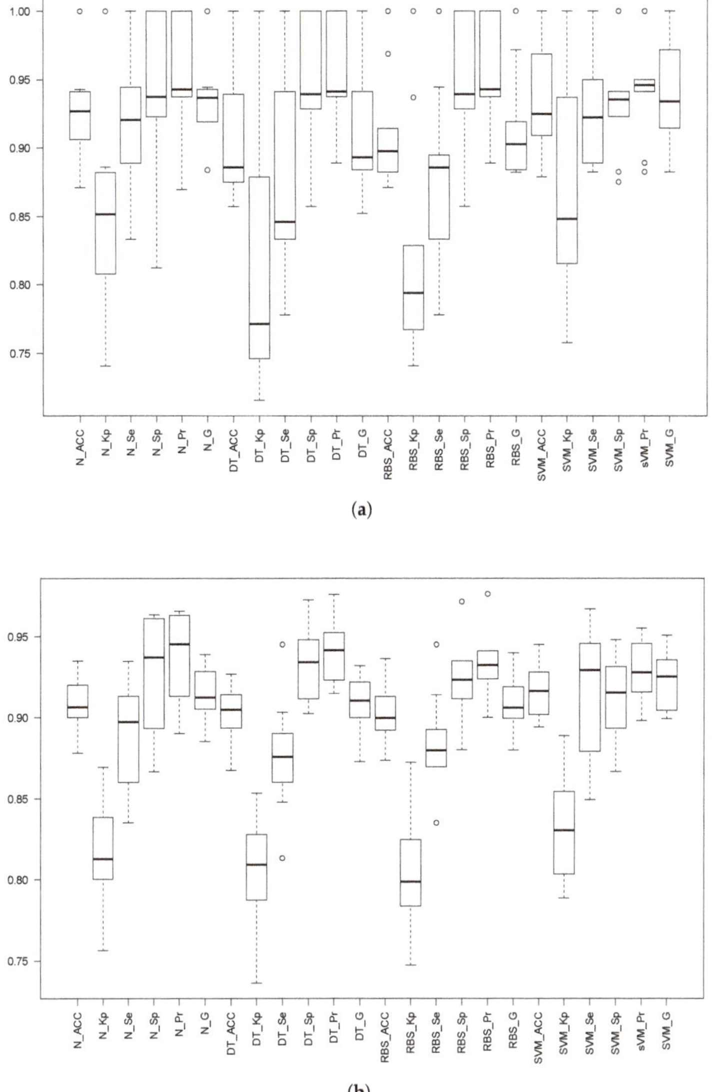

(a)

(b)

Figure 8. Box plots of the different statistics for the three models when the threshold is set to 2.5× *g*. The prefixes N_, SVM_, DT_ and RBS_ stand for the NN, SVM, Decision Trees C5.0 and Rule-Based System C5.0 models. The statistics are: Accuracy (Acc), Kappa factor (Kp), Sensitivity (Se), Specificity (Sp), Precision (Pr) and the Geometric mean (G), all of them computed using Equations (1) to (8). (**a**) Ten-fold cv; (**b**) 5 × 2 cv.

Table 7. Results obtained from the 10-fold cv when the threshold is set to $2.5\times g$: the different statistics are the Accuracy (Acc), Kappa factor (Kp), Sensitivity (Se), Specificity (Sp), Precision (Pr) and the Geometric mean (G), all of them computed using Equations (1) to (8). The models are feed forward NN, Support Vector Machine (SVM), decision trees learned with C5.0 (DT) and Rule-Bases systems learned with C5.0 (RBS).

	NN						DT					
Fold	Acc	Kp	Se	Sp	Pr	G	Acc	Kp	Se	Sp	Pr	G
1	0.9091	0.81564	0.92857	0.89474	0.86667	0.89709	0.78788	0.5777	0.85714	0.7368	0.70588	0.77784
2	0.8611	0.71154	0.86364	0.85714	0.90476	0.88396	0.88889	0.7534	1.00000	0.7143	0.84615	0.91987
3	0.9211	0.84034	0.83333	1.00000	1.00000	0.91287	0.94737	0.8939	0.88889	1.0000	1.00000	0.94281
4	0.9032	0.80503	1.00000	0.80000	0.84211	0.91766	0.87097	0.7406	0.93750	0.8000	0.83333	0.88388
5	0.9375	0.85520	0.91304	1.00000	1.00000	0.95553	0.81250	0.5915	0.78261	0.8889	0.94737	0.86106
6	0.9118	0.82353	0.88235	0.94118	0.93750	0.90951	0.94118	0.8824	0.94118	0.9412	0.94118	0.94118
7	0.8387	0.68041	0.75000	1.00000	1.00000	0.86603	0.80645	0.6092	0.75000	0.9091	0.93750	0.83853
8	0.8438	0.68750	0.78947	0.92308	0.93750	0.86031	0.87500	0.7470	0.84211	0.9231	0.94118	0.89026
9	0.9714	0.93783	0.92308	1.00000	1.00000	0.96077	0.91429	0.8073	0.76923	1.0000	1.00000	0.87706
10	0.8529	0.68401	0.86364	0.83333	0.90476	0.88396	0.88235	0.7323	0.95455	0.7500	0.87500	0.91391
mean	0.8951	0.78410	0.87471	0.92495	0.93933	0.90477	0.87269	0.7335	0.87232	0.8663	0.90276	0.88464
median	0.9062	0.81034	0.87299	0.93213	0.93750	0.90330	0.87868	0.7438	0.87302	0.8990	0.93934	0.88707
std	0.0442	0.08832	0.07245	0.07624	0.05949	0.03394	0.05534	0.1125	0.08635	0.1079	0.08982	0.05039

	RBS						SVM					
Fold	Acc	Kp	Se	Sp	Pr	G	Acc	Kp	Se	Sp	Pr	G
1	0.9091	0.8121	0.85714	0.9474	0.92308	0.88950	0.96970	0.93738	0.92857	1.0000	1.00000	0.96362
2	0.9444	0.8831	0.95455	0.9286	0.95455	0.95455	0.88889	0.77215	0.86364	0.9286	0.95000	0.90579
3	0.9474	0.8939	0.88889	1.0000	1.00000	0.94281	0.97368	0.94708	0.94444	1.0000	1.00000	0.97183
4	0.9032	0.8058	0.93750	0.8667	0.88235	0.90951	0.90323	0.80585	0.93750	0.8667	0.88235	0.90951
5	0.8750	0.7277	0.82609	1.0000	1.00000	0.90889	0.96875	0.92523	0.95652	1.0000	1.00000	0.97802
6	0.9412	0.8824	0.94118	0.9412	0.94118	0.94118	0.94118	0.88235	0.94118	0.9412	0.94118	0.94118
7	0.8710	0.7293	0.85000	0.9091	0.94444	0.89598	0.87097	0.73950	0.80000	1.0000	1.00000	0.89443
8	0.8125	0.6206	0.78947	0.8462	0.88235	0.83462	0.93750	0.87352	0.89474	1.0000	1.00000	0.94591
9	0.9143	0.8135	0.84615	0.9545	0.91667	0.88070	0.91429	0.80734	0.76923	1.0000	1.00000	0.87706
10	0.8824	0.7323	0.95455	0.7500	0.87500	0.91391	0.85294	0.68401	0.86364	0.8333	0.90476	0.88396
mean	0.9000	0.7901	0.88455	0.9144	0.93196	0.90716	0.92211	0.83744	0.88995	0.9570	0.96783	0.92713
median	0.9062	0.8090	0.87302	0.9349	0.93213	0.90920	0.92589	0.84043	0.91165	1.0000	1.00000	0.92534
std	0.0417	0.0875	0.05935	0.0762	0.04532	0.03516	0.04297	0.08965	0.06485	0.0629	0.04536	0.03753

Table 8. Results obtained from the 5×2 cv when the threshold is set to $2.5\times g$: the different statistics are the Accuracy (Acc), Kappa factor (Kp), Sensitivity (Se), Specificity (Sp), Precision (Pr) and the geometric mean (G), all of them computed using Equations (1) to (8). The models are feed forward NN, Support Vector Machine (SVM), decision trees learned with C5.0 (DT) and Rule-Based systems learned with C5.0 (RBS).

	NN						DT					
Fold	Acc	Kp	Se	Sp	Pr	G	Acc	Kp	Se	Sp	Pr	G
1	0.8966	0.7930	0.8989	0.8941	0.8989	0.8989	0.9310	0.8621	0.9101	0.9529	0.9529	0.9313
2	0.8395	0.6763	0.8105	0.8806	0.9059	0.8569	0.8580	0.7105	0.8526	0.8657	0.9000	0.8760
3	0.8757	0.7508	0.8587	0.8961	0.9081	0.8830	0.8876	0.7736	0.8913	0.8831	0.9011	0.8962
4	0.8503	0.7022	0.7935	0.9200	0.9241	0.8563	0.8862	0.7704	0.8913	0.8800	0.9011	0.8962
5	0.8970	0.7935	0.8602	0.9444	0.9524	0.9051	0.9091	0.8189	0.8495	0.9861	0.9875	0.9159
6	0.8421	0.6855	0.7912	0.9000	0.9000	0.8439	0.8421	0.6846	0.8132	0.8750	0.8810	0.8464
7	0.8084	0.6211	0.6667	0.9625	0.9508	0.7962	0.8383	0.6785	0.7586	0.9250	0.9167	0.8339
8	0.9290	0.8548	0.9381	0.9167	0.9381	0.9381	0.9112	0.8188	0.9175	0.9028	0.9271	0.9223
9	0.8862	0.7724	0.8652	0.9103	0.9167	0.8906	0.9162	0.8324	0.8876	0.9487	0.9518	0.9192
10	0.8935	0.7881	0.8316	0.9730	0.9753	0.9006	0.9053	0.8088	0.8947	0.9189	0.9341	0.9142
mean	0.8718	0.7438	0.8315	0.9198	0.9270	0.8770	0.8885	0.7759	0.8667	0.9138	0.9253	0.8952
median	0.8810	0.7616	0.8451	0.9135	0.9204	0.8868	0.8965	0.7912	0.8895	0.9109	0.9219	0.9052
std	0.0359	0.0706	0.0740	0.0308	0.0261	0.0398	0.0323	0.0646	0.0494	0.0397	0.0321	0.0332

Table 8. *Cont.*

	RBS						**SVM**					
Fold	**Acc**	**Kp**	**Se**	**Sp**	**Pr**	**G**	**Acc**	**Kp**	**Se**	**Sp**	**Pr**	**G**
1	0.9195	0.8392	0.8989	0.9412	0.9412	0.9198	0.9253	0.8509	0.8764	0.9765	0.9750	0.9244
2	0.8210	0.6381	0.8000	0.8508	0.8837	0.8408	0.88272	0.7619	0.8632	0.9105	0.9318	0.8967
3	0.8698	0.7381	0.8696	0.8701	0.8889	0.8792	0.9172	0.8341	0.8913	0.9481	0.9535	0.9219
4	0.8982	0.7945	0.9022	0.8933	0.9121	0.9071	0.8982	0.7970	0.8478	0.9600	0.9630	0.9036
5	0.8485	0.7000	0.7742	0.9444	0.9474	0.8564	0.9212	0.8416	0.8925	0.9583	0.9651	0.9281
6	0.8304	0.6622	0.7802	0.8875	0.8875	0.8321	0.8421	0.6836	0.8352	0.8500	0.8636	0.8493
7	0.8204	0.6430	0.7356	0.9125	0.9014	0.8143	0.8503	0.7026	0.7586	0.9500	0.9429	0.8458
8	0.9112	0.8214	0.8763	0.9583	0.9659	0.9200	0.9468	0.8909	0.9588	0.9306	0.9490	0.9539
9	0.9042	0.8082	0.8876	0.9231	0.9294	0.9083	0.8982	0.7963	0.8764	0.9231	0.9286	0.9021
10	0.8994	0.7984	0.8632	0.9460	0.9535	0.9072	0.8994	0.7996	0.8421	0.9730	0.9756	0.9064
mean	0.8723	0.7443	0.8388	0.9127	0.9211	0.8785	0.8981	0.7958	0.8642	0.9380	0.9448	0.9032
median	0.8840	0.7663	0.8664	0.9178	0.9208	0.8932	0.8988	0.7983	0.8698	0.9490	0.9512	0.9050
std	0.0392	0.0780	0.0603	0.0362	0.0303	0.0396	0.0328	0.0650	0.0511	0.0375	0.0328	0.0337

Table 9. Results obtained from the 5×2 cv when the threshold is set to $3.0\times g$: the different statistics are the Accuracy (Acc), Kappa factor (Kp), Sensitivity (Se), Specificity (Sp), Precision (Pr) and the geometric mean (G), all of them computed using Equations (1) to (8). The three different models are feed forward NN, Support Vector Machines (SVM), Decision Trees learned with C5.0 (DT) and Rule-Based Systems learned with C5.0 (RBS).

	NN						**DT**					
Fold	**Acc**	**Kp**	**Se**	**Sp**	**Pr**	**G**	**Acc**	**Kp**	**Se**	**Sp**	**Pr**	**G**
1	0.8781	0.7564	0.8352	0.9315	0.9383	0.8852	0.9268	0.8535	0.8901	0.9726	0.9759	0.9320
2	0.9302	0.8603	0.9032	0.9620	0.9655	0.9339	0.9070	0.8131	0.9032	0.9114	0.9231	0.9131
3	0.9203	0.8387	0.9032	0.9429	0.9546	0.9285	0.9141	0.8278	0.8710	0.9714	0.9759	0.9219
4	0.9075	0.8156	0.8571	0.9634	0.9630	0.9085	0.9249	0.8490	0.9451	0.9024	0.9149	0.9299
5	0.9042	0.8064	0.9130	0.8933	0.9130	0.9130	0.8922	0.7832	0.8804	0.9067	0.9205	0.9002
6	0.9053	0.8100	0.8913	0.9221	0.9318	0.9113	0.9053	0.8108	0.8696	0.9481	0.9524	0.9100
7	0.8795	0.7568	0.8901	0.8667	0.8901	0.8901	0.8675	0.7362	0.8132	0.9333	0.9367	0.8728
8	0.9000	0.8002	0.8602	0.9481	0.9524	0.9051	0.8941	0.7882	0.8602	0.9351	0.9412	0.8998
9	0.9102	0.8178	0.9348	0.8800	0.9053	0.9199	0.9042	0.8078	0.8804	0.9333	0.9419	0.9106
10	0.9349	0.8695	0.9130	0.9610	0.9655	0.9389	0.8935	0.7875	0.8478	0.9481	0.9512	0.8980
mean	0.9070	0.8132	0.8901	0.9271	0.9379	0.9135	0.90230	0.8057	0.8761	0.9362	0.9434	0.9088
median	0.9064	0.8128	0.8973	0.9372	0.9453	0.9122	0.9048	0.8093	0.8757	0.9342	0.9415	0.9103
std	0.0187	0.0376	0.0305	0.0356	0.0272	0.0176	0.0175	0.0345	0.0347	0.0247	0.0212	0.0174

	RBS						**SVM**					
Fold	**Acc**	**Kp**	**Se**	**Sp**	**Pr**	**G**	**Acc**	**Kp**	**Se**	**Sp**	**Pr**	**G**
1	0.9024	0.8041	0.8791	0.9315	0.9412	0.9096	0.9451	0.8888	0.9560	0.9315	0.9457	0.9508
2	0.9128	0.8246	0.9140	0.9114	0.9239	0.9189	0.8954	0.7905	0.8710	0.9241	0.9310	0.9005
3	0.9203	0.8398	0.8817	0.9714	0.9762	0.9278	0.9080	0.8125	0.9140	0.9000	0.9239	0.9189
4	0.9364	0.8724	0.9451	0.9268	0.9348	0.9399	0.9017	0.8035	0.8791	0.9268	0.9302	0.9043
5	0.8802	0.7586	0.8804	0.8800	0.9000	0.8902	0.9222	0.8421	0.9457	0.8933	0.9158	0.9306
6	0.8994	0.7987	0.8696	0.9351	0.9412	0.9047	0.9112	0.8205	0.9348	0.8831	0.9053	0.9199
7	0.8735	0.7473	0.8352	0.9200	0.9268	0.8798	0.9217	0.8406	0.9670	0.8667	0.8980	0.9319
8	0.9000	0.7989	0.8925	0.9091	0.9222	0.9072	0.8941	0.7887	0.8495	0.9481	0.9518	0.8992
9	0.8922	0.7838	0.8696	0.9200	0.9302	0.8994	0.9281	0.8544	0.9457	0.9067	0.9255	0.9355
10	0.8994	0.7987	0.8696	0.9351	0.9412	0.9047	0.9349	0.8692	0.9239	0.9481	0.9551	0.9394
mean	0.9017	0.8027	0.8837	0.9240	0.9338	0.9082	0.9162	0.8311	0.9187	0.9128	0.9282	0.9231
median	0.8997	0.7988	0.8798	0.9234	0.9325	0.9059	0.9165	0.8306	0.9294	0.9154	0.9279	0.9253
std	0.0184	0.0367	0.0293	0.0234	0.0194	0.0175	0.0171	0.0337	0.0396	0.0274	0.0189	0.0176

Recall that these results regard the feature extraction dataset obtained for the corresponding threshold. This means that, in this stage of the experiment, we are only considering that if a peak is found we could correctly label it to belong to the FALL or NOT_FALL class. Thus, this would allow us to choose the most suitable model, if enough evidence is found.

Table 10. Results obtained from the 5 × 2 cv when the threshold is set to 3.09290× *g*: the different statistics are the Accuracy (Acc), Kappa factor (Kp), Sensitivity (Se), Specificity (Sp), Precision (Pr) and the Geometric mean (G), all of them computed using Equations (1) to (8). The three different models are feed forward NN, Support Vector Machines (SVM), Decision Trees learned with C5.0 (DT) and Rule-Based Systems learned with C5.0 (RBS).

	NN						DT					
Fold	Acc	Kp	Se	Sp	Pr	G	Acc	Kp	Se	Sp	Pr	G
1	0.9226	0.8440	0.9239	0.9211	0.9341	0.9290	0.8988	0.7936	0.9565	0.8290	0.8713	0.9129
2	0.8810	0.7586	0.9130	0.8421	0.8750	0.8938	0.9286	0.8548	0.9674	0.8816	0.9082	0.9373
3	0.8810	0.7608	0.8696	0.8947	0.9091	0.8891	0.8333	0.6549	0.9674	0.6711	0.7807	0.8691
4	0.8750	0.7468	0.9022	0.8421	0.8737	0.8878	0.9048	0.8065	0.9457	0.8553	0.8878	0.9163
5	0.8988	0.7969	0.8804	0.9211	0.9310	0.9054	0.7798	0.5540	0.8152	0.7368	0.7895	0.8022
6	0.8869	0.7725	0.8804	0.8947	0.9101	0.8952	0.8810	0.7603	0.8804	0.8816	0.9000	0.8902
7	0.8988	0.7965	0.8913	0.9079	0.9214	0.9062	0.8691	0.7405	0.7935	0.9605	0.9605	0.8730
8	0.8810	0.7624	0.8370	0.9342	0.9390	0.8865	0.9226	0.8426	0.9674	0.8684	0.8990	0.9326
9	0.8691	0.7351	0.8913	0.8421	0.8723	0.8818	0.8929	0.7838	0.9022	0.8816	0.9022	0.9022
10	0.8750	0.7509	0.8261	0.9342	0.9383	0.8804	0.9167	0.8323	0.9130	0.9211	0.9333	0.9231
mean	0.8869	0.7725	0.8815	0.8934	0.9104	0.8955	0.8827	0.7623	0.9109	0.8487	0.8832	0.8959
median	0.8810	0.7616	0.8859	0.9013	0.9157	0.8915	0.8958	0.7887	0.9294	0.8750	0.8995	0.9075
std	0.0159	0.0320	0.0309	0.0380	0.0274	0.0147	0.0459	0.0935	0.0640	0.0856	0.0572	0.0403

	RBS						SVM					
Fold	Acc	Kp	Se	Sp	Pr	G	Acc	Kp	Se	Sp	Pr	G
1	0.9107	0.8200	0.9130	0.9079	0.9231	0.9181	0.9345	0.8671	0.9674	0.8947	0.9175	0.9421
2	0.8929	0.7847	0.8804	0.9079	0.9205	0.9002	0.8988	0.7955	0.9130	0.8816	0.9032	0.9081
3	0.8869	0.7694	0.9457	0.8158	0.8614	0.9025	0.9107	0.8200	0.9130	0.9079	0.9231	0.9181
4	0.8988	0.7936	0.9565	0.8290	0.8713	0.9129	0.9048	0.8069	0.9348	0.8684	0.8958	0.9151
5	0.8691	0.7387	0.8261	0.9211	0.9268	0.8750	0.9107	0.8192	0.9348	0.8816	0.9053	0.9199
6	0.9107	0.8196	0.9239	0.8947	0.9141	0.9189	0.8869	0.7730	0.8696	0.9079	0.9195	0.8942
7	0.8631	0.7290	0.7826	0.9605	0.9600	0.8668	0.9405	0.8790	0.9787	0.8947	0.9184	0.9478
8	0.9286	0.8545	0.9783	0.8684	0.9000	0.9383	0.8988	0.7951	0.9239	0.8684	0.8947	0.9092
9	0.9107	0.8196	0.9239	0.8947	0.9140	0.9189	0.9107	0.8183	0.9565	0.8553	0.8889	0.9221
10	0.9286	0.8562	0.9239	0.9342	0.9444	0.9341	0.9167	0.8326	0.9022	0.9342	0.9432	0.9225
mean	0.9000	0.7985	0.9054	0.8934	0.9135	0.9086	0.9113	0.8207	0.9294	0.8895	0.9110	0.9199
median	0.9048	0.8066	0.9239	0.9013	0.9172	0.9155	0.9107	0.8188	0.9294	0.8882	0.9114	0.9190
std	0.0224	0.0438	0.0602	0.0449	0.0300	0.0232	0.0162	0.0324	0.0325	0.0234	0.0164	0.0157

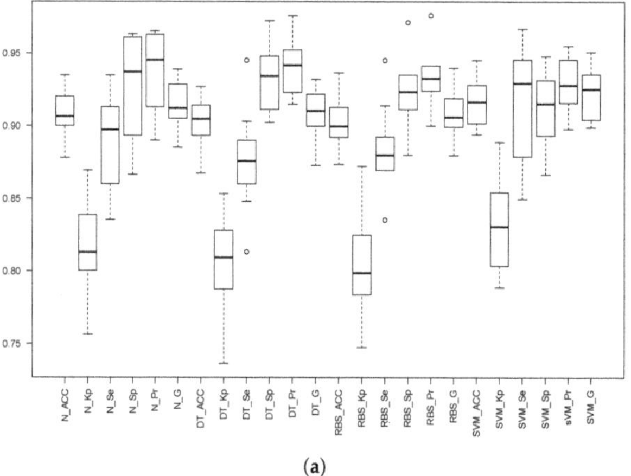

(a)

Figure 9. *Cont.*

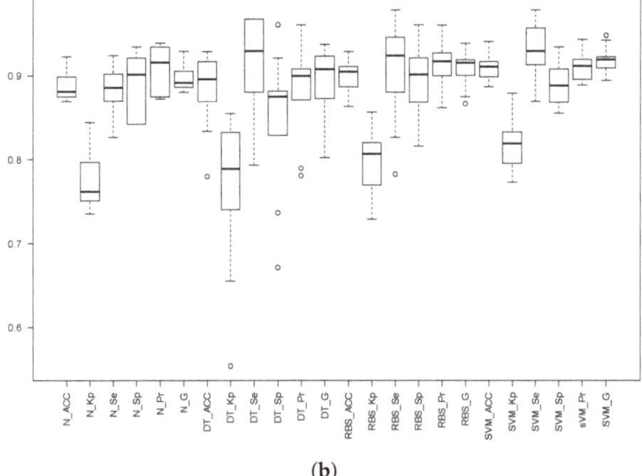

(b)

Figure 9. Box plots of the different statistics for the three models when the threshold is set to $3.0\times g$ (upper part) and $3.09290\times g$ (lower part) with the 5×2 cv. The prefixes N_, SVM_, DT_ and RBS_ stand for the NN, SVM, Decision Trees C5.0 and Rule-Based System C5.0 models. The statistics are: Accuracy (Acc), Kappa factor (Kp), Sensitivity (Se), Specificity (Sp), Precision (Pr) and the geometric mean (G), all of them computed using Equations (1) to (8). (**a**) $th = 3.0\times g$. (**b**) $th = 3.09290\times g$.

In general, the results for 10-fold cv are better due to the differences in the number of samples contained in the training and testing datasets; however, the same behavior of the statistics can be observed. This is the reason why only the results for 5×2 cv are shown in the remainder of this subsection.

We have statistically compared the different methods for each of the thresholds. To do so, we have used the analysis of variance and Tukey honest significance differences, both tools included in R. With a confidence level of 95%, it has been stated that:

- For *th*25, SVM outperforms in sensitivity the other methods. However, in the remainder of the classifier performance measurements, all the methods are comparable.
- For *th*3, all of the methods are comparable except when using the sensitivity. With this measurement, NN is outperformed by SVM, DT and RBS.
- For *th*309, all the methods are comparable for all the measurements.

As a conclusion of this stage, we can state that:

- The different models are totally comparable, and there is no evidence that one of the combinations outperforms the others.
- In this scenario of similar behavior, the DT or the RBS might be advisable due to their simplicity and tuning capability. However, SVM are at least as interesting as these two models.
- No threshold has been observed better than the others. The original threshold proposed in [33] is just in the middle compared with the performances obtained for *th*25 and *th*309.
- The decrease in the performance from the 10-fold cv to the 5×2 cv suggests that the validation results might be significantly worse, as the participants chosen for validation have not been presented to the models, representing the performance in real scenarios in the case of deploying the solution.

Henceforward, there is no clear winner from this comparison, neither with the threshold values, nor with the models. Thus, the next stage of the experimentation, which will evaluate the overall performance of the pair <threshold, model>, will be the definitive phase in this research.

4.4. Final Validation

In this stage, the performance of the whole solution will be evaluated. To do so, for each threshold, a model will be learned using the corresponding best parameter subset and the full training and testing datasets. With these models, the following algorithm is performed:

```
For each participant included in validation
For each TS from the current participant
If a peak is found using the currently chosen threshold
Extract the features
Predict the class using the corresponding model
Update the classifying statistics according to the TS label
Otherwise
Update the classifying statistics according to the TS label
```

The obtained results are included in Tables 11 and 12. The former shows the confusion matrices for each combination of threshold and model. The latter shows the classifying performance of the whole solution.

Table 11. Confusion matrices for the three analyzed thresholds and for each model type: feed forward NN, Decision Trees learned with C5.0 (DT), Rule-Based Systems learned with C5.0 (RBS) and Support Vector Machines (SVM).

Threshold 2.5												
	Reference			**Reference**			**Reference**			**Reference**		
NN	**Fall**	**Not Fall**	**DT**	**Fall**	**Not Fall**	**RBS**	**Fall**	**Not Fall**	**SVM**	**Fall**	**Not Fall**
Fall	10	47	**Fall**	10	20	**Fall**	10	42	**Fall**	8	18
Not Fall	2	250	**Not Fall**	2	277	**Not Fall**	2	245	**Not Fall**	4	279
Threshold 3.0												
	Reference			**Reference**			**Reference**			**Reference**		
NN	**Fall**	**Not Fall**	**DT**	**Fall**	**Not Fall**	**RBS**	**Fall**	**Not Fall**	**SVM**	**Fall**	**Not Fall**
Fall	12	52	**Fall**	11	18	**Fall**	11	29	**Fall**	10	12
Not Fall	0	245	**Not Fall**	1	279	**Not Fall**	1	268	**Not Fall**	2	285
Threshold 3.09290												
	Reference			**Reference**			**Reference**			**Reference**		
NN	**Fall**	**Not Fall**	**DT**	**Fall**	**Not Fall**	**RBS**	**Fall**	**Not Fall**	**SVM**	**Fall**	**Not Fall**
Fall	12	59	**Fall**	11	26	**Fall**	12	35	**Fall**	10	13
Not Fall	0	238	**Not Fall**	1	271	**Not Fall**	0	262	**Not Fall**	2	284

In our opinion, the confusion matrices obtained for the *th*25 threshold, independently of the model, show a performance where (i) the number of false alarms is higher for the NN and RBS and (ii) there are several undetected fall events. The relevance of an undetected fall event makes the *th*25 threshold the worst candidate.

Increasing the threshold has a clear impact on the number of undetected fall events. However, the false alarm number varies from one case to the other: the number of false alarms and the corresponding specificities suggest that further research is needed to tackle this problem. More importantly, for the *th*309, two of the models did detect all the fall events, which suggests this *th*309 threshold learned from the optimization stage may be considered the best solution.

Furthermore, the comparison of the two main models (NN and RBS) shows this latter as more robust and reliable as the number of false alarms is about one third of that reported for the NN.

Besides, the SVM performance is really good if we consider the small number of false alarms (showing a very good specificity indeed), although it was not able to detect all the falls.

Table 12. Results obtained for the best model for each threshold. Different statistics are shown: the Accuracy (Acc), Kappa factor (Kp), Sensitivity (Se), Specificity (Sp), Precision (Pr) and the Geometric mean (G), all of them computed using Equations (1) to (8). The models are feed forward NN, Decision Trees learned with C5.0 (DT), Rule-Bases Systems learned with C5.0 (RBS) and Support Vector Machines (SVM).

Threshold	Model	Acc	Kp	Se	Sp	Pr	G
	NN	0.8414	0.2412	0.8333	0.8418	0.1754	0.8375
2.5	DT	0.9288	0.4454	0.8333	0.9327	0.3333	0.8816
	RBS	0.8576	0.2662	0.8333	0.8586	0.1923	0.8459
	SVM	0.9288	0.3886	0.6667	0.9394	0.3077	0.7914
	NN	0.8317	0.2679	1.0000	0.8249	0.1875	0.9082
3.0	DT	0.9385	0.5096	0.9167	0.9394	0.3793	0.9280
	RBS	0.9029	0.3864	0.9167	0.9024	0.2750	0.9095
	SVM	0.9547	0.5664	0.8333	0.9596	0.4545	0.8942
	NN	0.8091	0.2386	1.0000	0.8013	0.1690	0.8952
3.09290	DT	0.9126	0.4146	0.9167	0.9125	0.2973	0.9146
	RBS	0.8867	0.3677	1.0000	0.8822	0.2553	0.9392
	SVM	0.9515	0.5484	0.8333	0.9562	0.4348	0.8927

However, there is no real evidence about how this solution would perform with elderly people because (i) the intensity level of the ADL is expected to be smaller for this population, which favors the solution, indeed, (ii) there are no real fall datasets with the sensor placed on one wrist, which go against this solution, and (iii) adapting the thresholds for each individual is not addressable in the current design. Furthermore, there would be differences between the evolution of the 3DACC TS for healthy elderly people and those obtained for, say, elderly people with impairments. These reflections lead us to conclude that a solution should be independent of the user intensity level and easier to tune and adapt to the current user. Moreover, gathering data from the elderly population would help in obtaining a more representative dataset. In those cases, like in faints, where there is not enough data, mimicking the faints with human-like flexible mannequins can also help.

5. Conclusions

This research focuses on fall detection for elderly people. Several solutions were studied, one of them was chosen for deployment and improvement with the premise of a reduced computational cost because it has to be implemented on wearable sensors. A threshold-based peak detection plus an NN stage to label the features extracted from the data has been extended with (i) an optimization stage to find the best threshold candidate, (ii) an SMOTE stage to balance the classes in the feature extraction domain and (iii) alternative classifiers with reduced computation and higher adaptability.

The experimentation includes several published datasets: the FARSEEING dataset that includes real falls gathered from a 3DACC placed on the lower back of patients suffering from some impairment illnesses, the UMA FALL including simulated falls and ADL with several sensors and locations, the DaLiac including ADL and the simulated epilepsy, including ADL and simulated seizures; these two latter datasets gathered the data from a 3DACC placed on a wrist. After a comparison of the falls included in FARSEEING and in UMA Fall, it has been found that simulating falls might not represent the real movements. Therefore, using simulated data might help in evaluating a solution, but extra research with data from real falls will be needed in order to validate a solution.

The threshold optimization introduced did not show a clear advantage with regard to neither the original proposed in [33], nor the manually chosen one. However, SVM, RBS and DT were found comparable for almost all the cases. Besides, SVM was the modeling technique that performed with better specificity, producing the smallest amount of false alarms.

More research is needed to find a solution that performs independently of the intensity level of the user. Furthermore, the relevance of the wrist orientation in the FD must be evaluated. Moreover, a dataset gathered from elderly people using the sensor on a wrist and including real falls is needed. Additionally, using mannequins would enrich the fall detection dataset. Finally, the use of different oracles for different types of falls, like faints, for instance, might be needed to cope with all the possible sources of fall events to detect. Perhaps introducing ensembles can enhance the final results, but always keeping in mind the battery life of the wearable smartwatches.

Author Contributions: José R. Villar, Samad Barri Khojasteh and Camelia Chira conceived of and designed the experiments. All the authors participated in performing the experiments, collecting, processing, organizing and analyzing the data of the experiments. José R. Villar and Camelia Chira wrote the paper. All the authors participated reading, improving and amending the paper.

Funding: This research has been funded by the Spanish Ministry of Science and Innovation, under Projects MINECO-TIN2014-56967-R and MINECO-TIN2017-84804-R. Furthermore, this research has been funded by the research contract No. 1996/12.07.2017, Internal Competition CICDI-2017 of Technical University of Cluj-Napoca, Romania.

Acknowledgments: The authors thank all participating men and women in the FARSEEING project, as well as all FARSEEING research scientists, study and data managers and clinical and administrative staff who made this study possible.

Conflicts of Interest: The authors declare no conflict of interest. The founding sponsors had no role in the design of the study; in the collection, analyses or interpretation of data; in the writing of the manuscript; nor in the decision to publish the results.

Abbreviations

The following abbreviations are used in this manuscript:

3DACC	Tri-Axial Accelerometer
Acc	Accuracy
ADL	Activity of Daily Living
AI	Artificial Intelligence
BLE	Bluetooth Low Energy
cv	Cross Validation
DT	Decision Tree
FD	Fall Detection
FN	False Negative
FP	False Positive
K	Cohen's Kappa measurement
ML	Machine Learning
NN	Neural network
RBS	Rule-Based System
Sen	Sensitivity
Spec	Specificity
SVM	Support Vector Machine
TS	Time Series
TP	True Positive
TN	True Negative
Std	Standard Deviation
AAMV	Absolute Acceleration Magnitude Module
ARI	Activity Radio Index
FFI	Free Fall Index
IDI	Impact Duration Index
MPI	Maximum Peak Index
MVI	Minimum Valley Index
PDI	Peak Duration Index
SCI	Step Count Index

References

1. Rubenstein, L. Falls in older people: Epidemiology, risk factors and strategies for prevention. *Age Ageing* **2006**, *35*, 37–41. [CrossRef] [PubMed]
2. Purch.com. Top Ten Reviews for Fall Detection of Seniors. Available online: http://www.toptenreviews.com/health/senior-care/best-fall-detection-sensors/ (accessed on 25 April 2018).
3. Bagala, F.; Becker, C.; Cappello, A.; Chiari, L.; Aminian, K.; Hausdorff, J.M.; Zijlstra, W.; Klenk, J. Evaluation of accelerometer-based fall detection algorithms on real-world falls. *PLoS ONE* **2012**, *7*, e37062. [CrossRef] [PubMed]
4. Igual, R.; Medrano, C.; Plaza, I. Challenges, issues and trends in fall detection systems. *BioMed. Eng. OnLine* **2013**, *12*, 24. [CrossRef] [PubMed]
5. Khan, S.S.; Hoey, J. Review of fall detection techniques: A data availability perspective. *Med. Eng. Phys.* **2017**, *39*, 12–22. [CrossRef] [PubMed]
6. Zhang, S.; Wei, Z.; Nie, J.; Huang, L.; Wang, S.; Li, Z. A review on human activity recognition using vision-based method. *J. Healthc. Eng.* **2017**, *2017*, 31. [CrossRef] [PubMed]
7. Kumari, P.; Mathew, L.; Syal, P. Increasing trend of wearables and multimodal interface for human activity monitoring: A review. *Biosens. Bioelectron.* **2017**, *90*, 298–307. [CrossRef] [PubMed]
8. Sabatini, A.M.; Ligorio, G.; Mannini, A.; Genovese, V.; Pinna, L. Prior-to- and post-impact fall detection using inertial and barometric altimeter measurements. *IEEE Trans. Neural Syst. Rehabil. Eng.* **2016**, *24*, 774–783. [CrossRef] [PubMed]
9. Sorvala, A.; Alasaarela, E.; Sorvoja, H.; Myllyla, R. A two-threshold fall detection algorithm for reducing false alarms. In Proceedings of the 6th International Symposium on Medical Information and Communication Technology (ISMICT), La Jolla, CA, USA, 25–29 March 2012.
10. Daher, M.; Diab, A.; Najjar, M.E.B.E.; Khalil, M.A.; Charpillet, F. Elder tracking and fall detection system using smart tiles. *IEEE Sens. J.* **2017**, *17*, 469–479. [CrossRef]
11. Bianchi, F.; Redmond, S.J.; Narayanan, M.R.; Cerutti, S.; Lovell, N.H. Barometric pressure and triaxial accelerometry-based falls event detection. *IEEE Trans. Neural Syst. Rehabil. Eng.* **2010**, *18*, 619–627. [CrossRef] [PubMed]
12. Zhang, T.; Wang, J.; Xu, L.; Liu, P. Fall detection by wearable sensor and one-class SVM algorithm. In *Intelligent Computing in Signal Processing and Pattern Recognition*; Lecture notes in control and information systems; Huang, D.S., Li, K., Irwin, G.W., Eds.; Springer: Berlin/Heidelberg, Germany, 2006; Volume 345, pp. 858–863.
13. Hakim, A.; Huq, M.S.; Shanta, S.; Ibrahim, B. Smartphone based data mining for fall detection: Analysis and design. *Procedia Comput. Sci.* **2017**, *105*, 46–51. [CrossRef]
14. Wu, F.; Zhao, H.; Zhao, Y.; Zhong, H. Development of a wearable-sensor-based fall detection system. *Int. J. Telemed. Appl.* **2015**, *2015*, 11. [CrossRef] [PubMed]
15. Bourke, A.; O'Brien, J.; Lyons, G. Evaluation of a threshold-based triaxial accelerometer fall detection algorithm. *Gait Posture* **2007**, *26*, 194–199. [CrossRef] [PubMed]
16. Huynh, Q.T.; Nguyen, U.D.; Irazabal, L.B.; Ghassemian, N.; Tran, B.Q. Optimization of an accelerometer and gyroscope-based fall detection algorithm. *J. Sens.* **2015**, *2015*, 8. [CrossRef]
17. Kangas, M.; Konttila, A.; Lindgren, P.; Winblad, I.; Jämsaä, T. Comparison of low-complexity fall detection algorithms for body attached accelerometers. *Gait Posture* **2008**, *28*, 285–291. [CrossRef] [PubMed]
18. Chaudhuri, S.; Thompson, H.; Demiris, G. Fall detection devices and their use with older adults: A systematic review. *J. Geriatr. Phys. Ther.* **2014**, *37*, 178–196. [CrossRef] [PubMed]
19. Jatesiktat, P.; Ang, W.T. An elderly fall detection using a wrist-worn accelerometer and barometer. In Proceedings of the 39th Annual International Conference of the IEEE Engineering in Medicine and Biology Society (EMBC), Seogwipo, South Korea, 11–15 July 2017; pp. 125–130.
20. Abbate, S.; Avvenuti, M.; Corsini, P.; Light, J.; Vecchio, A. Monitoring of human movements for fall detection and activities recognition in elderly care using wireless sensor network: A survey. In *Wireless Sensor Networks: Application—Centric Design*; Intech: London, UK, 2010; p. 22.
21. Bourke, A.; van de Ven, P.; Gamble, M.; O'Connor, R.; Murphy, K.; Bogan, E.; McQuade, E.; Finucane, P.; Olaighin, G.; Nelson, J. Evaluation of waist-mounted tri-axial accelerometer based fall-detection algorithms during scripted and continuous unscripted activities. *J. Biomech.* **2010**, *43*, 3051–3057. [CrossRef] [PubMed]

22. Bourke, A.K.; Klenk, J.; Schwickert, L.; Aminian, K.; Ihlen, E.A.F.; Mellone, S.; Helbostad, J.L.; Chiari, L.; Becker, C. Fall detection algorithms for real-world falls harvested from lumbar sensors in the elderly population: A machine learning approach. In Proceedings of the 38th Annual International Conference of the IEEE Engineering in Medicine and Biology Society (EMBC), Orlando, FL, USA, 16–20 August 2016; pp. 3712–3715.

23. Delahoz, Y.S.; Labrador, M.A. Survey on fall detection and fall prevention using wearable and external sensors. *Sensors* **2014**, *14*, 19806–19842. [CrossRef] [PubMed]

24. Medrano, C.; Plaza, I.; Igual, R.; Sánchez, Á.; Castro, M. The effect of personalization on smartphone-based fall detectors. *Sensors* **2016**, *16*, 117. [CrossRef] [PubMed]

25. Igual, R.; Medrano, C.; Plaza, I. A comparison of public datasets for acceleration-based fall detection. *Med. Eng. Phys.* **2015**, *37*, 870–878. [CrossRef] [PubMed]

26. Ngu, A.; Wu, Y.; Zare, H.; Polican, A.; Yarbrough, B.; Yao, L. Fall detection using smartwatch sensor data with accessor architecture. In *Lecture Notes in Computer Science, Proceedings of the International Conference on Smart Health ICSH, Hong Kong, China, 26–27 June 2017*; Chen, H., Zeng, D.D., Karahanna, E., Bardhan, I., Eds.; Springer: Berlin/Heidelberg, Germany, 2017; Volume 10347, pp. 81–93.

27. Kostopoulos, P.; Nunes, T.; Salvi, K.; Deriaz, M.; Torrent, J. F2D: A fall detection system tested with real data from daily life of elderly people. In Proceedings of the 17th International Conference on E-health Networking, Application Services (HealthCom), Boston, MA, USA, 14–17 October 2015; pp. 397–403.

28. Tasoulis, S.K.; Doukas, C.N.; Maglogiannis, I.; Plagianakos, V.P. Statistical data mining of streaming motion data for fall detection in assistive environments. In Proceedings of the 2011 Annual International Conference of the IEEE Engineering in Medicine and Biology Society, Boston, MA, USA, 30 August–3 September 2011; pp. 3720–3723.

29. Deutsch, M.; Burgsteiner, H. A smartwatch-based assistance system for the elderly performing fall detection, unusual inactivity recognition and medication reminding. In *Studies in Health Technology and Informatics*; Health Informatics Meets eHealth; IOS Press: Amsterdam, The Netherlands, 2016; Volume 223, pp. 259–266.

30. Casilari, E.; Oviedo-Jiménez, M.A. Automatic fall detection system based on the combined use of a smartphone and a smartwatch. *PLoS ONE* **2015**, *10*, e0140929. [CrossRef] [PubMed]

31. Vilarinho, T.; Farshchian, B.; Bajer, D.G.; Dahl, O.H.; Egge, I.; Hegdal, S.S.; Lønes, A.; Slettevold, J.N.; Weggersen, S.M. A Combined Smartphone and Smartwatch Fall Detection System. In Proceedings of the IEEE International Conference on Computer and Information Technology; Ubiquitous Computing and Communications; Dependable, Autonomic and Secure Computing; Pervasive Intelligence and Computing, Liverpool, UK, 26–28 October 2015; pp. 1443–1448.

32. Gjoreski, H.; Bizjak, J.; Gams, M. Using Smartwatch as Telecare and Fall Detection Device. In Proceedings of the 12th International Conference on Intelligent Environments (IE), London, UK, 14–16 September 2016; pp. 242–245.

33. Abbate, S.; Avvenuti, M.; Bonatesta, F.; Cola, G.; Corsini, P.; Vecchio, A. A smartphone-based fall detection system. *Pervasive Mob. Comput.* **2012**, *8*, 883–899. [CrossRef]

34. Casilari, E.; Santoyo-Ramón, J.A.; Cano-García, J.M. UMAFall: A multisensor dataset for the research on automatic fall detection. *Procedia Comput. Sci.* **2017**, *110*, 32–39. [CrossRef]

35. Leutheuser, H.; Schuldhaus, D.; Eskofier, B.M. Hierarchical, multi-sensor based classification of daily life activities: Comparison with state-of-the-art algorithms using a benchmark dataset. *PLoS ONE* **2013**, *8*, e75196. [CrossRef] [PubMed]

36. Villar, J.R.; Vergara, P.; Menéndez, M.; de la Cal, E.; González, V.M.; Sedano, J. Generalized models for the classification of abnormal movements in daily life and its applicability to epilepsy convulsion recognition. *Int. J. Neural Syst.* **2016**, *26*, 21. [CrossRef] [PubMed]

37. Chawla, N.V.; Bowyer, K.W.; Hall, L.O.; Kegelmeyer, W.P. SMOTE: Synthetic minority over-sampling technique. *J. Artific. Intell. Res.* **2002**, *16*, 321–357.

38. Vergara, P.M.; de la Cal, E.; Villar, J.R.; González, V.M.; Sedano, J. An IoT platform for epilepsy monitoring and supervising. *J. Sens.* **2017**, *2017*, 18. [CrossRef]

39. Villar, J.R.; González, S.; Sedano, J.; Chira, C.; Trejo-Gabriel-Galán, J.M. Improving human activity recognition and its application in early stroke diagnosis. *Int. J. Neural Syst.* **2015**, *25*, 1450036–1450055. [CrossRef] [PubMed]

40. Han, Y.; Park, K.; Hong, J.; Ulamin, N.; Lee, Y.K. Distance-constraint k-nearest neighbor searching in mobile sensor networks. *Sensors* **2015**, *15*, 18209–18228. [CrossRef] [PubMed]
41. R Development Core Team. *R: A Language and Environment for Statistical Computing*; R Foundation for Statistical Computing: Vienna, Austria, 2008; ISBN 3-900051-07-0.
42. Kuhn, M. The Caret Package. 2017. Available online: http://topepo.github.io/caret/index.html (accessed on 15 January 2018).

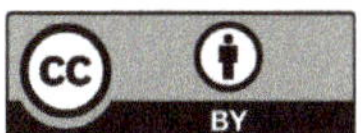 © 2018 by the authors. Licensee MDPI, Basel, Switzerland. This article is an open access article distributed under the terms and conditions of the Creative Commons Attribution (CC BY) license (http://creativecommons.org/licenses/by/4.0/).

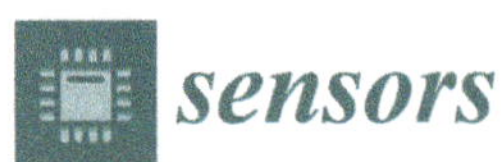 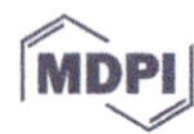

Article

A Telerehabilitation System for the Selection, Evaluation and Remote Management of Therapies

David Anton [1,*], Idoia Berges [2], Jesús Bermúdez [2], Alfredo Goñi [2] and Arantza Illarramendi [2]

[1] Department of Electrical Engineering & Computer Sciences, University of California, Berkeley, CA 94720, USA

[2] Department of Languages and Information Systems, University of the Basque Country UPV/EHU, 20018 Donostia-San Sebastián, Spain; idoia.berges@ehu.eus (I.B.); jesus.bermudez@ehu.eus (J.B.); alfredo@ehu.eus (A.G.); a.illarramendi@ehu.eus (A.I.)

* Correspondence: davidantonsaez@eecs.berkeley.edu; Tel.: +34-943-015-109

Received: 16 March 2018; Accepted: 4 May 2018; Published: 8 May 2018

Abstract: Telerehabilitation systems that support physical therapy sessions anywhere can help save healthcare costs while also improving the quality of life of the users that need rehabilitation. The main contribution of this paper is to present, as a whole, all the features supported by the innovative Kinect-based Telerehabilitation System (KiReS). In addition to the functionalities provided by current systems, it handles two new ones that could be incorporated into them, in order to give a step forward towards a new generation of telerehabilitation systems. The knowledge extraction functionality handles knowledge about the physical therapy record of patients and treatment protocols described in an ontology, named TRHONT, to select the adequate exercises for the rehabilitation of patients. The teleimmersion functionality provides a convenient, effective and user-friendly experience when performing the telerehabilitation, through a two-way real-time multimedia communication. The ontology contains about 2300 classes and 100 properties, and the system allows a reliable transmission of Kinect video depth, audio and skeleton data, being able to adapt to various network conditions. Moreover, the system has been tested with patients who suffered from shoulder disorders or total hip replacement.

Keywords: telerehabilitation; virtual therapy; Kinect; eHealth; telemedicine

---

1. Introduction

Traditional rehabilitation takes place in rehabilitation centers or hospitals, which requires that patients travel to their appointments. This travel is often associated with both time and financial costs [1]. An alternative rehabilitation method involves using telerehabilitation technologies, which allow rehabilitation services to be delivered directly to patients' homes [2]. Telerehabilitation systems have the potential of providing anywhere and anytime physiotherapy support for different groups of persons such as the elderly, disabled and sick, facilitating their contact with caregivers and improving their quality of life. Several studies indicate the therapeutic usefulness of telerehabilitation systems [3,4]; and tests based on virtual interaction have shown that these can be as effective as traditional treatments [5,6]. In addition, as the abandonment of classical rehabilitation sessions because of boredom or disinterest is relatively frequent, the motivating character of telerehabilitation systems is an important factor to consider. In this sense, several studies have found that Virtual Reality (VR) game-based telerehabilitation is perceived as enjoyable and engaging and that it can increase the intensity of rehabilitation and the patient's enjoyment [7–9]. Another advantage of telerehabilitation programs is the easy access of the healthcare professionals to the data collected from patients via the Internet and mobile devices [10–12]. Data collected via sensors during telerehabilitation sessions can be further processed to provide more effective health interventions [13,14]. Finally, telerehabilitation is significantly more time-efficient for both physiotherapists and patients, even when travel time to regular therapies is excluded [15].

A basic telerehabilitation system has at least one camera that allows a physiotherapist to see the patient and monitor the therapy directly (videoconferencing). More complex systems include sensors that can record the movements of the patient. Existing telerehabilitation systems are oriented toward the treatment of many pathologies. In a first approximation, they can be classified into three main groups. The first group comprises those systems that propose that users wear devices, such as [16–19]. Thus, the system for task-oriented games presented in [16] evaluates whether people with cognitive impairment can reach some predefined locations. The system presented in [17] uses smartphones' built-in inertial sensors to monitor exercise execution and to provide acoustic feedback on exercise performance and execution errors. The systems presented in [18,19] make use of sensorized garments and sensors, respectively, that are worn by patients for evaluating a series of exercises related to the upper limbs.

The second group includes those systems that advocate that users do not wear devices, but use low-cost non-intrusive tracking devices such as the Nintendo Wii Remote, Leap Motion or Kinect. The system based on the Nintendo Wii Remote presented in [20] uses an accelerometer to record in 3D and focuses on rehabilitation exercises of the upper limbs. The system presented in [21] uses a webcam and adaptive gaming for tracking finger and hand movement. Trackers are attached to some objects, and a webcam captures the patient's hand to generate some metrics that provide information about the quality, efficiency and skill of the patient. The system presented in [22] uses a Leap Motion device to conduct a video game-based therapy that evaluates the hand's ability and grasp force. Furthermore, Kinect has become one of the most widely-used tracking devices in telerehabilitation [23–36]. The device offers visual tracking without markers, which allows users to control and interact with applications. The data provided can be used to analyze movements, gestures and body postures and can assist in obtaining scores for medical analysis [23]. Among the Kinect-based systems that consider different pathologies, we can mention the following ones: Kinerehab [24], an occupational therapy system where patients can perform three different exercises: lift arms front, lift arms sides and lift arms up; a game aimed at training a dynamic postural control system [25] for people with Parkinson's disease; a 21-game prototype system [26] that evaluates upper body exercises for individuals with spinal cord injury; an upper limb rehabilitation system [27] for stroke survivors, and a similar system, but for people with cerebral palsy [28]; a full body gait analysis system [29]; and finally [30], where fine motor movements are evaluated (like hand and wrist movement) in patients with traumatic brain injury. In addition to the previous works, we would like to mention the system presented in [31], which explores the combined use of Kinect and inertial sensors in order to provide robust hand position tracking; and the Tele-MFAsT telerehabilitation system [32], which has been designed for remote motion and function assessment that facilitates streaming and visualization of data (video, depth, audio and skeleton data) from remotely-connected Microsoft Kinect devices. There are also some commercial solutions that make use of Kinect, such as [33–36], which allow physiotherapists to customize and monitor the therapy sessions of the patients and analyze their evolution. Nevertheless, they do not support both of the two innovative functionalities supported by the Kinect-based Telerehabilitation System (KiReS)–automatic recommendation of therapies and two-way teleimmersion—which we have designed, implemented and the interest in which has been tested.

Finally, in the third group, proposals that belong to the telerehabilitation robotics area can be found. According to [37], those systems are considered as cost-effective alternatives compared to clinic-based therapy, but still, some barriers need to be addressed in order to get a more widespread acceptance. In any case, clinical guidelines recommend these kinds of systems for the recovery of the lost functions in some pathologies such as acute/subacute or chronic strokes. For instance, we can mention the following: MOTORE++ [38], a rehabilitation robot that restores upper limb functionality by using a rolling device; HOMEREHAB [39], which tries to help people who suffer from hemiparesis regain movement of their weak arms and legs by making use of a floor-grounded haptic interface; a WAM robot [40], which is used for upper extremity rehabilitation of patients whose legs can move and which follows the patient trunk movement tracked by Kinect in real time; and those in [41,42], which use haptic sticks in a virtual environment with rehabilitation games for upper limb movement therapy and assessment.

The development of a telerehabilitation system requires interdisciplinary collaboration in order to achieve a good result. Thus, in addition to software and computer engineers for designing, modeling and implementing the system, the presence of experts in the field of rehabilitation, such as doctors and physiotherapists, is required. The role of the end users as active participants must also be taken into account during the whole process of the design, testing and deployment of new technologies. In this sense, we believe that for a telerehabilitation system to be considered as useful, it must be able to help physiotherapists in performing the following tasks: (1) selecting appropriated therapies for patients; (2) evaluating the therapies performed by the patients; and (3) managing those therapies in a remote way. The telerehabilitation system must also empower the patients in following their therapies by motivating them, so that they do not abandon them, as well as by providing the patients with feedback that allows an autonomous evaluation without the direct intervention of the physiotherapist during rehabilitation sessions.

The main emphasis of the majority of works previously mentioned is the evaluation of the therapies' tasks, and they only consider superficially other tasks such as the selection of adequate therapies. For this reason, we have built KiReS (Kinect TeleRehabilitation System), an innovative system that provides a solution for different tasks. KiReS can be a very useful system for both physiotherapists and patients. In the first case, KiReS can accompany them through the entire process of managing the rehabilitation of the patients (designing and selecting therapies, following patients' progress, communicating with patients in virtual environments). In the second case, KiReS can accompany patients in their rehabilitation process by motivating and informing them about their progress. In order to build our system, we have collaborated with physiotherapists to add the adequate expert knowledge to the system and with patients to validate their interest.

The rest of the paper is organized as follows. In Section 2, the main features of KiReS are shown: the workflow of activities, the modules of its architecture that support those activities and the specific methods implemented in those modules. In Section 3, the main results obtained from two real trials are described. Finally, in Sections 4 and 5, some discussion and conclusions are presented, respectively.

2. Materials and Methods

In this section, first, we show the main activities associated with the use of KiReS through a workflow represented using a UMLdiagram and, then, the architecture of the system that supports those activities. Next, the main methods applied in KiReS for selecting, evaluating and remotely managing therapies are explained briefly.

2.1. KiReS Workflow

The use of KiReS involves performing the activities shown in the UML activity diagram of Figure 1, which are executed by two human actors (physiotherapists and the patients) and by the data analyzer, which is a system actor that performs the data analytics processes.

With respect to the therapy selection, physiotherapists have to assign rehabilitation exercises to the patients (Assign Exercises). In order to do this, the exercises must have been previously created (Create New Exercises), along with adequate tests to obtain feedback from the patients (Create Tests). With respect to therapy evaluation, patients have to perform the assigned exercises, which are automatically monitored by KiReS (Perform Monitoring Exercises), and answer to the evaluation tests (Answer Rehabilitation Tests). After that, the data analyzer performs the data analysis with all the data generated during the patients' rehabilitation sessions (Data Analytics). The result of that data analytics is provided to the physiotherapists so that they can evaluate the evolution of the patients (Evaluate Data Analytics Results). With respect to the remote management of therapies, depending on the evolution of the patients, physiotherapists can choose to establish remote rehabilitation sessions in real time with the patients (Teleimmersion session). In addition to the activities, there are two important objects in this activity diagram: (a) the KiReSdb database, which stores the recorded rehabilitation exercises and tests, as well as the data generated by the patients while they perform the exercises and the answers that they give to the rehabilitation tests; and (b) the TRHONT ontology, which is used to help physiotherapists assign exercises and evaluate the results of the data analytics obtained from the data stored in KiReSdb.

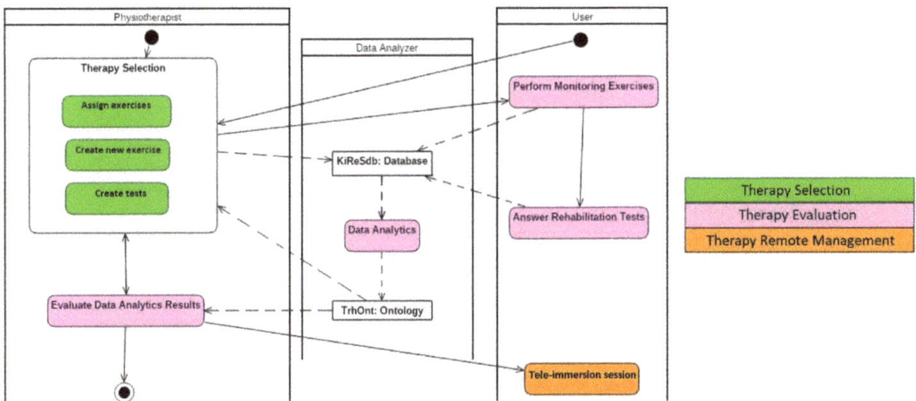

Figure 1. The Kinect-based Telerehabilitation System (KiReS) activity diagram.

2.2. KiReS Architecture

The architecture of KiReS (see Figure 2) is composed of three modules that support the main activities provided for the human actors (patients and physiotherapists) and the system actor (data analyzer): the Interface and Communications Module, the Recognition and Evaluation Module and the Knowledge Extraction Module. These modules implement the specific methods that are going to be explained in the following subsections, through which the activities defined in the KiReS workflow can be performed.

The Interface and Communications Module provides patients with friendly and helpful interfaces that include motivational features such as avatars in order to perform exercises defined in therapies or treatments. This module also provides physiotherapists with interfaces to define and create new exercises that can be included in therapies. Lastly, it also allows real-time teleimmersion sessions among patients and physiotherapists if required and is responsible for managing and transmitting all the data generated in those sessions.

The Recognition and Evaluation Module is responsible for monitoring the patients when they are performing the exercises defined in their therapies in front of the Kinect device. The module evaluates whether the patients are executing those exercises properly, by comparing them with the reference exercises recorded previously by the physiotherapists. The evaluation is made by an exercise recognition algorithm, which is applied to the data of the skeleton joints captured in real time by the Kinect. As a result, patients can receive appropriated feedback about how they are doing (through the aforementioned Interface and Communications Module).

The Knowledge Extraction Module is involved in the therapy selection process performed by physiotherapists. This module relies on the TRHONT ontology, which is used for reasoning and which is enriched with new knowledge extracted from the data generated during physiotherapy sessions (by the Recognition and Evaluation Module). Physiotherapists can also reevaluate patients and modify their therapies depending on such new generated knowledge.

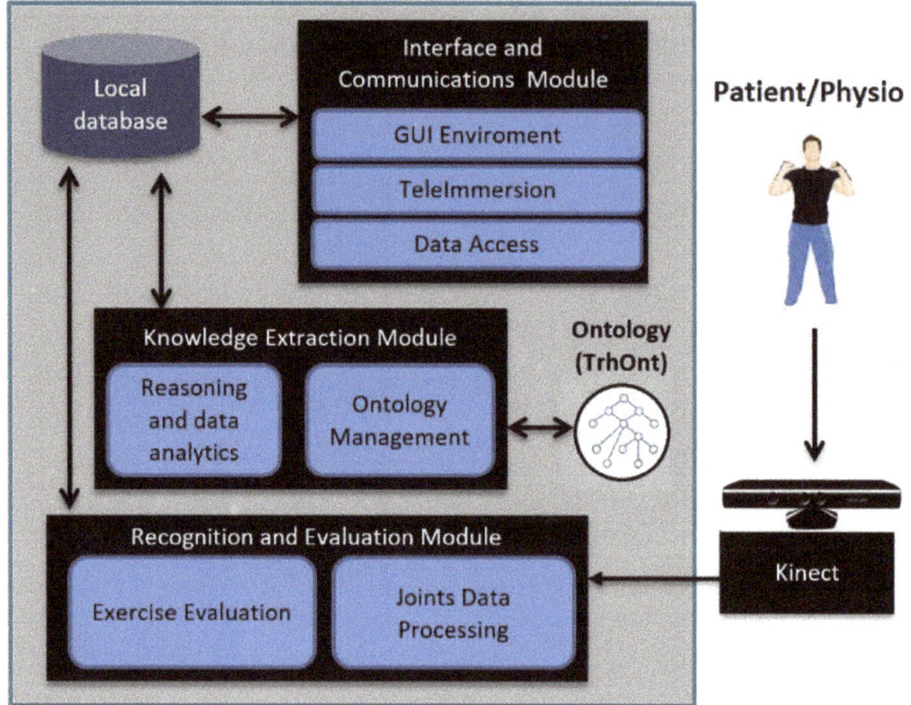

Figure 2. System architecture.

2.3. Therapy Selection Methods

In order to accomplish the activities associated with the therapy selection process, three methods are needed: Create New Exercise, Create Tests and Assign Exercises.

2.3.1. Create New Exercise

KiReS offers an interface for the physiotherapist that provides assistance for creating exercises step by step. Exercises can be created from scratch or can be reused if they are already recorded in the KiReS database. This interface is handled by the Interface and Communications Module of the system architecture (see Figure 2). In the exercise model used in KiReS, a body posture is the simplest element that composes an exercise and therefore necessary for the definition of any other structure. The physiotherapist performs the posture in front of the Kinect, and the system records it. Movements have an associated name to identify them and are defined with two postures (initial and final) and with the recording of the transition between those postures. The relevant joints that best represent the transition from the initial posture to the final posture are selected, recorded and stored. Data representation for the information concerning the name, the initial and final postures, the type of movement (e.g., flexion), the joint and the range of motion involved is added to the ontology to allow reasoning over movements.

Lastly, exercises are defined by assigning movements to them. Simple exercises can consist of just one movement, but complex exercises are a combination of basic movements that form a sequence. The exercise creation interface (see Figure 3) allows the physiotherapist to define the composition of an exercise. It shows a form to fulfill data about the exercise and two lists, one with the movements that have been assigned to that exercise and the other with the movements that are available to be added. Once stored in the system (in the database and in the ontology), the exercise will be available to be included in a therapy session.

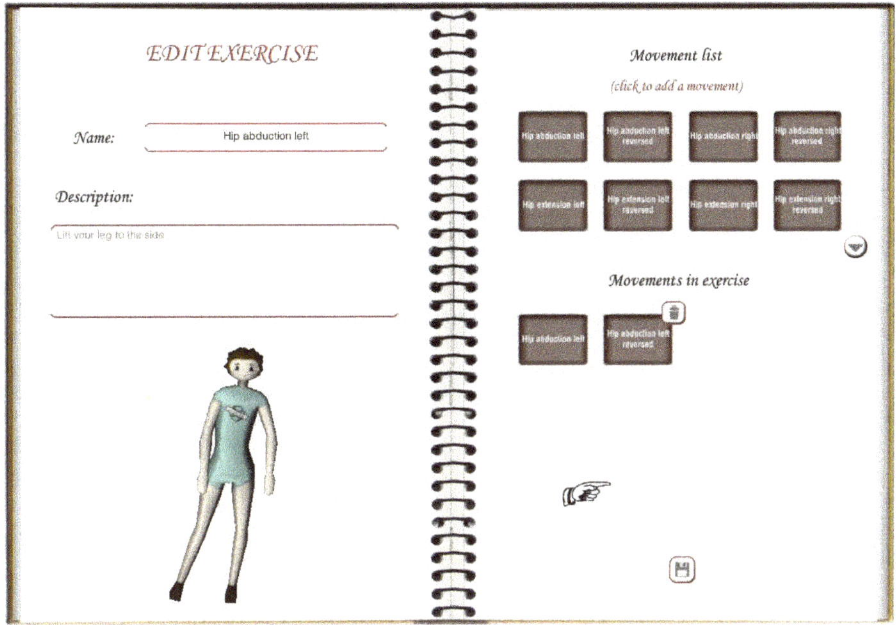

Figure 3. Interface for the physiotherapist.

2.3.2. Create Tests

Performance evaluation is an important factor in a therapy session. In the specialized literature, many user-oriented tests can be found. This kind of test is designed to be answered by the user after ending a therapy session. The answers of the user provide qualitative and quantitative information about their state. Answers to questions about daily life or pain suffered can provide useful feedback to the physiotherapist as a complement to the objective information that is automatically retrieved during exercise execution. Since these tests are widely used in physiotherapy sessions, we decided to incorporate in KiReS the functionality that supports them.

The Interface and Communications Module of the system architecture also provides the physiotherapists with assistance to create these tests. Our proposal includes the option of adding two types of subjective evaluation tests: auto-tests and the Visual Analogue Scale (VAS).

The auto-test interface is oriented to create, manage and evaluate auto tests. These auto tests include questions about different aspects of users' daily life, and the possible answers are valued differently depending on their severity. The tool to manage these tests lets the physiotherapist define the questions of the test and the possible answers with their scores. By default, the tests are evaluated by adding the scores of the provided answers and giving a final result, but the tool also allows the physiotherapist to define the type of function to be applied to the scores. For example, the system can count the number of answers with a certain score or give the result as a percentage depending on a fixed value. Once a test is defined, the physiotherapist can assign it to a therapy, so that the user will have to answer the test after ending a session.

Another evaluation tool used in physiotherapy that we have incorporated with KiReS is the Visual Analogue Scale (VAS). The VAS is a technique used to measure subjective phenomena like pain. It is a self-reporting device consisting of a line of a predetermined length that separates extreme boundaries of the phenomenon being measured [43]. The user sees the image A, on which they mark a point on the line between the "no pain" label and the "worst pain ever" label (see Figure 4). This datum is incorporated with the ontology and can be accessed by the physiotherapist for its analysis. As in the auto tests, the physiotherapist decides when to present the test to the user.

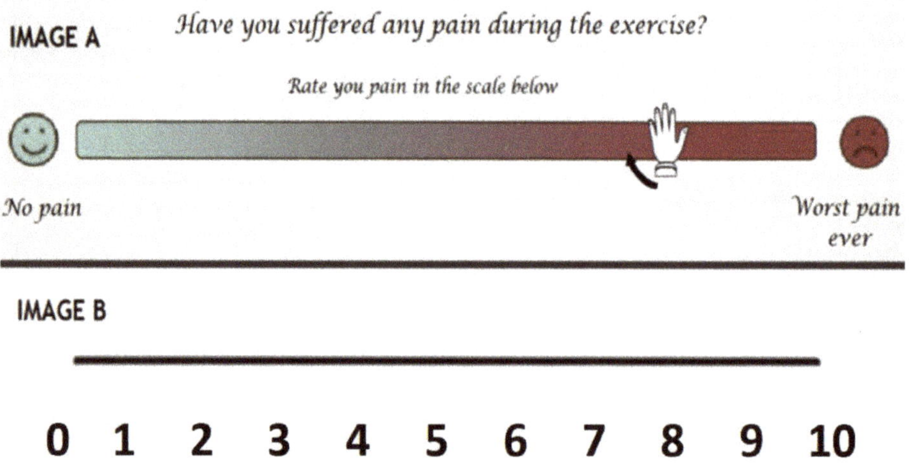

Figure 4. Visual Analogue Scale (VAS) example.

2.3.3. Assign Exercises

During the first visit to the physiotherapist, patients are physically evaluated and their patient record is created. Overall, the patient's record consists of information about personal and family data, symptoms, results of physical examination (joint movement), diagnoses, reported pain value and the recovering goals that are pursued, which cover several relevant aspects for the therapy. The patient's record will change over time as the patient advances in the therapy. Joint movement exploration information will be updated after each session with the data gathered from the Kinect to keep a record of the patient's evolution. Moreover, the information contained in the patient record is included in the TRHONT ontology. This ontology assists physiotherapists in recording and searching for information about the physical therapy record of a patient; identifying in which phase of a treatment protocol a patient is; and identifying which exercises are most suitable for a patient at some specific moment. Ontology reasoning plays a crucial role in these tasks. The TRHONT ontology is based on the Foundational Model of Anatomy (FMA) ontology [44] and is composed of four interrelated types of knowledge (personal data of patients, anatomy, movements and exercises and expert's domain). The components of this ontology have been designed and validated by collaborator physiotherapists to create a tool with the most relevant concepts for physiotherapy and therapy planning. The functionality to manage the TRHONT ontology is provided by the Knowledge Extraction Module of the system architecture (see Figure 2).

For example, in Figure 5, we show part of the knowledge stored for a fictional patient named John that has gone through a Total Hip Replacement (THR) surgery.

In general, rehabilitation therapies follow protocols that contain recommended exercises for a pathology classified in phases (e.g., see Table 1). Each phase contains the exercises to be performed, as well as the conditions that indicate when a patient is in that phase. These conditions are indicated, for example, in terms of the Range Of Motion (ROM) that patients achieve and the pain they report using a Visual Analogue Scale (VAS). Notice that exercises valid at any phase are appropriated also for subsequent phases: the physiotherapist can select them, for example, in order to warm the joint up.

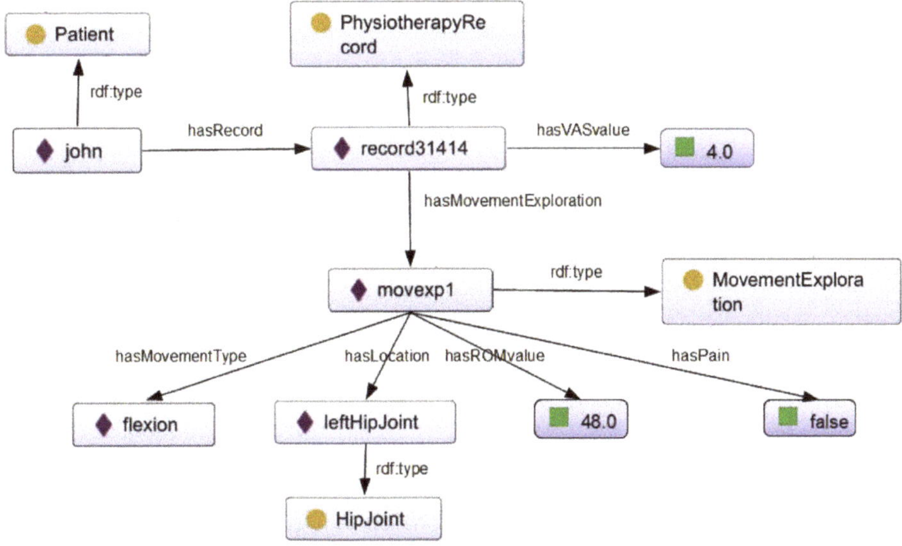

Figure 5. Knowledge excerpt about John contained in TRHONT.

Table 1. Conditions for the first two phases of a general protocol for Total Hip Replacement (THR protocol). ROM, Range Of Motion.

Phase	Recommended Exercises	Patient Classification
I	Hip Flexion ROM 60 Hip Abduction ROM 20 Hip Extension ROM 20 Soft Squats	(ROM Flexion < 60 OR ROM Abduction < 20 OR ROM Extension < 20) AND Moderate General Pain (VAS $\leq$ 6)
II	Hip Flexion ROM 90 Hip Abduction ROM 20 Hip Extension ROM 30 Soft Squats	(60 $\leq$ ROM Flexion AND 20 $\leq$ ROM Extension) AND (ROM Flexion < 90 OR ROM Abduction < 20 OR ROM Extension < 30) AND Mild General Pain (VAS $\leq$ 2)

The TRHONT ontology contains logical axioms for the description of treatment protocols, including their phases, exercises and movements that compose the exercises. For example, in Figure 6, we present the description of the 'Hip Flexion ROM 60' exercise recommended in Phase I of the THR protocol. This refers to exercises with flexion movements with a maximum ROM of 60.

Since the THR surgery protocol specifies that hip flexion exercises with movements up to 60° are suitable for patients in Phase I of that protocol, any specific exercise included in the TRHONT ontology that complies with the definition of `HipFlexionROM60` (e.g., a hip flexion with maximum ROM of 40) will be automatically classified as an exercise for that phase (`ExerPhase1THR`) and will be recommended for patients who are in Phase I of the protocol (represented by `PatientPhase1THR`).

In the case of John, a patient that had THR surgery, a reasoning process with the TRHONT ontology over the information known about him will classify him in Phase I of the THR protocol (see Figure 5), because he has reported a VAS value of 4.0 and has obtained an ROM value of 48.0 in the flexion movement exploration of his left hip joint. Therefore, KiReS will suggest as recommended a set of exercises described in the TRHONT ontology that comply with the types of exercises of Phase I of Table 1. Moreover, the system is flexible enough to allow the physiotherapist to specify rules for certain patients that will generate different sets of recommended/contraindicated exercises (e.g., 'John can perform hip extension exercises with ROM up to 25°'). As a result, a possible therapy plan for John could be the one in Figure 7. More details about the TRHONT ontology, which contains more than 2300 classes and 100 properties, can be found in [45].

```
HipFlexionROM60    ≡   Exercise and hasMovement only MovHipFlexionMax60
MovHipFlexionMax60 ≡   Movement and hasComponent some (Submovement
                       and hasLocation some HipJoint
                       and hasMovementType some Flexion
                       and hasROM.value[<= 60])
HipFlexionROM60    ⊑   ExerPhase1THR
PatientPhase1THR   ⊑   recommended some ExerPhase1THR
```

Figure 6. Axioms for ontology classes `HipFlexionROM60` and `MovHipFlexionMax60`.

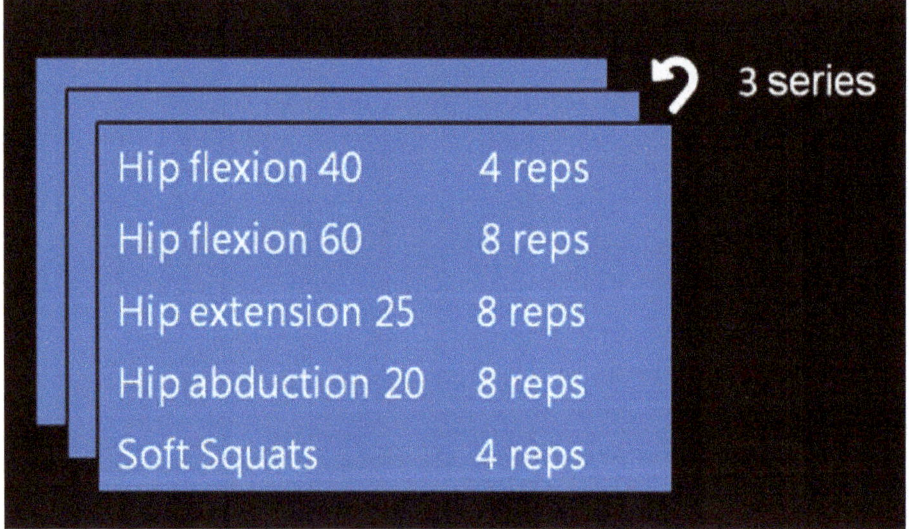

Figure 7. Therapy plan for John.

2.4. Therapy Evaluation Methods

In order to accomplish the activities associated with the therapy evaluation process, two methods are needed: Perform Monitoring Exercises and Data Analytics.

2.4.1. Perform Monitoring Exercises

The Interface and Communication Module of KiReS offers an interface (see Figure 8) that provides a game-like immersive experience that motivates and makes the therapy more enjoyable.

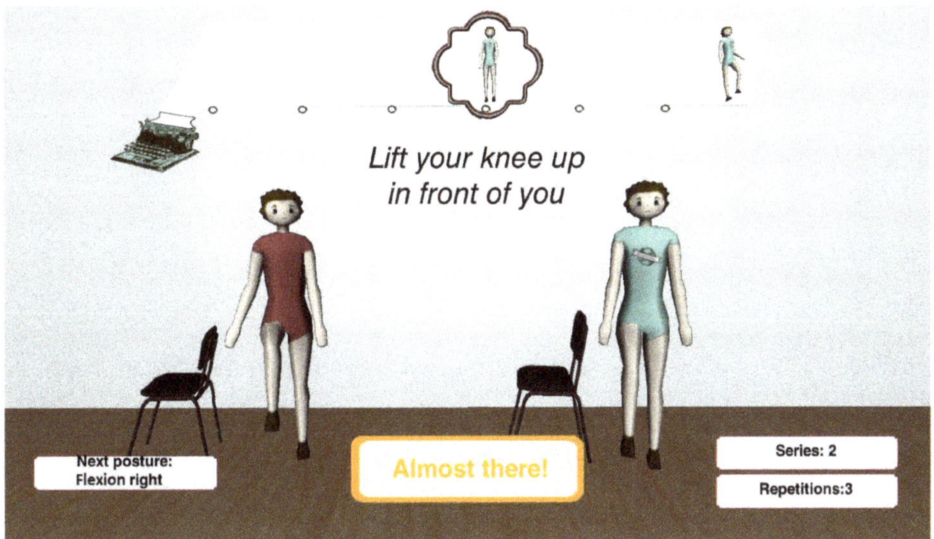

Figure 8. User interface.

The interface presents two 3D avatars to guide the patient. The avatar on the left provides guidance, by showing the posture the patient has to reach or the movement the patient has to do. The avatar on the right shows in real time the movement that the patient is performing. The interface also includes informative boxes at the bottom that provide information about the ongoing therapy session to the patient. The two boxes on the right show the number of series and repetitions left. When the patient has completed all the series, a session is finished. The box on the left shows the name of the next posture the patient has to reach. The box in the middle shows the 'state' of the current movement, and it is continuously updated by the exercise recognition algorithm in real time. Besides, when the patient is close to reaching a posture, the box indicates with a three-level color scale (red, yellow and green) how close they are from reaching the posture. In the upper center of the screen, there is a ribbon that shows the exercise as a list of postures that have to be reached in the current execution. This ribbon is updated as the patient completes exercises in order to show in every moment how many are left. Under this ribbon, a textual explanation of the exercise is displayed. In summary, the interface through the avatars and the boxes gives real-time information to the patient. This way, the system empowers and keeps the patients aware of their therapy.

The Recognition and Evaluation Module of the system architecture is responsible for monitoring the performance of the exercises included in the therapies assigned to the patients. It provides the implementation of the exercise recognition algorithm. An exercise is composed of a series of movements. These movements are characterized by an initial posture, a final posture and the angular trajectories of the limbs that are involved in the movement between the initial and final postures. For identifying each of the initial and final postures, a posture descriptor of 30 features (18 binary features that give information about the relative position in 3D of some joints and 12 features that represent the angles formed by the different limbs of the body) is generated. These descriptors are obtained from the skeleton structure provided by Kinect. Then, the new descriptors are classified by comparing them to previously-recorded and annotated posture descriptors. If the distance is less than a threshold value, the corresponding class is assigned. To represent the movement between both postures, the sequence of angular values of the limbs that are in a different position from the initial posture to the final posture is captured. The sequence is then compared to the previously-stored trajectory for that movement, and again, a similarity value is obtained. Finally, the algorithm analyzes the results of the performance of the exercise by taking into account the similarity values obtained in the previous step (see more details in [46]). The accuracy of the algorithm is around 94%.

2.4.2. Data Analytics

Once exercises are performed by patients, KiReS provides actionable information to physiotherapists and patients through the two submodules of the Knowledge Extraction module: the Ontology Management submodule and the Reasoning and Data Analytics submodule. Within the first submodule, the aforementioned TRHONT ontology assists physiotherapists in their daily tasks via reasoning supported by semantic technology.

Concerning data analytical functionalities, by analyzing the data retrieved from Kinect, the Reasoning and Data Analytics submodule of KiReS provides insight into a number of quantitative and qualitative measures (e.g., posture rating, exercise rating, balance, etc.) that can be useful for the physiotherapist to customize and adapt the patient's therapy and for the patients to be aware of their improvements. If the patient is not discharged, the physiotherapist will use this new information to modify the therapy.

For instance, KiReS allows the comparison of the results of one patient with the results obtained by other patients that fulfill some conditions. For example, in Figure 9, the exercise rating given by KiReS to several patients during the sessions they performed and the corresponding average rating compared to John's results (in blue) can be observed. In Figure 10, the performance, measured as the accuracy of achieving postures, can be found.

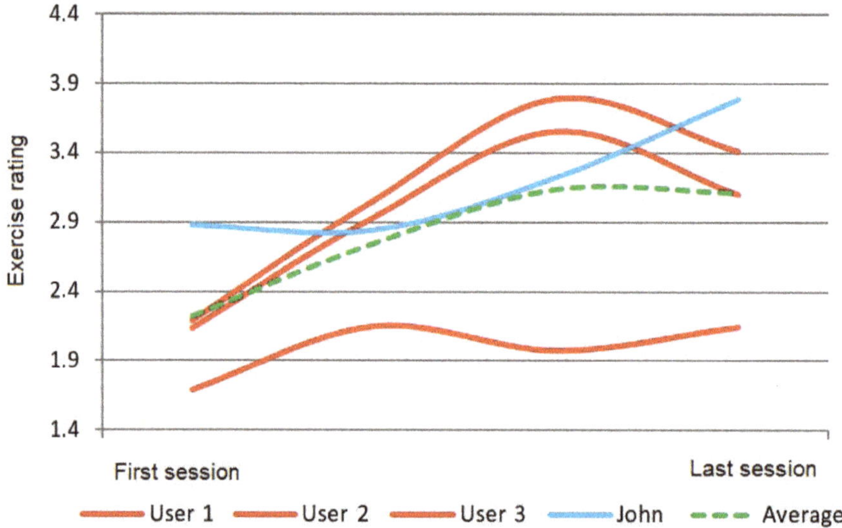

Figure 9. Performance over time (exercise rating).

Furthermore, other types of analysis are possible; for example, the analysis of the maximum, minimum and arc ranges the patient has achieved during shoulder exercises can be discovered by using the raw data of the body joints recorded with the Kinect on several executions of an exercise.

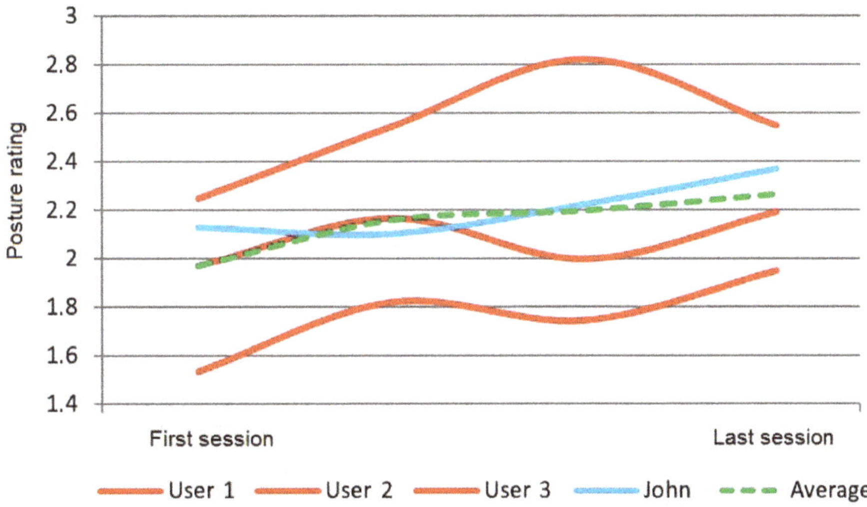

Figure 10. Performance over time (posture rating).

2.5. Therapy Remote Management Method

The only method required for the remote management of therapies is the teleimmersion session. This method, implemented in the Teleimmersion submodule of the Interfaces and Communications Module, allows a two-way real-time multimedia communication and interaction between two remote users (physiotherapist and patient) inside a virtual environment. This provides a convenient, effective and user-friendly experience when performing the telerehabilitation sessions. The submodule relies on a communication framework (called KinectRTC), based on WebRTC and the first version of Kinect.

Web Real-Time Communication (WebRTC) is an API (Application Programming Interface) that enables peer-to-peer audio, video and data sharing between peers in real time. WebRTC alleviates some of the issues in multimedia communication between various platforms and across different network configurations [47,48], and it manages congestion, data synchronization and multimedia buffering. Therefore, it has been widely adopted for video conferencing solutions and also integrated across several web browsers as a communication standard. Moreover, the implementation of secure communication protocols and platform independency makes WebRTC an ideal network framework for personal data, medical data and real-time interaction in remote locations, as all WebRTC components require mandatory encryption [49].

KinectRTC allows for real-time interaction between a physiotherapist and a patient inside a virtual environment, while also providing quantitative information on the patient's movement. It facilitates stable and secure transmission of video, audio and Kinect data (i.e., camera parameters, skeleton data and depth image) in real time between two sites. More precisely, KinectRTC relays on a P2P architecture consisting of three main modules. The Peer Connection Management Module is in charge of managing the connection of peers. The Data Communication Module controls the streaming of data between peers. Finally, the 3D Data Retrieval Module provides access to multimedia streams and data structures necessary for visualization.

By integrating this framework with the other capabilities presented, KiReS is able to provide remotely quantitative information on the patient's movement, which includes the 3D data points of the relevant joints of the patient's skeleton. KiReS integrates a specific interface for remote interaction where local and remote video are displayed and avatars are animated with the streamed skeleton data to show real-time motion (see Figure 11). The 3D avatars on the center represent the remote (red avatar) and the local user (green avatar), respectively, and the remote and local video streams are depicted in the upper part of the interface. This interface allows the physiotherapist to interact with the patients by performing specific exercises directly in front of them. Moreover, at the same time, it makes it possible for the physiotherapist to observe the patient's movements and correct them in real time. The Teleimmersion submodule, whose technical details are explained in depth in [50], provides a reliable streaming solution for Kinect video, audio and skeleton data, being able to adapt to various network conditions by taking advantage of WebRTC multimedia streaming performance, which helps keep the latencies of audio and video within a range that guaranties an acceptable Quality of Service (QoS).

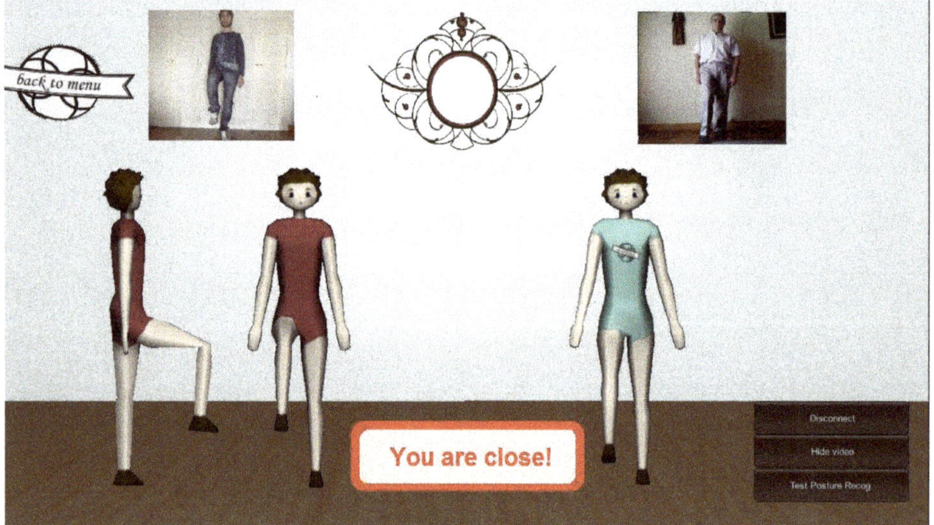

Figure 11. Teleimmersion in KiReS.

3. Results

In order to retrieve the patients' subjective perceptions, we used a Likert scale questionnaire that consisted of 13 questions about the session with five possible answers from one (strongly disagree) to five (strongly agree). The questions were divided into three categories: the system; the user experience; and the interface (see Figure 12). There was a yes/no question asking whether the patients had previously heard about telerehabilitation and also an open-ended question in which patients could write any opinion or suggestion they had about their experience with KiReS.

That questionnaire was answered by the patients that took part in two real trials after they completed each exercise session. One trial was held in a rehabilitation center in Bilbao (Spain) and the other one at Queen Elizabeth II Jubilee Hospital in Brisbane (Australia). The objective of these trials was to validate KiReS in order to evaluate the satisfaction of patients with the system. Prior to the sessions, the physiotherapists that assisted these trials designed the adequate therapy for each of the participants based on their pathologies, severity of their physical limitations and intended intensity of the recovery session. Using the KiReS tools, the physiotherapist combined exercises and established the number of series and repetitions, as well as some difficulty parameters (hold time, pain evaluation, waiting periods, etc).

Aside from the pathologies that the patients suffered, all the trials carried out during this work shared some common aspects: prior to commencing the session, the system was presented to each of the participants, and a brief explanation of the objectives and achievements of the project was given, along with a tutorial about how the system works and the elements that they were going to find in the interface during the therapy session. After that, the participants began the exercises they were assigned. Ethical clearance was provided by the relevant institutional review boards, and those participating in the study signed an informed consent form including a privacy protection statement, which was written with the endorsement of the respective institutions.

If this is your first visit, have you ever heard about telehealth or telerehabilitation?

System	1	2	3	4	5
1 This system could help with my rehabilitation.					
2 This telehealth exercise session is as good as a usual exercise session.					
3 I think this system would help me do my exercises at home.					

User experience	1	2	3	4	5
4 I am satisfied with the telehealth exercise session.					
5 I would like to use this system again.					
6 It was easy using the system.					
7 Getting used to exercising with the system was hard for me.					
8 The telehealth system worked well.					

Interface	1	2	3	4	5
9 I liked the way that the system looked.					
10 The system helped me to perform the exercises.					
11 It is useful to see my movements on the screen.					
12 The instructions to perform the exercises helped me.					
13 The system was confusing to use.					

Figure 12. Questionnaire.

3.1. Shoulder Disorder Patients (Bilbao)

A physiotherapist from the rehabilitation center selected 11 patients that agreed to participate in a rehabilitation session. All patients suffered from shoulder disorders in only one of their arms and had been going to rehabilitation for at least one month. The ages of the patients were in a range from 32 to 58, with 45 being the average. A physiotherapist recorded a set of exercises appropriate for patients with shoulder disorders based on standard therapy protocols. This resulted in a set of 11 different exercises. These exercises were a combination of 27 postures and 16 movements (these 16 movements were also reversed, making a total of 32 movements) that the physiotherapist recorded, and using our managing tools, he combined them into the mentioned 11 exercises.

In Figure 13, we present a boxplot with the answers to each one of the 13 questions of the questionnaire (Figure 12). Each boxplot shows the mean value (red dot), the minimum value, the maximum value and the values of the interquartile ranges (IQR) Q1 (the middle value in the first half of the rank-ordered answers), Q2 (the median) and Q3 (the middle value in the second half of the rank-ordered answers). Questions of that questionnaire were classified into three categories (system, user experience and interface), and their mean values were 3.77, 3.59 and 4.05, respectively, which can be interpreted as 'quite agree' taking into account that one meant 'strongly disagree' and five 'strongly agree'. Therefore, we can say globally that the patients were moderately satisfied with the system and showed interest in using it. In the open-ended question, some of them wrote down an answer; two of the patients commented that they 'liked the system' and that it was 'a positive experience'; another one stated that 'with some adjustments it will be useful'; and one asked for 'a bigger font in the interface'. Their feedback provided new insight into how the interface and the interactions with KiReS were affecting user experience, and we used this input to further improve the system.

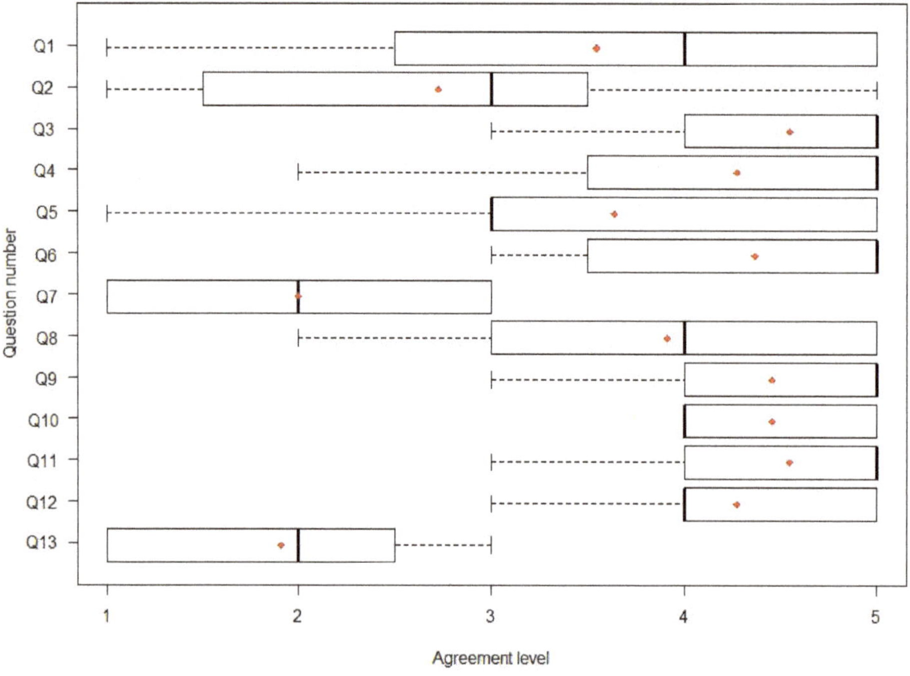

Figure 13. Questionnaire results from user experience at the telerehabilitation center in Bilbao: median, mean (red dot) and IQR.

Informed consent was obtained from all individual participants included in the study. The Asepeyo Medical Board also approved the study design, protocols and procedures.

3.2. Hip Replacement Patients (Brisbane)

In this trial, a full deployment of KiReS was made with a group of patients that had THR surgery. The inclusion criteria for the selection of the participants were: having undergone primary THR in the last four months, full weight-bearing or weight-bearing as tolerated and normal mentation. The exclusion criteria were: revision THR, restricted weight-bearing postoperatively and having co-morbidities preventing participation in a rehabilitation program. The ages of patients were in a range from 33 to 67, with 56 being the average. Most of them (five of seven) had hip replacement surgery in their left hip. Patients were invited by their treating physiotherapist to participate in the study. Nineteen questionnaires were retrieved in total from participants. None of the patients reported that they had heard about telerehabilitation or telemedicine before. Participants reported that the main negative features of the system were the size of the font and the structure of the interface, which some of them found distracting, as they considered that some of the elements were not useful.

With respect to the satisfaction results, we can mention that mean scores of 4.71 for the system and 4.4 for the user experience category were obtained (Figure 14). We also found that the evaluation of those patients who tested the system with the improved new interface (Figure 15) was higher (4.77) than with the original interface (4.43) and significantly different ($X^2 = 6.6347$, df = 2, $p = 0.03625$).

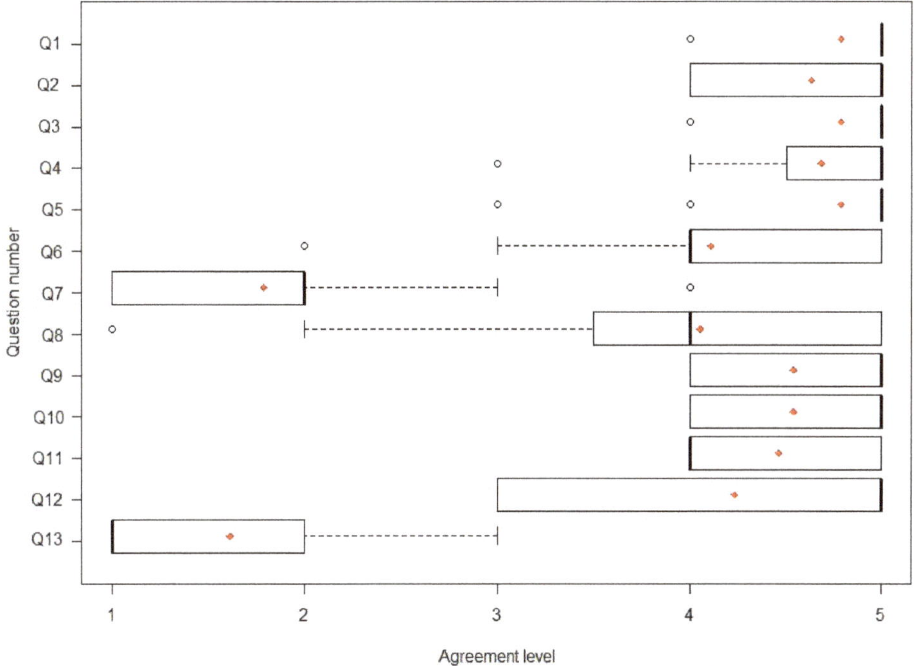

Figure 14. Questionnaire results from user experience at the hospital in Brisbane with the original interface: median, mean (red dot) and IQR.

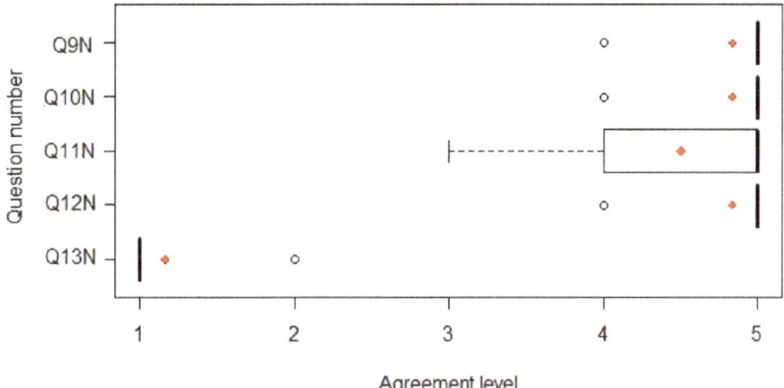

Figure 15. Questionnaire results from user experience at the hospital in Brisbane with the new interface: median, mean (red dot) and IQR.

Informed consent was obtained from all individual participants included in the study. This study was approved by The Office of the Metro South Human Research Ethics Committee, HREC Reference Number: HREC/13/QPAH/235, date of approval: 24 March 2014.

4. Discussion

There is a growing interest in developing telerehabilitation systems oriented toward the treatment of different pathologies, both physical and cognitive. Our telerehabilitation system, KiReS (Kinect TeleRehabilitation System), allows people to perform physical telerehabilitation sessions anytime in different environments. The main contribution of KiReS and what differentiates it from other systems is not only that it tackles the evaluation of the patient's evolution, but also helps physiotherapists in their daily tasks such as: storing and consulting patient records and exercises, assigning exercises, analyzing the evolution of patients and sometimes conducting two-way teleimmersion sessions. We have not found any system that provides all those functionalities altogether.

During the development of KiReS, we collaborated with physiotherapists in order to introduce adequate expert knowledge into the system, and with patients in order to validate their interest. In summary, the main goals pursued when building the KiReS system were: (1) Friendly and helpful interaction with the system: KiReS combines the use of a non-wearable motion control device with motivational interfaces based on avatars and dynamic exercise guiding, since rehabilitation depends largely on the patient's motivation and compliance to be successful. Furthermore, KiReS facilitates physiotherapists with an interface that, on the one hand, provides an easy way to define new exercises based on the therapy protocols they typically use; and on the other hand, also facilitates the task of developing tests. (2) Provision of smart data: KiReS uses different techniques to provide actionable information. It manages a novel domain ontology that provides a reference model for the representation of the physiotherapy-related information that is needed for the whole physiotherapy treatment of a patient, from when they step for the first time into the physiotherapist's office, until they are discharged. The ontology also allows the representation of patients' reports, therapy exercises, movements and evidence-based rehabilitation knowledge; and favors reasoning capabilities over therapy data for the selection of exercises and the notification of events to the therapist. This type of information is not provided by current systems, and it has been recognized as very interesting by the consulted physiotherapists. Moreover, it is able to convert low-level recorded Kinect data into qualitative measures (e.g., posture rating, exercise rating, balance, etc.) that can be useful for the physiotherapists to customize and adapt patients' therapy and for the patients to be aware of their improvements. (3) Monitoring of rehabilitation sessions: KiReS incorporates an algorithm that evaluates online performed exercises and assesses if they have been properly executed by comparing the obtained results with the recorded reference data. Automatic exercise assessment is something relevant since in home-oriented telerehabilitation systems, it is crucial that the patient is autonomously evaluated without the direct intervention of the physiotherapist during rehabilitation sessions. (4) Provision of a teleimmersion mechanism: KiReS supports a facility that allows 3D transmission of body postures and movements provided by Kinect. It facilitates stable and secure transmission of video, audio and Kinect data in real time between two peers. Thus, physiotherapists can display exercise performance remotely to the patients while also being able to observe their performance. Moreover, the patients can communicate to the physiotherapist any question or concerns about their performance. Streaming performance results showed how the combination of an open source real-time networking framework, such as WebRTC, and the Kinect camera can provide the next step in remote physical therapy with the reliable transmission of diverse medical data.

As previously mentioned, the recognition algorithm was experimentally validated by using some datasets created by five healthy volunteers. Once KiReS was operative, we tested it with real patients in two different scenarios: a rehabilitation center in Bilbao and at a hospital in Brisbane. In the first case, the system was tested with eleven patients who suffered from shoulder disorders. A physiotherapist recorded a set of exercises to be executed, and after that, the patients participated in a rehabilitation session. The accuracy of the exercise recognition algorithm was 88.14%. In the case of Brisbane, the same procedure was followed: a physiotherapist prepared the set of exercises to be performed, and seven patients that had had THR surgery participated in several rehabilitation sessions. KiReS categorized 91.88% of the exercises performed by the patients as being correct.

Finally, when we tested KiReS with patients, we also debriefed them about the system and other aspects related to telemedicine applied to their pathology. In this sense, we found that only very few of them had heard about the concept of telerehabilitation. Even though our test was oriented toward checking the functionality and usability of our telerehabilitation system and gathering the impressions of the patients, we found it relevant that the patients had neither knowledge about telerehabilitation, nor about the benefits that these systems can provide to them. Furthermore, the trials with patients showed some aspects that we consider relevant about the patients' interaction and experience with the system. First, we found that the interaction with the Kinect was easy to learn for the patients and that they thought the system comfortable to interact with. Second, they perceived the system as a useful complement to their regular therapy sessions, which can enhance healthcare assistance. However, they considered it less effective than ordinary sessions. This is nevertheless the objective of telerehabilitation, to be complementary to traditional therapy, making it more accessible, but without replacing the traditional rehabilitation. Third, the patients showed interest in using the system again and manifested being satisfied with the experience. Finally, patients found the 3D avatars a helpful source of information, and they rated the interface and interaction with the system in a positive way. In summary, the trials showed that the system can provide benefits for the patients and the interest they have in this kind of technology, but new studies in which larger populations would participate are needed to find the best balance between traditional rehabilitation and telerehabilitation so that the results and user experience with the system can keep improving.

Limitations

Though it was announced that the Kinect device itself was discontinued, Microsoft still provides support for Kinect SDK developers [51]. Furthermore, according to Microsoft, "Microsoft is working with Intel to provide an option for developers looking to transition from the Kinect for Windows platform". Intel RealSense cameras [52] or Orbbec cameras [53] are an alternative to the Kinect, as they provide similar features.

From the point of view of our system, even though our current implementation relies on the Kinect for motion tracking, other depth camera devices such as those mentioned above could be integrated with it. Skeleton tracking is the main requirement for a 3D camera to be compatible with the presented system. As the system is designed to be modular, updating the Joints Data Processing module (shown in Figure 2) would be the main change necessary for such an integration. Other modules would suffer only minimal changes. For instance, the Recognition and Evaluation and the Knowledge Extraction Modules would a priori only require a new mapping of variables to fit the skeleton provided by a different tracking device. The interface would probably require an update to accommodate the new device's SDK. In our experience, however, a depth camera's SDK usually provides a similar framework to give access to color images, depth images, etc. The Teleimmersion Module would not have to change if joint data and depth images were stored in the local database (see Figure 2) by using the same format as before. Therefore, integration in this respect would be straightforward.

5. Conclusions

The goal of the system presented in this paper was to go a step further in the development of telerehabilitation systems and to show how new relevant functionalities can be incorporated with them, which can serve as a great help to patients and physiotherapists. Thus, the system incorporates methods that allow creating new exercises and tests in a friendly way; helping physiotherapists in the task of assigning the adequate exercises and in the task of evaluating the evolution of patients; empowering patients in their rehabilitation process, allowing them to perform exercises in an autonomous way and providing immediate feedback about how they are performing them; and finally, to perform the exercises in real time, remotely, in a virtual environment.

The results obtained so far using KiReS show its suitability for telerehabilitation and a good quality user experience. The patients who used it found that the interaction with it was friendly; they considered it as a complement to their therapy that can improve medical attention; and they showed a predisposition to using the system again. KiReS can be extended and as future work we plan to enhance the information KiReS retrieves by adding bio-signal tracking devices. Thus, it would be possible to extend the reasoning and data analysis capabilities of the system with these new inputs.

Author Contributions: All authors participated in the definition and design of the system and in the discussion of its relevant aspects. D.A., A.G. and A.I. were involved in the development and the deployment of the telerehabilitation system. I.B. and J.B. designed and implemented the ontology. D.A. designed the experiments and was involved in data collection and interpretation during the trials. All authors wrote the manuscript and read and approved the final manuscript.

Funding: This research was funded by the Spanish Ministry of Economy and Competitiveness grant number FEDER/TIN2016-78011-C4-2R.

Acknowledgments: Authors thank Jon Torres-Unda and Jesús Seco for their valuable collaboration with physiotherapy-related aspects and for their feedback about KiReS. Some parts of this paper are available in an earlier PhD thesis publication, accessible in the following repository of the University of the Basque Country UPV/EHU: https://addi.ehu.es/handle/10810/16068.

Conflicts of Interest: The authors declare no conflict of interest. The founding sponsors had no role in the design of the study; in the collection, analyses or interpretation of data; in the writing of the manuscript; nor in the decision to publish the results.

References

1. Dávalos, M.E.; French, M.T.; Burdick, A.E.; Simmons, S.C. Economic evaluation of telemedicine: Review of the literature and research guidelines for benefit–cost analysis. *Telemed. e-Health* **2009**, *15*, 933–948. [CrossRef] [PubMed]

2. Botsis, T.; Demiris, G.; Pedersen, S.; Hartvigsen, G. Home telecare technologies for the elderly. *J. Telemed. Telecare* **2008**, *14*, 333–337. [CrossRef] [PubMed]

3. Tousignant, M.; Moffet, H.; Boissy, P.; Corriveau, H.; Cabana, F.; Marquis, F. A randomized controlled trial of home telerehabilitation for post-knee arthroplasty. *J. Telemed. Telecare* **2011**, *17*, 195–198. [CrossRef] [PubMed]

4. Cason, J. A pilot telerehabilitation program: Delivering early intervention services to rural families. *Int. J. Telerehabil.* **2009**, *1*, 29–38. [CrossRef] [PubMed]

5. Weiss, P.L.; Sveistrup, H.; Rand, D.; Kizony, R. Video capture virtual reality: A decade of rehabilitation assessment and intervention. *Phys. Ther. Rev.* **2009**, *14*, 307–321. [CrossRef]

6. Frederix, I.; Hansen, D.; Coninx, K.; Vandervoort, P.; Vandijck, D.; Hens, N.; Craenenbroeck, E.V.; Driessche, N.V.; Dendale, P. Effect of comprehensive cardiac telerehabilitation on one-year cardiovascular rehospitalization rate, medical costs and quality of life: A cost-effectiveness analysis. *Eur. J. Prev. Cardiol.* **2016**, *23*, 674–682. [CrossRef] [PubMed]

7. Rizzo, A.S.; Kim, G.J. A SWOT analysis of the field of virtual reality rehabilitation and therapy. *Presence Teleoper. Virtual Environ.* **2005**, *14*, 119–146. [CrossRef]

8. Lewis, G.N.; Woods, C.; Rosie, J.A.; Mcpherson, K.M. Virtual reality games for rehabilitation of people with stroke: Perspectives from the users. *Disabil. Rehabil. Assist. Technol.* **2011**, *6*, 453–463. [CrossRef] [PubMed]

9. Cikajlo, I.; Rudolf, M.; Goljar, N.; Burger, H.; Matjačić, Z. Telerehabilitation using virtual reality task can improve balance in patients with stroke. *Disabil. Rehabil.* **2012**, *34*, 13–18. [CrossRef] [PubMed]

10. Bidargaddi, N.; Sarela, A. Activity and heart rate-based measures for outpatient cardiac rehabilitation. *Methods Inf. Med.* **2008**, *47*, 208–216. [CrossRef] [PubMed]

11. Fan, Y.J.; Yin, Y.H.; Xu, L.D.; Zeng, Y.; Wu, F. IoT-Based Smart Rehabilitation System. *IEEE Trans. Ind. Inform.* **2014**, *10*, 1568–1577.

12. Hamida, S.T.B.; Hamida, E.B.; Ahmed, B. A new mHealth communication framework for use in wearable WBANs and mobile technologies. *Sensors* **2015**, *15*, 3379–3408. [CrossRef] [PubMed]

13. Rolim, C.O.; Koch, F.L.; Westphall, C.B.; Werner, J.; Fracalossi, A.; Salvador, G.S. A Cloud Computing Solution for Patient's Data Collection in Health Care Institutions. In Proceedings of the 2010 Second International Conference on eHealth, Telemedicine, and Social Medicine, Sint Maarten, The Netherlands, 10–16 February 2010; pp. 95–99.

14. Benharref, A.; Serhani, M.A. Novel Cloud and SOA-Based Framework for E-Health Monitoring Using Wireless Biosensors. *IEEE J. Biomed. Health Inform.* **2014**, *18*, 46–55. [CrossRef] [PubMed]

15. Koh, G.; Ho, W.; Koh, Y.Q.; Lim, D.; Tay, A.; Yen, S.C.; Kumar, Y.; Wong, S.M.; Cai, V.; Cheong, A.; et al. A Time Motion Analysis of Outpatient, Home and Telerehabilitation Sessions From Patient and Therapist Perspectives. *Arch. Phys. Med. Rehabil.* **2017**, *98*, e28. [CrossRef]

16. Llorens, R.; Gil-Gomez, J.A.; Mesa-Gresa, P.; Alcaniz, M.; Colomer, C.; Noe, E. BioTrak: A comprehensive overview. In Proceedings of the 2011 International Conference on Virtual Rehabilitation (ICVR), Zurich, Switzerland, 27–29 June 2011; pp. 1–6.

17. Spina, G.; Huang, G.; Vaes, A.; Spruit, M.; Amft, O. COPDTrainer: A smartphone-based motion rehabilitation training system with real-time acoustic feedback. In Proceedings of the 2013 ACM International Joint Conference on Pervasive and Ubiquitous Computing, Zurich, Switzerland, 9–12 September 2013; pp. 597–606.

18. Giorgino, T.; Tormene, P.; Maggioni, G.; Pistarini, C.; Quaglini, S. Wireless Support to Poststroke Rehabilitation: MyHeart's Neurological Rehabilitation Concept. *IEEE Trans. Inf. Tech. Biomed.* **2009**, *13*, 1012–1018. [CrossRef] [PubMed]

19. Holden, M.K.; Dyar, T.A.; Dayan-Cimadoro, L. Telerehabilitation using a virtual environment improves upper extremity function in patients with stroke. *IEEE Trans. Neural Syst. Rehabil. Eng.* **2007**, *15*, 36–42. [CrossRef] [PubMed]

20. Martin-Moreno, J.; Ruiz-Fernandez, D.; Soriano-Paya, A.; Berenguer-Miralles, V.J. Monitoring 3D movements for the rehabilitation of joints in physiotherapy. In Proceedings of the 2008 30th Annual International Conference of the IEEE Engineering in Medicine and Biology Society, Vancouver, BC, Canada, 20–25 August 2008; pp. 4836–4839.

21. Lockery, D.; Peters, J.F.; Ramanna, S.; Shay, B.L.; Szturm, T. Store-and-Feedforward Adaptive Gaming System for Hand-Finger Motion Tracking in Telerehabilitation. *IEEE Trans. Inf. Tech. Biomed.* **2011**, *15*, 467–473. [CrossRef] [PubMed]

22. Iosa, M.; Morone, G.; Fusco, A.; Castagnoli, M.; Fusco, F.R.; Pratesi, L.; Paolucci, S. Leap motion controlled video game-based therapy for rehabilitation of elderly patients with subacute stroke: A feasibility pilot study. *Top. Stroke Rehabil.* **2015**, *22*, 306–316. [CrossRef] [PubMed]

23. Blumrosen, G.; Miron, Y.; Intrator, N.; Plotnik, M. A Real-Time Kinect Signature-Based Patient Home Monitoring System. *Sensors* **2016**, *16*, 1965. [CrossRef] [PubMed]

24. Chang, Y.J.; Chen, S.F.; Huang, J.D. A Kinect-based system for physical rehabilitation: A pilot study for young adults with motor disabilities. *Res. Dev. Disabil.* **2011**, *32*, 2566–2570. [CrossRef] [PubMed]

25. Galna, B.; Jackson, D.; Schofield, G.; McNaney, R.; Webster, M.; Barry, G.; Mhiripiri, D.; Balaam, M.; Olivier, P.; Rochester, L. Retraining function in people with Parkinson's disease using the Microsoft kinect: Game design and pilot testing. *J. Neuroeng. Rehabil.* **2014**, *11*, 60. [CrossRef] [PubMed]

26. Gotsis, M.; Lympouridis, V.; Turpin, D.; Tasse, A.; Poulos, I.C.; Tucker, D.; Swider, M.; Thin, A.G.; Jordan-Marsh, M. Mixed reality game prototypes for upper body exercise and rehabilitation. In Proceedings of the 2012 IEEE Virtual Reality Workshops (VRW), Costa Mesa, CA, USA, 4–8 March 2012; pp. 181–182.

27. Pastor, I.; Hayes, H.A.; Bamberg, S.J. A feasibility study of an upper limb rehabilitation system using kinect and computer games. In Proceedings of the 2012 Annual International Conference of the IEEE Engineering in Medicine and Biology Society, San Diego, CA, USA, 28 August–1 September 2012; pp. 1286–1289.

28. Chang, Y.J.; Han, W.Y.; Tsai, Y.C. A Kinect-based upper limb rehabilitation system to assist people with cerebral palsy. *Res. Dev. Disabil.* **2013**, *34*, 3654–3659. [CrossRef] [PubMed]

29. Gabel, M.; Gilad-Bachrach, R.; Renshaw, E.; Schuster, A. Full body gait analysis with Kinect. In Proceedings of the 2012 Annual International Conference of the IEEE Engineering in Medicine and Biology Society, San Diego, CA, USA, 28 August–1 September 2012; pp. 1964–1967.

30. Venugopalan, J.; Cheng, C.; Stokes, T.H.; Wang, M.D. Kinect-based rehabilitation system for patients with traumatic brain injury. In Proceedings of the 2013 35th Annual International Conference of the IEEE Engineering in Medicine and Biology Society (EMBC), Osaka, Japan, 3–7 July 2013; pp. 4625–4628.

31. Tian, Y.; Meng, X.; Tao, D.; Liu, D.; Feng, C. Upper limb motion tracking with the integration of IMU and Kinect. *Neurocomputing* **2015**, *159*, 207–218. [CrossRef]

32. Kurillo, G.; Han, J.J.; Nicorici, A.; Bajcsy, R. Tele-MFAsT: Kinect-based tele-medicine tool for remote motion and function assessment. *Stud. Health Technol. Inform.* **2014**, *196*, 215–221. [PubMed]

33. Jintronix. Jintronix Rehabilitation System. Available online: http://www.jintronix.com/ (accessed on 17 April 2018).

34. VirtualRehab. Available online: http://www.virtualrehab.info/ (accessed on 17 April 2018).

35. DoctorKinetic. Available online: http://www.doctorkinetic.com (accessed on 17 April 2018).

36. VAST.Rehab. VAST.Rehab: Rehabilitation with Bio-Feedback. Available online: http://www.virtual-reality-rehabilitation.com (accessed on 17 April 2018).

37. Colombo, R.; Sanguineti, V. Rehabilitation Robotics: Technology and Applications. In *Rehabilitation Robotics*; Colombo, R., Sanguineti, V., Eds.; Academic Press: London, UK, 2018; pp. xix–xxvi.

38. Saracino, L.; Avizzano, C.A.; Ruffalde, E.; Cappiello, G.; Curto, Z.; Scoglio, A. Motore++ A portable haptic device for domestic rehabilitation. In Proceedings of the 42nd Annual Conference of the IEEE Industrial Electronics Society, Florence, Italy, 23–26 October 2016.

39. Díaz, I.; Catalan, J.M.; Badesa, F.J.; Justo, X.; Lledo, L.D.; Ugartemendia, A.; Gil, J.J.; Díez, J.; García-Aracil, N. Development of a robotic device for post-stroke home tele-rehabilitation. *Adv. Mech. Eng.* **2018**, *10*, 1–8. [CrossRef]

40. Bai, J.; Song, A.; Xu, B.; Nie, J.; Li, H. A Novel Human-Robot Cooperative Method for Upper Extremity Rehabilitation. *Int. J. Soc. Robot.* **2017**, *9*, 265–275. [CrossRef]

41. Song, A.; Wu, C.; Ni, D.; Li, H.; Qin, H. One-therapist to three-patient telerehabilitation for the upper limb after stroke. *Int. J. Soc. Robot.* **2016**, *8*, 319–329. [CrossRef]

42. Pareto, L.; Johanssong, B.; Ljungberg, C.; Zeller, S.; Sunnerhagen, K.S.; Rydmark, M.; Broeren, J. Telehealth with 3D games for stroke rehabilitation. *Int. J. Disabil. Hum. Dev.* **2011**, *10*, 373–377. [CrossRef]

43. Miller, M.D.; Ferris, D.G. Measurement of subjective phenomena in primary care research: The Visual Analogue Scale. *Fam. Pract. Res. J.* **1993**, *13*, 15–24. [PubMed]

44. Golbreich, C.; Grosjean, J.; Darmoni, S.J. The Foundational Model of Anatomy in OWL 2 and its use. *Artif. Intell. Med.* **2013**, *57*, 119–132. [CrossRef] [PubMed]

45. Berges, I.; Anton, D.; Bermudez, J.; Goñi, A.; Illarramendi, A. TrhOnt: Building an ontology to assist rehabilitation processes. *J. Biomed. Semant.* **2016**, *7*, 1–21. [CrossRef] [PubMed]

46. Anton, D.; Goñi, A.; Illarramendi, A. Exercise Recognition for Kinect-based Telerehabilitation. *Methods Inf. Med.* **2015**, *54*, 145–155. [PubMed]

47. Bertin, E.; Cubaud, S.; Tuffin, S.; Cazeaux, S.; Crespi, N.; Beltran, V. WebRTC, the day after. In Proceedings of the 17 th International Conference on Intelligence in Next Generation Networks, ICIN, Venice, Italy, 15–16 October 2013; pp. 46–52.

48. Johnston, A.B.; Burnett, D.C. *WebRTC: APIs and RTCWEB Protocols of the HTML5 Real-Time Web*; Digital Codex LLC: St. Louis, MO, USA, 2012.

49. Jang-Jaccard, J.; Nepal, S.; Celler, B.; Yan, B. WebRTC-based video conferencing service for telehealth. *Computing* **2014**, *98*, 169–193. [CrossRef]

50. Anton, D.; Kurillo, G.; Goñi, A.; Illarramendi, A.; Bajcsy, R. Real-time communication for Kinect-based telerehabilitation. *Future Gener. Comput. Syst.* **2017**, *75*, 72–81. [CrossRef]

51. Microsoft. Kinect for Windows. Available online: https://developer.microsoft.com/en-us/windows/kinect (accessed on 3 May 2018).

52. Intel. Intel Real Sense. Available online: https://realsense.intel.com/stereo/ (accessed on 3 May 2018).

53. Orbbec. Available online: https://orbbec3d.com/products/ (accessed on 3 May 2018).

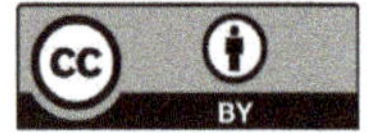
© 2018 by the authors. Licensee MDPI, Basel, Switzerland. This article is an open access article distributed under the terms and conditions of the Creative Commons Attribution (CC BY) license (http://creativecommons.org/licenses/by/4.0/).

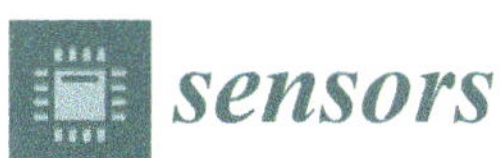 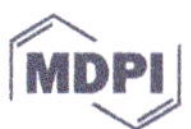

Article

Biomechanical Gait Variable Estimation Using Wearable Sensors after Unilateral Total Knee Arthroplasty

Ik-Hyun Youn [1,*], Jong-Hoon Youn [2], Joseph A. Zeni [3] and Brian A. Knarr [4]

[1] Division of Navigation & Information Systems, Mokpo National Maritime University, Mokpo 58628, Korea
[2] Department of Computer Science, University of Nebraska Omaha, Omaha, NE 68182, USA; jyoun@unomaha.edu
[3] Department of Physical Therapy, University of Delaware, Newark, DE 19716, USA; jzenijr@udel.edu
[4] Department of Biomechanics, University of Nebraska Omaha, Omaha, NE 68182, USA; bknarr@unomaha.edu
* Correspondence: iyoun@mmu.ac.kr; Tel.: +82-61-240-7283

Received: 7 April 2018; Accepted: 11 May 2018; Published: 15 May 2018

Abstract: Total knee arthroplasty is a common surgical treatment for end-stage osteoarthritis of the knee. The majority of existing studies that have explored the relationship between recovery and gait biomechanics have been conducted in laboratory settings. However, seamless gait parameter monitoring in real-world conditions may provide a better understanding of recovery post-surgery. The purpose of this study was to estimate kinematic and kinetic gait variables using two ankle-worn wearable sensors in individuals after unilateral total knee arthroplasty. Eighteen subjects at least six months post-unilateral total knee arthroplasty participated in this study. Four biomechanical gait variables were measured using an instrumented split-belt treadmill and motion capture systems. Concurrently, eleven inertial gait variables were extracted from two ankle-worn accelerometers. Subsets of the inertial gait variables for each biomechanical gait variable estimation were statistically selected. Then, hierarchical regressions were created to determine the directional contributions of the inertial gait variables for biomechanical gait variable estimations. Selected inertial gait variables significantly predicted trial-averaged biomechanical gait variables. Moreover, strong directionally-aligned relationships were observed. Wearable-based gait monitoring of multiple and sequential kinetic gait variables in daily life could provide a more accurate understanding of the relationships between movement patterns and recovery from total knee arthroplasty.

Keywords: biomechanical gait variable estimation; inertial gait variable; total knee arthroplasty; wearable sensors

---

1. Introduction

Osteoarthritis (OA) of the knee is a common disease that impacts functional mobility and quality of life for many individuals [1,2]. Total Knee Arthroplasty (TKA) is the most common surgical treatment for end-stage OA. By replacing the impaired knee joint with implants, knee joint function and quality of life can be improved [2]. Since a primary goal of TKA is to regain ambulatory function, assessment of recovery after unilateral TKA using biomechanical gait variables can be useful clinical indicators. Monitoring the improvement of functional performance after TKA usually includes examining flexion and adduction knee moments and directional ground reaction forces [3]. Typically, studies on gait patterns before and after TKA use overground force plates and optical motion capture systems to collect biomechanical data [4]. While these instruments produce valid biomechanical data, they are constrained to laboratory settings and may not reflect real-world mobility patterns.

Wearable sensor-based continuous gait analysis is a promising alternative that can address the limitations of laboratory-based biomechanical evaluations [5]. Wearable devices are getting smaller and smarter, and wearables are easy to use and do not interfere with the natural behavior of the subject. Thus, wearable sensor-based gait analysis is one of the most promising methods for quantifying gait patterns in real-world conditions. Acceleration data from wearable sensors can also provide kinetic attributes outside of the laboratory setting. Monitoring multiple and sequential kinetic parameters using wearables in real-world conditions may lead to a more accurate understanding of the relationship between movement patterns and recovery from TKA.

Given the potential of wearable sensor-based gait analysis and the importance of gait outcomes post-TKA, the purpose of this study was to estimate biomechanical gait metrics using two wearable sensors in individuals after unilateral TKA. Biomechanical variables related to initial loading behavior (the initial 10% of the gait cycle) were selected since they are correlated with OA progression [6]. Concurrently, multiple inertial gait variables including a temporal parameter and kinetic parameters were extracted using wearable sensors. Then, the inertial gait variables were used to develop statistical prediction models of the selected biomechanical gait variables, such as moments and ground reaction forces, in the TKA population. Two main contributions of the present work are: (1) a generic method for linear inertial gait variable extraction; and (2) statistical models for estimation of important biomechanical gait variables.

2. Materials and Methods

The framework in Figure 1 outlines the entire method of this study from data collection to estimation model development. Due to the importance of the initial loading characteristics during the initiative gait cycle of the TKA population [6], gait variables related to initial loading behavior were carefully considered when both biomechanical and inertial gait variables were selected. Feature selection was performed to obtain statistically meaningful inertial gait variable subsets, and hierarchical linear regressions were created to determine the directional contributions of inertial gait variables to the key biomechanical gait variables of the TKA population.

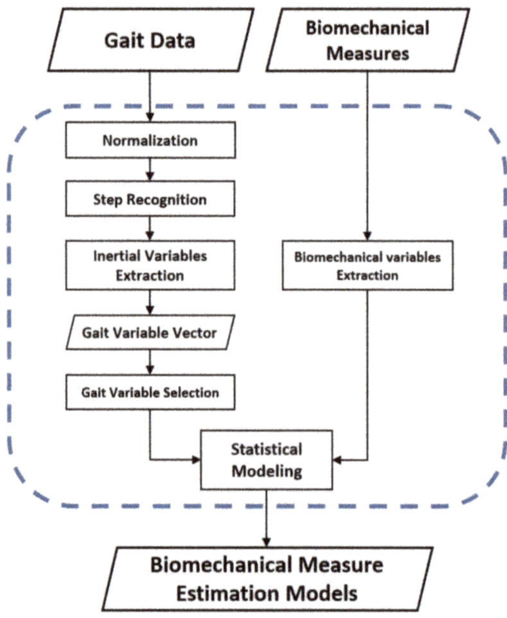

Figure 1. Framework for developing proposed biomechanical measure estimation models.

2.1. Data Description

Data were acquired in the Neuromuscular Biomechanics Laboratory at the University of Delaware. An instrumented split-belt treadmill (Bertec Corp, Columbus, OH, USA) and an 8-camera motion capture system (Motion Analysis Corp, Santa Rosa, CA, USA) were used to collect kinetic and kinematic gait variables. Concurrently, two accelerometers (Noraxon USA, Scottsdale, AZ, USA) were attached above the lateral malleoli using elastic bands to collect three-dimensional acceleration data. The sampling frequency of acceleration data was 200 Hz. Figure 2 demonstrates the orientation of both wearable sensors. For both legs, the X-axis of the sensors pointed up to the shank, but the Y-axis and Z-axis orientations pointed in different directions on the left and right legs. The biomechanical data from the force place, and the cameras and inertial data from the wearables, were synched via hardware trigger. Biomechanical gait variables and inertial gait variables were computed using Visual 3D (C-Motion, Bethesda, MD, USA) and custom software developed in the MATLAB 9.0 (Mathworks, Natick, MA, USA) environment, respectively.

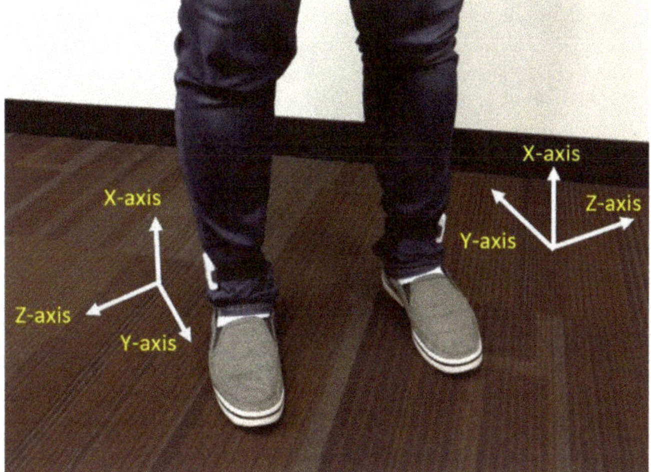

Figure 2. Wearable sensor orientation on both legs.

2.2. Participants and Protocol

Eighteen subjects (1.71 ± 0.08 m, 87.1 ± 17.5 kg, 66.5 ± 7.7 years) after unilateral TKA participated in this study. The study was approved by the Institutional Review Board at the University of Delaware. Each participant signed an informed consent before commencing protocols. Participants at least six months post-unilateral TKA were recruited (Table 1). Each subject conducted a 6-m walk test to determine a self-selected walking speed. Then, each participant was instructed to walk at a self-selected, comfortable walking speed on the instrumented split-belt treadmill for one minute. Participants walked 1.11 (± 0.19) m/s during the one-minute walk test.

Table 1. Participants' characteristics.

Characteristics	Mean (Standard Deviation)
n	18
Female/male	9/9
Age (years)	66.5 (7.7)
Body Mass Index (BMI, kg/m^2)	29.5 (4.9)
Height (cm)	171.4 (8.4)
Weight (kg)	87.1 (17.5)

2.3. Normalization

Kinetic and kinematic gait variables are often affected by the height and weight of the subjects. Acceleration from the lower limb may also be affected by these same factors. To minimize the confounding effects of patient anthropometric differences, we normalized both biomechanical and inertial gait variables by relevant factors. In prior research, Moisio et al. found that normalization methods were highly effective in reducing individual differences [7]. To normalize personal differences, kinetic and kinematic gait signals were divided by weight, and acceleration data were divided by height.

2.4. Biomechanical Gait Variable Extraction

In this session, we present information on the processes used to obtain the biomechanical gait variables of interest from laboratory instruments. Biomechanical gait variables included kinetic parameters such as knee moments and ground reaction forces. The process of feature extraction is detailed below. In this study, we focused on initial loading behavior-related inertial gait variables as important recovery indicators for the population. Loading characteristics during gait are important as they are correlated with OA progression [6]. To address the loading patterns, relevant kinetic biomechanical gait variables were measured including the maximum knee flexion moment (KFM), the maximum knee adduction moment (KAM), the first peak of vertical ground reaction force (vGRF) [8,9]. Additionally, the maximum anterior ground reaction force (aGRF) was included since the parameter has been used for various knee moment studies [10]. Although aGRF has less association with initial loading, the prediction of aGRF was expected to provide us information about the validity of our approach.

Each step was first recognized by the point where 20% of the maximum vertical ground reaction force occurred [11]. Then, intended patterns (i.e., maximum or first peak maximum) were recognized to obtain targeted biomechanical gait variables (Table 2 and Figure 3). Since both the average and symmetry of biomechanical gait variables are important indicators for unilateral TKA [12,13], the four biomechanical gait variables from each step were then summarized in terms of average and symmetry across the one-minute trial. On average, 103 (±27.4) steps were included from the trial. Symmetry was calculated for each stride, and data from all steps were averaged when calculating average parameters.

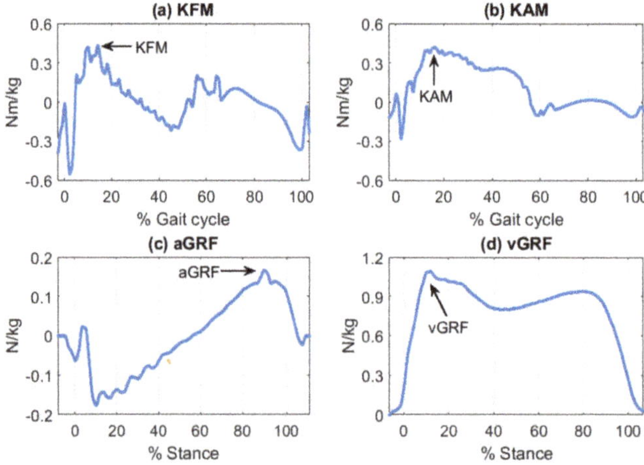

Figure 3. Kinetic biomechanical gait variables: weight-normalized. (**a**) Knee flexion moment (KFM); (**b**) knee adduction moment (KAM); (**c**) anterior/posterior ground reaction forces (aGRF); (**d**) vertical ground reaction force (vGRF).

Table 2. Biomechanical gait variable properties.

Purpose	Acronym	Description
Knee Flexion Moment	KFM	Maximum anterior knee moment
Knee Adduction Moment	KAM	Maximum lateral knee moment
Anterior Ground Reaction Force	aGRF	Maximum anterior direction GRF
Vertical Ground Reaction Force	vGRF	Maximum first vertical GRF

2.5. Inertial Gait Variable Extraction

Anterior directional acceleration was selected for accurate gait event recognition since the anterior dimensional motion of the lower limbs was dominant over the two other dimensions from an ankle-worn sensor perspective. Each heel-strike action generated a dramatic peak in the anterior directional acceleration; this peak was a clear indicator of the initial loading within a gait cycle (Figure 4a). The identified peaks were compared to the vertical ground reaction force data to validate the accuracy of acceleration-based gait event detection (Figure 4b). The described methodology was applied to each ankle sensor individually. Once individual step recognition was complete, the recognized peaks from the two sensors and raw acceleration data were merged together to obtain data on step cycles.

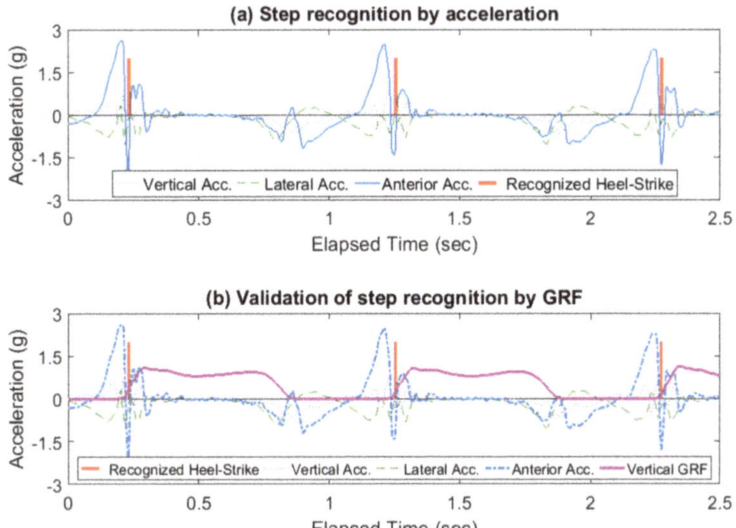

Figure 4. Step detection and validation with recognized heel-strikes. (**a**) Step detection using acceleration in the anterior/posterior direction; (**b**) validation of step recognition using the ground reaction force in the vertical direction. Note that the intervals between recognized heel-strikes indicate stride cycles.

Eleven gait variables were extracted to estimate the magnitude, impulse, and angles of initial loading from 3D-acceleration data. Since the focus of this study was on the initial loading characteristics of TKA patients, the inertial motion of the lower limbs following heel-strike (HS) was analyzed. Characteristics from the initial 10% of the stance phase of the gait cycle, the initial 10% of the directional impulse of the gait cycle, and the maximum directional acceleration at HS were extracted. Additionally, whole step vector magnitude, ankle angle variation in the lateral and anterior directions, and step time were computed to explain the characteristics of the whole step cycle (Table 3).

The vectors of the basic gait variables from each step were summarized in terms of average and symmetry for each trial. The trial-averaged inertial gait variables were applied to estimate the biomechanical gait variables. Since bilateral gait symmetry has gained more attention, particularly in the unilateral TKA population [9,13], the basic gait variables were used to calculate symmetry. The Symmetry Index (SI) proposed by Robinson et al. was applied to assess the symmetry of inertial gait variables [14]. To apply the concept of SI for TKA patients, SI was defined in the study as the difference between the non-surgical limb from the surgical limb, rather than the difference between the left limb and the right limb.

Table 3. Inertial gait variable properties.

Purpose	Acronym	Description	Method
Step magnitude	VM	Whole step vector magnitude	Residual acceleration during the step
Initial step magnitude	VM10	Step magnitude of initial 10% of the step time	Initial 10% of residual acceleration during the step
Directional magnitude of initial loading	MAG-L	Lateral heel-strike magnitude	Maximum lateral acceleration at HS
	MAG-V	Vertical heel-strike magnitude	Maximum vertical acceleration at HS
	MAG-A	Anterior heel-strike magnitude	Maximum anterior acceleration at HS
Directional impulse of initial loading	IMP-L	Lateral heel-strike impulse	SD of lateral acceleration during initial 10% of step
	IMP-V	Vertical heel-strike impulse	SD of vertical acceleration during initial 10% of step
	IMP-A	Anterior heel-strike impulse	SD of anterior acceleration during initial 10% of step
Directional ankle angle variation during stance phase	ANG-L	Ankle angle change to the gravity in the lateral direction during the stance phase	SD of sensor local angle change in lateral direction during stance phase
	ANG-A	Ankle angle change to the gravity in the anterior direction during the stance phase	SD of sensor local angle change in lateral direction during stance phase
Temporal parameter	ST	Step time	HS-to-HS time

HS is heel-strike; SD is standard deviation.

2.6. Data Analysis

To quantify the relationships between all independent (i.e., eleven inertial gait variables) and dependent variables (i.e., four biomechanical gait variables), a Pearson Correlation analysis was conducted. For the statistical analysis, the eleven inertial gait variables were categorized by directional perspectives, i.e., lateral, anterior, vertical, and inclusive inertial gait variables (Table 4).

Table 4. Directional categories of inertial gait variables.

Directional Category	Description	Variable
Inclusive	Non-directional variables	VM, VM10, ST
Lateral	Lateral variables	MAG-L, IMP-L, ANG-L
Vertical	Vertical variables	MAG-V, IMP-V
Anterior	Anterior variables	MAG-A, IMP-A, ANG-A

To avoid overfitting the estimation models, subsets of eleven inertial gait variables were carefully selected for each of the four biomechanical gait variables as a preprocessing method. Stepwise regression was applied to systematically select relevant inertial gait variables for the four biomechanical gait variables [15]. The automatic procedure of stepwise regression of feeding all useful inertial variables helped us to reduce the amount of mutual information (i.e., non-overlapping) among eleven independent variables- with smaller subset sizes. The stepwise regression criterion for variable inclusion was an increase in the adjusted R^2 value. To improve the robustness of the model, k-fold cross-validation [16] was applied with k = 10. In k-fold cross-validation, 18 participants were randomly partitioned into 10 subfolders. A single subfolder was retained as the validation data for testing the model, and the remaining nine subfolders were used as training data. The cross-validation process was then repeated 10 times, with each subfolder used exactly once as the validation data. The procedure was intended to make estimation models robust enough to be for unseen TKA patients' gait data and to improve the overall validity of model predictions.

To determine the directional contributions to biomechanical measures, hierarchical linear regressions were used [16]. Specifically, selected inertial variables in each directional category were added to the regression models in steps as discussed in [17]. This procedure provided information regarding which directional inertial variables had the most predictive power on the biomechanical variable estimation models. Separate regressions were conducted for each of the four biomechanical gait variables. Primary axis inertial variables were entered into the regressions at the first step. For example, KFM was knee moment in the anterior–posterior direction, so the anterior direction inertial variables from feature selection outcomes were added to the KFM estimation regression model in the first step. Then, the vertical and lateral inertial variables were entered in the second and third steps, respectively. For all hierarchical regressions, the inclusive inertial variables were entered at the last step. The order of hierarchical regression steps was determined in a cyclic way depending on directional aspects of target biomechanical variables. For example, to establish the KFM estimation model, anterior variables were entered first, then vertical and lateral inertial variables were additionally entered first, then vertical and lateral inertial variables were additionally entered, respectively. Inclusive variables were always entered last. The significance of each model and the significant change in R^2 at each step were evaluated. The change in R^2 provided increased predictive power through the addition of certain directional inertial variables at each regression step.

3. Results

Overall, ten inertial variables were significantly correlated with KFM, aGRF, and vGRF (Table 5). Only the step time (ST) was not significantly correlated with any biomechanical variables. In particular, the vertical heel-strike impulse (IMP-V) was solely correlated with KAM. The selected inertial gait variable subsets for each of the four biomechanical gait variables are listed in Tables 6 and 7.

Table 5. Pearson correlation coefficient between inertial and biomechanical variables.

	KFM	KAM	aGRF	vGRF
VM	0.63 **	-	0.74 **	0.62 **
VM10	0.60 **	-	0.79 **	0.67 **
MAG-L	-	-	0.51 *	-
MAG-V	-	-	0.52 *	-
MAG-A	0.73 **	-	0.74 **	0.55 **
IMP-L	0.59 **	-	0.74 **	0.54 *
IMP-V	-	−0.58 **	-	-
IMP-A	0.51 *	-	0.65 **	0.58 **
ANG-L	0.47 *	-	0.61 **	0.58 **
ANG-A	0.60 **	-	0.71 **	0.66 **
ST	-	-	-	-

** Correlation is significant at the 0.01 level; * correlation is significant at the 0.05 level; those with significance greater than 0.05 were removed.

For the trial-averaged biomechanical variable prediction models, no lateral inertial variables were selected for KFM and aGRF, and none of the vertical inertial variables were selected for KAM and vGRF (Table 6). ST was selected for all four biomechanical variable estimations, although ST was not significantly correlated with them in the Pearson Correlation analysis results. For the trial symmetry of biomechanical variable prediction models, the lateral and vertical magnitude variables (i.e., MAG-L, and MAG-V) were selected except the anterior magnitude variable (i.e., MAG-A) (Table 7). The inclusive variables were relatively less frequently selected for symmetry prediction models. The robustness and generalizability of the estimation models were improved by reducing the dimensionality of the inertial gait variables.

Table 6. Feature selection results for average prediction.

Biomechanical Variable	Selected Inertial Gait Variables			
	Lateral	Vertical	Anterior	Inclusive
KFM	None	MAG-V	ANG-A	ST
KAM	IMP-L, MAG-L ANG-L	None	MAG-A	VM10 ST
aGRF	None	MAG-V IMP-V	MAG-A ANG-A	ST
vGRF	IMP-L, MAG-L ANG-L	None	IMP-A	VM10 ST

Table 7. Feature selection results for symmetry prediction.

Biomechanical Variable	Selected Inertial Gait Variables			
	Lateral	Vertical	Anterior	Inclusive
KFM	MAG-L IMP-L	MAG-V	IMP-A ANG-A	VM, VM10, ST
KAM	MAG-L	MAG-V IMP-V	IMP-A	None
aGRF	MAG-L	MAG-V	ANG-A	VM
vGRF	MAG-L	MAG-V	ANG-A	None

The hierarchical linear regression results demonstrated a strong indication that the proposed wearable sensor-derived acceleration data could assist in quantifying biomechanical gait measures. In Tables 8 and 9, the average and symmetry of the biomechanical variables were predicted using the selected inertial variables.

Each individual table contains the prediction results for 17 subjects. One subject (71-year-old male, BMI 31.6) was excluded from the analysis due to a distinctly abnormal gait pattern characterized by heel-strikes with overtly large vertical ground reaction forces. The subject was identified as an outlier based on the median absolute deviation measure. By removing this subject, the average and symmetry of the vGRF prediction showed a more reasonable prediction power. Regarding the average prediction results, all four biomechanical variables were significantly predicted using the selected subsets of inertial variables. Directional contributions were identified. For instance, aGRF was primarily related to the anterior axis, and the anterior inertial gait variables predicted most of the outcomes (i.e., 0.467 of 0.697 as adj. R^2). Similar directional alignments were observed from KFM and KAM. Although vGRF was significantly predicted, there was no such directional alignment because none of the vertical inertial variables were selected. In the symmetry prediction outcomes, the selected inertial variables were significantly correlated with the symmetry of KFM. The effect of the uncommon walking subject was also trivial, so the exclusion of the subject did not change the results. Specifically, the symmetry of vGRF was substantially affected by the uncommon walking subject. The subject caused strongly biased gait variables and abnormally increased adj. R^2 values of up to 0.919. By removing the subject, adj. R^2 was adjusted by 0.547.

Table 8. Hierarchical linear regressions for averages of biomechanical gait variables.

(a) Average Knee Flexion Moment (KFM)

Step	All subjects			Excluding outlier	
	R	Adj. R^2	ΔR^2	Adj. R^2	ΔR^2
Anterior	0.605	0.326	0.326	0.350	0.350
Vertical	0.740	0.486	0.160	0.442	0.092
Lateral	0.740	0.486	0.000	0.442	0.000
Inclusive	0.773	0.510	0.024	0.455	0.014

(b) Average Knee Adduction Moment (KAM)

Step	All subjects			Excluding outlier	
	R	Adj. R^2	ΔR^2	Adj. R^2	ΔR^2
Lateral	0.664	0.321	0.321	0.319	0.319
Anterior	0.756	0.441	0.120	0.432	0.113
Vertical	0.756	0.441	0.000	0.432	0.000
Inclusive	0.867	0.615	0.175	0.614	0.182

(c) Average Anterior Ground Reaction Force (aGRF)

Step	All subjects			Excluding outlier	
	R	Adj. R^2	ΔR^2	Adj. R^2	ΔR^2
Anterior	0.728	0.467	0.467	0.486	0.486
Vertical	0.846	0.629	0.162	0.614	0.128
Lateral	0.846	0.629	0.000	0.614	0.000
Inclusive	0.887	0.697	0.067	0.677	0.063

(d) Average Vertical Ground Reaction Force (vGRF)

Step	All subjects			Excluding outlier	
	R	Adj. R^2	ΔR^2	Adj. R^2	ΔR^2
Vertical	0.000	0.000	0.000	0.000	0.000
Lateral	0.738	0.446	0.446	0.377	0.377
Anterior	0.748	0.425	−0.020	0.417	0.040
Inclusive	0.857	0.589	0.164	0.463	0.046

Table 9. Hierarchical linear regressions for symmetry of biomechanical gait variables.

(a) Symmetry Knee Flexion Moment (KFM)

Step	All subjects			Excluding outlier	
	R	Adj. R^2	ΔR^2	Adj. R^2	ΔR^2
Anterior	0.680	0.391	0.391	0.373	0.373
Vertical	0.704	0.387	−0.004	0.431	0.058
Lateral	0.811	0.515	0.128	0.564	0.132
Inclusive	0.969	0.882	0.368	0.873	0.309

(b) Symmetry Knee Adduction Moment (KAM)

Step	All subjects			Excluding outlier	
	R	Adj. R^2	ΔR^2	Adj. R^2	ΔR^2
Lateral	0.126	−0.046	−0.046	−0.055	−0.055
Anterior	0.173	−0.100	−0.054	−0.115	−0.060
Vertical	0.733	0.395	0.494	0.379	0.495
Inclusive	0.733	0.395	0.000	0.499	0.120

Table 9. *Cont.*

(c) Symmetry Anterior Ground Reaction Force (aGRF)					
Step	**All subjects**			**Excluding outlier**	
	R	**Adj. R^2**	**ΔR^2**	**Adj. R^2**	**ΔR^2**
Anterior	0.308	0.038	0.038	0.083	0.083
Vertical	0.488	0.136	0.098	0.014	−0.069
Lateral	0.501	0.090	−0.046	0.162	0.148
Inclusive	0.560	0.103	0.013	0.364	0.202

(d) Symmetry Vertical Ground Reaction Force (vGRF)					
Step	**All subjects**			**Excluding outlier**	
	R	**Adj. R^2**	**ΔR^2**	**Adj. R^2**	**ΔR^2**
Vertical	0.626	0.354	0.354	0.165	0.165
Lateral	0.765	0.529	0.175	0.222	0.057
Anterior	0.797	0.522	−0.007	0.473	0.251
Inclusive	0.971	0.919	0.397	0.547	0.074

4. Discussion

The goal of this study was to estimate kinematic and kinetic gait metrics using two ankle-worn wearable sensors in individuals after unilateral TKA. Overall, we found that our novel method of extracting unique features from 3D accelerations was capable of predicting key biomechanical measure in a post-TKA population.

Compared to previous studies which focused on predicting knee loads post-TKA, our results demonstrated a greater predictive power. Rivière et al. focused on isolated clinical measures, such as limb alignment ($R^2 < 0.13$) [3], and Vahtrick et al. investigated limb strength ($R^2 < 0.32$) [4]. The results of this study indicate that wearable sensors can be used to predict key knee loading [1,2] variables important to recovery post-TKA with greater power than basic clinical measures. This may be due to the more direct nature of wearable accelerometry during gait, versus indirect measures of predisposition (limb alignment) or capacity (strength) that do not take into account an individual's active movement and muscle coordination during the specific task of gait.

The outcomes of the regression models indicated that inertial gait features significantly estimated all four biomechanical gait features. Interestingly, the temporal parameter of step time was not significantly correlated with any biomechanical variables of interest, whereas most of the inertial variables showed moderate to significant correlations with biomechanical variables. In particular, as the anterior direction motion of ankle-worn sensors was predominant over the other two directions, many inertial variables were significantly corrected with aGRF.

The primary axes of biomechanical variables were related to selected inertial variables. However, it was difficult to explain the connection between response and predictor variables due to the complex nature of gait. Notably, lateral and vertical heel-strike magnitude and anterior stance phase angle variation were commonly selected for symmetry prediction models, and inclusive variables were considered to be less important predictor variables. Our results imply that wearable sensor-based data that explains overall step timing were not useful to estimate the symmetry of biomechanical variables.

Knee flexion moment was primarily predicted by vertical inertial gait variables. It is likely that vertical inertial variables are related to limb impact during heel strike. The impact may be partially controlled by knee flexion, with an increase in knee flexion during weight acceptance serving to soften the impact but subsequently, increasing peak knee flexion moment. On the other hand, knee adduction moment was primarily predicted by lateral inertial gait variables. Gait modifications including increased step width, increased trunk sway, and toe-in gait have been shown to be effective for reducing the knee adduction moment in a healthy population. It is likely that individuals post-TKA may adapt similar strategies to reduce the knee adduction moment because of pain or functional compensations. It is reasonable to believe that such gait adaptations may be evidenced through lateral inertial gait variables, given the changes in side-to-side movement (i.e., swaying, wide steps).

5. Conclusions

The proposed models and biomechanical gait variable estimation results provided evidence that inertial measurements can be used to reasonably estimate conventional biomechanical metrics. Although cross-validation was applied, generalization to the TKA population could be limited due to the small sample size of the study. Future work will examine the relationship between additional kinematic and kinetic variables and inertial variables to characterize changes over time and to expand to additional populations and biomechanical metrics.

Author Contributions: I.-H.Y. and J.-H.Y. conceived and designed the paper; J.A.Z. and B.A.K. designed the experiments, contributed to data analysis and reviewed the paper.

Funding: The authors acknowledge support from the National Institute of Health (NIH) grants NIH P30-GM103333 and NIH P20-GM109090.

Conflicts of Interest: The authors declare no conflict of interest.

References

1. Komnik, I.; Weiss, S.; Pagani, C.F.; Potthast, W. Motion analysis of patients after knee arthroplasty during activities of daily living—A systematic review. *Gait Posture* **2015**, *41*, 370–377.
2. Pozzi, F.; Snyder-Mackler, L.; Zeni, J. Relationship between biomechanical asymmetries during a step up and over task and stair climbing after total knee arthroplasty. *Clin. Biomech.* **2015**, *30*, 78–85.
3. Rivière, C.; Ollivier, M.; Girerd, D.; Argenson, J.N.; Parratte, S. Does standing limb alignment after total knee arthroplasty predict dynamic alignment and knee loading during gait? *Knee* **2017**, *24*, 627–633.
4. Vahtrik, D.; Gapeyeva, H.; Ereline, J.; Pääsuke, M. Relationship between leg extensor muscle strength and knee joint loading during gait before and after total knee arthroplasty. *Knee* **2014**, *21*, 216–220.
5. Chen, S.; Lach, J.; Lo, B.; Yang, G. Toward pervasive gait analysis with wearable sensors: A systematic review. *IEEE J. Biom. Health Inf.* **2016**, *20*, 1521–1537.
6. Hatfield, G.L.; Stanish, W.D.; Hubley-Kozey, C.L. Three-Dimensional biomechanical gait characteristics at baseline are associated with progression to total knee arthroplasty. *Arth. Care Res.* **2015**, *67*, 1004–1014.
7. Moisio, K.C.; Sumner, D.R.; Shott, S.; Hurwitz, D.E. Normalization of joint moments during gait: A comparison of two techniques. *J. Biomech.* **2003**, *36*, 599–603.
8. Burnett, D.R.; Campbell-Kyureghyan, N.H.; Cerrito, P.B.; Quesada, P.M. Symmetry of ground reaction forces and muscle activity in asymptomatic subjects during walking, sit-to-stand, and stand-to-sit tasks. *J. Electromyogr. Kinesiol.* **2011**, *21*, 610–615.
9. Burnett, D.R.; Campbell-Kyureghyan, N.H.; Topp, R.V.; Quesada, P.M. Biomechanics of lower limbs during walking among candidates for total knee arthroplasty with and without low back pain. *BioMed Res. Int.* **2015**. [CrossRef]
10. Ueno, R.; Ishida, T.; Ymanaka, M. Quadriceps force and anterior tibial force occur obviously later than vertical ground reaction force: A simulation study. *BMC Musculoskeletal Disord.* **2017**, *18*, 467–481.
11. Bertani, A.; Cappello, A.; Benedetti, M.; Simoncini, L.; Catani, F. Flat foot functional evaluation using pattern recognition of ground reaction data. *Clin. Biomech.* **1999**, *14*, 484–493.
12. Milner, C.E. Interlimb asymmetry during walking following unilateral total knee arthroplasty. *Gait Posture* **2008**, *28*, 69–73.
13. Zeni, J.; Abujaber, S.; Pozzi, F.; Raisis, L. Relationship between strength, pain, and different measures of functional ability in patients with End-Stage hip osteoarthritis. *Arthr. Care Res.* **2014**, *66*, 1506–1512.
14. Nigg, B.; Robinson, R.; Herzog, W. Use of force platform variables to quantify the effects of chiropractic manipulation on gait symmetry. *J. Manipulative Physiol. Ther.* **1987**, *10*, 172–176.
15. Boulet, S.; Boudot, E.; Houel, N. Relationships between each part of the spinal curves and upright posture using multiple stepwise linear regression analysis. *J. Biomech.* **2016**, *49*, 1149–1155.

16. Masse, F.; Gonzenbach, R.; Paraschiv-Ionescu, A.; Luft, A.R.; Aminian, K. Wearable barometric pressure sensor to improve postural transition recognition of mobility-impaired stroke patients. *IEEE Trans. Neural Syst. Rehab. Eng.* **2016**, *24*, 1210–1217.
17. Rebar, A.L.; Elavsky, S.; Maher, J.P.; Doerksen, S.E.; Conroy, D.E. Habits predict physical activity on days when intentions are weak. *J. Sport Exerc. Psychol.* **2014**, *36*, 157–165.

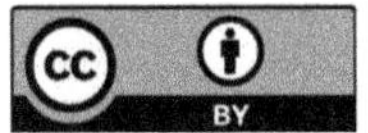

© 2018 by the authors. Licensee MDPI, Basel, Switzerland. This article is an open access article distributed under the terms and conditions of the Creative Commons Attribution (CC BY) license (http://creativecommons.org/licenses/by/4.0/).

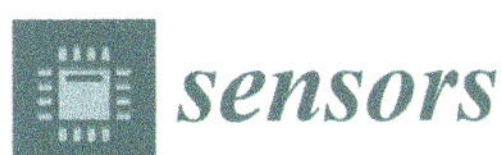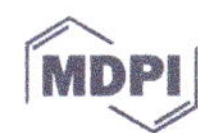

sensors

Article

Recognition of a Person Wearing Sport Shoes or High Heels through Gait Using Two Types of Sensors

Marcin Derlatka [1,*] and Mariusz Bogdan [2]

[1] Department of Biocybernetics and Biomedical Engineering of the Faculty of Mechanical Engineering at Bialystok University of Technology, 15-351 Bialystok, Poland
[2] Department of Automatic Control and Robotics of the Faculty of Mechanical Engineering at Bialystok University of Technology, 15-351 Bialystok, Poland; m.bogdan@pb.edu.pl
* Correspondence: m.derlatka@pb.edu.pl; Tel.: +48-571-443-044

Received: 9 April 2018; Accepted: 18 May 2018; Published: 21 May 2018

Abstract: Biometrics is currently an area that is both very interesting as well as rapidly growing. Among various types of biometrics the human gait recognition seems to be one of the most intriguing. However, one of the greatest problems within this field of biometrics is the change in gait caused by footwear. A change of shoes results in a significant lowering of accuracy in recognition of people. The following work presents a method which uses data gathered by two sensors: force plates and Microsoft Kinect v2 to reduce this problem. Microsoft Kinect is utilized to measure the body height of a person which allows the reduction of the set of recognized people only to those whose height is similar to that which has been measured. The entire process is preceded by identifying the type of footwear which the person is wearing. The research was conducted on data obtained from 99 people (more than 3400 strides) and the proposed method allowed us to reach a Correct Classification Rate (CCR) greater than 88% which, in comparison to earlier methods reaching CCR's of <80%, is a significant improvement. The work presents advantages as well as limitations of the proposed method.

Keywords: biometrics; human gait recognition; ground reaction forces; Microsoft Kinect; high heels; fusion data; ensemble classifiers

---

1. Introduction

In the world of constantly developing technology biometrics occupies a special place. Biometrics understood as the recognition of a particular person is already in use in forensic [1,2] as well as commercially (by ATMs, for example). Among the various field of biometrics the human gait is especially intriguing [3,4]. It is the result of a coordinated cooperation between the nervous and the musculoskeletal systems and it is accepted that after maturity all the way to advanced age it generally remains unchanged. As early as the 1970s research had shown that the way a person moves is to a great degree individual and allows the identification of a person [5]. A number of works dealing with the subject of identifying people in relation to the way they move have been published since that time [6–10]. Connor and Ross categorized these studies on the basis of sensors used to obtain measurements and divided them into methods using [11]:

- video cameras [12,13],
- the measurement of pressure exerted by a person's foot on the ground [14–16],
- accelerometers and other wearable devices [17–19],
- audio [20,21].

Works connected with the biometrics of the human gait mainly concentrate on creating systems guaranteeing the highest accuracy possible. Of course, the methodology which allows this relies directly on the character of the registered data. In case of signals recorded using video sensors the Gait Energy Image (GEI) representation has been successfully employed. GEI is obtained through a simple average of silhouettes during walking. Modifications of this method which improve GEI effectiveness [22] are also utilized. Wavelet transform [23], fuzzy logics [24] or dynamic time warping (DTW) [25,26] are some methods which are used to preprocess measured time series.

When it comes to classifiers hidden Markov models (HMM) [27], support vectors machine (SVM) [28], k-nearest neighbors [29,30], neural networks [31] or deep learning [32] are often utilized. Additionally, to improve the quality of obtained results, ensemble classifiers are being used more and more often [33,34]. These are systems which consist of several homogeneous or heterogeneous classifiers used for the realization of the same classification task. A decision of a set of classifiers is made on the basis of decisions reached by individual classifiers, for example, on the basis of the majority vote.

The most frequent sets of classifiers seen in biometrics are those which, to identify a person, simultaneously use various types of biometrics. Most often encountered works combine two or more varying biometrics. The recognition of people on the basis of face and palm print [35], face and gait [36] or shape of hand and palm print [37] can be seen as examples of bimodal biometrics. The use of multi-biometrics can be found in the work of [38]. It is also possible to encounter biometric systems utilizing a single human feature in which the input to classifiers is obtained through bagging [39] or boosting [40]. The measurement of that same phenomenon is less often gained through various sensors. To recognize gait in their work Hoffman et al. [21] used visual RGB image sequence, depth image sequence and four channel audios. In [41] to human gait recognition the GRFs and some anthropometric features obtained from Kinect have been used. The obtained results showed that in the majority of examined scenarios combining information from sensors varying in physical character improved recognition results.

Regardless which measuring methods are used to preprocess data or classifiers the quality of biometric systems based on the way a person moves is still greatly influenced by the footwear the subject is wearing. From biomechanical point of view the greatest change becomes visible in regard to the movement of women wearing high-heeled shoes. According to [42] an increase in the height of the heel in a woman's shoe causes a decrease in her walking speed and the length of her stride while keeping nearly an identical cadence. In [43] it has been noticed that the increase in the height of the heel causes an increase of extreme values of all components of ground reaction force. Additionally, Barton et al. [44] showed that heel lifts exerted greater muscle activity before and after the heel strike. Significant rise in the activity range of muscles of the lower limbs was also observed in [45]. Of course, the way a person moves walking in high-heeled shoes is also influenced by that person's experience. In [46] it has been shown that a change of footwear has a greater impact on the way a person walks if the subject is less experienced. Similarly, de Oliveira et al. [47] recoded the influence of high-heeled shoes on lumbar lordosis and pelvis position dependent on how often such footwear was worn. In case of experienced users hyperlordosis and pelvic anteversion was noted while in inexperienced users rectification of the lumbar spine and pelvic retroversion was reported. It must also be mentioned that in Simonssen's et al. work no significant difference in the electromyographic activity of muscles (EMG) or joint movements between experienced and inexperienced high heels users has been recorded [45].

When it comes to biometrics problems connected with the impact of footwear change on the accuracy of identifying people is not often brought up. Using an RGB camera Sakar et al. [48] studied a group of 122 people mainly men of which slightly more than half walked in two different types of shoes (sneakers, sandals, high heels, etc.). Unfortunately, during the experiment various people could walk in different types of footwear, therefore, the conclusion of the article stating that a change in footwear has little impact on the accuracy of identifying people is of limited value. Bouchrika and Nixon [49] noticed that the influence of footwear on the correct recognition of a person depends on its type. Although their study was performed on a group consisting of only 20 people (440 video sequences) their results showed that Correct Classification Rate (CCR) falls from 83.33% in trainer shoes to only 46% in flip flops. Gafurov et al. [50] utilized data from accelerometers to identify a group of 30 men with each of them walking in four different types of shoes. In case of limiting data to a particular type of footwear Equal Error Rate (EER) was from 1.6 to 6.1%. However, inclusion of all types of shoes caused a significant decrease in the system's accuracy and EER increased in range from 16.4 to 23.6%. Connor conducted barefoot gait recognition and shod-foot recognition when the shoe used in training was the same or different from the test shoe. In the first instance EER was 2.1% (15 people) and in the second it ranged from 11.4 to 15.9% (13 people) with a study group consisting mainly of men.

Studies in which high-heeled shoes are considered are even rarer. In his work Kim [51] used a motion capture system (Vicon, Oxford, UK) to identify people from a group of 10 (160 gait strides) who walked in four types of shoes having various heel heights. The results obtained for the greatest difference in heel height allowed identification in only 72.5% of cases. Cronin [42] conducted a study on a group of 125 people on the basis of data obtained from a video camera. This research concerned, among others, the impact of the type of footwear on the accuracy of a system for the identification of people. Types of shoes taken into account in the study included: normal shoes, formal shoes (high-heeled shoes for females and dress shoes for males) and casual wear (slippers). CCR for those individual shoe types was respectively: 81.25%, 78.84% and 80.65%. In [46] the ground reaction force and ensemble classifiers have been used to identify people with consideration for three research scenarios. The first one examined only gait in sport shoes, the second assumed that the learning set contains data describing gait only in sport shoes and the testing set also includes data from movement in high heels, while the third permitted both types of footwear in both sequences. The percentage of accurate recognition was respectively 98.87%, 69.21% and 98.96%.

A review of literature shows that there is a significant gap in works connected to human gait recognition related to the recognition of the gait of women walking in high-heeled shoes. This became our motivation for this paper to project a biometric system which will, with high accuracy, identify women walking in high-heeled footwear on the basis of data gathered through two sensors: force plates and Microsoft Kinect. The additionally presented biometric system has been validated through a secondary study performed on a selected sub-group of subjects.

2. Basics of Human Gait

Typical gait of people is distinctive in the coordinated, repeatable movement of the trunk and limbs used to move the body, maintain it in a vertical position with the least possible expansion of energy. While walking the lower limbs function as supports and a means of propulsion. They work in an alternating manner and their movements are cyclical which means that the same movements are performed in particular time increments. From the biomechanical point of view the human gait is perceived as a spatial, cyclical motion act in which the center of gravity of the torso is momentarily shifted beyond the support plane of the lower limbs to, within the next stage, regain balance along with performance of forward movements in the direction of stepping. The forward progression of the body begins at the moment when the bearing foot leaves the ground with the simultaneous raising of the heel and the shifting up of the entire body's center of gravity. At the same time, the second, unburdened limb swings forward until its heel touches the ground. In effect there is the lowering of the foot with the simultaneous shifting of body mass. During the performance of these alternating movements the trailing leg becomes the leading leg and vice versa.

Within the biomechanical gait analysis it has been accepted that the walking cycle is measured from the moment the heel of one lower limb touches the ground (in respect to physiological gait) to the moment until it touches the ground again. During this time both limbs go through the support phase and the swing phase in which the limb is shifted above the ground. The support phase lasts approximately 60% of the entire cycle and can be broken down into the following sub-phases:

- The Initial Contact (IC)—in this phase the foot comes into contact with the ground. In a typical gait the initial contact is made with the heel which is the reason this phase is often also called the Heel Strike (HS).
- The Loading Response (LR)—the foot is rotated forward to maintain the speed of the body's forward momentum and cause its full contact with the ground. LR lasts from IC until the moment the toes of the other foot lose contact with the ground. This sub-phase completes the double-support phase where both legs touch the ground. LR lasts from 0 to approximately 10% of the entire cycle.
- The Midstance (MSt)—begins the single support phase. It is the phase lasting from the time the toes of the opposite foot lose contact with the ground and the moment when the body weight is aligned over the forefoot. The analyzed foot lies flat on the ground. It is the period from about 10 to 30% of the entire time of the gait cycle.
- The Terminal stance (TSt)—starts with the heel-off, followed by the limb bending forward and the trail leg (opposite leg) becomes the leading leg. The phase ends with the initial contact of the opposite leg. TSt lasts from 30 to approximately 50% of the gait cycle.
- The Preswing (PSw)—begins with IC of the opposite leg and finishes with the toe off of the analyzed lower limb. Interval: 50–60% of gait cycle.

The transfer phase lasts about 40% of the entire gait cycle and can be divided into the following sub-phases:

- The Initial swing (ISw)—begins with the lifting of the foot off the ground. Thanks to the bending of the limb in the knee and the hip the foot is shifted forward. This phase ends when the swinging foot is opposite the stance limb. It is assumed that this phase lasts from 60 to 73% of the gait cycle.
- The Mid swing (MSw)—This phase begins when the swing foot is opposite the stance leg and ends when the moving limb is forward and the tibia is vertical. This phase lasts from 73 to 87% of the gait cycle.
- The Terminal swing (TSw)—is the last phase of the swing which ends with the initial contact of the leg being analyzed. This phase lasts from 87 to 100% of the gait cycle.

During walking it is possible to see a change in the distance between the top of the person's head and the ground. The maximum distance is measured during the midstance and the minimum distance occurs during the double-support phase. According to [52] the difference between those two distances can be as much as 9.5 cm.

3. Materials and Method

3.1. Sensors and Measured Data

3.1.1. Force Plate

The force generated during walking between the foot and the ground is called the ground reaction force or GRF. To measure this force plates made by the Kistler Company (Winterthur, Switzerland) utilize four piezoelectric sensors located in the corners of the platform. The signal measured by the sensors is employed to represent three components of GRF: anterior-posterior F_x, vertical F_y and lateral F_z.

Maximum values for the vertical component F_y correspond to the moments of: transferring the entire body weight onto the analyzed limb (first maximum—maximum of the overload phase) and the load of the forefoot (the heel is not in contact with the ground) right before the toes off (the second maximum—maximum of propulsion). In a typical gait these maximum values reach approximately 120% of body weight. This is the result of the dynamics of the phenomenon and the need of maintaining balance while walking. Hence the value of the reaction forces is greater than the force of gravity (weight). Half way through the supporting phase the entire active surface of the foot is in contact with the ground. This is a period of unloading (minimum of the unloading phase) and the decrease in the force value to below 100% can be seen on the Figure 1 The anterior-posterior Fx component consists of two phases. During the first its value is negative when it is opposite to the direction of movement. It is the result of the deceleration of the analyzed lower limb. The minimum of the deceleration phase is most often reached right before the occurrence of the maximum of the overloading phase for the vertical Fy component. Similarly, during the second phase the anterior-posterior component shows positive values. It is then that the process of acceleration begins concluded by pushing off the ground with the toes. During this entire interval the turn of the Fx force corresponds to the direction of movement. The maximum of the acceleration phase occurs in the initial phase of push the toe offs. This happens right after the maximum of propulsion for the vertical Fy component. The value of the Fx component is equal to zero at the moment when the analyzed limb passes the trail leg. This more or less corresponds to the moment of the minimum of the unloading phase for the vertical Fy component. Extreme values of the Fx component reach approximately 20% of the weight of the test subject.

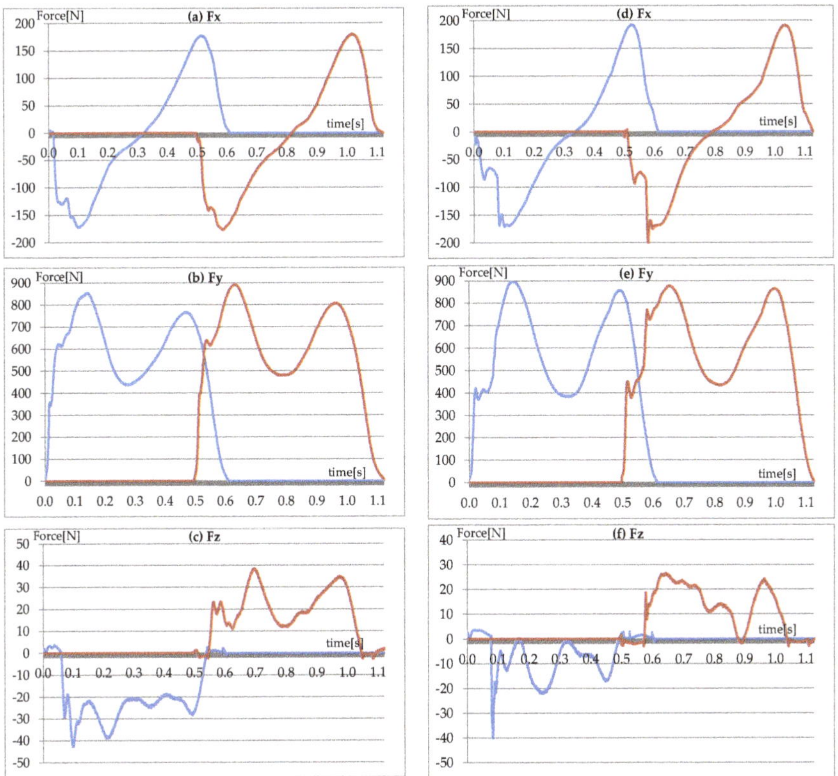

Figure 1. Components of GRF in: (**a,d**) anterior/posterior; (**b,e**) vertical; (**c,f**) medial/lateral direction of the left lower limb (blue line) and of the right one (red line) in sport shoes (**a–c**) and high heels (**d–f**). Data derived from the same subject.

The value of the lateral Fz component depends on the limb being analyzed. Assuming that movement occurs in the direction determined by the orientation of the Fx force than the values of the Fz component will be positive for the left leg and negative for the right leg. The exceptions include the moment of initial contact and the moment when the toes leave the ground where the foot is slightly supinated. The value of the Fz force depends on the manner in which the test subject places his feet. This force should be greater both in the event of pronation as well as the abduction of the foot. Extremes for Fz use the same nomenclature as those for the vertical Fy component; maximum of the overloading phase, minimum of the unloading phase and maximum of the propulsion phase. The values of these forces are about 10% of the body weight of the test subject.

Measurements made as part of this study were performed using two Kistler platforms with the dimensions of 60 cm × 40 cm registering data with a frequency of 960 Hz.

3.1.2. Microsoft Kinect v2

Kinect from Microsoft (Redmond, Wa, USA) in the v2 version (Xbox One) is the successor of Kinect v1 (Xbox 360). Due to the price and opportunities offered (sensor set: RGB camera, depths, directional microphones—Figure 2a), similarly to the previous version, it is very popular: It has found a wide application in various types of applications related to, among others, object recognition and reconstruction, 3D reconstruction and many others [53–55]. In the case of human recognition based on gait, it significantly expanded the approach area in methods based on a model description (model-based approaches) [56–59]. This is related to the ease of obtaining information about depth and skeletal data without the need for implementation computationally complex processing algorithms and video analysis algorithms. Kinect v2 sensor allows tracking and construction of virtual 3D skeleton in real time (Figure 2b). In 2014, Microsoft released the Kinect for Windows SDK 2.0 version. The SDK software [60] contains the NUI Skeleton library, which allows obtaining information about the location of the 25 parts of the body (joints) relative to the sensor (Figure 2b).

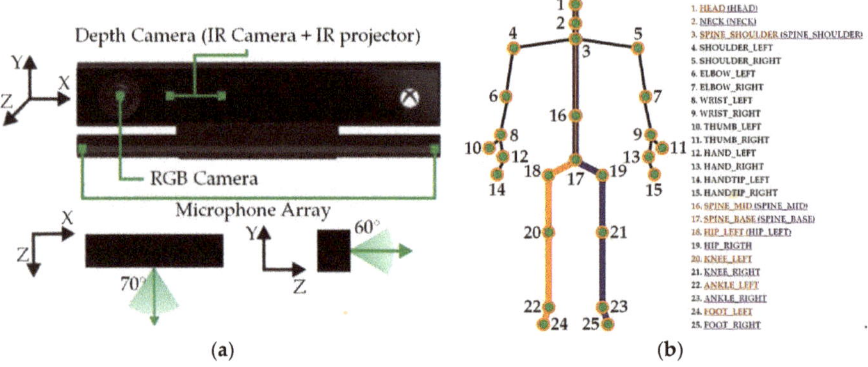

Figure 2. Microsoft Kinect v2: (**a**) Kinect structure and visual field marking; (**b**) the location of 25 parts of the body in Kinect v2.

In Table 1, the Kinect v2 features relevant from the point of view of the performed measurements are listed. In general, the individual Kinect v2 parameters and thus the skeleton tracking accuracy has been improved in relation to the previous generation of the sensor. In addition, the ability to register the number of skeletal joints has been increased by 5.

Along with the improvement of individual sensor parameters, the method of depth measurement has a great influence on the quality of the skeleton tracking as well. In Kinect v2, unlike in Kinect v1 (the technology used is based on structured lighting, pattern deflection and triangulation), Time of Flight technology—ToF (ToF camera) is used. The ToF system is based on the measurement of the return time of the infrared electromagnetic radiation beam reflected from the illuminated object. Thanks to these combined treatments (improvement of parameters + new method), the quality of skeleton tracking has been improved in relation to Kinect v1 [61,62] (lower image degradation due to lighting effect, higher quality and accuracy of depth image, reduction by $\frac{1}{4}$ of blur caused by motion and much larger field of view).

Table 1. Technical specification of the Kinect v2 sensor.

Feature	Kinect v2
Color camera	1920 × 1080 × 16 bit per pixel 16:9 YUY2; 30 Hz (15 Hz in low light, HD)
Depth camera	512 × 424 × 16 bits per pixel 16-bit ToF depth sensor IR can now be used at the same time as colour
Working range	Only one configuration: 0.5 m to 8 m; Quality degrades after 4.5 m
Angular field of view	60° vertical; 70° horizontal
Skeletal joints	25 joints tracked; 5 more than the Kinect for Windows V1: Neck, left and right Thumbs and Hand Tips
Maximum skeletal tracking	6 with joints (renamed to Bodies)
Method of depth measurement	Time of Flight

For the needs of the research, an (C#) application was created. The application is based on the official 2.0 Microsoft SDKs (Software Development Kits, freely available for Kinect v2) and it allows the following activities:

- simultaneous capture of image data stream from the RGB camera and depth camera of the Kinect controller;
- skeletal tracking;
- the choice of image resolution from RGB camera and a depth camera;
- a description of the figure movement—calculating and displaying the registered figure;
- displaying graphs from earlier collected data;
- recording specific (significant) parameters and status of tracked points (joints) to an Excel file (.xlsx or .cs extension) or notepad (.txt extension), including registration time (DateAndTime::Now, .Net Framework).

For the purposes of this article, it was decided to choose only the body height (selected anthropometric characteristic). It should be noted that static data are fixed i.e., it is not dependent on the type of human gait (it is often of non-constant speed and non-constant frequency) and on its characteristics (speed of locomotion, stride length, etc.). In the course of the research, it was found that, unlike Kinects v1, Kinects v2 do not interfere with each other, which makes it possible to freely adjust them in relation to each other. In addition, the application gave a preview of the entire skeleton. "Bones" can take two colours: blue—for those correctly detected and yellow—when the sensor is not able to accurately determine the position of a joint (Figure 3).

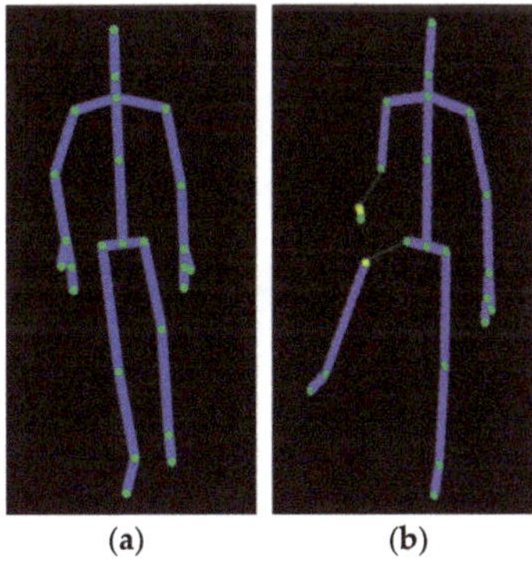

(a)   (b)

Figure 3. Preview of the user's skeleton when: (**a**) all joints are properly tracked; (**b**) Kinect is not able to determine the position of certain joints.

The .txt file saved all information related to the tracking of the person, including skeleton joint tracking states (fully tracked, inferred, or not tracked). Skeleton joint tracking was used in offline processing. To determine the length of individual body parts, only joints (Figure 2b additionally denotes sections that were taken into account when determining the body height—dark purple and orange lines) classified as fully tracked were taken into account. Therefore, in order to be able to determine, for example, the length of the right lower limb as fully tracked, there had to be joints marked: 19 (hip right) and 21 (knee right) (see Figure 2b).

For the lower limbs, especially in areas deviating from the optical axis (in the areas at the border of the sensor's field of view) during the movement, the need to use information from both sensors was emphasized. Individual points enabling the determination of sections of the lower limbs were determined based on their correct detection (skeleton joint tracking states: fully tracked). In the case of detection errors of the body part (or body parts) of one of the lower limb, to calculate the body height, the correctly determined body part was taken from the correspondent part of the other leg and from the values determined by the second Kinect. If the above conditions were not met, the algorithm was to omit this measurement. However, in the conducted studies, such a case did not occur. In a situation in which both Kinect sensors correctly detected individual body parts, the average value for the given body part was determined. Due to the bandwidth required by Kinect v2, each sensor was connected to a separate computer with identical technical specifications (Windows 10 OS, Intel Core i7-4700MQ, 16 GB RAM, Kinect SDK 2.0). The application was simultaneously run by one user on two computers using two computer mice with shortcut connection. It required a relatively simple interference in the construction of a computer mouse. It was about detecting the left mouse button pressed (then the contacts are shorted and the current flows in the system) and sending the pulse with the cable to the second mouse (that is passing the current despite the fact that there was no short-circuit), which corresponded to almost simultaneous pressing the left mouse button on the second mouse same time. The delay caused by the propagation time by the cable connecting the two mice in comparison to the operating frequency of Kinect v2 was not significant. Almost simultaneous starting of the applications allows to treat both measurements as synchronized in time. Because during one experiment Kinect registered more than one step, even possible time shifts in the time course would have a much smaller impact on the average body height than the type of shoes in which the measured person was moving. It is also worth noting that the registration of the time of registration (DateAndTime::Now, .Net Framework) enabled full control over the offline synchronization of measured data (measurements). The measurement results of body height of people while walking in sport shoes and high-heeled shoes have been presented in Figure 4.

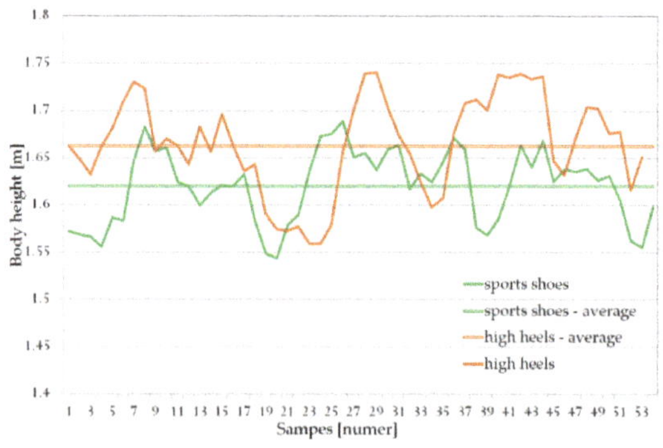

Figure 4. Changes in body height during walking.

Figure 4 shows the dynamic change in body height during walking (the relationship expressed in meters). This change is caused by, among others, the previously mentioned natural change in human body height during the gait cycle. In addition, the entire measurement is burdened with quite a big error, which in selected moments reaches a value of a few centimeters. However, it should be emphasized that this error does not significantly affect the results obtained. The location of Kinects during the measurement makes it possible to register more than one gait cycle so that the received average values are close to the actual ones. The average body height value determined with two Kinects, in the case of walking in sports footwear, was 162.1 cm (actual measured body height 160.9 cm). However, in the case of the same person walking in high heels, the average body height value was 166.1 cm with the actual measured height of 166.7 cm.

The difference in the average value of body height of people walking in sport shoes and high-heeled footwear has been presented on the graph below (Figure 5). The Shapiro-Wilk test showed that the presented data exhibits normal distribution. Statistical analysis was performed using Statistics 13.5, and the statistical significance was set at $p < 0.05$.

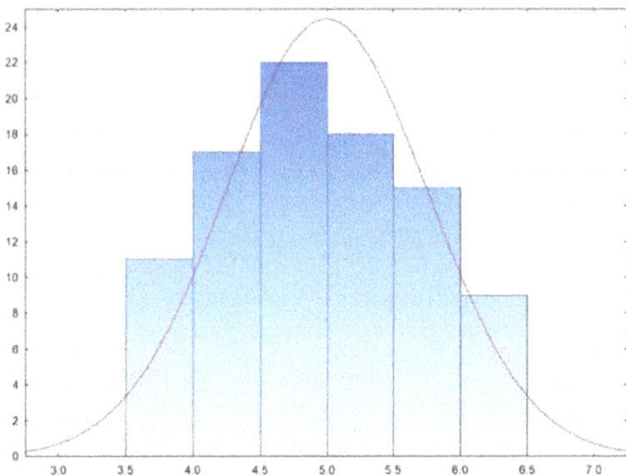

Figure 5. Histogram of the difference in the body height of people walking in sport shoes and high-heeled footwear with a height of 8–10 cm; average value = 4.988 cm; σ = 0.7504 cm.

The average difference in the body height of a person walking in high heels with a heel height of 8–10 cm and in sport shoes was less than 5 cm. This difference is not equal to the heel height which is caused both by the thickness of the sport shoes' soles as well as the inaccuracy of measurements made using Microsoft Kinect v2. It should be said that that the desired result of the proposed method is not the actual height of the person being measured but rather the ability to differentiate between individuals and dependence on the type of the footwear which the person is wearing. The most important is the fact that assumed range of differences of ±3σ will allow consideration of all cases occurring in the data set.

3.2. Data Processing

Ground reaction forces registered using force plates made by the Kistler Company are in the form of time series: $x_1, x_2, \ldots, x_n$, where n is the number of samples. Generally, the duration of the supporting phase for various steps differs which is the reason that the representation of the gait cycle consists of time series of varying lengths. Therefore, to determine GRF similarities of various gait cycles a well-known algorithm of dynamic time warping (DTW) was used. DTW calculates an optimal warping path which allows the transformation of one time series (the one being analyzed) into a different one (referential). The cost of such transformation is smaller if the two time series being compared are similar. Hence the cost of imitation has been utilized as the measure of distance.

Within this work fragments concerning phases were chosen from obtained GRF's: Mid stance and Terminal stance separately for each leg. The duration of individual phases has been presumed in accordance to the values presented in Section 2. We assume that $\rho_{v,s}$ signifies a distance between two time series describing the GRF in the v phase of the gait cycle for the s limb. This distance has been calculated using the following formula:

$$P_{v,s} = \sum_{m=1}^{M} \text{DTW}_m \tag{1}$$

where DTW_m is the distance between two time series calculated for the m component of GRF. M is equal to the number of considered components. In this work we made use of all components therefore $M = 3$.

Additionally, the distance of the entire stride without dividing it into individual phases or limbs has also been determined (in that case $M = 6$ in Equation (1)). This resulted in 5 distances: $\rho_{MSt,L}$; $\rho_{TSt,L}$; $\rho_{MSt,R}$; $\rho_{TSt,R}$; ρ_{Stride}.

3.3. Data Fusion

Measurements made using devices described above can be presented as a six element vector:

$$V = [\rho_{MSt,L}; \rho_{TSt,L}; \rho_{MSt,R}; \rho_{TSt,R}; \rho_{Stride}; BH] \tag{2}$$

where $\rho_{MSt,L}$ is the distance between two time series calculated for the left lower limb during Mid Stance phase; $\rho_{MSt,R}$—the distance between two time series calculated for the right lower limb during Mid Stance phase; $\rho_{TSt,L}$—the distance between two time series calculated for the left lower limb during Terminal Stance, $\rho_{TSt,R}$—the distance between two time series calculated for the right lower limb during Terminal Stance, ρ_{Stride}—the distance calculated for both legs without division into phases, BH—subject's body height.

The data is in the form of individual values hence there was no need to synchronize measurements between those obtained from the force plates and those from the Microsoft Kinect devices. The method of identifying people proposed by this work is carried out in two stages and utilizes data from sensors mentioned above. Within the first phase there is the recognition of the type of footwear which the test subject is wearing. Then, as part of the second phase, through the consideration of data from vector V the actual identification process occurs.

Identification of footwear was done using the vertical and the anterior-posterior components of GRF of both legs generated during the LR phase of the gait cycle. The decision was made after an analysis of time series' values of that phase. To develop the input vector for the classifier the coefficients of a polynomial of 5th degree that fits the $F_{c,s} = f(\text{time})$ best in a least-squares sense: $[a_{c,s,5};$ $a_{c,s,4}; a_{c,s,3}; a_{c,s,2}; a_{c,s,1}; a_{c,s,0}]$ where c—designates a component of GRF, $c \in \{x,y\}$ and s—defines the limb $s \in \{L,R\}$ were utilized [63]. The choice of the polynomial to the 5th degree was dictated, on the one hand by the accuracy of representing the time series and, on the other, by the possibility of overfitting the classifier in the event of the input space being too large. As a result an input vector consisting of 24 elements was obtained. 10-fold cross-validation was used to bulid the classifier where the registered inputs from the same person were always within the same set.

The aforementioned second phase of identification started from the results of footwear recognition of the test subject. In the event where a classifier determined that the person was walking in high heels than a correction of that person's height was made. On the basis of the data presented in Figure 4 the average value of the difference in the height of a person walking in sports shoes or in high-heeled shoes is 4.988 cm ($\sigma = 0.7504$ cm). Since this is a certain approximation of a phenomenon the rounded up value of 5 cm and the acceptable deviation of ± 2 cm (which is a value only slightly lower than $\pm 3\sigma$) were used in subsequent calculations:

$$BH_{norm} = \begin{cases} BH_{measured} & \text{if } y = 0 \\ BH_{measured} - 5 & \text{if } y = 1 \end{cases} \tag{3}$$

where BH_{norm} is the height after modification; $BH_{measured}$ is the person's height measured using the Microsoft Kinect v2 device; y is the value of classifier output ($y = 1$ for high-heeled footwear and $y = 0$ for sport shoes).

The resulting BH_{norm} was used to limit the number of potential recognized people present in the data base through not taking into consideration for the final solution those women whose body height differed by more than ± 2 cm. Hence all subsequent calculations were performed on a 'Reduced Database'. The scheme of the experiment is presented in Figure 6.

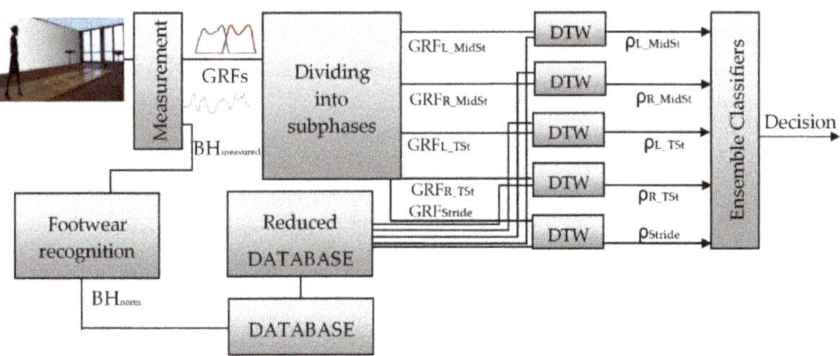

Figure 6. The scheme of the experiment.

3.4. Human Recognition

The recognition of people comes down to the issue of classification where the number of classes is equal to the number of people present in the database (people who, for example, have access to resources). Since DTW allows the designation of the distance between two time series it is natural to use a classifier like k-Nearest Neighbor (kNN). On the basis of the affiliation of its nearest neighbors to the k classes kNN makes a decision about assigning the considered subject to one of the classes.

Since after preprocessing we obtained 5 distances it only seemed natural to utilize an ensemble of classifiers which consisted of 5 k-NN classifiers. K labels defining the affiliation to nearest classes of 'points' within a state space are delivered to the inputs of every database classifier. The decision of the entire set of classifiers was made on the basis of a weighted vote (weights based on rank order). The weighted value connected to every label depended on rank R in a particular base classifier. The final decision was the class label with the largest total of weights:

$$cl = \arg\max\left(\sum_{j=1}^{5} w_j \cdot d_{j,i}\right) \tag{4}$$

where cl—class label; k—the number of neighbors, $w_j = [w_1, \ldots, w_R, \ldots, w_k]$—weights, which are calculated from the following formula:

$$w_R = \frac{k+1-R}{k} \tag{5}$$

where R—indicates the rank for j-th classifier, $R = \{1, 2, \ldots, k\}$. $d_{j,i}$—decision of the j-th classifier, which indicates the k nearest neighbors, $d_{j,i} \in \{0,1\}$. If j-th classifier chooses class i then $d_{j,i} = 1$ otherwise $d_{j,i} = 0$.

It was accepted that a person is unrecognized (which meant that the person was not in the database) if at least two classes had the same total weight or if the final total was smaller than the arbitrarily chosen threshold Th. In those cases the person was given a 'NONE' label. The accepted threshold permits a minimum required level of similarity to consider the person being scrutinized as identified.

3.5. The Study Group

The study was carried out at the Bialystok University of Technology on a group of 99 women aged 21.48 ± 1.17 with a body weight of 61.90 ± 11.07 kg and a body height of 166.41 ± 5.74 cm. All participants were informed about the aim and course of the experiment and signed a consent form. During the research the women walked through a measuring path with two hidden force plates manufactured by the Kistler Company. The participants were not informed about the presence or about the location of the plates nor about having to step on one. In the event when the test subject did not tread on the platform or stepped on its edge the measurement was repeated with a slight adjustment of the starting point of the test. Additionally, two Microsoft Kinect v2 devices were used to record the person's body height. The devices were placed more or less symmetrically in relation to the walking path of the test subject who moved toward them. The two devices were not concealed in any way (Figure 7).

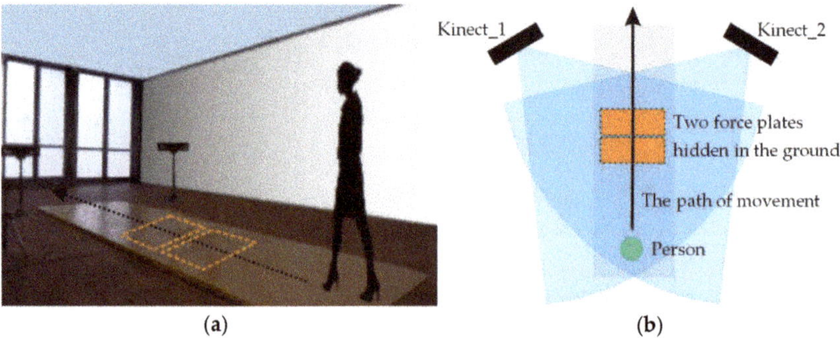

Figure 7. Diagram of human gait measurement: (**a**) a perspective view; (**b**) a view from above.

Each of the analyzed subjects walked in their own footwear: sports shoes and high heeled shoes with the heel height specified to be from 8 to 10 cm. Testing with both types of footwear was conducted on the same day. During the experiment, after every 10 gait strides with a single person there was a short, 1–2 min, break to avoid the subject becoming tired. 14 to 20 gait cycles were carried out for each type of footwear with every participant. In total 3402 strides were recorded (1874 cycles for sport shoes and 1528 cycles for high heels).

Additionally, to ensure the robustness of the proposed method, a secondary study was performed on a group of 6 women. The selected ladies were tested after a period ranging from 3 to 12 months from the date of the first test. During the second test the women, for the most part (5 of the 6), used the same footwear as during the first series of tests. In the first series of tests 201 strides were recorded for this sub-group and as the results of the secondary testing 203 strides were recorded. In respect to this sub-group the selected footwear recognition classifier (see Figure 6) was trained on data describing the gait of all 93 people taking part in the experiment.

Since the set of people who participated in secondary test is relatively small obtained results of recognition may not be representative. Hence these results will be compared in relation to the sub-group of the selected 6 women (meaning the recognition results on the basis of the 1st test vs. the 2nd test) and discussed separately.

4. Results

Testing of classifiers which made the identification of footwear was conducted with the help of the WEKA software and the cumulative results obtained for test runs have been presented in Table 2.

Parameters characterizing gait in high heels was selected as the relevant class, and sensitivity and specificity were calculated using the following formulas:

$$Sensitivity = \frac{TP}{(TP + FN)} \cdot 100\% \tag{6}$$

$$Specificity = \frac{TN}{(TN + FP)} \cdot 100\% \tag{7}$$

where *TP*—the number of true positives (correctly recognized strides of people walking in high heels); *FN*—the number of false negatives (gait strides of people walking in high heels which have been recognized as gait strides of people walking in sport shoes); *TN*—the number of true negatives (correctly recognized gait strides of people walking sport shoes); *FP*—the number of false positives (gait strides of people walking in sport shoes which have been recognized as gait strides of people walking in high heels).

Table 2. The average value of Correct Classification Rate, Sensitivity and Specificity ± SD for different types of classifiers.

Type of Classifier	CCR	Sensitivity	Specificity
kNN	95.27 ± 4.11	90.98 ± 7.18	98.71 ± 2.09
Naïve Bayes	93.81 ± 4.76	91.85 ± 6.46	95.70 ± 5.68
SVM	**96.43 ± 3.09**	**95.80 ± 5.51**	**96.82 ± 4.80**
ANN	96.13 ± 4.14	96.07 ± 5.97	96.09 ± 3.85
Random Forest	95.77 ± 3.62	94.10 ± 6.15	97.26 ± 3.19
Deep ANN	93.94 ± 6.13	95.87 ± 5.20	91.97 ± 11.82

The best results were seen with the SVM classifier while the worst were seen with the Naive Bayes. A high CCR value was also obtained using the feedforward neural network. However, a higher standard deviation caused the authors to utilize SVM in further work. A very high specificity value was reached by the kNN classifier ($k = 3$, city blocks) but its lowest sensitivity value caused it to be excluded from further work. Slightly higher specificity than sensitivity values for all classifiers were an expected result and stemmed from the fact that walking in high-heeled footwear is characterized by a greater variability within classes than walking in sport shoes. It is also worth mentioning that CCR of most classifiers oscillated around 95–96%.

The following scenarios were considered within the framework of this study:

(a) Data contained only the gait of people wearing sport shoes and used solely measurements from force plates;

(b) Data within the training set contained only gait in sport shoes while the testing set included all other data but the classification was done solely on the basis of GRF (without Microsoft Kinect v2 measurements);

(c) Same as in point (a) but with identification of footwear type and body height of the person being identified;

(d) Same as in point (b) but with identification of footwear type and body height of the person being identified (as described in Materials and Methods);

(e) Same as in point (d) but with the assumption that the identification of footwear will be at 100% accuracy.

In order to enable the comparison of gathered results with the outcomes of other authors randomly selected results for varying number of people from 10 to 90 in increments of 10 (10, 20, 30, . . . , 90) as well as for all people participating in the experiment were presented. In order to reduce the impact of randomness on results the tests were repeated 10 times for every group of people. On the basis of preliminary studies the number of considered nearest neighbors k equaled to 5. Number of gait cycles in the testing set varied and depended on the number of people considered in a particular test.

Assumptions defined in scenario (d) were applied in respect to the sub-group of women with whom secondary testing was performed. In this case, the training set was data from all 99 people, drawn in accordance with the methodology described in subsection 3.5. The testing set was data from the second series of the experiment.

The results presented below assume the acceptance of the most liberal strategy where $Th = 0$. Data in tables (Tables 3 and 4) a presents Correct Classification Rates, False Rejected Rates (FRR) and False Accepted Rates (FAR). Figure 8 consists of the ROC curve for scenarios (a), (b) and (d).

Data from the table above should be treated as a reference in relation to the proposed method. Results achieved in scenario (a) confirm that in cases where the training set as well as the testing set contained measurements of gait in the same type of footwear then the accuracy of classification is very high and only single cycles are assigned to other people. It should be added that in the majority of bad classifications the weighted total has a value which is significantly lower than in cases of correct classifications. Therefore, in establishing the value of the threshold Th it is very easy to reduce the error value of FAR with the obvious increase in the error of FRR. In turn, data from scenario (b) demonstrates that the usefulness of gait biometrics with such a drastic change of footwear type is small even with relatively small data sets.

Table 3. Correct Classification Rate, False Rejected Rate and False Accepted Rate for the reference scenarios: (a) and (b).

No. of Sub.	Scenario (a)			Scenario (b)		
	CCR	FRR	FAR	CCR	FRR	FAR
10	99.09	0	0.91	92.70	0	7.90
20	99.21	0.04	0.04	86.81	0.27	12.92
30	98.60	0	0	83.92	0.23	15.86
40	98.53	0	0	81.49	0.39	18.12
50	98.45	0.06	0.06	77.27	0.56	22.17
60	97.86	0.08	0.08	75.48	0.48	24.04
70	98.15	0.04	0.04	74.98	0.65	24.37
80	97.96	0.06	0.06	73.53	0.69	25.78
90	97.73	0.11	0.11	72.20	0.75	27.05
99	97.74	0.06	0.06	71.62	0.73	27.65

Table 4. Correct Classification Rate, False Rejected Rate and False Accepted Rate for scenarios: (c), (d) and (e).

No. of Sub.	Scenario (c)			Scenario (d)			Scenario (e)		
	CCR	FRR	FAR	CCR	FRR	FAR	CCR	FRR	FAR
10	97.93	0.58	1.49	95.38	0.82	3.80	97.48	0	2.52
20	95.82	0.31	3.87	94.63	0.59	4.78	98.13	0	1.87
30	97.29	0.03	2.67	92.76	1.16	6.08	96.28	0.04	3.68
40	97.06	0.02	2.91	92.72	0.71	6.56	95.77	0.11	4.12
50	96.68	0.06	3.26	90.93	0.70	8.37	95.91	0.05	4.38
60	96.22	0.03	3.75	90.62	0.56	8.83	93.85	0.06	6.09
70	96.57	0.03	3.40	89.83	0.66	9.51	93.29	0.10	6.61
80	96.71	0.05	3.24	89.14	0.60	10.26	93.19	0.13	6.68
90	96.64	0.02	3.34	88.70	0.58	10.71	92.27	0.16	7.57
99	96.47	0.01	3.52	88.27	0.59	11.14	91.42	0.17	8.41

The goal of scenario (c) was to show the impact of the effect of the classifier recognizing footwear which the person being tested was wearing. Obviously, since this classifier does not have 100% correct classifications the results here are less accurate than those from scenario (a). They are also quite surprising since increasing the number of people within a group has practically no impact on the final results. The differences between particular amounts of people result from the random character of selecting these people to the given group. Additionally, some badly classified standards find their way into the training set (gallery) and do not influence the results negatively. It must also be added that our observations are confirmed by the spread of CCR between individual samples for particularly small sets.

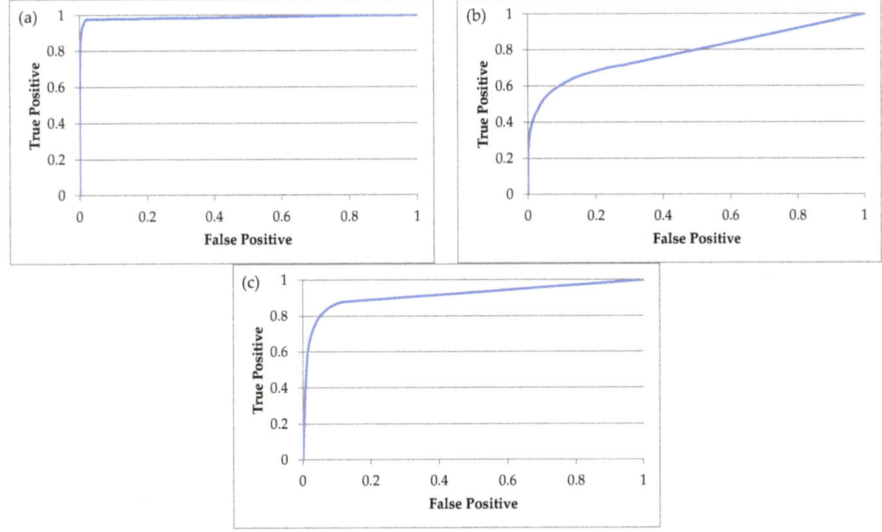

Figure 8. The ROC curves in case of 99 subjects for: (**a**) scenario (a) AUC = 0.987; (**b**) scenario (b) AUC = 0.789; (**c**) scenario (d) AUC = 0.921. AUC = Area Under Curve.

The effectiveness of the proposed method is most aptly demonstrated by the values obtained with scenario (d). The larger the group of participants the greater the difference between values of scenario (b) and (d). The relatively small CCR value for a group of 10 people may cause concern but similar to the other scenarios it is the result of the random selection of people for the group (in individual samples CCR varied from 90.84 to 98.48%). Scenario (e) presented results in cases where the classifier identifying footwear type worn by the test subject worked with 100% accuracy. It shows the potential of the presented method and suggests the best results which could be obtained on the basis of measurements gathered in this study and without changing applied base classifiers.

In relation to the sub-group of 6 women who took part both in the first series of tests as well as in secondary testing the footwear recognition classifier correctly identified 95.02% and 97.04% of footwear in recorded walking cycles. These values are at similar levels to those presented in Table 2. The recognition accuracy of people from this group after the application of the procedure described in scenario (d) has been presented in Table 5.

Table 5. Correct Classification Rate, False Rejected Rate and False Accepted Rate for subgroup of six women for the first and second series of tests.

Experiment	CCR	FRR	FAR
First test	92.06	0.06	7.88
Second test	91.53	0.07	8.40

The resulting values show that there was only a slight decrease in the accuracy of people recognition on the basis of gait data recorded a few months later. It is smaller from the expected and natural for behavioral biometrics. It is worth pointing out that the higher than average level of footwear recognition worn by the person subjected to the tests plays a certain positive role in all of this. Because this phenomenon may be incidental then, in general, a CCR below 91% for a given group of people should be expected. Generally, it must be said that the proposed biometric system turned out to be relatively resistant to the passing of time.

5. Discussion

The obtained results are already very good. Results shown in scenario (b) are noticeably better in comparison to [46]. It is the effect of reducing the number of base classifiers through excluding classifiers operating on data from the first and last gait sub-phases registered through the platform (loading response and pre swing). GRF values in those phases are relatively low. This, in many cases, causes the intra-individual variability to be greater than inter-individual variability which, in turn, leads to low values of CCR in base classifiers responsible for recognizing people on the basis of time series of those phases and, in consequence, impacts negatively the recognition accuracy of the entire team of classifiers.

Results gained through the use of the proposed method (scenario (d)) are considerably better than those reported in work of other authors dealing with similar topics [51,64,65]. They are, in fact, superior also because, for example, Connor tested only men and gait in men's formal footwear does not significantly vary from walking in sport shoes which, as has been shown in [51], has a smaller impact on classification results. In turn, in the work of Connie et al. the test set used data describing the gait of both women as well as men, however, lack of information about the percentage of women in the study group and the large number of participants (125) makes comparison of results difficult. Nevertheless, it does seem that the presented method would achieve better results with a similar group of people. It is also worth mentioning that in two of these works different measuring systems were utilized: motion capture system [51] and video cameras [65]. Similar signals were considered in Connor's work but were additionally augmented with spatial features and signals derived from high-resolution sensing floor tile.

Unfortunately the method being discussed also possesses limitations. Its weaknesses undoubtedly include the tightly defined heel height. In real situations and with the number of people being considered it would be highly probable that there would be people who would wear shoes with lower heels. The direct application of the proposed method and the reduction of the body height of such a person could have caused not being able to properly identify her. Such cases would require the algorithm to be altered either through adding another type of footwear as a potential class recognized in the first stage of the method or through replacing the classifier with an approximator generating on its output a particular value by which the person's body height would need to be modified.

6. Conclusions

Within this article we have presented the workings of a biometric system dependent on the type of footwear worn by women—sport shoes or high heels. It has been shown that in cases where gait in high heels is not included in the learning set of the ensemble classifiers then the accuracy of the biometric system is lower even with a relatively small study group than the precision of the same system with a large group of women walking only in sport shoes. However, the obtained results are very good and demonstrated a significant improvement in the quality of a biometric system in comparison to reports currently available in literature. The robustness of the proposed method is especially worthy of attention.

Further work in this area can be carried out in two directions. First, the database needs to be enhanced with data presenting the gait of men and women in several different types of footwear.

Secondly it is necessary to seek feature extraction methods or classifications which will improve the results presented within this study.

Author Contributions: M.D. and M.B. conceived and designed the experiments; M.D. and M.B. performed the experiments; M.D. analyzed the data; Both authors took part in writing the paper.

Funding: This work was co-financed by Ministry of Science and Higher Education of Poland within the frame of projects (no. S/WM/1/2017 and S/WM/1/2016).

Conflicts of Interest: The authors declare no conflict of interest. The founding sponsors had no role in the design of the study; in the collection, analyses, or interpretation of data; in the writing of the manuscript, and in the decision to publish the results.

References

1. Bouchrika, I.; Goffredo, M.; Carter, J.; Nixon, M. On using gait in forensic biometrics. *J. Forensic Sci.* **2011**, *56*, 882–889. [CrossRef] [PubMed]
2. Jain, A.K.; Ross, A. Bridging the gap: From biometrics to forensics. *Philos. Trans. R. Soc. B* **2015**, *370*, 20140254. [CrossRef] [PubMed]
3. Matovski, D.S.; Nixon, M.S.; Carter, J.N. Gait recognition. In *Computer Vision*; Springer: New York, NY, USA, 2014; pp. 309–318. [CrossRef]
4. Boulgouris, N.V.; Hatzinakos, D.; Plataniotis, K.N. Gait recognition: A challenging signal processing technology for biometric identification. *IEEE Signal Process. Mag.* **2005**, *22*, 78–90. [CrossRef]
5. Cutting, J.E.; Kozlowski, L.T. Recognizing friends by their walk: Gait perception without familiarity cues. *Bull. Psychon. Soc.* **1977**, *9*, 353–356. [CrossRef]
6. Lee, L.; Grimson, W.E.L. Gait analysis for recognition and classification. In Proceedings of the Fifth IEEE International Conference on Automatic Face & Gesture Recognition, Washington, DC, USA, 21 May 2002; pp. 155–162. [CrossRef]
7. Bashir, K.; Xiang, T.; Gong, S. Gait recognition without subject cooperation. *Pattern Recognit. Lett.* **2010**, *31*, 2052–2060. [CrossRef]
8. Xu, D.; Huang, Y.; Zeng, Z.; Xu, X. Human gait recognition using patch distribution feature and locality-constrained group sparse representation. *IEEE Trans. Image Process.* **2012**, *21*, 316–326. [CrossRef] [PubMed]
9. Kim, D.; Paik, J. Gait recognition using active shape model and motion prediction. *IET Comput. Vis.* **2010**, *4*, 25–36. [CrossRef]
10. Alotaibi, M.; Mahmood, A. Improved gait recognition based on specialized deep convolutional neural network. *Comput. Vis. Image Underst.* **2017**, *164*, 103–110. [CrossRef]
11. Connor, P.; Ross, A. Biometric recognition by gait: A survey of modalities and features. *Comput. Vis. Image Underst.* **2018**, *167*, 1–27. [CrossRef]
12. Zeng, W.; Wang, C.; Yang, F. Silhouette-based gait recognition via deterministic learning. *Pattern Recognit.* **2014**, *47*, 3568–3584. [CrossRef]
13. Lv, Z.; Xing, X.; Wang, K.; Guan, D. Class energy image analysis for video sensor-based gait recognition: A review. *Sensors* **2015**, *15*, 932–964. [CrossRef] [PubMed]
14. Li, Y.; Zhang, D.; Zhang, J.; Xun, L.; Yan, Q.; Zhang, J.; Gao, Q.; Xia, Y. A Convolutional Neural Network for Gait Recognition Based on Plantar Pressure Images. In Proceedings of the Chinese Conference on Biometric Recognition, Beijing, China, 28–29 October 2017.
15. Moustakidis, S.P.; Theocharis, J.B.; Giakas, G. Subject recognition based on ground reaction force measurements of gait signals. *IEEE Trans. Syst. Man Cybern. Part B Cybern.* **2008**, *38*, 1476–1485. [CrossRef] [PubMed]
16. Vera-Rodriguez, R.; Mason, J.S.; Fierrez, J.; Ortega-Garcia, J. Comparative analysis and fusion of spatiotemporal information for footstep recognition. *IEEE Trans. Pattern Anal. Mach. Intell.* **2013**, *35*, 823–834. [CrossRef] [PubMed]
17. Yang, G.; Tan, W.; Jin, H.; Zhao, T.; Tu, L. Review wearable sensing system for gait recognition. *Cluster Comput.* **2018**, 1–9. [CrossRef]
18. Sprager, S.; Juric, M.B. Inertial sensor-based gait recognition: A review. *Sensors* **2015**, *15*, 22089–22127. [CrossRef] [PubMed]

19. Zhang, Y.; Pan, G.; Jia, K.; Lu, M.; Wang, Y.; Wu, Z. Accelerometer-based gait recognition by sparse representation of signature points with clusters. *IEEE Trans. Cybern.* **2015**, *45*, 1864–1875. [CrossRef] [PubMed]

20. Geiger, J.T.; Kneißl, M.; Schuller, B.W.; Rigoll, G. Acoustic gait-based person identification using hidden Markov models. In Proceedings of the 2014 Workshop on Mapping Personality Traits Challenge and Workshop, Istanbul, Turkey, 12 November 2014; ACM: New York, NY, USA, 2014; pp. 25–30. [CrossRef]

21. Hofmann, M.; Geiger, J.; Bachmann, S.; Schuller, B.; Rigoll, G. The tum gait from audio, image and depth (gaid) database: Multimodal recognition of subjects and traits. *J. Vis. Commun. Image Represent.* **2014**, *25*, 195–206. [CrossRef]

22. Li, W.; Kuo, C.C.J.; Peng, J. Gait recognition via GEI subspace projections and collaborative representation classification. *Neurocomputing* **2018**, *275*, 1932–1945. [CrossRef]

23. Xue, Z.; Ming, D.; Song, W.; Wan, B.; Jin, S. Infrared gait recognition based on wavelet transform and support vector machine. *Pattern Recognit.* **2010**, *43*, 2904–2910. [CrossRef]

24. Yao, Z.M.; Zhou, X.; Lin, E.D.; Xu, S.; Sun, Y.N. A novel biometric recognition system based on ground reaction force measurements of continuous gait. In Proceedings of the Third Conference on Human System Interactions (HSI 2010), Rzeszow, Poland, 13–15 May 2010; pp. 452–458. [CrossRef]

25. Ahmed, F.; Paul, P.P.; Gavrilova, M.L. DTW-based kernel and rank-level fusion for 3D gait recognition using Kinect. *Vis. Comput.* **2015**, *31*, 915–924. [CrossRef]

26. Wang, T.; Gong, S.; Zhu, X.; Wang, S. Person re-identification by video ranking. In Proceedings of the European Conference on Computer Vision, Zurich, Switzerland, 6–12 September 2014; Springer: Cham, Switzerland, 2014; pp. 688–703. [CrossRef]

27. Nickel, C.; Busch, C. Classifying accelerometer data via hidden markov models to authenticate people by the way they walk. *IEEE Aerosp. Electron. Syst. Mag.* **2013**, *28*, 29–35. [CrossRef]

28. Samà, A.; Ruiz, F.J.; Agell, N.; Pérez-López, C.; Català, A.; Cabestany, J. Gait identification by means of box approximation geometry of reconstructed attractors in latent space. *Neurocomputing* **2013**, *121*, 79–88. [CrossRef]

29. Arora, P.; Srivastava, S. Gait recognition using gait Gaussian image. In Proceedings of the 2015 2nd International Conference on Signal Processing and Integrated Networks (SPIN), Noida, India, 19–20 February 2015; pp. 791–794. [CrossRef]

30. Choi, S.; Youn, I.H.; LeMay, R.; Burns, S.; Youn, J.H. Biometric gait recognition based on wireless acceleration sensor using k-nearest neighbor classification. In Proceedings of the 2014 International Conference on Computing, Networking and Communications (ICNC), Honolulu, HI, USA, 3–6 February 2014; pp. 1091–1095. [CrossRef]

31. Arora, P.; Srivastava, S.; Singhal, S. Analysis of gait flow image and gait Gaussian image using extension neural network for gait recognition. *Int. J. Rough Sets Data Anal.* **2016**, *3*, 45–64. [CrossRef]

32. Wu, Z.; Huang, Y.; Wang, L.; Wang, X.; Tan, T. A comprehensive study on cross-view gait based human identification with deep cnns. *IEEE Trans. Pattern Anal. Mach. Intell.* **2017**, *39*, 209–226. [CrossRef] [PubMed]

33. Derlatka, M.; Bogdan, M. Ensemble kNN classifiers for human gait recognition based on ground reaction forces. In Proceedings of the 2015 8th International Conference on Human System Interactions (HSI), Warsaw, Poland, 25–27 June 2015; pp. 88–93. [CrossRef]

34. Guan, Y.; Li, C.T.; Roli, F. On reducing the effect of covariate factors in gait recognition: A classifier ensemble method. *IEEE Trans. Pattern Anal. Mach. Intell.* **2015**, *37*, 1521–1528. [CrossRef] [PubMed]

35. Farmanbar, M.; Toygar, Ö. Feature selection for the fusion of face and palmprint biometrics. *SIVP* **2016**, *10*, 951–958. [CrossRef]

36. Xing, X.; Wang, K.; Lv, Z. Fusion of gait and facial features using coupled projections for people identification at a distance. *IEEE Signal Process. Lett.* **2015**, *22*, 2349–2353. [CrossRef]

37. Charfi, N.; Trichili, H.; Alimi, A.M.; Solaiman, B. Bimodal biometric system for hand shape and palmprint recognition based on SIFT sparse representation. *Multimed. Tools Appl.* **2017**, *76*, 20457–20482. [CrossRef]

38. Poh, N.; Ross, A.; Lee, W.; Kittler, J. A user-specific and selective multimodal biometric fusion strategy by ranking subjects. *Pattern Recognit.* **2013**, *46*, 3341–3357. [CrossRef]

39. Casale, P.; Pujol, O.; Radeva, P. Personalization and user verification in wearable systems using biometric walking patterns. *Pers. Ubiquit. Comput.* **2012**, *16*, 563–580. [CrossRef]

40. Zhang, Z.; Yi, D.; Lei, Z.; Li, S.Z. Regularized transfer boosting for face detection across spectrum. *IEEE Signal Process. Lett.* **2012**, *19*, 131–134. [CrossRef]
41. Derlatka, M.; Bogdan, M. Fusion of static and dynamic parameters at decision level in human gait recognition. In Proceedings of the International Conference on Pattern Recognition and Machine Intelligence, Warsaw, Poland, 30 June–3 July 2015; Springer: Cham, Switzerland, 2015; pp. 515–524. [CrossRef]
42. Cronin, N.J. The effects of high heeled shoes on female gait: A review. *J. Electromyogr. Kinesiol.* **2014**, *24*, 258–263. [CrossRef] [PubMed]
43. Blanchette, M.G.; Brault, J.R.; Powers, C.M. The influence of heel height on utilized coefficient of friction during walking. *Gait Posture* **2011**, *34*, 107–110. [CrossRef] [PubMed]
44. Barton, C.J.; Coyle, J.A.; Tinley, P. The effect of heel lifts on trunk muscle activation during gait: A study of young healthy females. *J. Electromyogr. Kinesiol.* **2009**, *19*, 598–606. [CrossRef] [PubMed]
45. Simonsen, E.B.; Svendsen, M.B.; Nørreslet, A.; Baldvinsson, H.K.; Heilskov-Hansen, T.; Larsen, P.K.; Alkjær, T.; Henriksen, M. Walking on high heels changes muscle activity and the dynamics of human walking significantly. *J. Appl. Biomech.* **2012**, *28*, 20–28. [CrossRef] [PubMed]
46. Derlatka, M. Human gait recognition based on ground reaction forces in case of sport shoes and high heels. In Proceedings of the 2017 IEEE International Conference on INnovations in Intelligent SysTems and Applications (INISTA), Gdynia, Poland, 3–5 July 2017; pp. 247–252. [CrossRef]
47. De Oliveira Pezzan, P.A.; João, S.M.A.; Ribeiro, A.P.; Manfio, E.F. Postural assessment of lumbar lordosis and pelvic alignment angles in adolescent users and nonusers of high-heeled shoes. *J. Manip. Physiol. Ther.* **2011**, *34*, 614–621. [CrossRef] [PubMed]
48. Sarkar, S.; Phillips, P.J.; Liu, Z.; Vega, I.R.; Grother, P.; Bowyer, K.W. The humanid gait challenge problem: Data sets, performance, and analysis. *IEEE Trans. Pattern Anal. Mach. Intell.* **2005**, *27*, 162–177. [CrossRef] [PubMed]
49. Bouchrika, I.; Nixon, M.S. Exploratory factor analysis of gait recognition. In Proceedings of the 8th IEEE International Conference on Automatic Face & Gesture Recognition, (FG '08), Amsterdam, The Netherlands, 17–19 September 2008; pp. 1–6. [CrossRef]
50. Gafurov, D.; Snekkenes, E.; Bours, P. Improved gait recognition performance using cycle matching. In Proceedings of the 2010 IEEE 24th International Conference on Advanced Information Networking and Applications Workshops (WAINA), Perth, WA, Australia, 20–23 April 2010; pp. 836–841. [CrossRef]
51. Kim, M.; Kim, M.; Park, S.; Kwon, J.; Park, J. Feasibility Study of Gait Recognition Using Points in Three-Dimensional Space. *Int. J. Fuzzy Log. Intell. Syst.* **2013**, *13*, 124–132. [CrossRef]
52. Perry, J.; Burnfield, J. *Gait Analysis: Normal and Pathological Function*, 2nd ed.; Slack Inc.: Thorofare, NJ, USA, 2010; ISBN 13 9781556427664.
53. Pham, T.T.D.; Nguyen, H.T.; Lee, S.; Won, C.S. Moving object detection with Kinect v2. In Proceedings of the IEEE International Conference on Consumer Electronics-Asia (ICCE-Asia), Seoul, Korea, 26–28 October 2016; pp. 1–4. [CrossRef]
54. Cho, H.; Yeon, S.; Choi, H.; Doh, N. Detection and Compensation of Degeneracy Cases for IMU-Kinect Integrated Continuous SLAM with Plane Features. *Sensors* **2018**, *18*, 935. [CrossRef] [PubMed]
55. Fankhauser, P.; Bloesch, M.; Rodriguez, D.; Kaestner, R.; Hutter, M.; Siegwart, R. Kinect v2 for mobile robot navigation: Evaluation and modeling. In Proceedings of the 2015 International Conference on Advanced Robotics (ICAR), Istanbul, Turkey, 27–31 July 2015; pp. 388–394. [CrossRef]
56. Cippitelli, E.; Gasparrini, S.; Spinsante, S.; Gambi, E. Kinect as a tool for gait analysis: Validation of a real-time joint extraction algorithm working in side view. *Sensors* **2015**, *15*, 1417–1434. [CrossRef] [PubMed]
57. Mentiplay, B.F.; Perraton, L.G.; Bower, K.J.; Pua, Y.H.; McGaw, R.; Heywood, S.; Clark, R.A. Gait assessment using the Microsoft Xbox One Kinect: Concurrent validity and inter-day reliability of spatiotemporal and kinematic variables. *J. Biomech.* **2015**, *48*, 2166–2170. [CrossRef] [PubMed]
58. Dolatabadi, E.; Taati, B.; Mihailidis, A. Concurrent validity of the Microsoft Kinect for Windows v2 for measuring spatiotemporal gait parameters. *Med. Eng. Phys.* **2016**, *38*, 952–958. [CrossRef] [PubMed]
59. Springer, S.; Seligmann, G.Y. Validity of the Kinect for gait assessment: A focused review. *Sensors* **2016**, *16*, 194. [CrossRef] [PubMed]
60. Kinect for Windows sdk 2.0. Available online: https://www.microsoft.com/en-us/download/details.aspx?id=44561 (accessed on 9 April 2018).
61. Sell, J.; O'Connor, P. The xbox one system on a chip and kinect sensor. *IEEE Micro* **2014**, *34*, 44–53. [CrossRef]

62. Wasenmüller, O.; Stricker, D. Comparison of kinect v1 and v2 depth images in terms of accuracy and precision. In Proceedings of the Asian Conference on Computer Vision, Taipei, Taiwan, 20–24 November 2016; Springer: Cham, Switzerland, 2016; pp. 34–45. [CrossRef]

63. Derlatka, M. Human gait recognition based on signals from two force plates. In Proceedings of the International Conference on Artificial Intelligence and Soft Computing, Zakopane, Poland, 29 April–3 May 2012; Springer: Berlin/Heidelberg, Germany, 2012; pp. 251–258. [CrossRef]

64. Connor, P.C. Comparing and combining underfoot pressure features forshod and unshod gait biometrics. In Proceedings of the 2015 IEEE International Symposium on Technologies for Homeland Security (HST), Waltham, MA, USA, 14–16 April 2015; pp. 1–7. [CrossRef]

65. Connie, T.; Goh, M.; Ong, T.S.; Toussi, H.L.; Teoh, A.B.J. A challenging gait database for office surveillance. In Proceedings of the 2013 6th International Congress on Image and Signal Processing (CISP), Hangzhou, China, 16–18 December 2013; Volume 3, pp. 1670–1675. [CrossRef]

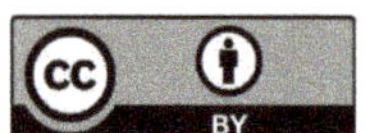

© 2018 by the authors. Licensee MDPI, Basel, Switzerland. This article is an open access article distributed under the terms and conditions of the Creative Commons Attribution (CC BY) license (http://creativecommons.org/licenses/by/4.0/).

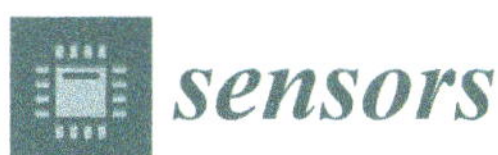 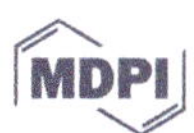

Article

Dynamical Properties of Postural Control in Obese Community-Dwelling Older Adults [†]

Christopher W. Frames [1,2], Rahul Soangra [3], Thurmon E. Lockhart [1,*], John Lach [4], Dong Sam Ha [5], Karen A. Roberto [6] and Abraham Lieberman [2]

[1] School of Biological and Health Systems Engineering, Arizona State University, Tempe, AZ 85281, USA; cframes@asu.edu

[2] Muhammad Ali Parkinson Center (MAPC), Barrow Neurological Institute, St. Joseph's Hospital and Medical Center, Phoenix, AZ 85013, USA; abraham.lieberman@dignityhealth.org

[3] Department of Physical Therapy, Crean College of Health and Behavioral Sciences, Chapman University, Orange, CA 92866, USA; soangra@chapman.edu

[4] Department of Electrical and Computer Engineering, University of Virginia, Charlottesville, VA 22904, USA; jlach@virginia.edu

[5] The Bradley Department of Electrical and Computer Engineering, Virginia Polytechnic Institute and State University, Blacksburg, VA 24061, USA; ha@vt.edu

[6] Center for Gerontology, Virginia Polytechnic Institute and State University, Blacksburg, VA 24061, USA; kroberto@vt.edu

* Correspondence: Thurmon.Lockhart@asu.edu; Tel.: +1-540-257-3058

[†] The paper is an extension of our paper published in Lockhart, T.; Soangra, R.; Frames, C.; Lach, J. Fall risks assessment among community dwelling elderly using wearable wireless sensors. In Proceedings of the Signal Processing, Sensor/Information Fusion, and Target Recognition, Baltimore, MD, USA, 20 June 2014.

Received: 10 March 2018; Accepted: 22 May 2018; Published: 24 May 2018

Abstract: Postural control is a key aspect in preventing falls. The aim of this study was to determine if obesity affected balance in community-dwelling older adults and serve as an indicator of fall risk. The participants were randomly assigned to receive a comprehensive geriatric assessment followed by a longitudinal assessment of their fall history. The standing postural balance was measured for 98 participants with a Body Mass Index (BMI) ranging from 18 to 63 kg/m^2, using a force plate and an inertial measurement unit affixed at the sternum. Participants' fall history was recorded over 2 years and participants with at least one fall in the prior year were classified as fallers. The results suggest that body weight/BMI is an additional risk factor for falling in elderly persons and may be an important marker for fall risk. The linear variables of postural analysis suggest that the obese fallers have significantly higher sway area and sway ranges, along with higher root mean square and standard deviation of time series. Additionally, it was found that obese fallers have lower complexity of anterior-posterior center of pressure time series. Future studies should examine more closely the combined effect of aging and obesity on dynamic balance.

Keywords: obesity; postural control; nonlinear

---

1. Introduction

Obesity is a growing health problem in older adults [1]. In 2012, approximately 35% of the population above the age of 60 years was considered obese [2]. By 2015, 75% of adults were estimated to be overweight, in which 41% were classified as obese [2–4]. Obesity is a complex multifactorial disease associated with risk factors for various diseases and medical complications, including cardiovascular disease [5], atrial fibrillation [6], depression [7–9], stroke [8], and a reduction in quality of life [1,2]. Along with the multisystem deterioration that accompanies old age, obesity comports functional decline, sensory deficits [10–16], and significantly reduced mass-relative lower extremity strength that precipitates falls [17,18]. Compounding the age-related decrements are obesity's increased mechanical demands that not only increase system constraints, but also prompt an interminable state of physiological and biomechanical compromise: compensatory adaptations to offset the excess trunk mass. It has been reported that obese adults carry an anteriorly displaced center of mass that elicits greater trunk extension while standing in an effort to counteract the excessive weight and maintain balance [19–22]. As a result, studies show that postural control elicits behavior modifications associated with greater fall risk and injuries [22,23], including increased postural sway area, range, and velocity [19–21]. However, not all of literature coincides with these findings, in fact, many studies contradict this and are not explicitly synonymous with fall incidence and injuries [24–26], indeed, the literature is rife with contradictions. Some researchers report that obesity necessitates additional balance control constraints that ultimately reduce stability [17,27,28] others report that obesity's effect on balance is minimal [29,30], merely providing protection from fall-related injuries [24,26].

The ambiguity may be a consequence of the limitations involved in traditional analysis techniques and the lack of consideration for the multifactorial nature of human postural control. Standard variability analysis techniques comprise of linear statistical measures estimating amplitude of center of pressure (COP) excursions. COP displacements equate in linear manner with arbitrary fluctuations in which putative randomness is averaged out, ignoring the time-dependent evolution of the system's dynamics. A more comprehensive view of postural stability may require the addition of nonlinear measures to characterize the temporal dynamics of the COP time series and evince the underlying motor control processes involved. In this context, the focus of stability is appropriated from the amount of variability in the signal—standard deviation (SD), root mean square (RMS)—to the organization of variability.

To quantify the dynamical properties of postural stability, several nonlinear measures expressed as time series of COP trajectories in both force plate and inertial measurement units (IMU) were employed. Over the last two decades regulatory statistics from nonlinear dynamics, have been used extensively in COP time series analyses to measure neuromuscular connections (feedback) and the subtle changes in postural control [31,32]. By observing the evolution of the postural control system, entropy measures can estimate specific feedback mechanisms and spontaneous properties of interconnected neurons, in which a weak, or degraded neuromuscular system, can be characterized by increased regularity in the physiological time series [33,34]. Furthermore, entropy measures are believed to provide a direct measurement of feedback among neuromuscular connections. Lower entropy indicates high predictability and regularity of time series data whereas high entropy values indicate unpredictability and random variation [33,35].

Weight gain in obesity may alter fractal properties of the motor function. Detrended Fluctuation Analysis (DFA) is a useful technique to characterize the long-range correlations of a time series and provides complementary insight and also reveals the underlying complexity into the multifactorial nature of human postural control. The present study utilizes, both forceplates and inertial sensors to evaluate postural sway which is characterized by sway area (elliptical and circular area) and mean power frequency (MPF), standard deviation (SD), root mean square (RMS), range, mean COP velocity and path length of COP signals. However, an increase in body mass may induce subtle impairments in balance and without obviously detectable unsteadiness.

This study is an extended version of our previous study [3] and has explored the responsiveness of linear and nonlinear postural measures to evaluate the effects of increased body weight on postural stability and fall risk in obese community-dwelling elderly adults.

2. Materials and Methods

Ninety-eight community-dwelling older adults participated in the study. Demographics of population are provided in Table 1, anthropometric information in Table 2 and gender ratio in Table 3. This sample size was selected to provide smaller confidence interval on the estimated error rate when classifying fallers and non-fallers [36]. Study participants were divided into three groups based on their BMI: normal ($19 \leq$ BMI < 25 kg/m^2), overweight ($25 \leq$ BMI < 30 kg/m^2), and obese (BMI ≥ 30 kg/m^2) [36]. Fall history was recorded, retrospectively, for 2-years with emphasis on fall frequency and characteristics of the falls. Any person with at least one fall in the prior year was classified as a faller and the others as non-fallers; demographics of participants is shown in Tables 1–3. The study was conducted in four separate senior community centers throughout Virginia, using the IMU and force plate on four different days. This study was approved by the Virginia Tech Institutional Review Board (VT-IRB) and was conducted in collaboration with Northern Virginia Fall Prevention Coalition (NVFPC) and INOVA Hospital. All participants provided written consent which was approved by VT_IRB prior to their participation. All measurements were performed barefoot in quiet standing, looking in the forward direction, with their foot placement standardized. For postural stability, the participants were asked to stand in two visual conditions: eyes open (EO) and eyes closed (EC). Each measurement lasted for 60 s and was repeated twice. The sampling rate inertial sensors and forceplate was 100 Hz. A rest of 3 min was provided between each measurement. For the analysis, the COP trajectory was separated into its mediolateral, ML and anteroposterior, AP, components. BMI was calculated for each participant based on his/her height and weight. The recorded COP signals were filtered using a fourth-order low-pass Butterworth filter, with a cut-off frequency of 5 Hz to eliminate measurement noise. Given the limited data length, measurements began a few seconds after the informed start of the trial and ended a few seconds before the informed termination of the trial. All analysis was performed using custom Matlab routines (The Mathworks, Version 2015a). A mixed effect MANOVA model was used, with participants being the random effect. Because the design was unbalanced, we used restricted maximum likelihood (REML) as the fitting method using JMP (JMP®, Pro 10.0.2. SAS Institute Inc., Cary, NC, USA, 1989–2007).

Methods for entropy and detrended fluctuation analysis are provided below similar to our previous study [3].

Table 1. Demographics of the subject population.

Health Status	Faller (F)	Non-Faller (NF)
Non-obese (NOB)	14	20
Obese (OB)	8	22
Overweight (OW)	10	24

Table 2. Age, height, weight and BMI ratio of each group.

	Fall Risk			
	Faller		Non-Faller	
	NOB	**OB**	**NOB**	**OB**
Age (years)	76.82 ± 6.87	72.29 ± 4.72	77.41 ± 8.49	72.68 ± 7.40
Height (m)	1.71 ± 0.06	1.61 ± 0.07	1.67 ± 0.11	1.64 ± 0.05
Weight (kg)	79.14 ± 8.18	80.77 ± 21.98	67.26 ± 12.41	87.66 ± 21.05
BMI (kg/m^2)	26.85 ± 2.08	31.27 ± 8.09	24.29 ± 2.16	32.65 ± 7.62

Table 3. Gender ratio for each group.

Gender	Fall Risk		Weight Status		
	F	**NF**	**NOB**	**OB**	**OW**
Female	12	53	21	19	25
Male	6	27	13	11	9

We hereby provide information pertaining to non-linear analysis performed similar to our previous work [3]. Approximate entropy (ApEn) quantifies the ensemble amount of randomness, or irregularity [37]. Here in this study, we employ ApEn as measure of complexity to quantify COP time series based non-linear variability during quiet standing in community-dwelling older adults. Some of the earlier research has reported that ApEn is sensitive enough too and can detect subtle changes in COP variability which may not be apparent in traditional biomechanical measures of postural stability [31,38], such as COP area, sway velocity, path length etc. The concept of Approximate Entropy (ApEn) was firstly reported by Pincus [39]. Although ApEn can be computed for any timeseries, here, we explain the approach of ApEn estimation as applied to center of pressure (COP) timeseries data. ApEn works on logarithmic likelihood such that the patterns of the nearby data have similar pattern. For example a sequence of total N numbers of COP time series e.g., COPx(1), COPx(2),..., COPx(N). To compute ApEn, m-dimensional vector sequences p_m (i) were constructed from the COP time series like [p_m (1), p_m (2),..., p_m (N − m + 1)], where the index i can take values ranging from 1 to N − m + 1. Where the distance between two vectors p_m (i) and p_m (j) is defined as $|p_m (j) - p_m (i)|$,

$$C_i^m(d) = \frac{1}{N - m + 1} \text{ such that } |P_m(j) - P_m(i)| < d \tag{1}$$

where m is the pattern length selected as 2, d is the similarity coefficient which has been set to 0.2% of the standard deviation of total length of COP data [33]. These constants have previously yielded statistically reliable and reproducible results. $C_i^m(d)$ is considered as the mean of the fraction of patterns of length m that resemble the pattern of the same length that begins at index i. ApEn is computed as:

$$\text{ApEn}(N, m, d) = (N - m + 1)^{-1} \sum_{i=1}^{N-(m-1)} \ln C_i^m(d) - (N - m)^{-1} \sum_{i=1}^{N-m} \ln C_i^{m+1}(d) \tag{2}$$

ApEn is a unitless value between 0 and 2 [37]. Smaller ApEn values indicate a higher probability of regular repeating sequences and less complex timeseries. An ApEn value of zero, depicts that the time series is perfectly repeatable (for example periodic sinewave), whereas, the value of 2 is produced by random time series, for which repeating sequences only occur by chance (example Gaussian noise). Thus, the input parameters for the ApEn calculation were (1) a pattern length (m) of 2 data points; (2) a tolerance window normalized to 0.2 times the standard deviation of individual time series. The pattern length (m) and tolerance level (r) were chosen as per previous research using COP [31,32,40].

Signal regularity was also quantified using sample entropy (SaEn). SaEn indexes the regularity of a time series by calculating the probability that having a repeated signal for a window length m, will remain similar for m + 1 data points—excluding any self-matches and within a matching tolerance r. The greater SaEn values delineate irregularity and rate generation of new information, in which a set of similar points are considered unique as they will likely not be followed by a similar set of matching points within a specified tolerance r. Higher SaEn values are considered part of a healthy, robust system able to adapt to challenges and unexpected perturbations. Lower values are associated with greater regularity of the time series, in which there is a greater likelihood that sets of matching epochs in a time series will be followed by another match within a specified tolerance r. Lower values denote a possible rigid, disease state unable to adapt to challenges. For the present study, SaEn was computed with the COP time series and the increment of the COP time series in both the AP and ML directions. Parameters m and r were chosen according to the procedure described by Lake et al. Ramdani et al. (2011) obtaining m = 3 and r = 0.25 for both directions [6,41,42].

$$\text{SaEn}(N, m, r) = \ln \left[\frac{\sum_{i=1}^{N-(m-1)} C_i^m(r)}{\sum_{i=1}^{N-m} C_i^{m+1}(r)} \right] \tag{3}$$

Multiscale entropy (MSE) is a regularity measure that quantifies the information content of postural fluctuations over a range of physiologically relevant time scales while sample entropy is computed for every consecutive coarse-grained time series. The entropy values are then plotted as a function of the time scales in which the area under the curve reveals the signal's complexity index (CI). A complex signal is associated with a time evolution with a rich structure on multiple scales. For white noise, which is irregular on small time scales but not structurally complex, the entropy decreases for larger time scales. For a complex signal, such as pink $1/f$ noise, the entropy remains high on different scales. For the computation of MSE the input parameters $m = 3$ and $r = 0.25$ were chosen similar to the SaEn algorithm as shown in Figure 1b.

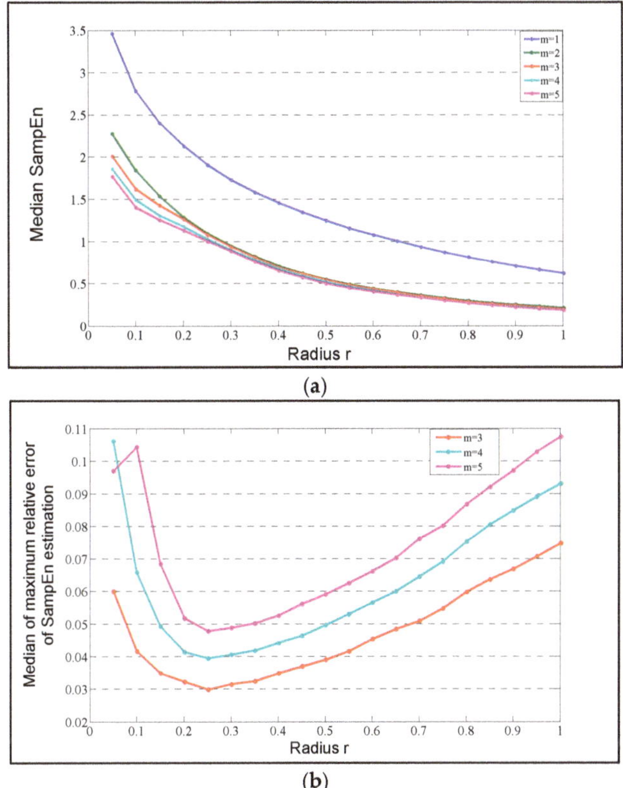

Figure 1. (**a**) Median over all the center of pressure (COP) AP time series; (**b**) The lowest curve is obtained for $m = 3$ as it shows a minimum that is lower than 0.05. This minimum is reached for $r = 0.25$ for both AP and ML directions.

Detrended fluctuation analysis (DFA) is a nonlinear analysis tool used to detect long range correlations in time series with nonstationarity [43]. Firstly, intrinsic trends are removed as trends could mislead for long range correlations. DFA provides insights into scaling behavior of natural variability in time series. The COP time series are also non-stationary [44,45]. Time series data is systematically divided into segments of different lengths (scales). Fluctuation analysis is then performed as sum of the residuals squared divided by segment length. Finally, a log-log plot of the average error (fluctuation) versus segment length (scale) is performed. The slope of this plot is the scaling exponent α (DFA parameter). Pure random walk has α as 1.5 and white noise α is 0.5 [46]. DFA is computed in two steps:

The time series $B(k)$ is shifted by the mean $<B>$ and integrated (cumulatively summed),

$$y(k) = \sum_{i=1}^{k} [B(i) - <B>] \tag{4}$$

Then segmented into windows of various sizes Δn

In each segmentation the integrated data is locally fit to a polynomial $y_{\Delta n}(k)$ and mean-squared residual $F(\Delta n)$ (fluctuations) with N as total number of data points

$$F(\Delta n) = \sqrt{\frac{1}{N} \sum_{k=1}^{N} [y(k) - y_{\Delta n}(k)]^2} \tag{5}$$

$F^2(\Delta n)$ is the average of the summed squares of the residual in windows. DFA procedure tests for self-similarity or fractal properties at different resolutions (windows sizes).

$$F(\Delta n) = C(\Delta n)^{\alpha} \tag{6}$$

where C is a constant and α is estimated from a least-square fit.

$$\ln(F(\Delta n)) = \propto \ln(\Delta n) + \ln(C) \tag{7}$$

This scaling coefficient α is a measure of correlation in the noise and an estimate of the Hurst exponent H.

The median of the maximum relative error $Q(m,r)$ of the *SaEn* calculation as a function of $r = 0.25$ and $m = 3$.

3. Results

3.1. Linear Measures

Significant differences were observed in a multitude of linear force plate measures comparing obese fallers and obese non-fallers: Sway area (95% confidence ellipse, $p = 0.0008$, $F = 7.39$; circular area, $p < 0.0001$, $F = 9.80$), mean velocity ($p = 0.001$, $F = 6.51$), and mean path length of COP ($p = 0.001$, $F = 6.51$); the eyes-open (EO) vs eyes-closed (EO) condition afforded similar results (Figure 2). Obese fallers demonstrated significantly higher sway range (p-value $= 0.001$, $F = 7.44$), RMS values (p-value $= 0.002$, $F = 6.62$) and SD values (p-value $= 0.002$, $F = 6.62$) from the force plate COP time series. Significant statistical variability between obese fallers and obese non-fallers was similarly observed utilizing the IMU: Sway area (ellipse area, $p = 0.003$, $F = 5.89$; and circular area $p < 0.0002$, $F = 8.97$), mean velocity ($p = 0.011$, $F = 4.56$), mean radius ($p < 0.0001$, $F = 10.47$) (Table 4) and mean path length of COP ($p = 0.011$, $F = 4.56$). Further traditional postural stability parameters with eyes open and eyes closed condition are shown in Table 5.

Similarly, sway range (p-value $= 0.002$, $F = 6.22$), RMS-value (p-value $= 0.001$, $F = 7.19$) and SD-values (p-value $= 0.004$, $F = 5.86$) were significantly higher in obese fallers from IMU time series. Mean power frequency (MPF) of the time series in eyes closed condition were found to be significantly higher than in eyes open condition (p value < 0.0001, $F = 23.89$) for all elderly participants.

3.2. Nonlinear Measures

The α scaling exponent from DFA utilizing both the force plate and IMU signals, did not reach significance for any of the fall and obese conditions, respectively. However, the general trend was that in the eyes open condition, α was higher than in the eyes closed condition. Anterior-posterior COP times series were found to have significantly higher persistence than in mediolateral direction time series (Figure 3). It was also seen (Table 6) that obese fallers had higher persistence than non-obese and overweight.

Regarding COP fluctuations taken from the force plate, approximate entropy ($p < 0.0001$, $F = 2957.9$) in the AP direction was significantly lower than in the ML direction in obese as well as in non-obese and overweight older adults (Figure 3). Whereas, scaling exponent (alpha) (p-value = 0.03, $F = 4.75$) in the AP direction was significantly higher than ML direction in obese as well as in non-obese and overweight elderly persons. Sample entropy in the AP direction during the eyes open condition was found to be significantly lower in obese fallers ($p = 0.007$, $F = 4.95$) than other non-obese and overweight elderly persons (Figure 3).

COP signals from the IMU revealed that approximate entropy ($p < 0.0001$, $F = 2857.7$) in the AP direction was significantly lower than in the ML direction in the obese participants as well as in the non-obese and overweight elderly individuals (Figure 4). Whereas, the scaling exponent (alpha) (p-value < 0.0001, 54.37) in the AP direction was significantly higher than ML direction in obese as well as in non-obese and overweight elderly individuals. Sample entropy in AP direction was found to be significantly lower in obese fallers ($p = 0.015$, $F = 4.21$) than other non-obese and overweight elderly individuals (Figures 4 and 5). Figure 6 shows discriminative parameters for obesity.

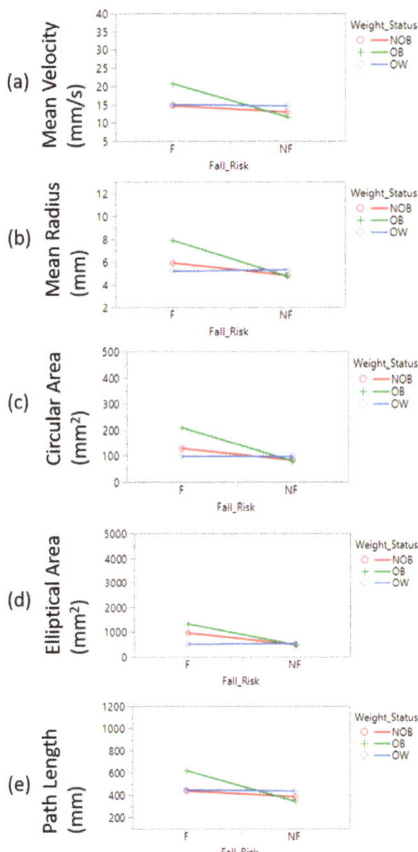

Figure 2. Linear measures of postural stability (**a**) Mean Velocity; (**b**) Mean Radius; (**c**) Circular area; (**d**) Elliptical area; (**e**) COP Path length.

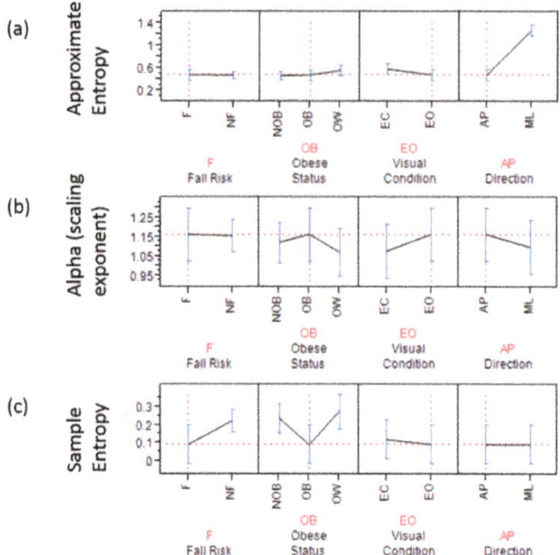

Figure 3. Forceplate signal based non-linear analysis showing (**a**) approximate entropy; the graph highlights (dashed red line) obese fallers have significantly lower complexity in anterior posterior direction with eyes open condition; (**b**) scaling exponent α and; the graph highlights (dashed red line) that obese fallers have significantly higher scaling exponents in anterior posterior direction during eyes open condition (**c**) sample entropy is significantly lower for AP time series derived from forceplate for fallers with obesity in eyes open condition (red dashed lines).

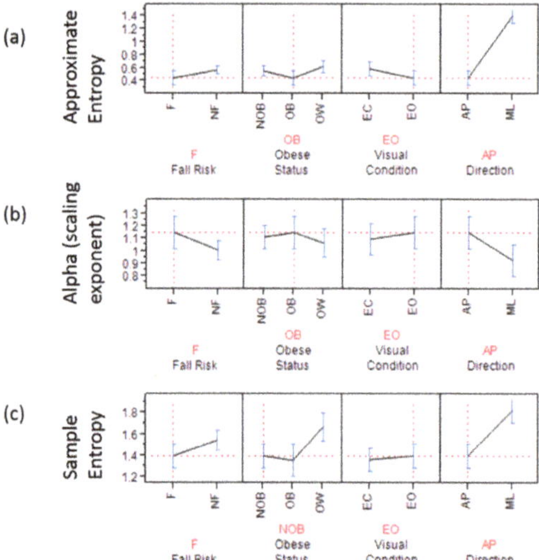

Figure 4. Inertial measurement units (IMU) based nonlinear analysis showing (**a**) approximate entropy; The graph highlights (dashed red-line) approximate entropy is significantly lower in obese fallers in anterior posterior direction during eyes open double limb stance; (**b**) scaling exponent α and; The graph highlights (dashed red-line) that the scaling exponent is significantly higher for obese fallers in anterior posterior direction during eyes open double limb stance; (**c**) sample entropy; The graph highlights (red dashed line) that fallers who were non-obese showed significantly lower complexity (measured by sample entropy)for AP time series derived from IMU.

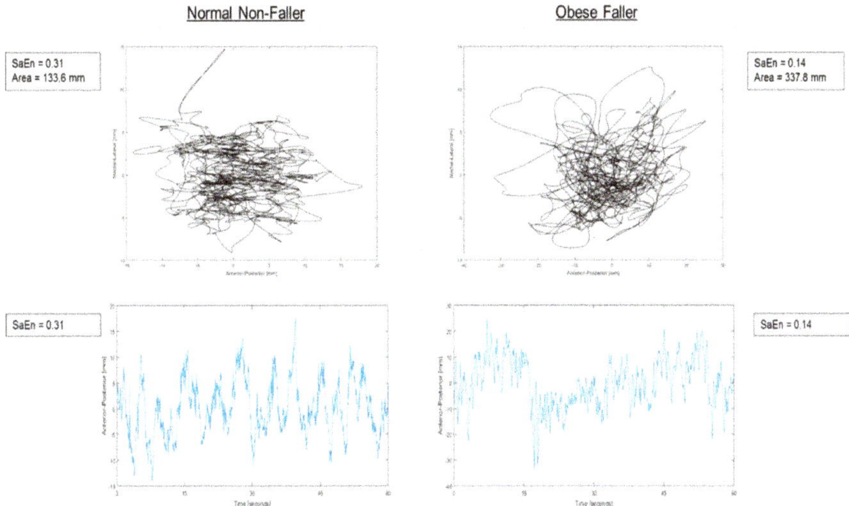

Figure 5. Ensemble patterns of postural stability of fallers and non-fallers exhibiting fallers with larger area of sway with lower sample entropy.

Table 4. Means and standard deviations of force plate parameters.

	NOB		OB		OW	
	F	**NF**	**F**	**NF**	**F**	**NF**
Area [1]	9.69 ± 1.20	4.91 ± 3.57	13.36 ± 7.30	4.92 ± 3.90	5.19 ± 4.96	5.41 ± 3.52
Range AP [2]	34.29 ± 14.44	26.53 ± 8.68	51.78 ± 20.77	26.73 ± 10.48	29.24 ± 13.47	30.49 ± 7.58
Range ML [2]	15.40 ± 10.66	11.31 ± 5.36	17.42 ± 4.12	11.41 ± 6.39	11.31 ± 8.06	11.18 ± 5.54
RMS AP	6.20 ± 2.25	5.13 ± 1.87	8.87 ± 3.33	5.18 ± 2.06	5.60 ± 2.32	5.93 ± 1.82
RMS ML	3.05 ± 1.95	2.18 ± 1.15	3.53 ± 0.86	2.10 ± 1.21	2.15 ± 1.63	2.06 ± 0.94
SD AP	6.20 ± 2.25	5.13 ± 1.87	8.87 ± 3.33	5.19 ± 2.06	5.60 ± 2.32	5.94 ± 1.82
SD ML	3.05 ± 1.95	2.18 ± 1.15	3.53 ± 0.86	2.10 ± 1.21	2.16 ± 1.63	2.07 ± 0.94
MPF AP	0.36 ± 0.05	0.38 ± 0.06	0.38 ± 0.05	0.37 ± 0.05	0.40 ± 0.05	0.40 ± 0.06
MPF ML	0.39 ± 0.06	0.40 ± 0.07	0.38 ± 0.07	0.39 ± 0.06	0.42 ± 0.08	0.40 ± 0.06
DFA α AP	1.12 ± 0.16	1.14 ± 0.16	1.16 ± 0.23	1.15 ± 0.18	1.07 ± 0.15	1.09 ± 0.16
DFA α ML	1.37 ± 0.13	1.33 ± 0.12	1.40 ± 0.09	1.37 ± 0.10	1.30 ± 0.15	1.35 ± 0.12
ApEn AP	0.47 ± 0.12	0.54 ± 0.18	0.48 ± 0.14	0.48 ± 0.14	0.56 ± 0.12	0.52 ± 0.17
ApEn ML	0.55 ± 0.23	0.57 ± 0.23	0.44 ± 0.13	0.60 ± 0.26	0.62 ± 0.17	0.57 ± 0.21
SaEn AP	0.23 ± 0.22	0.25 ± 0.21	0.09 ± 0.03	0.22 ± 0.18	0.28 ± 0.21	0.19 ± 0.14
SaEn ML	0.23 ± 0.22	0.25 ± 0.21	0.09 ± 0.03	0.22 ± 0.18	0.28 ± 0.20	0.19 ± 0.14
MSE AP	3.41 ± 1.03	4.13 ± 1.51	3.73 ± 1.68	3.33 ± 1.13	4.18 ± 0.98	4.09 ± 1.52
MSE ML	3.41 ± 1.30	3.24 ± 1.03	3.17 ± 1.17	3.42 ± 1.51	3.58 ± 1.16	3.68 ± 1.27

[1] 95% confidence ellipse area (cm^2); [2] units in cm.

Table 5. Mean and standard deviations of forceplate measures during Eyes Open and Eyes Closed conditions.

	Weight Status					
	NOB		OB		OW	
	Eyes Closed	**Eyes Open**	**Eyes Closed**	**Eyes Open**	**Eyes Closed**	**Eyes Open**
MPF	0.42 ± 0.07	0.39 ± 0.06	0.42 ± 0.08	0.38 ± 0.06	0.44 ± 0.07	0.41 ± 0.07
RMS	4.54 ± 2.65	4.06 ± 2.38	5.12 ± 3.93	4.33 ± 2.91	4.51 ± 2.51	3.97 ± 2.47
Range	24.66 ± 15.03	21.36 ± 13.14	26.08 ± 18.76	23.22 ± 16.69	24.00 ± 13.69	20.68 ± 12.42
DFA	0.99 ± 0.19	1.06 ± 0.21	1.04 ± 0.23	1.09 ± 0.21	0.98 ± 0.19	1.05 ± 0.18
ApEn	0.63 ± 0.21	0.54 ± 0.20	0.58 ± 0.18	0.52 ± 0.20	0.63 ± 0.17	0.56 ± 0.18
MSE	4.34 ± 1.74	3.58 ± 1.28	4.20 ± 1.58	3.40 ± 1.34	4.55 ± 1.59	3.89 ± 1.31

Table 6. Means and standard deviations of IMU parameters.

	NOB		OB		OW	
	F	NF	F	NF	F	NF
Area [1]	40.17 ± 34.11	41.24 ± 43.69	68.87 ± 20.91	27.20 ± 14.16	32.83 ± 21.30	27.36 ± 15.74
Range AP [2]	0.36 ± 0.05	0.36 ± 0.04	0.37 ± 0.07	0.36 ± 0.04	0.38 ± 0.05	0.36 ± 0.05
Range ML [2]	1.58 ± 0.92	1.32 ± 0.44	2.17 ± 0.66	1.38 ± 0.50	1.16 ± 0.37	1.43 ± 0.55
RMS AP	1.74 ± 1.01	1.41 ± 0.42	2.49 ± 0.57	1.47 ± 0.57	1.23 ± 0.38	1.63 ± 0.62
RMS ML	8.19 ± 5.19	7.01 ± 2.26	12.45 ± 2.75	6.89 ± 2.17	6.41 ± 2.30	7.06 ± 2.19
SD AP	1.11 ± 0.21	1.11 ± 0.16	1.15 ± 0.22	1.01 ± 0.19	1.06 ± 0.12	1.05 ± 0.18
SD ML	1.26 ± 0.10	1.29 ± 0.12	1.27 ± 0.09	1.31 ± 0.09	1.36 ± 0.02	1.27 ± 0.09
MPF AP	1.40 ± 0.31	1.54 ± 0.27	1.35 ± 0.19	1.54 ± 0.21	1.67 ± 0.11	1.47 ± 0.21
MPF ML	8.43 ± 2.28	9.23 ± 2.25	7.84 ± 1.96	9.20 ± 2.04	10.71 ± 1.40	8.21 ± 2.28
DFA α AP	0.44 ± 0.07	0.41 ± 0.05	0.43 ± 0.04	0.41 ± 0.05	0.44 ± 0.07	0.42 ± 0.06
DFA α ML	0.49 ± 0.21	0.55 ± 0.32	0.62 ± 0.15	0.44 ± 0.13	0.54 ± 0.34	0.42 ± 0.13
ApEn AP	0.56 ± 0.28	0.59 ± 0.33	0.75 ± 0.18	0.52 ± 0.18	0.61 ± 0.34	0.47 ± 0.14
ApEn ML	3.12 ± 1.52	3.93 ± 3.50	3.87 ± 0.70	2.51 ± 0.64	3.57 ± 2.41	2.62 ± 1.09
SaEn AP	0.96 ± 0.25	0.95 ± 0.14	0.93 ± 0.22	0.95 ± 0.15	0.88 ± 0.24	0.97 ± 0.16
SaEn ML	1.40 ± 0.04	1.39 ± 0.04	1.41 ± 0.04	1.42 ± 0.03	1.39 ± 0.08	1.41 ± 0.03
MSE AP	1.82 ± 0.15	1.82 ± 0.14	1.82 ± 0.12	1.90 ± 0.10	1.86 ± 0.21	1.88 ± 0.09
MSE ML	12.60 ± 2.00	12.48 ± 1.71	12.01 ± 1.32	12.57 ± 1.36	12.64 ± 1.97	12.78 ± 1.28

[1] 95% confidence ellipse area (cm^2); [2] units in cm.

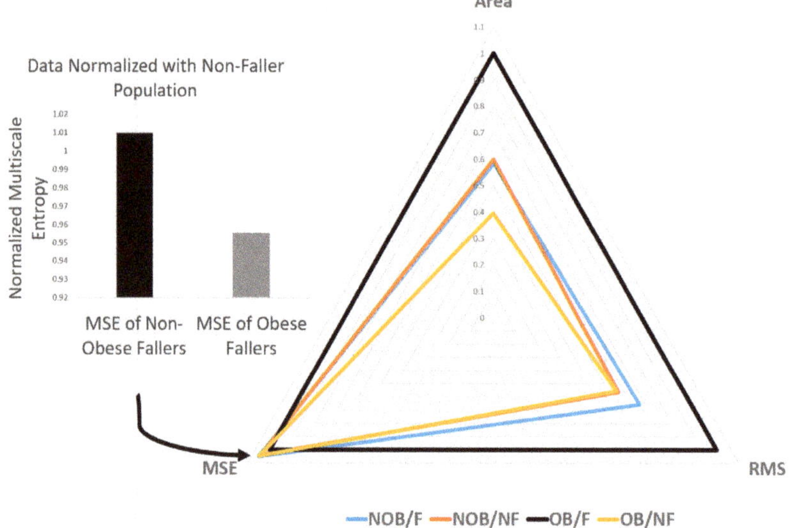

Figure 6. Radar plot of significant discriminative parameters.

4. Discussion

The present study investigated the effects of obesity on fall risk in community-dwelling older adults, utilizing nonlinear analyses on signals acquired from force plate and IMU measurements. It was hypothesized that body weight-related factors increased fall risk in obese older adults identified by linear and nonlinear measures of postural sway. A significant increase in linear parameters (mean radius, ellipse area, sway range, RMS, SD) was identified for obese older adults. Nonlinear regularity measures through sample entropy revealed that the presence of obesity and fall risk had loss of complexity (lower sample entropy values) in eyes open condition in AP sway signals (Figures 3c and 6).

It was also found that obese fallers (Table 6) had higher persistence than non-obese and overweight older adults. Complexity in the ML direction of COP time series was significantly higher in obese participants than that in non-obese and overweight community-dwelling elderly people [46–48].

Statistical variability, such as range and standard deviation, reflect the overall magnitude of COP displacement without considering the temporal structure of COP time series. However, nonlinear measures of postural signals reveal subtle temporal properties of signals which are not detected in obese individuals through a traditional linear approach [27,28,31]. Traditionally, greater COP displacements in anterior posterior and medial-lateral directions have been linked with less stability and consequently, pathology [49]. Although implicated, as the biological systems are intrinsically complex and the linear analysis alone may not account for the time-dependent evolution of the complex system hidden within the time series of COP displacements. As such, an increased excursion of COP may not be an indicator of deficient postural control system, rather, it may be a healthy, vigilant adaptable system capable of adapting to unexpected perturbations for balance maintenance.

In the present study, entropy-based estimations of organizational variability delineate the adaptive capacity of obese participants to maintain balance (lower ApEn and SaEn values indicate greater regularity and decreased complexity). These results are in agreement with previous studies linking aging and pathology [3,47]. It was also found that movements were constrained in the AP direction compared to the ML direction leading to less complex, more stable response modes—a more regular sway pattern with closed-loop short term dependencies to restore balance. Hence, the motor system is probably unable to adjust to the demands inherent to obesity and overweight characteristics, therefore movements transition to a more rigid postural control behavior (repeated patterns and decreased complexity) in the AP direction that diminish both adaptability and stability. In essence, the increase in regularity and possible decrease in complexity may be a result of impaired feedback control or impaired proprioception [50] leading to a reduced adaptive capacity of the postural system [48]. Obese or overweight individuals make hyper activation of plantar mechanoreceptors due to continuous pressure of supporting a large mass, which leads to reduced plantar sensitivity [28,51]. Moreover, the firing of postural muscles may follow an adaptive strategy to reduce joint loads in obese elderly persons that diminish postural stability. Fractal analysis of the COP time series revealed relatively marginal differences in obese fallers versus non-obese and overweight fallers in both the AP and ML directions which were not found to be statistically significant. Obese fallers generally had higher α values in the eyes-open condition (1.23 vs. 1.22) relative to eyes-closed conditions, without reaching significance. From a biomechanics perspective, it may also be due to inability of elderly people to control and accelerate center of mass (COM) over base of support, perhaps due to lack of strength and degradation of type II fibers in skeletal muscles. While muscle strength was not objectively measured in this study, it has been documented that many older people have relatively weaker tibialis anterior and vastus lateralis muscle strength compared to that of healthy adults [52,53]. Obesity is also found related with lower level of physical activity and impaired cardiorespiratory fitness and knee strength compared to lean counterparts [54], possibly impairing obese persons' ability to correct a shift in the body's center of mass and effectively prevent from falling. Probably an increased postural sway could be an adaptive strategy in obese individuals to provide additional stability under conditions of weakness in muscles involved for postural control. Age-related deterioration of sensory and neuromuscular control mechanisms could have definitely added to this problem. Degradation of balance shows that fall risk is increased in those with higher BMI.

Obese elderly persons adopt compensatory strategies, despite their report of having no difficulty in performing the same task as lean counterparts [55]. We assume several mechanisms might have accounted for poor postural balance in obese older adults. First, as body mass of various segments increases, the energy and the strength required to bring the COM over the base of support increases correspondingly similar to when ambulating [56,57]. This may lead to extra biomechanical burden in lower extremity joints to maintain balance, thus obese elderly individuals are liable to adopt an adaptive strategy during quiet standing (perhaps a more closely posture or rigid fixed system with reduction in system degrees of freedom). Secondly, undoubtedly aging is associated with progressive muscle loss (specifically Type II fiber) and which could have resulted in muscular weakness and fat infiltration [58].

These methods build on narrative descriptions of variability in obesity-related postural control by quantifying qualities of postural control, such as complexity. Complexity can be described by the regularity of the pattern of variability and by the number of strategies used over time. In combination, linear and nonlinear analysis quantify postural control to provide a more complete understanding of the adaptive strategies used in postural control than either method could provide alone. The strength of the conclusions of this study must be tempered by the study's limitations. The older participants were aware that they were participating in a fall risk assessment protocol. This could be a bias in the population studied. They may be conscious of the environment and their performance may have been affected by the environment. We tested balance of community-dwelling older adults in four different community centers, and the environment of data collection may also have been a confound in this study. The community center setting in which data were obtained for this study provided a familiar environment for the older participants. At the same time, the non-laboratory setting limited the scope of this data. Howsoever, such analyses may provide insight as to the potential fall risk associated with elderly obese participants.

5. Conclusions

Obesity in older adults is recognized as an important issue with fall risk implications. However, little is known about the relationship between obese elderly persons and their gait characteristics. With fractal analysis, we have not found differences between the results from faller/non-faller and obese/non-obese/overweight groups under EO and EC conditions using both the instruments force plate COP and IMU COP. This indicates that DFA is not able to elucidate the role played by body weight and faller/on-faller status. Although α was found to be higher for the AP direction and for the EO condition, which shows that COP trajectories are more persistence in AP direction and in EO condition (Table 6). With obesity, ApEn revealed a change in the randomness of COP oscillations that occurred in eyes open (EO) visual condition in anterior-posterior direction. Obese elderly persons were found to have significantly lower randomness in the AP direction (or lower entropy) ($p < 0.0001$, $F = 2957.9$).

The present study suggests that the body-weight influences postural balance in obese elderly individuals and both traditional biomechanical parameters as well as non-linear measures could help detect fall risk in persons who are obese. Our results are consistent with recent findings by Rossi-Izquierdo et al. [59]. Inertial sensors can be used to detect fall risk caused by higher body mass in elderly individuals. Indeed, our findings indicate that a change in temporal structure of COP variability as seen by ApEn and SaEn can detect postural changes due to obesity in elderly persons and IMUs may serve as alternative instrument in assessing this. Although implicated, further studies are warranted to elucidate the dynamics of fall recovery to provide comprehensive interpretations of fall risks in the aging population.

Author Contributions: T.E.L., J.L., K.A.R. and D.S.H. conceived and designed the experiments; R.S. and C.W.F. performed the experiments; R.S. along with C.W.F. analyzed the data wrote the manuscript with support from T.E.L. and A.L. All authors discussed the results and contributed to the final manuscript.

Funding: This research was supported by the National Science Foundation-Information and Intelligent Systems (IIS) and Smart and Connected Health (1065442, and 1547466, and secondary 1065262).

Acknowledgments: We would like to thank Misha Pavel and Wendy Nilsen for their encouragement in the development of wireless health monitoring systems and fostering the support of wearable wireless health monitoring systems.

Conflicts of Interest: The authors declare no conflict of interest.

Ethical Statements: All subjects gave their written consent for inclusion before they participated in the study. The study was conducted in accordance with the Declaration of Helsinki, and the protocol was approved by the Institutional Review Board, Virginia Tech (VT-IRB#11-1088).

References

1. Mokdad, A.H.; Bowman, B.A.; Ford, E.S.; Vinicor, F.; Marks, J.S.; Koplan, J.P. The continuing epidemics of obesity and diabetes in the United States. *JAMA* **2001**, *286*, 1195–1200. [CrossRef] [PubMed]
2. Wang, Y.; Beydoun, M.A. The Obesity Epidemic in the United States Gender, Age, Socioeconomic, Racial/Ethnic, and Geographic Characteristics: A Systematic Review and Meta-Regression Analysis. *Epidemiol. Rev.* **2007**, *29*, 6–28. [CrossRef] [PubMed]
3. Lockhart, T.; Frame, C.; Soangra, R.; Lach, J. *Fall Risk Prediction Using Wearable Wireless Sensors*; SPIE Newsroom: Bellingham, WA, USA, 2014.
4. Ogden, C.L.; Carroll, M.D.; Curtin, L.R.; McDowell, M.A.; Tabak, C.J.; Flegal, K.M. Prevalence of overweight and obesity in the United States, 1999–2004. *JAMA* **2006**, *295*, 1549–1555. [CrossRef] [PubMed]
5. Wilson, P.W.; D'Agostino, R.B.; Sullivan, L.; Parise, H.; Kannel, W.B. Overweight and obesity as determinants of cardiovascular risk: The Framingham experience. *Arch. Intern. Med.* **2002**, *162*, 1867–1872. [CrossRef] [PubMed]
6. Wang, T.J.; Parise, H.; Levy, D.; D'Agostino, R.B., Sr.; Wolf, P.A.; Vasan, R.S.; Benjamin, E.J. Obesity and the risk of new-onset atrial fibrillation. *JAMA* **2004**, *292*, 2471–2477. [CrossRef] [PubMed]
7. Luppino, F.S.; de Wit, L.M.; Bouvy, P.F.; Stijnen, T.; Cuijpers, P.; Penninx, B.W.; Zitman, F.G. Overweight, obesity, and depression: A systematic review and meta-analysis of longitudinal studies. *Arch. Gen. Psychiatry* **2010**, *67*, 220–229. [CrossRef] [PubMed]
8. Strazzullo, P.; D'Elia, L.; Cairella, G.; Garbagnati, F.; Cappuccio, F.P.; Scalfi, L. Excess body weight and incidence of stroke: Meta-analysis of prospective studies with 2 million participants. *Stroke* **2010**, *41*, e418–e426. [CrossRef] [PubMed]
9. Kopelman, P.G. Obesity as a medical problem. *Nature* **2000**, *404*, 635–643. [CrossRef] [PubMed]
10. Bray, G.A. Medical consequences of obesity. *J. Clin. Endocrinol. Metab.* **2004**, *89*, 2583–2589. [CrossRef] [PubMed]
11. Ferraro, K.F.; Su, Y.P.; Gretebeck, R.J.; Black, D.R.; Badylak, S.F. Body mass index and disability in adulthood: A 20-year panel study. *Am. J. Public Health* **2002**, *92*, 834–840. [CrossRef] [PubMed]
12. Peeters, A.; Bonneux, L.; Nusselder, W.J.; de Laet, C.; Barendregt, J.J. Adult obesity and the burden of disability throughout life. *Obes. Res.* **2004**, *12*, 1145–1151. [CrossRef] [PubMed]
13. Metzger, J.S.; Catellier, D.J.; Evenson, K.R.; Treuth, M.S.; Rosamond, W.D.; Siega-Riz, A.M. Patterns of objectively measured physical activity in the United States. *Med. Sci. Sports Exerc.* **2008**, *40*, 630–638. [CrossRef] [PubMed]
14. Reynolds, S.L.; Saito, Y.; Crimmins, E.M. The impact of obesity on active life expectancy in older American men and women. *Gerontologist* **2005**, *45*, 438–444. [CrossRef] [PubMed]
15. Jenkins, K.R. Obesity's effects on the onset of functional impairment among older adults. *Gerontologist* **2004**, *44*, 206–216. [CrossRef] [PubMed]
16. Fontaine, K.R.; Barofsky, I. Obesity and health-related quality of life. *Obes. Rev.* **2001**, *2*, 173–182. [CrossRef] [PubMed]
17. Corbeil, P.; Simoneau, M.; Rancourt, D.; Tremblay, A.; Teasdale, N. Increased risk for falling associated with obesity: Mathematical modeling of postural control. *IEEE Trans. Neural Syst. Rehabil. Eng.* **2001**, *9*, 126–136. [CrossRef] [PubMed]
18. Fjeldstad, C.; Fjeldstad, A.S.; Acree, L.S.; Nickel, K.J.; Gardner, A.W. The influence of obesity on falls and quality of life. *Dyn. Med.* **2008**, *7*, 4. [CrossRef] [PubMed]
19. Hasselkus, B.R.; Shambes, G.M. Aging and postural sway in women. *J. Gerontol.* **1975**, *30*, 661–667. [CrossRef] [PubMed]
20. Era, P.; Heikkinen, E. Postural sway during standing and unexpected disturbance of balance in random samples of men of different ages. *J. Gerontol.* **1985**, *40*, 287–295. [CrossRef] [PubMed]

21. Baloh, R.W.; Fife, T.D.; Zwerling, L.; Socotch, T.; Jacobson, K.; Bell, T.; Beykirch, K. Comparison of static and dynamic posturography in young and older normal people. *J. Am. Geriatr. Soc.* **1994**, *42*, 405–412. [CrossRef] [PubMed]

22. Fernie, G.R.; Gryfe, C.I.; Holliday, P.J.; Llewellyn, A. The relationship of postural sway in standing to the incidence of falls in geriatric subjects. *Age Ageing* **1982**, *11*, 11–16. [CrossRef] [PubMed]

23. Maki, B.E.; Holliday, P.J.; Topper, A.K. A prospective study of postural balance and risk of falling in an ambulatory and independent elderly population. *J. Gerontol.* **1994**, *49*, M72–M84. [CrossRef] [PubMed]

24. Flegal, K.M.; Williamson, D.F.; Pamuk, E.R.; Rosenberg, H.M. Estimating deaths attributable to obesity in the United States. *Am. J. Public Health* **2004**, *94*, 1486–1489. [CrossRef] [PubMed]

25. Owusu, W.; Willett, W.; Ascherio, A.; Spiegelman, D.; Rimm, E.; Feskanich, D.; Colditz, G. Body anthropometry and the risk of hip and wrist fractures in men: Results from a prospective study. *Obes. Res.* **1998**, *6*, 12–19. [CrossRef] [PubMed]

26. Compston, J.E.; Watts, N.B.; Chapurlat, R.; Cooper, C.; Boonen, S.; Greenspan, S.; Pfeilschifter, J.; Silverman, S.; Díez-Pérez, A.; Lindsay, R.; et al. Obesity is not protective against fracture in postmenopausal women: GLOW. *Am. J. Med.* **2011**, *124*, 1043–1050. [CrossRef] [PubMed]

27. Handrigan, G.A.; Corbeil, P.; Simoneau, M.; Teasdale, N. Balance control is altered in obese individuals. *J. Biomech.* **2010**, *43*, 383–384. [CrossRef] [PubMed]

28. Hue, O.; Simoneau, M.; Marcotte, J.; Berrigan, F.; Dore, J.; Marceau, P.; Marceau, S.; Tremblay, A.; Teasdale, N. Body weight is a strong predictor of postural stability. *Gait Posture* **2007**, *26*, 32–38. [CrossRef] [PubMed]

29. Blaszczyk, J.W.; Cieslinska-Swider, J.; Plewa, M.; Zahorska-Markiewicz, B.; Markiewicz, A. Effects of excessive body weight on postural control. *J. Biomech.* **2009**, *42*, 1295–1300. [CrossRef] [PubMed]

30. Teasdale, N.; Hue, O.; Marcotte, J.; Berrigan, F.; Simoneau, M.; Dore, J.; Marceau, P.; Marceau, S.; Tremblay, A. Reducing weight increases postural stability in obese and morbid obese men. *Int. J. Obes.* **2007**, *31*, 153–160. [CrossRef] [PubMed]

31. Cavanaugh, J.T.; Guskiewicz, K.M.; Giuliani, C.; Marshall, S.; Mercer, V.; Stergiou, N. Detecting altered postural control after cerebral concussion in athletes with normal postural stability. *Br. J. Sports Med.* **2005**, *39*, 805–811. [CrossRef] [PubMed]

32. Cavanaugh, J.T.; Guskiewicz, K.M.; Giuliani, C.; Marshall, S.; Mercer, V.S.; Stergiou, N. Recovery of postural control after cerebral concussion: New insights using approximate entropy. *J. Athl. Train.* **2006**, *41*, 305–313. [PubMed]

33. Pincus, S. Approximate entropy (ApEn) as a complexity measure. *Chaos* **1995**, *5*, 110–117. [CrossRef] [PubMed]

34. Pincus, S.M. Approximate entropy as a measure of irregularity for psychiatric serial metrics. *Bipolar Disord.* **2006**, *8*, 430–440. [CrossRef] [PubMed]

35. Khandoker, A.H.; Palaniswami, M.; Begg, R.K. A comparative study on approximate entropy measure and poincare plot indexes of minimum foot clearance variability in the elderly during walking. *J. Neuroeng. Rehabil.* **2008**, *5*, 4. [CrossRef] [PubMed]

36. Bartlett, S.A.; Maki, B.E.; Fernie, G.R.; Holliday, P.J.; Gryfe, C.I. On the classification of a geriatric subject as a faller or nonfaller. *Med. Biol. Eng. Comput.* **1986**, *24*, 219–222. [CrossRef] [PubMed]

37. Pincus, S.M. Approximate entropy as a measure of system complexity. *Proc. Natl. Acad. Sci. USA* **1991**, *88*, 2297–2301. [CrossRef] [PubMed]

38. Harbourne, R.T.; Stergiou, N. Nonlinear analysis of the development of sitting postural control. *Dev. Psychobiol.* **2003**, *42*, 368–377. [CrossRef] [PubMed]

39. Pincus, S.M.; Goldberger, A.L. Physiological time-series analysis: What does regularity quantify? *Am. J. Physiol.* **1994**, *266*, H1643–H1656. [CrossRef] [PubMed]

40. Vaillancourt, D.E.; Newell, K.M. The dynamics of resting and postural tremor in Parkinson's disease. *Clin. Neurophysiol.* **2000**, *111*, 2046–2056. [CrossRef]

41. Pincus, S.M. quantifying complexity and regularity of neurobiological systems. In *Methods in Neurosciences*; Michael, L.J., Johannes, D.V., Eds.; Academic Press: Cambridge, MA, USA, 1995; Volume 28, pp. 336–363.

42. Richman, J.S.; Moorman, J.R. Physiological time-series analysis using approximate entropy and sample entropy. *Am. J. Physiol. Heart Circ. Physiol.* **2000**, *278*, H2039–H2049. [CrossRef] [PubMed]

43. Peng, C.K.; Buldyrev, S.V.; Havlin, S.; Simons, M.; Stanley, H.E.; Goldberger, A.L. Mosaic organization of DNA nucleotides. *Phys. Rev. E Stat. Phys. Plasmas Fluids Relat. Interdiscip. Top.* **1994**, *49*, 1685–1689. [CrossRef]
44. Carroll, J.P.; Freedman, W. Nonstationary properties of postural sway. *J. Biomech.* **1993**, *26*, 409–416. [CrossRef]
45. Loughlin, P.J.; Redfern, M.S.; Furman, J.M. Nonstationarities of postural sway. *IEEE Eng. Med. Biol. Mag.* **2003**, *22*, 69–75. [CrossRef] [PubMed]
46. Peng, C.K.; Havlin, S.; Hausdorff, J.M.; Mietus, J.E.; Stanley, H.E.; Goldberger, A.L. Fractal mechanisms and heart rate dynamics. Long-range correlations and their breakdown with disease. *J. Electrocardiol.* **1995**, *28*, 59–65. [CrossRef]
47. Lipsitz, L.A.; Goldberger, A.L. Loss of 'complexity' and aging. Potential applications of fractals and chaos theory to senescence. *JAMA* **1992**, *267*, 1806–1809. [CrossRef] [PubMed]
48. Manor, B.; Costa, M.D.; Hu, K.; Newton, E.; Starobinets, O.; Kang, H.G.; Peng, C.K.; Novak, V.; Lipsitz, L.A. Physiological complexity and system adaptability: Evidence from postural control dynamics of older adults. *J. Appl. Physiol. (1985)* **2010**, *109*, 1786–1791. [CrossRef] [PubMed]
49. Melzer, I.; Oddsson, L.I. Altered characteristics of balance control in obese older adults. *Obes. Res. Clin. Pract.* **2016**, *10*, 151–158. [CrossRef] [PubMed]
50. Dutil, M.; Handrigan, G.A.; Corbeil, P.; Cantin, V.; Simoneau, M.; Teasdale, N.; Hue, O. The impact of obesity on balance control in community-dwelling older women. *Age* **2013**, *35*, 883–890. [CrossRef] [PubMed]
51. Wu, X.; Madigan, M.L. Impaired plantar sensitivity among the obese is associated with increased postural sway. *Neurosci. Lett.* **2014**, *583*, 49–54. [CrossRef] [PubMed]
52. Murray, M.P.; Gardner, G.M.; Mollinger, L.A.; Sepic, S.B. Strength of isometric and isokinetic contractions: Knee muscles of men aged 20 to 86. *Phys. Ther.* **1980**, *60*, 412–419. [CrossRef] [PubMed]
53. Hurley, M.V.; Rees, J.; Newham, D.J. Quadriceps function, proprioceptive acuity and functional performance in healthy young, middle-aged and elderly subjects. *Age Ageing* **1998**, *27*, 55–62. [CrossRef] [PubMed]
54. Duvigneaud, N.; Matton, L.; Wijndaele, K.; Deriemaeker, P.; Lefevre, J.; Philippaerts, R.; Thomis, M.; Delecluse, C.; Duquet, W. Relationship of obesity with physical activity, aerobic fitness and muscle strength in Flemish adults. *J. Sports Med. Phys. Fit.* **2008**, *48*, 201–210.
55. Naugle, K.M.; Higgins, T.J.; Manini, T.M. Obesity and use of compensatory strategies to perform common daily activities in pre-clinically disabled older adults. *Arch. Gerontol. Geriatr.* **2012**, *54*, e134–e138. [CrossRef] [PubMed]
56. Ko, S.; Stenholm, S.; Ferrucci, L. Characteristic gait patterns in older adults with obesity—Results from the Baltimore Longitudinal Study of Aging. *J. Biomech.* **2010**, *43*, 1104–1110. [CrossRef] [PubMed]
57. Messier, S.P.; Legault, C.; Loeser, R.F.; van Arsdale, S.J.; Davis, C.; Ettinger, W.H.; DeVita, P. Does high weight loss in older adults with knee osteoarthritis affect bone-on-bone joint loads and muscle forces during walking? *Osteoarthr. Cartil.* **2011**, *19*, 272–280. [CrossRef] [PubMed]
58. Delmonico, M.J.; Harris, T.B.; Visser, M.; Park, S.W.; Conroy, M.B.; Velasquez-Mieyer, P.; Boudreau, R.; Manini, T.M.; Nevitt, M.; Newman, A.B.; et al. Longitudinal study of muscle strength, quality, and adipose tissue infiltration. *Am. J. Clin. Nutr.* **2009**, *90*, 1579–1585. [PubMed]
59. Rossi-Izquierdo, M.; Santos-Pérez, S.; Faraldo-García, A.; Vaamonde-Sánchez-Andrade, I.; Gayoso-Diz, P.; Del-Río-Valeiras, M.; Lirola-Delgado, A.; Soto-Varela, A. Impact of obesity in elderly patients with postural instability. *Aging Clin. Exp. Res.* **2016**, *28*, 423–428. [CrossRef] [PubMed]

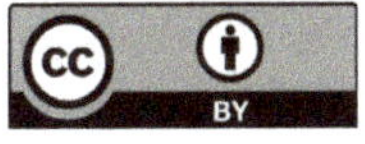

© 2018 by the authors. Licensee MDPI, Basel, Switzerland. This article is an open access article distributed under the terms and conditions of the Creative Commons Attribution (CC BY) license (http://creativecommons.org/licenses/by/4.0/).

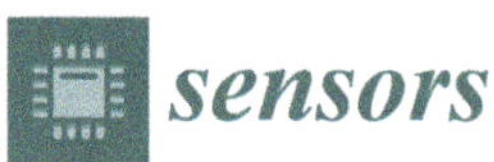 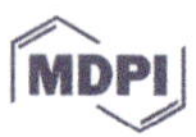

Article

Estimation of Temporal Gait Parameters Using a Human Body Electrostatic Sensing-Based Method

Mengxuan Li, Pengfei Li, Shanshan Tian, Kai Tang and Xi Chen *

State Key Laboratory of Mechatronics Engineering and Control, Beijing Institute of Technology, Beijing 100081, China; formlmx@126.com (M.L.); pfli@bit.edu.cn (P.L.); shanshanbit@126.com (S.T.); tangkai0205@163.com (K.T.)
* Correspondence: chenxi@bit.edu.cn; Tel.: +86-010-6891-8017

Received: 3 April 2018; Accepted: 25 May 2018; Published: 28 May 2018

Abstract: Accurate estimation of gait parameters is essential for obtaining quantitative information on motor deficits in Parkinson's disease and other neurodegenerative diseases, which helps determine disease progression and therapeutic interventions. Due to the demand for high accuracy, unobtrusive measurement methods such as optical motion capture systems, foot pressure plates, and other systems have been commonly used in clinical environments. However, the high cost of existing lab-based methods greatly hinders their wider usage, especially in developing countries. In this study, we present a low-cost, noncontact, and an accurate temporal gait parameters estimation method by sensing and analyzing the electrostatic field generated from human foot stepping. The proposed method achieved an average 97% accuracy on gait phase detection and was further validated by comparison to the foot pressure system in 10 healthy subjects. Two results were compared using the Pearson coefficient r and obtained an excellent consistency ($r = 0.99$, $p < 0.05$). The repeatability of the purposed method was calculated between days by intraclass correlation coefficients (ICC), and showed good test-retest reliability (ICC = 0.87, $p < 0.01$). The proposed method could be an affordable and accurate tool to measure temporal gait parameters in hospital laboratories and in patients' home environments.

Keywords: electrostatic field sensing; gait measurement; temporal parameters

---

1. Introduction

Human gait is a coordinated and rhythmic periodic motion produced by an integrated control of nerve and muscle systems, which is mainly dictated by body features and health conditions. The gait cycle can be defined as the time interval between two initial contacts of the same foot. The initial contact (IC) and separate events (SE) segment the gait cycle into gait phases and provide temporal gait parameters. Temporal gait parameters are essential in many gait analysis applications [1], such as (1) the evaluation of rehabilitation status in patients [2,3]; (2) the recognition of daily life activities [4]; and (3) distinguishing between a normal and pathological gait [5].

The technological devices used to acquire human gait can be classified into two categories: those based on non-wearable sensors and those based on wearable sensors [6]. Non-wearable sensor systems require lab-based facilities where the sensors are located and capture data on the gait while the subject walks on a certain space. Typical representatives of non-wearable sensors systems are the foot pressure plate [7] and the optical motion capture system. They are often used as the gold standard for measuring gait parameters. However, these measurement methods still have a certain degree of limitation when it comes to commercial measurement products, which are generally expensive. For example, the market price of the pressure plate is about $2000. Non-commercial laboratory self-made measurement equipment has relatively complex components such as the walkway in Reference [8]. More than 18,432 sensors arranged under a rubber pad were used for parameter acquisition. They are bulky and only suited to capture human gait in a confined space. The optical motion capture system has the disadvantage of light interference and uses complicated processing algorithms. Furthermore, laboratory settings are unable to represent the daily environment. For this reason, the subject who is performing the test will change their inherent gait rhythm due to the fact that they may feel conditioned by the specialist and the experiment system. The above defects greatly restrict the extensive usage of these methods, especially in developing countries.

In contrast, wearable sensor systems make it possible to analyze data outside the laboratory and capture gait parameters during a person's daily activities. The wearable sensor systems use sensors attached to several parts of the body such as the ankles, knees, or waist. Different types of sensors are used to capture gait signals and extract gait parameters. These include accelerometers [9], gyroscopic sensors [10], electromyography [11], and more. These gait analysis platforms are widely considered to be viable alternatives and are made possible by the recent progress of integrated circuits and sensing technology. The prospect of these sensors is to simplify gait analysis, making it relatively cheaper and no longer constricted to use in a laboratory. Accelerometers and other inertial sensors have been widely used in gait events estimation [12], gait action recognition [13], and gait analysis because they are miniaturized, low powered, durable, inexpensive, highly mobile, and readily available [14–18]. Clearly, low-cost wearable accelerometer sensors can be easily integrated into the acts of daily living and are beneficial for pre-diagnostic and rehabilitation monitoring [19]. With the online gait event detection algorithm embedded into this device, it simplified the analysis and acquisition of the gait parameters. This analysis may include operations such as the segmentation of gait signals into gait cycles, the estimation of temporal gait parameters [20], and the calculation of gait asymmetry, gait variability, and gait stability [21].

However, accelerometers are susceptible to researchers' placement skill and minor variations in the attachment site. The same sensor placed in five anatomical foot locations could obtain different evaluation accuracies of gait parameters [22]. Moreover, installation error will also lead to an inaccuracy of the gait parameter measurement. Unlike accelerometers, careful placement of the sensor on the body segments is not mandatory when using gyroscopic sensors [10]. When using the sensor output of different positions of the tester especially on the shank and thighs, more than 90% of the temporal gait parameters' measurement accuracy can be obtained [23]. However, these wearable sensors share a defect, in that they all require devices to be placed on the subject's body, which may be uncomfortable or obtrusive. Moreover, wireless systems usually store data on SD cards or transmit data through Bluetooth or Zigbee devices to personal computers, which demands a high energy consumption. The most commonly used energy sources are lithium batteries and, if gait is to be monitored over a long period of time, the capacity of the batteries may be a problem.

Due to this background, there is a need for affordable non-wearable and long-time monitoring technologies for gait analysis, which may be capable of continuously monitoring gait parameters during daily activities and reducing the stress and anxiety in testers subjected to gait studies. Such systems can accurately acquire a certain number of gait parameters and identify changes in gait patterns. Due to this, specialists can use the information to predict adverse events and diagnose early symptoms of some specific diseases, which encourages timely medical interventions. Accordingly, these technologies can complement traditional gait analysis systems.

Actually, electrostatic field sensing (EFS) technology may be an effective solution to this problem. The use of a non-contact EFS method for gait measurement has become a hot topic in recent years. In Reference [24], Koichi Kurita measured the electrostatic signals when walking with the electrostatic induction method and a correlation analysis of the gait signals was implemented by combining with the frequency domain information of the signal. We established the human body equivalent capacitance model through theoretical derivation, verified the correctness of the model through simulation, and measured the gait signal [25]. Previous studies on the human body electrostatic sensing method have proven that the gait signal can be obtained by the EFS method. However, no studies have explored how to extract the temporal parameters from the gait signal nor conducted an investigation on the validity and repeatability of this method.

In this study, an algorithm for extracting temporal gait parameters in the EFS gait signal was suggested. The effectiveness of the method was verified by comparison with the results of the foot pressure system. The repeatability of the EFS method was calculated between days by intraclass correlation coefficients (ICC), and showed a good test-retest reliability. The rest of the paper is organized as follows. In Section 2, we present the principle of the EFS method, the details of the system setup, the algorithm, and the data collection procedures. In Section 3, we briefly show the results and the error comparison of two measurement methods. In Section 4, we discuss the results of the validation and repeatability study. The paper is concluded in Section 5, with final remarks and future research directions.

2. Method

2.1. Principle of Electrostatic Field Sensing

The human body becomes charged with static electricity due to the creation of friction between the body and clothing [26–28]. Furthermore, friction, contact, and separation between the human foot and ground during walking also charges the human body [29–31]. The phenomenon of the human body becoming electrically charged leads to a corresponding change in the electric field around the human body with the foot movement during walking [32,33]. Based on this, we established an equivalent capacitance model of the human body and the surrounding environment [25]. When the human body is in a certain space, due to a certain amount of charge on the body, the human body and the surrounding environment produces an equivalent capacitance—including the left and right foot capacitance C_{f1} and C_{f2}—to the ground when standing still and C_{ri} ($i = 1, 2, ...$) between other parts of the human body and the surrounding environment, which together constitute the total capacitance of the human body (Equation (1)), where $C_f = C_{f1} + C_{f2} = 2\varepsilon_s S_s / d_e$. Here, ε_s, S_s, and d_e are the dielectric constant of the shoe sole, the equivalent area of the floor capacitance formed by the shoe sole and ground, and the thickness of the shoe sole. The human body equivalent capacitance model is shown in Figure 1a.

$$C_h = C_f + \sum_{i=1}^{\infty} C_{ri} \tag{1}$$

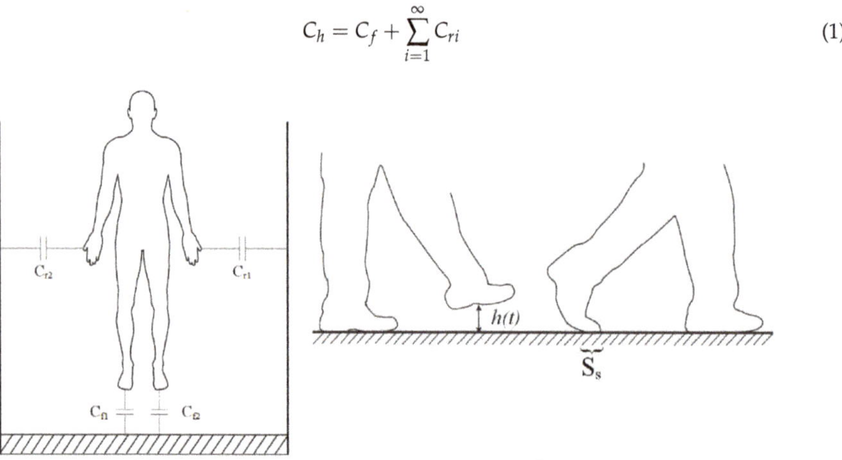

Figure 1. Schematic diagram of the human body movement capacitance model. (**a**) Schematic diagram of the human body equivalent capacitance; (**b**) Foot movement capacitance diagram.

Suppose the human body charge is Q_B and the two feet alternately leave the ground during walking. Then the capacitance between the foot and the ground is equivalent to C_f in series with a capacitance that changes based on the height of the foot from the ground. Although C_f cannot be measured directly, the law of human foot movement can be obtained through the analysis of changes in the induced current because the changes in capacitance caused by human body movement are directly related to the electrostatic induction current signal. Figure 1b shows two typical foot states in the process of the human body walking. In the figure, the height function of the foot from the ground in walking is defined as $h(t)$, the equivalent area function of the plate capacitor formed by the foot and the ground is S_s, and the air dielectric constant is ε_a. The induced potential of the human body can be expressed by the equation below.

$$U_B = Q_B \cdot \frac{\varepsilon_a S_s + h(t)C_f}{C_f \varepsilon_a S_s} \tag{2}$$

Assume the coupling capacitance between the human body and the induction electrode is C. Then, the charge Q induced by the induction electrode can be defined as below.

$$Q = C(U_B - V) \tag{3}$$

where V is the induced potential on the induction electrode. Then, the induced current I flowing through the induction electrode can be deduced from the above equation.

$$I = \frac{dQ}{dt} = C\frac{dU_B}{dt} \propto \frac{1}{S_s}\frac{d}{dt}(h(t)) - \frac{h(t)}{S_s^2}\frac{dS_s}{dt} \tag{4}$$

Here, we assume that the human body is a good conductor. Equation (4) shows that when the tester walks in the vicinity of the induction electrode, the change in the induced current caused by human body movement can be measured under non-contact conditions. The temporal gait parameters can be obtained by analyzing the induced current waveform.

2.2. Instrumentation and Configurations

2.2.1. Electrostatic Field Sensing Measurement Installation

The induced current is generated on the induction electrode when the charged human body moves in the vicinity of the induction electrode of the measurement installation. The induced current is then converted to an observable voltage signal (conversion rate of 10 mV/pA), which is shown in Figure 2 through I–V conversion via the sampling resistor R_s (R_s is 10 GΩ). The voltage signal is then amplified by an operational amplifier (op-amp) for observation. Since the voltage signal obtained by this measurement method is easily disturbed by the power frequency voltage of the grid, we designed a low-pass filter with a cutoff frequency of 20 Hz before the analog-to-digital (A/D) conversion. Subsequently, the analog signal is converted into the digital signal through A/D for data acquisition and processing. The sampling rate adopted in this paper is 1 kHz. The digital signal obtained after A/D sampling is sent to a personal computer for data processing through the 2.4 GHz data transmission module.

EFS is a passive detection method. Its only response is to the changes of the surrounding electric field. The electric field disturbance caused by human foot movement is a low-frequency electric field with a typical frequency of 1~2 Hz. Based on this, we designed a low-pass filter with a cutoff frequency of 20 Hz to eliminate the influence of the high-frequency electric field on our measurement installation. When the measurement installation is carried out in a room with various kinds of measuring instruments and personal computers, the low-pass filter can effectively filter the interference of the high-frequency electric field produced by the electrical apparatus and the frequency of the power grid and can effectively obtain the low-frequency electric field signal produced by human motion.

In order to avoid the influence of other individuals on the electric field tester, it is necessary to ensure that no other personnel walk in the effective measurement range of the measurement installation.

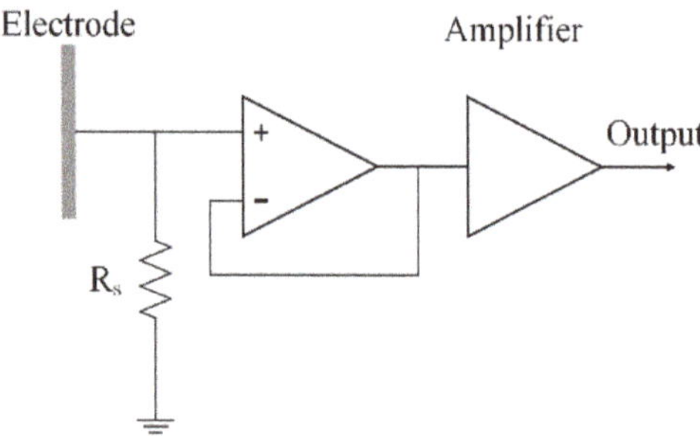

Figure 2. Schematic diagram of the I–V conversion part of the electrostatic measurement installation.

In the experiment, it is observed that the induced current flowing through the induction electrode is inversely proportional to the distance between the human body and the induction electrode. After repeated adjustment of the measurement installation sensitivity, the effective measurement distance of installation was adjusted to 3 m so that it can effectively measure the human body gait electrostatic signal without electric field interference by external equipment. In addition, the intensity of the induced current is related to the angle between the human body and the induction plate. The test results show that when the coronal plane of the human body is parallel to the electrode, the induced current is at a maximum level, as shown in Figure 3a. The induced current signal will be weakened when the angle between the human body and the induction plate changes, but the reduced amplitude change is not significant. A diagram illustrating the electrostatic measurement installation is shown in Figure 3a. The prototype of the electrostatic measurement installation is shown in Figure 3b.

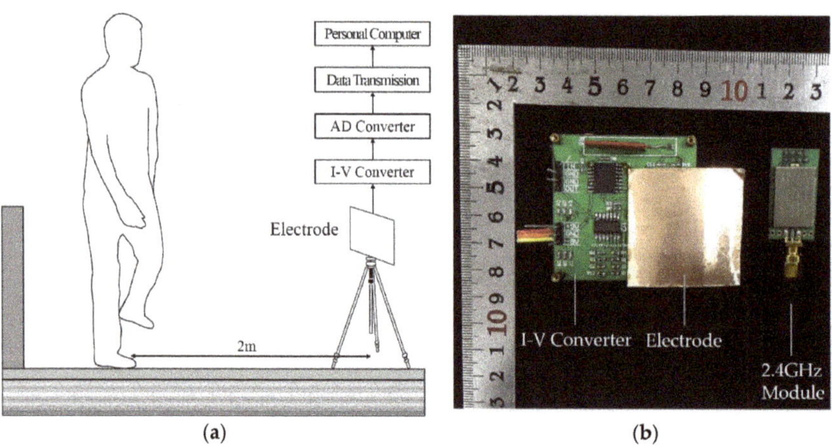

Figure 3. Illustration diagram and prototype of electrostatic measurement installation. (**a**) Illustration diagram of electrostatic measurement installation; (**b**) prototype of electrostatic measurement installation.

2.2.2. Foot Pressure Measurement System

In the design in Reference [34], we established a foot pressure system using two FSR406 pressure sensors of Interlink Electronics. This sensor features a low thickness (<0.05 inches), high dynamic response speed, insensitivity to temperature changes, resistance to high overload, and other advantageous characteristics.

Two pressure sensors with an effective area of 1.5 inches × 1.5 inches are fixed to the bottom of the insoles with medical tape and the insoles are cut from the transparent folder according to the foot bottom contour. One of the sensors is fixed in the front of the insole and roughly positioned under the toes while the other sensor is fixed in the rear part of the insole and roughly positioned under the heel. The two pressure sensors are connected in parallel and are actually used as a single pressure sensor. The system is powered by a 5 V battery. The two sensors are connected in series with the divider resistance and the changes in voltage values caused by pressure change are amplified by the operational amplifier before output. Experimental results show that the signal output is in the range of 0~2.5 V. The conditioning circuit together with the battery is fixed on the tester's legs. The signal output after A/D conversion is sent to a personal computer for data processing with a 2.4 GHz data transmission module.

2.3. Algorithm Development

2.3.1. Pressure-Based Foot Events Calculation Algorithm

The algorithm employed to determine the initial contact and separate events of the gait is divided into three steps. Since the pressure sensor output voltage is proportional to the foot pressure, we first determine the pressure time zone when the human foot is in the stance phase using the output voltage threshold. Afterward, we search for the minimum pressure signal near the threshold point, which is an important reference for determining the initial contact and separate events of the gait. Lastly, the time point determined in the previous step is compensated to determine the final contact and separation moments. The specific algorithm is described as follows. (1) Determine the time zone of the gait stance phase according to the rising and falling edges of the signal. The monotonically increasing signal above the fixed threshold can be determined as a rising edge and the monotonically reducing signal below the fixed threshold can be determined as a falling edge. In this paper, the threshold selected is 1 V, which is much smaller than the full load output of the pressure sensor when the foot fully contacts the ground and is much larger than the no load output; (2) Find out the minimum value of the signal in the rising and falling edges of the signal. With the human body walking movement, the output value of the pressure sensor under no load may drift. Therefore, we cannot use a fixed output value as the standard by which one can judge a moment. To find out the minimum value, we can derive the signal and find out the zero point from the peak point of the derivative, as shown in Figure 4b; (3) Lastly, the contact and separation moments are corrected by the local minimum point of the signal. The specific offset is 3% of the difference between the local maximum value and the local minimum value of the voltage signal in a gait cycle, and the local minimum point obtained in the previous step is shifted. The signal output, its derivative, and local minimum values, as well as the gait contact and separation moments determined by the offset during a test, are shown in Figure 4.

2.3.2. Electrostatic Signal-Based Foot Events Calculation Algorithm

In one test process, the time-domain waveform obtained by the electrostatic sensing system is shown in Figure 5.

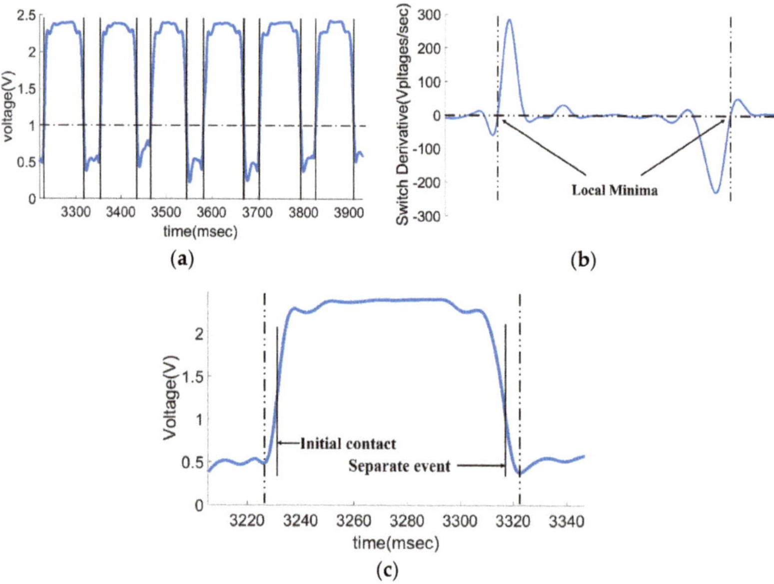

Figure 4. The process extracting the start and end moments of the support phase from the data measured by the foot pressure test system. (**a**) Pressure data time-domain waveform measured at normal speed by the foot pressure system as well as the rising edge and the falling edge of the signal from the threshold judgment; (**b**) signal local minimum point determined through the derivation of the signal in one cycle; (**c**) the initial contact and separate event of the gait cycle obtained by offsetting the minimum point.

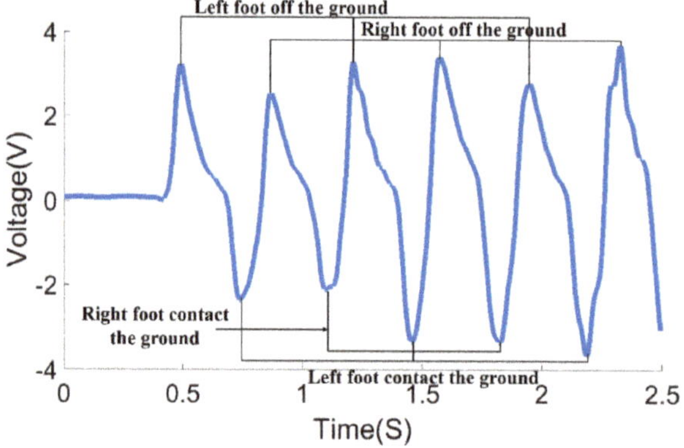

Figure 5. Time-domain waveform of electrostatic sensing signal.

Figure 5 shows the changes in body potential as the human body comes in contact with and is separated from the ground during stepping movements. The time-domain waveform includes the time parameters during the stepping movement. It can be determined using Equation (4) that the denominator of the left term is S_s and the denominator of the right term is S_s^2. Therefore, the right-hand term affects slightly more than the induced current I and the left-hand term mainly affects the induced current I. For example, when the right foot toe is about to leave the ground, the equivalent area S_s between the sole and the ground decreases. The distance $h(t)$ between the right foot and the ground increases, so the induced current through the induction electrode increases when the right foot leaves the ground. The rate of change of $h(t)$ is at the maximum level and the electrostatic signal reaches the local maximum level. Therefore, the results are consistent with the forecast from Equation (4). Subsequently, the induced current decreases as the lifting speed slows down. In the latter part of the swing phase, $h(t)$ decreases rapidly and leads to the decrease of the induced current, which is consistent with the prediction made by the left side of Equation (4). The equivalent area S_s of the heel contact area increases, which results in a rapid decrease in the induced current. Therefore, Equation (4) can effectively describe the variation trend of the induced current obtained on the induction electrode during the step process. The peak of the time-domain waveform of the electrostatic signal coincides with the moments when the foot separates from the initial contact with the ground. The moments of foot separation from and initial contact with the ground can be obtained by extracting the corresponding peak information.

2.4. Subjects

The current study was approved by the institutional academic board. A total of 10 testers participated in the gait measurement (seven are male and three are female). They have an average weight of 64.8 kg (weight range: 45~77 kg), and an average height of 1.7 m (height range: 1.58~1.79 m). Exclusion criteria included neurological or lower extremities conditions, respiratory or cardiovascular problems, insanity or mental disorder, and pregnancy. All subjects were informed of the purpose as well as the methods and instructions to complete the experiment measuring temporal gait parameters and all subjects signed informed consent paperwork.

2.5. Experimental Conditions

In the experiment, the insoles carrying the foot pressure system were placed under the right foot of the testers. The battery and conditioning circuit were fixed to the middle of the calf using the elastic band and the testers wore their own shoes to ensure the most natural movement. At the same time, the testers needed to keep the coronal plane parallel to the electrostatic induction electrode (shown in Figure 3) during walking. Testers were required to carry out the stepping movement at a slow, normal, and fast pace. An electronic metronome was used to assist testers in completing this process. In the course of the experiment, the testers were required to implement each type of pace continuously for at least 20 s in order to collect enough gait data. Since the human body needs to have an adjustment period before entering a steady step, 2 s at the beginning and 2 s at the end of each data point were removed to ensure data validity. Lastly, 300 valid gait cycle data were obtained from the EFS installation and the foot pressure system. At the same time, to rule out the effect of temperature and humidity on the electrostatic sensing method, the whole experiment was carried out at a laboratory temperature of 25 °C and relative humidity (RH) of 55%.

2.6. Analysis

The concurrent validity of temporal gait parameters obtained by the EFS method and by the foot pressure system was assessed using Pearson correlation coefficients. In addition, intraclass correlation coefficients (ICC) (2,1) (two-way random effect, single measure model) were used to assess the test-retest reliability of the temporal gait parameters obtained by the electrostatic sensing method between day 1 and day 8. All analyses were conducted with $p < 0.05$ as the significance level and performed using SPSS Version20.0 (IBM Corporation, Armonk, NY, USA). For the Pearson coefficient r, an excellent relationship was considered if r was greater than 0.90, a good relationship if r was between 0.8 and 0.89, a fair relationship if r was between 0.7 and 0.79, and a poor relationship if r was below 0.70 [35]. Regarding the ICC, it was considered excellent if the ICC was greater than 0.90, good if the ICC was between 0.75 and 0.90, moderate if the ICC was between 0.50 and 0.75, and poor if the ICC was below 0.50. The data processing and the algorithms were implemented in Matlab (R2016b, MathWorks Inc., Natick, MA, USA).

3. Results

According to the principle in Section 2.3, we utilized Matlab to process the data from the foot pressure system and the EFS method. We extracted the initial contact (IC) and separate events (SE) according to the proposed algorithm. The measurement error of the EFS method was verified with the date measured by the foot pressure system. Data analysis showed that, in the judgment of initial contact (IC) with the ground, the measurement error of the EFS method is in the range of ±40 ms (mean value: -1.5 ± 15 ms). In the judgment of separate events (SE) from the ground, the measurement error of the EFS method is also within ±40 ms (mean value: -1.3 ± 15 ms).

We counted the difference between moments obtained by the EFS method and the foot pressure system in 300 cycles of 10 testers, the statistical histogram of which is shown in Figure 6a,b.

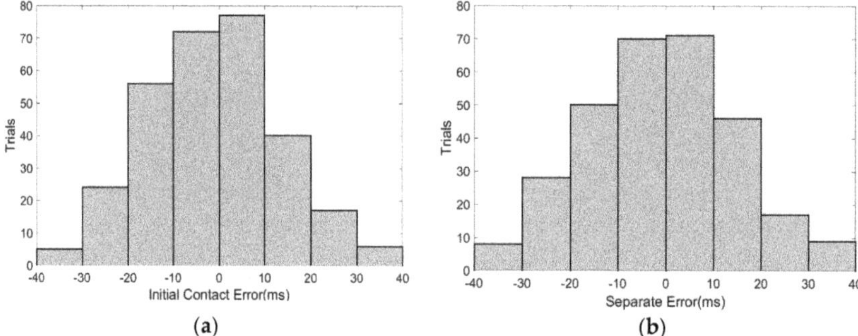

Figure 6. Measurement error of the moments of foot contact with and separation from the ground by the electrostatic field sensing (EFS) method. (**a**) Initial contact (IC) error statistical histogram; (**b**) separate events (SE) error statistical histogram.

Once gait events are identified, gait cycle (T_g), stance phase duration (T_s), swing phase duration (T_w), and gait cadence (C) can be calculated, as shown in Equations (5)–(8).

$$T_g = IC(m+1) - IC(m) \tag{5}$$

$$T_s = SE(n) - IC(m) \tag{6}$$

$$T_w = IC(m+1) - SE(n) = T_g - T_s \tag{7}$$

$$C = \frac{60}{T_g} \times 2 \quad (\text{Steps/Min}) \tag{8}$$

The ratio of T_s over T_g (R_S) and the ratio of T_w over T_g (R_W) are then computed. These ratios should represent approximately 60% of the stance phase duration ($R_S \approx 60\%$) and 40% of the swing phase duration ($R_W \approx 40\%$) if a person has a healthy gait.

Therefore, the gait cycle (T_g) of 10 testers at three different motion speeds are calculated and counted. The gait cycle (T_g) measured by the foot pressure system during high-speed, normal-speed, and slow-speed movement are 990 ± 120 ms (range: 870~1153 ms), 1198 ± 110 ms (range 1088~1398 ms), and 1498 ± 75 ms (range: 1358~1697 ms), respectively. The gait cycle derived from the 10 testers is illustrated separately in Figure 7.

We measured the error of the EFS method in the gait cycle (T_g) measurement with the foot pressure system. The error and the error percentage during high-speed, normal-speed, and low-speed movement are -0.2 ± 18 ms (range of ±45 ms) and $0.05 \pm 2\%$ (range of $\pm4\%$), 0.3 ± 18 ms (range ±39 ms) and $0.04 \pm 2\%$ (range of $\pm3\%$), and 1 ± 13 ms (range of ±30 ms) and $0.07 \pm 1\%$ (range of $\pm2\%$), respectively. This showed an average accuracy rate of 97%.

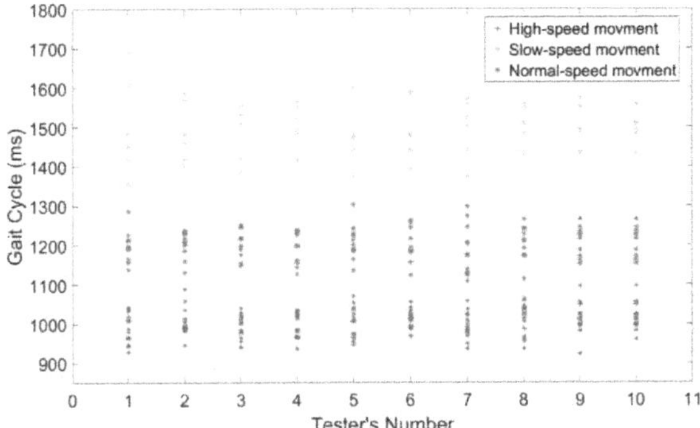

Figure 7. Gait cycle of the 10 testers.

The EFS-derived estimate of the gait cycle (T_g) agreed with the foot pressure system over the entire range of walking rates (see Figure 8). The two estimates of the gait cycle (T_g) were strongly correlated (Pearson's correlation coefficient $r = 0.99$). This confirmed the high reliability of the electrostatic sensing-based estimate of the gait cycle.

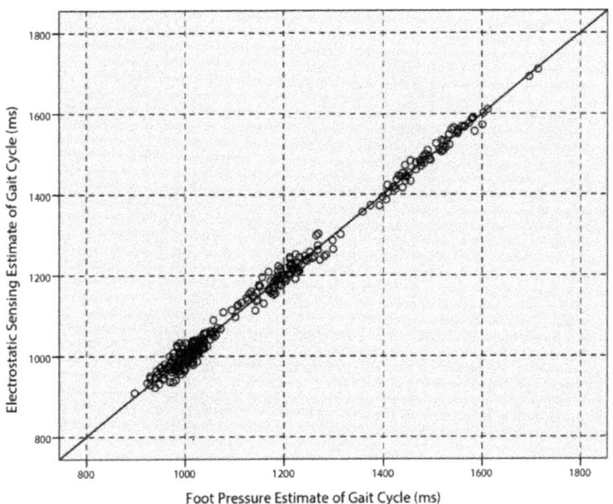

Figure 8. Gait cycle (T_g) obtained by the EFS method and the foot pressure system.

Table 1 shows the statistical results of the electrostatic field sensing (EFS) method and the foot pressure system of the other three temporal gait parameters. The concurrent validity of the EFS method and the foot pressure system showed that the two methods obtained excellent correlation in these three gait parameters.

Apart from these results, further validation showed that the average R_S for the EFS method is $60.49 \pm 2.45\%$. This value is in accordance with the norm gait parameters in which the stance phase lasts approximately 60% of the gait cycle for healthy individuals. Based on these results, it can be deduced that the proposed method can accurately determine temporal gait parameters.

Table 1. The statistical results of the EFS method and the foot pressure system with the Pearson coefficient value of three gait parameters ($p < 0.05$).

Gait Parameters	EFS Result	Foot Pressure Result	Pearson Coefficient r
Stance phase duration (T_s)	741.83 ± 117.97	775.03 ± 125.68	0.98
Swing phase duration (T_w)	431.32 ± 94.12	396.58 ± 94.10	0.99
Gait cadence (C)	102.53 ± 15.34	102.66 ± 15.42	0.99

The test-retest reliability of the EFS method on the first and eighth days shows that the ICC is 0.87 ($p < 0.001$). The scatter plot of the gait cycle measured using the EFS method for the first day and the eighth day is shown in Figure 9. The ICC values of the remaining gait parameters are illustrated in Table 2.

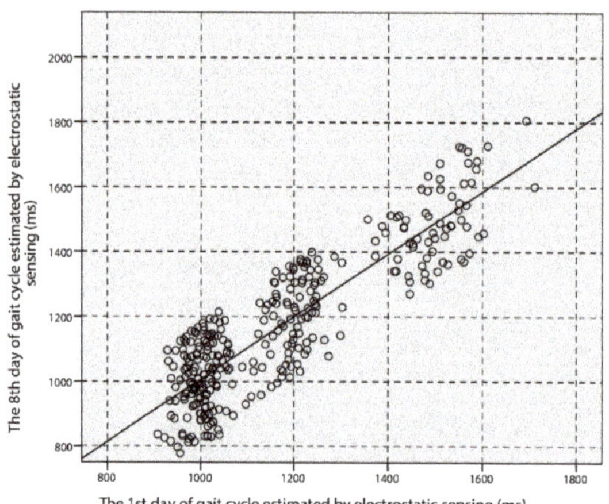

Figure 9. EFS method estimation of the gait cycle for day 1 and day 8.

Table 2. The statistical results of the EFS method results on the first and eighth days as well as the intraclass correlation coefficient (ICC) values of gait parameters.

Gait Parameters	Day 1	Day 8	ICC	p
Stance phase duration (T_s)	741.83 ± 117.97	805.56 ± 120.64	0.86	<0.001
Swing phase duration (T_w)	431.32 ± 94.12	458.79 ± 102.35	0.87	<0.001
Gait cadence (C)	102.53 ± 15.34	95.23 ± 16.49	0.85	<0.001

4. Discussions

Most existing gait event measurement methods rely on mechanical or kinetic parameters derived from an optical motion capture system and force plate. However, these devices rely on professional analyses to obtain gait parameters and can only operate in a confined space. These methods also require testers to control walking speeds and step length to ensure that the subject's foot always comes in contact with the force plate. Data obtained from these methods cannot be fully reflected in a natural human gait. On the other hand, wearable sensors can meet gait measurement needs under non-laboratory conditions. However, they all require placing sensors on the subject's body, which may be uncomfortable or obtrusive. Therefore, a low-cost, non-wearable EFS method can be a promising alternative for monitoring and determining gait temporal parameters of individuals outside the laboratory environment.

Previous research [25,33] employed the EFS method to detect sports motion signals and presented a method to recognize the moments of foot contact with a separation from the ground. However, the study of extracting temporal gait parameters forming the FES signal has not been explored. In addition, the credibility and test-retest repeatability of this method has not been verified. An algorithm for extracting temporal gait parameters from gait EFS signals was presented in this paper. The measuring error of the EFS method was calibrated with the foot pressure system. The study results showed that temporal gait parameters could be identified through EFS signals in the stepping gait and two important gait cycle parameters (initial contact and separate event) could be detected with high accuracy. Based on these detected results, six types of temporal gait parameters were calculated. These calculated parameters fit well with the results measured by the foot pressure system.

Our proposed EFS method manifested excellent correlation coefficients to the foot pressure system's results ($r = 0.99$, $p < 0.05$) and test-retest reliability (ICC = 0.87, $p < 0.001$) across an eight-day test-retest interval. These results indicate that the suggested EFS method may be a reliable measure of temporal gait parameters.

Kluge et al. employed an inertial measurement system to evaluate temporal gait parameters [36]. Two Shimmer3 sensors, which contained a three-axis gyroscope and a three-axis accelerometer worn only on the feet, obtained the temporal gait parameters. A state-of-the-art algorithm was used to extract the temporal gait parameters. The concurrent validity of the proposed system was compared with an external camera-based system. Even though their method obtained satisfactory precision in measuring stride time, the error was 5.4% when measuring the stance time. Contrary to the results of Kluge et al., our method has an average of 3% error in measuring stance time, which shows better measurement accuracy. Moreover, the method by Kluge et al. is a contact measuring system, which may reduce the comfort of the tester.

Cheng et al. used a wearable microphone-sensor-based system to collect footstep sound signals during walking [37]. Based on this system, a gait analysis algorithm was proposed for estimating the temporal parameters of gait. Although the purposed method used a non-contact acoustic signal detection method, the ambient sound noise and sound delay affected the measurement accuracy. The results showed that only 94.52% of the average accuracy could be obtained when measuring initial contact. In addition, although a non-contact microphone sensor was used, the tester still was required to wear the measurement system when testing. Our method uses the variable electrostatic field information to obtain the gait signal, which has a higher signal-to-noise ratio with a smaller time delay.

Yong developed a low-cost wearable wireless ultrasonic sensor system for estimating three-dimensional displacement to extract temporal gait parameters [38]. The lightweight and miniaturized sensor design could make the patient more unconstrained. Their system had only 3% measurement error when measuring the stride duration, which basically is the same accuracy as that achieved with our electrostatic sensing method. However, this ultrasonic-based gait parameter measurement method relied on a complex signal processing algorithm and lacked a visual representation of the gait signal. In our study, the induced current signal is strongly correlated with the gait and the algorithm for extracting the temporal gait parameters is simple.

The results showed that the EFS method can accurately measure the initial and separate events of walking as well as effectively obtain temporal gait parameters. The limitation of this study is that we only used a single sensor to estimate gait parameters. A single sensor has a certain effective measurement range and cannot capture gait parameters beyond the effective measurement range. The present algorithm can only analyze a single tester's gait data and cannot analyze the gait data of multiple testers in the effective measurement range simultaneously. Moreover, we lack gait data of real neurological patients. However, if the patient is able to completely lift his feet off the ground in the gait cycle, our method could capture gait events and then calculate the gait parameters. The differences between gait parameters could be used to diagnose related neurological diseases.

Despite this limitation, our low-cost, wireless, non-wearable method and estimation algorithm were proven to be effective and valuable for calculating temporal gait parameters.

With the rise of telemedicine, medical measurement systems will lead to major change. Clinicians and researchers are working toward long-distance measurement methods to monitor human gait parameters and provide remote diagnosis and guidance. This method could assist health professionals to monitor patients' behavior and prescribe corrective action when performing their activities of daily living. Although the method presented in this article is capable of detecting several gait parameters, we will also investigate the potential of expanding this method to extract more gait information or automatically start the measurement to complete the data capture and gait analysis when the patients enter the effective sensing area.

5. Conclusions

In this study, we presented a temporal gait parameters estimation method based on EFS, which uses human walking-generated electrostatic field information. For the first time, the temporal gait parameters were obtained based on electrostatic field sensing. By comparing the results with those obtained by a foot pressure system, the validity and test-retest reliability were verified. Due to the advantages of non-wearable, low-cost, long-term uninterrupted measurement, the proposed method could provide an affordable and accurate tool for conducting human gait parameters measurement in clinical laboratories and patients' home environments.

Author Contributions: M.L. designed the algorithm, performed the experiments, and analyzed and wrote the corresponding paragraphs. X.C. and P.L. initiated and supervised the entire research project. K.T. and S.T. analyzed the data. M.L. and X.C. drafted and revised the manuscript. All the authors read and approved the final version of the manuscript.

Acknowledgments: This work was financially supported by grants from National Natural Science Foundation of China (#51407009, #51777010, #51707008, #U1630130).

Conflicts of Interest: The authors declare no conflict of interest.

References

1. Mohammed, S.; Samé, A.; Oukhellou, L.; Kong, K.; Huo, W.; Amirat, Y. Recognition of gait cycle phases using wearable sensors. *Rob. Auton. Syst.* **2016**, *75*, 50–59. [CrossRef]
2. Tunca, C.; Pehlivan, N.; Ak, N.; Arnrich, B.; Salur, G.; Ersoy, C. Inertial sensor-based robust gait analysis in non-hospital settings for neurological disorders. *Sensors (Switzerland)* **2017**, *17*, 825. [CrossRef] [PubMed]
3. Alaqtash, M.; Yu, H.; Brower, R.; Abdelgawad, A.; Sarkodie-Gyan, T. Application of wearable sensors for human gait analysis using fuzzy computational algorithm. *Eng. Appl. Artif. Intell.* **2011**, *24*, 1018–1025. [CrossRef]
4. Mannini, A.; Sabatini, A.M. Gait phase detection and discrimination between walking-jogging activities using hidden Markov models applied to foot motion data from a gyroscope. *Gait Posture* **2012**, *36*, 657–661. [CrossRef] [PubMed]
5. Mariani, B.; Rouhani, H.; Crevoisier, X.; Aminian, K. Quantitative estimation of foot-flat and stance phase of gait using foot-worn inertial sensors. *Gait Posture* **2013**, *37*, 229–234. [CrossRef] [PubMed]
6. Muro-de-la-Herran, A.; García-Zapirain, B.; Méndez-Zorrilla, A. Gait analysis methods: An overview of wearable and non-wearable systems, highlighting clinical applications. *Sensors (Switzerland)* **2014**, *14*, 3362–3394. [CrossRef] [PubMed]
7. Abdul Razak, A.H.; Zayegh, A.; Begg, R.K.; Wahab, Y. Foot plantar pressure measurement system: A review. *Sensors (Switzerland)* **2012**, *12*, 9884–9912. [CrossRef] [PubMed]
8. Wearing, S.C.; Reed, L.F.; Urry, S.R. Agreement between temporal and spatial gait parameters from an instrumented walkway and treadmill system at matched walking speed. *Gait Posture* **2013**, *38*, 380–384. [CrossRef] [PubMed]
9. González, I.; Fontecha, J.; Hervás, R.; Bravo, J. Estimation of Temporal Gait Events from a Single Accelerometer through the Scale-Space Filtering Idea. *J. Med. Syst.* **2016**, *40*, 1–10. [CrossRef] [PubMed]

10. Gouwanda, D.; Gopalai, A.A.; Khoo, B.H. A Low Cost Alternative to Monitor Human Gait Temporal Parameters-Wearable Wireless Gyroscope. *IEEE Sens. J.* **2016**, *16*, 9029–9035. [CrossRef]

11. Wentink, E.C.; Schut, V.G.H.; Prinsen, E.C.; Rietman, J.S.; Veltink, P.H. Detection of the onset of gait initiation using kinematic sensors and EMG in transfemoral amputees. *Gait Posture* **2014**, *39*, 391–396. [CrossRef] [PubMed]

12. Boutaayamou, M.; Denoël, V.; Brüls, O.; Demonceau, M.; Maquet, D.; Forthomme, B.; Croisier, J.L.; Schwartz, C.; Verly, J.G.; Garraux, G. Algorithm for Temporal Gait Analysis Using Wireless Foot-Mounted Accelerometers. In *International Joint Conference on Biomedical Engineering Systems and Technologies*; Springer: Cham, Switzerland, 2016; pp. 236–254.

13. Ngo, T.T.; Makihara, Y.; Mukaigawa, Y.; Mukaigawa, Y.; Yagi, Y. Similar gait action recognition using an inertial sensor. *Pattern Recognit.* **2015**, *48*, 1289–1301. [CrossRef]

14. Washabaugh, E.P.; Kalyanaraman, T.; Adamczyk, P.G.; Claflin, E.S.; Krishnan, C. Validity and repeatability of inertial measurement units for measuring gait parameters. *Gait Posture* **2017**, *55*, 87–93. [CrossRef] [PubMed]

15. González, I.; López-Nava, I.H.; Fontecha, J.; Muñoz-Meléndez, A.; Pérez-SanPablo, A.I.; Quiñones-Urióstegui, I. Comparison between passive vision-based system and a wearable inertial-based system for estimating temporal gait parameters related to the GAITRite electronic walkway. *J. Biomed. Inform.* **2016**, *62*, 210–223. [CrossRef] [PubMed]

16. Caldas, R.; Mundt, M.; Potthast, W.; Buarque de Lima Neto, F.; Markert, B. A systematic review of gait analysis methods based on inertial sensors and adaptive algorithms. *Gait Posture* **2017**, *57*, 204–210. [CrossRef] [PubMed]

17. Bötzel, K.; Marti, F.M.; Rodríguez, M.Á.C.; Plate, A.; Vicente, A.O. Gait recording with inertial sensors—How to determine initial and terminal contact. *J. Biomech.* **2016**, *49*, 332–337. [CrossRef] [PubMed]

18. Khandelwal, S.; Wickström, N. Novel methodology for estimating Initial Contact events from accelerometers positioned at different body locations. *Gait Posture* **2018**, *59*, 278–285. [CrossRef] [PubMed]

19. Mertz, L. Convergence Revolution Comes to Wearables: Multiple Advances are Taking Biosensor Networks to the Next Level in Health Care. *IEEE Pulse* **2016**, *7*, 13–17. [CrossRef] [PubMed]

20. Yang, S.; Zhang, J.T.; Novak, A.C.; Brouwer, B.; Li, Q. Estimation of spatio-temporal parameters for post-stroke hemiparetic gait using inertial sensors. *Gait Posture* **2013**, *37*, 354–358. [CrossRef] [PubMed]

21. Toebes, M.J.; Hoozemans, M.J.; Furrer, R.; Dekker, J.; van Dieën, J.H. Associations between measures of gait stability, leg strength and fear of falling. *Gait Posture* **2015**, *41*, 76–80. [CrossRef] [PubMed]

22. Anwary, A.R.; Yu, H.; Vassallo, M. Optimal Foot Location for Placing Wearable IMU Sensors and Automatic Feature Extraction for Gait Analysis. *IEEE Sens. J.* **2018**, *18*, 2555–2567. [CrossRef]

23. Taborri, J.; Palermo, E.; Rossi, S.; Cappa, P. Gait partitioning methods: A systematic review. *Sensors (Switzerland)* **2016**, *16*, 66. [CrossRef] [PubMed]

24. Kurita, K.; Fujii, Y.; Shimada, K. A new technique for touch sensing based on measurement of current generated by electrostatic induction. *Sens. Actuators A Phys.* **2011**, *170*, 66–71. [CrossRef]

25. Chen, X.; Zheng, Z.; Cui, Z.; Zheng, W. A novel remote sensing technique for recognizing human gait based on the measurement of induced electrostatic current. *J. Electrostat.* **2012**, *70*, 105–110. [CrossRef]

26. Chubb, J.N. A Standard proposed for assessing the electrostatic suitability of materials. *J. Electrostat.* **2007**, *65*, 607–610. [CrossRef]

27. Castle, G.S.P. Contact charging between insulators. *J. Electrostat.* **1997**, *40–41*, 13–20. [CrossRef]

28. Watanabe, H.; Ghadiri, M.; Matsuyama, T.; Long Ding, Y.; Pitt, K.G. New instrument for tribocharge measurement due to single particle impacts. *Rev. Sci. Instrum.* **2007**, *78*. [CrossRef]

29. Gady, B.; Schleef, D.; Reifenberger, R.; Rimai, D.; DeMejo, L. Identification of electrostatic and van der Waals interaction forces between a micrometer-size sphere and a flat substrate. *Phys. Rev. B* **1996**, *53*, 8065–8070. [CrossRef]

30. Forward, K.M.; Lacks, D.J.; Sankaran, R.M. Charge segregation depends on particle size in triboelectrically charged granular materials. *Phys. Rev. Lett.* **2009**, *102*, 1–4. [CrossRef] [PubMed]

31. Ficker, T. Charging by walking. *J. Phys. D Appl. Phys.* **2006**, *39*, 410. [CrossRef]

32. Kurita, K.; Ueta, S. A new motion control method for bipedal robot based on noncontact and nonattached human motion sensing technique. *IEEE Trans. Ind. Appl.* **2011**, *47*, 1022–1027. [CrossRef]

33. Kurita, K. Novel non-contact and non-attached technique for detecting sports motion. *Meas. J. Int. Meas. Confed.* **2011**, *44*, 1361–1366. [CrossRef]

Sensors **2018**, *18*, 1737

34. Hausdorff, J.M.; Ladin, Z.; Wei, J.Y. Footswitch system for measurement of the temporal parameters of gait. *J. Biomech.* **1995**, *28*, 347–351. [CrossRef]
35. Zhu, M.; Huang, Z.; Ma, C.; Li, Y. An objective balance error scoring system for sideline concussion evaluation using duplex kinect sensors. *Sensors (Switzerland)* **2017**, *17*, 2398. [CrossRef] [PubMed]
36. Kluge, F.; Gaßner, H.; Hannink, J.; Pasluosta, C.; Klucken, J.; Eskofier, B.M. Towards mobile gait analysis: Concurrent validity and test-retest reliability of an inertial measurement system for the assessment of spatio-temporal gait parameters. *Sensors (Switzerland)* **2017**, *17*, 1522. [CrossRef] [PubMed]
37. Wang, C.; Wang, X.; Long, Z.; Yuan, J.; Qian, Y.; Li, J. Estimation of temporal gait parameters using a wearable microphone-sensor-based system. *Sensors (Switzerland)* **2016**, *16*, 2167. [CrossRef] [PubMed]
38. Qi, Y.; Soh, C.B.; Gunawan, E.; Low, K.S.; Thomas, R. Estimation of spatial-temporal gait parameters using a low-cost ultrasonic motion analysis system. *Sensors (Switzerland)* **2014**, *14*, 15371–15386. [CrossRef] [PubMed]

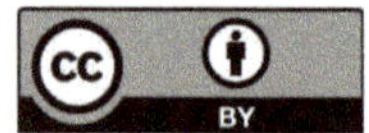

© 2018 by the authors. Licensee MDPI, Basel, Switzerland. This article is an open access article distributed under the terms and conditions of the Creative Commons Attribution (CC BY) license (http://creativecommons.org/licenses/by/4.0/).

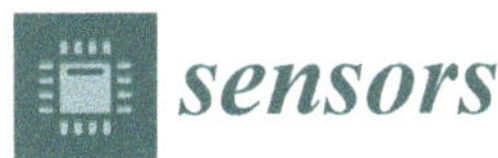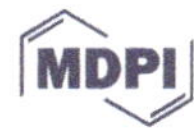

Article

Toward Smart Footwear to Track Frailty Phenotypes—Using Propulsion Performance to Determine Frailty

Hadi Rahemi [1,2,†], **Hung Nguyen** [1,†], **Hyoki Lee** [1,3] and **Bijan Najafi** [1,*]

1   Interdisciplinary Consortium on Advanced Motion Performance (iCAMP), Michael E. DeBakey Department of Surgery, Baylor College of Medicine, Houston, TX 77030, USA; rahemi@circulationconcepts.com (H.R.); hung.nguyen@bcm.edu (H.N.); Lee.hyoki@gmail.com (H.L.)
2   Circulation Concepts Inc., Houston, TX 77030, USA
3   BioSensics LLC, Watertown, MA 02472, USA
*   Correspondence: Najafi.Bijan@gmail.com; Tel.: +1-713-798-7536
†   These authors contributed equally to the manuscript.

Received: 31 March 2018; Accepted: 25 May 2018; Published: 1 June 2018

Abstract: Frailty assessment is dependent on the availability of trained personnel and it is currently limited to clinic and supervised setting. The growing aging population has made it necessary to find phenotypes of frailty that can be measured in an unsupervised setting for translational application in continuous, remote, and in-place monitoring during daily living activity, such as walking. We analyzed gait performance of 161 older adults using a shin-worn inertial sensor to investigate the feasibility of developing a foot-worn sensor to assess frailty. Sensor-derived gait parameters were extracted and modeled to distinguish different frailty stages, including non-frail, pre-frail, and frail, as determined by Fried Criteria. An artificial neural network model was implemented to evaluate the accuracy of an algorithm using a proposed set of gait parameters in predicting frailty stages. Changes in discriminating power was compared between sensor data extracted from the left and right shin sensor. The aim was to investigate the feasibility of developing a foot-worn sensor to assess frailty. The results yielded a highly accurate model in predicting frailty stages, irrespective of sensor location. The independent predictors of frailty stages were propulsion duration and acceleration, heel-off and toe-off speed, mid stance and mid swing speed, and speed norm. The proposed model enables discriminating different frailty stages with area under curve ranging between 83.2–95.8%. Furthermore, results from the neural network suggest the potential of developing a single-shin worn sensor that would be ideal for unsupervised application and footwear integration for continuous monitoring during walking.

Keywords: frailty; gait; artificial neural network; propulsion; aging; wearable sensor; walking; smart footwear

---

1. Introduction

By 2060, it is predicted that 1 in 4 Americans will be over 65 or older [1]. The surge of the aging population could be medically translated into an increase in geriatric condition and syndromes, such as frailty. Frailty syndrome is the loss in physiological reserve of a person and it is highly prevalent in older population. It has been shown to be an indicator of increased fall risk in older adults [2–4], a predictor of adverse outcomes of medical intervention [5–8], and it is associated with reduced quality of life [9]. Furthermore, frailty may result in an increase in healthcare cost with higher readmission cost and more specialist and emergency visits [10].

In recent years, multiple tools have been developed to capture age-related markers that might be indicators of decreased physiological reserve and diminished resistance to stressors [11,12].

For example, Fried et al. [13] initially hypothesized five frailty phenotypes, including shrinking, weakness, slowness, exhaustion, and low activity. Using these phenotypes, they then categorized an individual as either non-frail (zero phenotype is present), pre-frail (one or two phenotypes are present), or frail (three or more phenotypes are present). These phenotypes were then validated through a Cardiovascular Health Study [13], with cohorts of over five thousand participants that were followed over a seven-year period. This frailty classification was developed and recognized as "Fried Criteria" or "Frailty Phenotypes" and has been widely used to assess frailty in clinical setting. However, one of the drawbacks of the Fried Criteria is that some of the criteria are based on self-report (e.g., exhaustion, low activity, and shrinking); therefore, it is semi-objective and it requires trained personnel to conduct the assessment, especially when evaluating patients with cognitive impairment. Furthermore, since assessment using Fried Criteria provides categorical values to describe frailty, its sensitivity to ascertain the effectiveness of any intervention (e.g., nutrition, exercise, etc.), side effects of an intervention (e.g., medication, frailty induced by offloading boot, etc.), or frailty trajectories over time is limited [14,15].

Recent studies have suggested that gait speed is the strongest indicator to predict adverse outcomes, such as mobility disability, falls, or hospitalization, as described in a systematic review by Schwenk et al. [16]. Despite this fact, little efforts have been done to extract other gait related parameters that could describe different frailty phenotypes. Recently, there has been an increase in the utility of using wearable inertial sensors, which are often embedded with accelerometer and gyroscope, to measure frailty stages [17–28] with the potential implications of reducing burden on the medical staff, objectively assessing frailty, and monitoring changes in frailty over time. These studies attempted to quantify key physical frailty phenotypes, as described by Fried et al. (e.g., slowness, weakness, exhaustion, low activity, and shrinking), using wearable technologies and incorporating different functional performance test scenarios. These wearable technologies have the potential to remotely screen and/or track changes in frailty stages, including facilitating in-place and remote assessment, which can provide continuous and unsupervised monitoring for patients who have limited access to the clinics for assessment and follow ups. The development of simplified and innovative gait-related metrics that are sensitive to identifying frailty phenotypes can help to promote the integration of sensors in smart footwear devices (e.g., smart socks, smart brace, smart insoles, smart shoes, smart offloading boots, etc.) to help assess frailty during daily living activity such as walking. Currently, there is an emphasis on the technological development of embedding sensor into wearable, such as shoes [29,30] and insole [31], to monitor gait performance for health monitoring in geriatric [32] patients and people with movement disorders [33–36]. However, few studies have highlighted the use gait parameters to assess frailty.

Assessment of gait parameter, such as walking speed, can give rise to accurate classification of frailty in older adults [16]. Previous studies have shown that tracking sensor-derived gait parameters, such as maximum swing velocity of the shank [27], gait speed [37,38], and gait variability [39] could be used for classification of non-frail, pre-frail, and frail older adults; yet, few have examined the role of the gait parameters during the propulsion phase of walking in frailty assessment. During this phase of walking, the body is generating the majority of the push-off force to propel the body forward. It is estimated that the force that is generated during the propulsion phase accounts for more than 85% of the metabolic cost during a gait cycle [40]. Therefore, assessment of the propulsion phase might provide clinically-relevant correlation with the stage of frailty in a person.

The deterioration of gait performance during the propulsion phase can embody the five frailty phenotypes that were proposed by Fried et al. [13]. For example, the weakness in propulsive muscle group is similar to grip force decline mentioned in the weakness phenotype [41]. The loss of muscles mass (due to atrophy or dystrophy) may be correlated to shrinking phenotype (i.e., unintentional weight loss). As the result of weakness and muscle loss, the push-off force during the propulsion phase may be reduced, and this could have resulted in a reduction in gait speed, which is indicative of slowness phenotype [39], as well as physical fatigue (exhaustion phenotype) [42]. In addition to muscle weakness, the loss of propulsion could also be attributed to the reduction in the range of motion (ROM) as a result of the decline in joint flexibility. Toosizadeh et al. [19] had demonstrated that the elbow flexibility was significantly correlated with walking time, weakness, exhaustion, and low activity in the upper extremity. However, in the lower extremity, the joint stiffness not only affects the propulsion through the changes in flexion and extension of the ankle joint [43], but it also contributes to changes in ankle eversion and inversion, as well as tibia pronation and supination. These pieces of evidence suggest that gait parameters during the propulsion phase may be reliable indicators of physical frailty. Therefore, we designed a study to examine the role of gait parameters during the stance, swing, and propulsion phase to predict physical frailty. We hypothesize that gait parameters during the propulsion phase could be strong indicators of frailty status in the at-risk population. In addition, an artificial intelligence (AI) model was used to determine the reliability of the model to predicting the frailty status using a single-sensor system.

2. Materials and Methods

2.1. Participants

This is a cohort observational study. Participants were enrolled from geriatric outpatient clinical visits or community dwelling older adult settings. Inclusion criteria included older adults with age $\geq$55 years without significant gait or balance disorders, which may limit their ability to walk 20 m without aid. Therefore, participants who were able to walk with an assistive device, such as cane, were also included in the study. Our cutoff age was less than 65 years since we did not exclude those with chronic medical condition (e.g., diabetes mellitus, peripheral arterial disease, HIV, etc.), in whom geriatric symptoms were reported at earlier age [44–46]. Exclusion criteria were sign of severe cognitive impairment, which was evaluated using Mini-Mental State Examination (MMSE) [47]. Participants with MMSE score $\leq$16 and those who were unable or unwilling to consent were excluded from the study. Participants who met the eligibility criteria signed the written consent form. This study was approved by the local institutional review boards (IRBs).

2.2. Frailty Phenotype Assessment

Frailty was assessed using the frailty phenotype assessment that was developed by Fried et al. [13] based on the five phenotypes. These phenotypes are: shrinking, weakness, exhaustion, slowness, and low activity. Shrinking is characterized by an unintentional weight loss of 4.54 kg (10 lbs.) or more in the past year. Weakness was measured using a digital hand dynamometer (Camry Scale Store, City Industry, CA, USA). Participants were stratified for the presence of weakness phenotype using the lowest quintile (20%), based on gender and body mass index (BMI). Self-report exhaustion was evaluated using questions adopted from the Center for Epidemiologic Studies Depression questionnaire (CES-D). A 4.57 m (15 ft) walking test was used to measure slowness. Slowness was quantified by stratifying the walking speed by the slowest quintile based on gender and height. Self-reported level of physical activities was measured using the Minnesota Leisure Time Activity questionnaire [48]. Similar to self-report exhaustion and weakness, participants were stratified based on the lowest quintile.

Participants were classified by three level of frailty (non-frail, pre-frail, and frail) based on number of phenotypes presence in the participants. Non-frail participants exhibited zero phenotype. Pre-frail participants exhibited 1 to 2 of the five phenotypes. Participants were classified as frail if they had three or more phenotypes.

2.3. Sensor-Based Gait Assessment

Participants were asked to perform one trial of a 4.57 m (15 ft) free and unobstructed single walking task (i.e., straight walking along a path) at their self-selected pace. Gait data during the single walking task were collected using the two LEGSys^{TM} inertial sensors (Biosensics LLC, Watertown, MA, USA) worn on the left and right lower shin (Figure 1a). Three-dimensional angular velocity data were collected at the sampling rate of 100 Hz wirelessly via Bluetooth. The x-axis of the sensor was aligned along the tibia. The angular velocity of the shin in the sagittal plane was calculated by using the *z*-component of the gyroscope (mediolateral axis). Typical angular velocity of the shin in the sagittal plane during a gait cycle is shown in Figure 1b. The gait cycle was segmented and extracted using the gyroscope data based on algorithms that were presented in previous studies [49–52]. Briefly, peak detection of the angular velocity in the sagittal plane (about the mediolateral axis) was used to identify the three phases of the gait cycle: swing phase, stance phase, and propulsion phase. Separate gait cycle data were extracted using the gyroscope data on the left and right lower shin. Participants with at least two gait cycles on each leg were included in the analysis. The average of each gait parameter during single walking task was calculated for each participants.

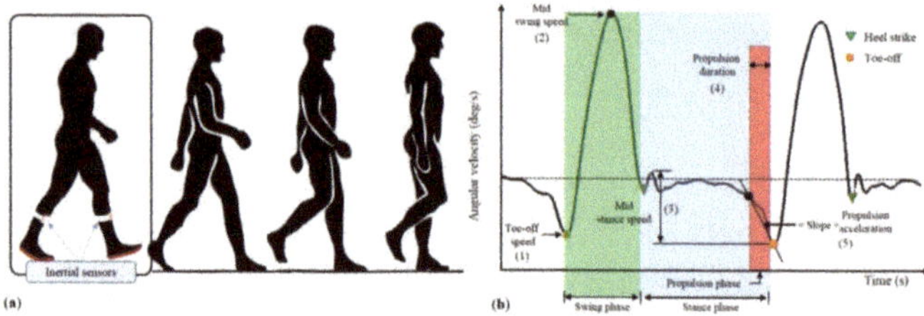

Figure 1. (**a**) Two wearable inertial sensors (LEGSys™, BioSensics LLC) were attached to the left and right lower shin of the participant during a single walking task. The propulsion phase happens toward the end of the stance phase of the gait cycle. It is segmented between heel-off and toe-off. (**b**) Typical angular velocity profile of gait cycle in the sagittal plane derived from the inertial sensor during single walking task. The definition of each gait parameters are detailed in Table 1.

Based on suggested evidences, six gait parameters during the stance, swing, and propulsion phase were identified in the analysis to investigate their power to predict frailty status based on single walking task. These parameters are: toe-off speed, mid swing speed, mid stance speed, propulsion duration, propulsion acceleration, and speed norm. The visual description of these parameters during a gait cycle is shown in Figure 1b. The propulsion phase was defined as the initiation from heel-off to toe-off. This was segmented by detecting the steepest slope from toe-off to a stance position where heel-off begins. The toe-off speed was defined as the magnitude of the angular velocity at toe-off, while mid swing was the magnitude of the angular velocity at mid swing. The mid stance speed was defined as the magnitude of the largest difference in angular velocity during the stance phase (from heel-strike to toe-off). The propulsion duration was defined as the time difference from heel-off to toe-off. The angular acceleration was defined as the change in angular velocity (slope) during the propulsion phase. The speed norm was defined as the magnitude of the vector sum of the angular velocity in the frontal and transverse plane. The definition of these gait parameters is summarized in Table 1.

Table 1. Definition of the sensor-derived gait parameters.

Sensor-Derived Gait Parameters	Unit	Description
Toe-off speed	degree/s	Magnitude of angular velocity at toe-off (Figure 1b, 1)
Mid swing speed	degree/s	Magnitude of angular velocity at mid swing (Figure 1b, 2)
Mid stance speed	degree/s	The magnitude of maximum range of the angular velocity during stance phase (Figure 1b,3)
Propulsion duration	second (s)	Duration of time from heel-off to toe-off in a gait cycle (Figure 1b, 4)
Propulsion acceleration	degree/s^2	The average angular acceleration (slope) during the propulsion phase (Figure 1b, 5)
Speed norm	degree/s	The magnitude of the vector sum of the angular velocity in the transverse and frontal plane

The mean, standard deviation, and coefficient of variation were calculated for all of the sensor-derived gait parameters. Toe-off, mid swing, and mid stance speed denote rotation in the sagittal plane.

2.4. Neural Network Model

A predictive model using a selected set of parameters was constructed using an Artificial Neural Network (ANN) algorithm (JMP^{TM}, Cary, NC, USA) to assess its accuracy in predicting frailty status (Figure 2). This algorithm may help to evaluate whether a single-sensor system could be optimized to assess frailty in unsupervised setting. A k-fold cross validation study was designed where the participants were randomly separated into two groups: training data set and validation data set. The ANN network was constructed using 8-fold with 5 layers of hidden nodes. In the eight-fold scenario, participants were randomly divided into eight subsets ($n = 20$), where each subset was used as a validation set and the remaining participants ($n = 141$) was used as training data set. This process was repeated eight times using each subset as the validation data set. A hyperbolic tangent (TanH) activation function was used to represent the neuron that mapped the inputs to the outputs. Six selected gait parameters were used as the input layers to predict the frailty status of the validation data set after training. Participants were classified as either non-frail, pre-frail, or frail. The receiver of characteristic (ROC) curve [53,54] was generated for the validation set to assess the accuracy of the algorithm to correctly classify each frailty stage for the participants in the validation set. It was generated by plotting the true positive rate (sensitivity) against the false positive rate (1-specificity) for each frailty stage. The accuracy of the classification for each stage was measured by calculating the area under the ROC curve (AUC) [55]. The AUC represents the probability that a random participant from each group (non-frail, pre-frail, and frail) is correctly classified. An area of 1 represents a perfect classification of the frailty stage based on the algorithm and an area of 0.5 denotes a randomized classification. The robustness of the model was evaluated by calculating the 95% confidence interval using bootstrapping. With bootstrapping, a new training and validation set was randomly resampled from the population. The AUC for predicting frailty stages (non-frail, pre-frail, and frail) was recalculated for each resampled data set. The process was repeated 500 times. A 95% confidence interval of the classification of the non-frail, pre-frail, and frail was calculated using the bootstrapping results. The results from the AUC imply that we are 95% confident in predicting the stage of frailty of the participants by monitoring proposed gait parameters, such as propulsion duration and propulsion time during walking.

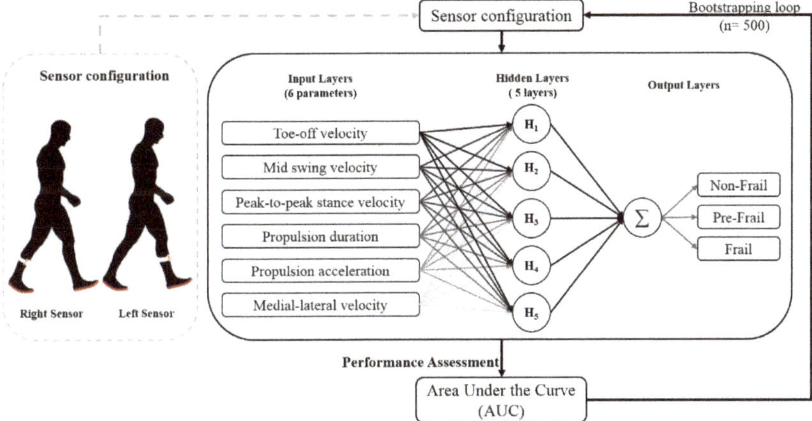

Figure 2. An eight-fold cross validation model with five hidden layers Artificial Neural Network was constructed to test the reliability and accuracy of classifying the frailty status of the participants in the study. Six selected gait parameters were identified and used as inputs to the model. The performance of the model was evaluated using the area under the curve. A 95% confidence interval was calculated to assess the reliability of the prediction.

2.5. Statistical Analysis

Chi-squared test (χ^2) was used to analyze the pairwise comparison of categorical variables, such as gender and fallers (faller vs. non-faller), in the non-frail, pre-frail, and frail group. The demographic, clinical characteristic, and gait parameters were analyzed using analysis of variance (ANOVA) and post hoc Game-Howell contrast was used for pairwise comparison assuming for unequal size and unequal variance. For comparison across three groups in ANOVA, the effect size eta squared (η^2) was calculated [56]. The eta squared measures the proportion of variance in the dependent variables across different groups. Eta squared of 0.01 is considered to be small, 0.06 is medium, and 0.14 is large. These values are interpreted using percentage by multiplying the value by 100. For pairwise comparison, the effect size was calculated using Cohen's effect size (d) [57]. Cohen's effect size of 0.2 is considered to be small, 0.5 is medium, and 0.8 is large. The mean and the standard deviation were reported, unless otherwise noted. A univariate analysis of covariance (ANCOVA) was used to characterize the performance of these parameters among three groups, while adjusting for age, gender, and BMI. Linear regression model was used to analyze the relationship between the gait parameters and the frailty phenotypes, as proposed by Fried et al. [13]. The Spearman's rho was used to calculate the correlation between the gait parameters and the frailty phenotypes [58]. For statistical analysis, the level of significance was set at alpha = 0.050.

3. Results

3.1. Demographic and Clinical Data

Using the inclusion criteria, 161 participants were selected for the study. Using Fried criteria, 30.4% ($n = 49$) of the participants were classified as non-frail, 57.2% ($n = 92$) was noted as pre-frail, and 12.4% ($n = 20$) were classified as frail [13] (Table 2). Chi-squared analysis showed that there were no significant differences between gender and fallers among the three groups. Age, which is often associated with frailty status, was matched among the non-frail (mean $\pm$ standard deviation, 71.2 $\pm$ 12.1 years old), pre-frail (74.6 $\pm$ 10.3 years old), and frail group (76.5 $\pm$ 14.3 years old). There were significant differences in weight between the non-frail versus pre-frail group ($p = 0.030$, d = 0.41) and pre-frail versus frail group ($p = 0.003$, d = 0.70); however, BMI was only significantly different between non-frail and pre-frail group ($p = 0.030$, d = 0.43). Pairwise comparison of cognitive performance showed significant differences in the MMSE score between frail versus non-frail ($p = 0.009$, d = 0.62) and frail versus pre-frail ($p = 0.049$, d = 0.46). Depression was significantly different in the frail group as compared to non-frail ($p = 0.001$, d = 1.17) and pre-frail ($p = 0.001$, d = 0.88). Non-frail participants had significantly less concern for fall when compared to the pre-frail ($p = 0.001$, d = 0.60) and frail group ($p = 0.019$, d = 1.72). Lastly, pre-frail individual exhibited more comorbidities than non-frail ($p = 0.006$, d = 1.27); however, there was no significant difference with frail individuals.

Table 2. Demographic and clinical characteristic of participants.

Characteristic	Non-Frail (N) ($n = 49$)	Pre-Frail (P) ($n = 92$)	Frail (F) ($n = 20$)	*p*-Value (η^2)	Pairwise Comparison *p*-Value (d)		
					N-P	N-F	P-F
Gender [+]							
Male *n* (%)	17 (34.7)	41 (44.6)	7 (35.0)		0.260	0.981	0.433
Female *n* (%)	32 (65.3)	51 (55.4)	13 (65.0)				
Age [a], years	71.2 ($\pm$12.1)	74.6 ($\pm$10.3)	76.5 ($\pm$14.3)	0.141 (0.025)	0.230 (0.31)	0.340 (0.41)	0.850 (0.17)
Height, m	1.66 ($\pm$0.09)	1.67 ($\pm$0.12)	1.60 ($\pm$0.12)	**0.023 (0.046)**	0.970 (0.04)	0.082 (0.66)	**0.052 (0.64)**
Weight, kg	73.5 ($\pm$15.5)	81.5 ($\pm$21.2)	67.6 ($\pm$14.3)	**0.003 (0.070)**	**0.030 (0.41)**	0.271 (0.31)	**0.002 (0.70)**
BMI, kg/m^2	26.5 ($\pm$5.3)	29.2 ($\pm$6.5)	26.5 ($\pm$5.4)	**0.025 (0.046)**	**0.030 (0.43)**	0.990 (0.02)	0.131 (0.43)
History of fall [+] *n* (%)	14 (28.6)	38 (20.7)	7 (35.0)		0.973	0.392	0.394
Cognition performance (MMSE)	29.0 ($\pm$1.3)	28.5 ($\pm$1.7)	27.4 ($\pm$3.2)	**0.032 (0.069)**	0.278 (0.19)	**0.009 (0.62)**	**0.049 (0.46)**
Depression (CES-D)	7.0 ($\pm$7.0)	9.0 ($\pm$8.0)	16.6 ($\pm$6.8)	**0.001 (0.15)**	0.215 (0.17)	**0.001 (1.17)**	**0.001 (0.88)**
Concerns for falls (FES-I)	20.9 ($\pm$3.8)	28.8 ($\pm$11.9)	34.1 ($\pm$17.0)	**0.001 (0.15)**	**0.001 (0.60)**	**0.019 (1.72)**	0.486 (0.43)
# of comorbidity	2.0 ($\pm$1.7)	3.4 ($\pm$2.0)	4.8 ($\pm$1.9)	**0.002 (0.166)**	0.071 (0.39)	**0.006 (1.27)**	0.125 (0.65)

[+] Gender and history of fall were evaluated using chi-squared (χ^2). [a] The mean $\pm$ standard deviation is presented here, unless denoted otherwise. *n* represents the number of sample in each group. Post hoc Games-Howell test was used for pairwise comparison with alpha = 0.050. For three group comparisons, the effect size eta squared (η^2) was calculated. Statistical significant interaction are highlighted with bold type.

3.2. Sensor-Based Assessment of Frailty

The selected gait parameters (e.g., propulsion duration, propulsion acceleration, mid stance speed, speed norm, toe-off speed, and mid swing speed) were evaluated using data from the left and right sensor separately. The results are summarized in Table 3. ANOVA was used to analyze the discriminating power of the selected parameters to differentiate among non-frail, pre-frail, and frail group. The results showed that there were significant differences among the three groups for all of the selected parameters with $p < 0.001$ and effect size eta squared (η^2) was between 0.09–0.24. This indicates that the selected gait parameters accounted for between 9.0–24.0% of the variance in the sample. Propulsion related parameters, such as propulsion duration, propulsion acceleration, and toe-off speed all demonstrated significant correlations among the three groups when using only the left or right sensor worn on the shin.

Gait performance data from the right sensor demonstrated that the frail group had longer propulsion duration when compared to the pre-frail (difference = +34%, $p = 0.035$, d = 1.01) and non-frail group (+57%, $p = 0.003$, d = 1.55). The propulsion acceleration was also significantly lower in the frail group as compared to the pre-frail (+54%, $p = 0.002$, d = 0.87) and non-frail (+84%, $p < 0.001$, d = 1.28). The toe-off speed was also significantly reduced in frail individuals when compared to pre-frail (+43%, $p = 0.038$, d = 0.65) and non-frail group (+66%, $p = 0.00$, d = 0.58). The mid swing speed was significantly lower in the frail group when compared to the non-frail (+46%, $p < 0.001$, d = 1.63) and pre-frail (+25%, $p = 0.007$, d = 0.84) group. The mid stance speed (non-frail vs. pre-frail) and speed norm (pre-frail vs. frail) yielded no statistical significance; however, there was a reduction in both velocities between groups, 11% and 24%, respectively. Using data from the sensor that was worn on the left shin, only the pairwise comparison of the propulsion duration between the frail and non-frail yielded no statistical significance ($p = 0.071$); however the effect size was large (d = 1.81).

The sensitivity of these gait parameters to age, gender, and BMI were investigated using a univariate analysis of covariance to account for these covariates. The results are shown in Figure 3. Age, sex, and BMI did not alter the effect on the performance of these gait parameters. Thus, the sensor-derived gait parameters remain significantly different among the three groups.

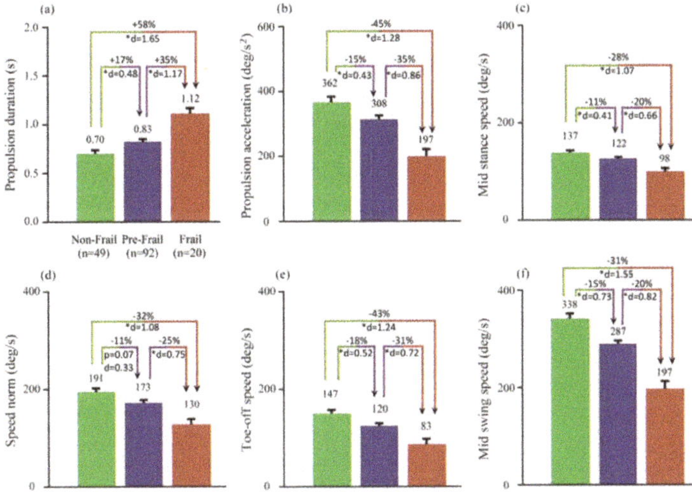

Figure 3. Result of univariate analysis of covariance for the six gait parameters (**a–f**) adjusting for gender, age, and BMI for the right sensor. * indicates statistical significance with alpha = 0.050. Percentage differences and Cohen's effect size (d) were also calculated in each pairwise comparison.

Table 3. Sensor-derived gait parameters during single walking task across three groups.

Gait Parameters	Group	Mean ± Std	*p*-Value (η^2)	Pairwise Comparison		
				Group	*p*-Value (*d*)	Mean Difference 95% CI
Right Sensor						Lower — Upper
Propulsion duration (s)	Non-frail	0.70 ± 0.11	**<0.001 (0.20)**	N-P	<0.001 (0.62)	−0.19 / −0.55
	Pre-frail	0.83 ± 0.23		N-F	0.003 (1.55)	−0.67 / −0.14
	Frail	1.11 ± 0.46		P-F	0.036 (1.00)	−0.55 / −0.17
Propulsion acceleration (deg/s^2)	Non-frail	366.6 ± 137.5	**<0.001 (0.13)**	N-P	0.035 (0.46)	3.4 / 115.8
	Pre-frail	306.0 ± 125.4		N-F	<0.001 (1.28)	90.6 / 243.1
	Frail	198.7 ± 109.8		P-F	0.002 (0.87)	38.8 / 175.8
Mid stance speed (deg/s)	Non-frail	137.6 ± 42.2	**<0.001 (0.10)**	N-P	0.075 (0.42)	−1.2 / 32.2
	Pre-frail	122.1 ± 34.5		N-F	<0.001 (0.99)	16.6 / 62.2
	Frail	98.2 ± 32.3		P-F	0.016 (0.70)	4.0 / 43.8
speed norm (deg/s)	Non-frail	196.4 ± 53.5	**<0.001 (0.11)**	N-P	0.025 (0.46)	2.7 / 49.0
	Pre-frail	170.6 ± 57.7		N-F	0.003 (1.12)	22.2 / 112.1
	Frail	129.2 ± 3.6		P-F	0.067 (0.68)	−2.4 / 85.1
Toe-off speed (deg/s)	Non-frail	149.4 ± 48.2	**<0.001 (0.13)**	N-P	0.003 (0.58)	9.4 / 52.1
	Pre-frail	118.6 ± 55.3		N-F	<0.001 (1.32)	31.4 / 101.9
	Frail	82.7 ± 56.1		P-F	0.038 (0.65)	1.8 / 70.1
Mid swing speed (deg/s)	Non-frail	336.9 ± 63.3	**<0.001 (0.20)**	N-P	<0.001 (0.73)	21.2 / 76.0
	Pre-frail	288.3 ± 69.0		N-F	<0.001 (1.63)	61.9 / 151.9
	Frail	230.0 ± 74.8		P-F	0.007 (0.84)	15.0 / 101.7
Left Sensor						
Propulsion duration (s)	Non-frail	0.69 ± 0.10	**<0.001 (0.17)**	N-P	<0.001 (0.94)	−0.21 / −0.65
	Pre-frail	0.83 ± 0.25		N-F	0.004 (4.02)	−0.63 / −0.12
	Frail	1.07 ± 0.45		P-F	0.071 (1.83)	−0.50 / 0.19
Propulsion acceleration (deg/s^2)	Non-frail	382.8 ± 115.3	**<0.001 (0.12)**	N-P	0.007 (0.60)	15.8 / 121.0
	Prefrail	314.4 ± 142.3		N-F	<0.001 (2.21)	82.2 / 242.9
	Frail	220.3 ± 126.5		P-F	0.016 (0.94)	15.4 / 172.8
Mid stance speed (deg/s)	Non-frail	144.1 ± 34.9	**<0.001 (0.10)**	N-P	0.037 (0.33)	0.8 / 31.9
	Pre-frail	127.8 ± 40.8		N-F	<0.001 (1.32)	18.6 / 64.9
	Frail	102.4 ± 35.8		P-F	0.023 (0.68)	3.1 / 47.8
Speed norm (deg/s)	Non-frail	198.8 ± 54.8	**<0.001 (0.12)**	N-P	0.041 (0.37)	0.8 / 48.6
	Pre-frail	174.1 ± 60.5		N-F	<0.001 (1.56)	36.4 / 101.9
	Frail	129.6 ± 48.9		P-F	0.004 (0.85)	13.4 / 75.4
Toe-off speed (deg/s)	Non-frail	154.2 ± 53.8	**0.001 (0.08)**	N-P	0.061 (0.34)	−0.8 / 47.6
	Pre-frail	130.8 ± 64.4		N-F	<0.001 (1.37)	25.9 / 93.8
	Frail	94.4 ± 51.8		P-F	0.027 (0.66)	3.6 / 69.3
Mid swing speed (deg/s)	Non-frail	347.6 ± 58.9	**<0.001 (0.24)**	N-P	<0.001 (0.78)	29.7 / 82.4
	Pre-frail	291.6 ± 69.2		N-F	<0.001 (2.59)	72.4 / 176.3
	Frail	223.2 ± 85.8		P-F	0.007 (1.19)	17.3 / 119.4

N = Non-frail, P = Pre-frail, and F = Frail. Effect size among the three groups were calculated using eta squared (η^2) for ANOVA analysis. For pairwise comparison, the Cohen's effect size (d) was calculated. Statistical significances were evaluated using alpha = 0.050 and highlighted with bold font. The pairwise confidence interval of the mean difference (Mean Difference 95% CI) is also present here.

Correlation of the selected parameters with frailty phenotypes that were proposed by Fried et al. [13] were analyzed using Spearman's correlation (*rho*). The correlation and the statistical results are summarized in Table 4. Using only the data from the right worn sensor, the results demonstrated that propulsion related parameters were highly correlated with several phenotypes. For example, propulsion duration was positively correlated with weakness (*rho* = 0.360, *p* < 0.001), slowness (*rho* = 0.684, *p* < 0.001), and exhaustion (*rho* = 0.237, *p* = 0.023). The propulsion acceleration was negatively correlated with weakness (*rho* = −0.257, *p* = 0.013) and slowness (*rho* = −0.645, *p* < 0.001). The mid stance speed was only correlated to slowness (*rho* = −0.553, *p* < 0.001); however, the speed norm was negatively correlated to weakness (*rho* = −0.330, *p* = 0.001), slowness (*rho* = −0.543, *p* < 0.001), exhaustion (*rho* = −0.248, *p* = 0.017), and low activity (*rho* = −0.212, *p* = 0.043). Speed norm was correlated to all frailty phenotype except shrinking. Toe-off speed was negatively correlated to weakness (*rho* = −0.402, *p* < 0.001), slowness (*rho* = −0.646, *p* < 0.001), and exhaustion (*rho* = −0.205, *p* = 0.050). Lastly, mid swing speed was negatively correlated to weakness (*rho* = −0.358, *p* < 0.001) and slowness (*rho* = −0.784, *p* < 0.001). Similar results were also observed when using data from the sensor that was worn on the left shin.

Table 4. Correlations between Fried phenotypes and sensor-derived gait parameters.

Gait Parameters	Shrinking		Weakness		Slowness		Exhaustion		Low Activity	
Right Sensor	*rho*	*p*-Value	*rho*	*p*-Value	*rho*	*p*-Value	*rho*	*p*-Value	*rho*	*p*-Value
Propulsion duration (s)	0.181	0.085	**0.360**	**<0.001**	**0.684**	**<0.001**	**0.237**	**0.023**	0.154	0.142
Propulsion acceleration (deg/s^2)	−0.141	0.180	**−0.257**	**0.013**	**−0.645**	**<0.001**	−0.200	0.056	−0.168	0.109
Mid stance speed (deg/s)	−0.068	0.520	−0.183	0.081	**−0.589**	**<0.001**	−0.129	0.219	−0.091	0.390
Speed norm (deg/s)	0.061	0.561	**−0.330**	**0.001**	**−0.543**	**<0.001**	**−0.248**	**0.017**	**−0.212**	**0.043**
Toe-off speed (deg/s)	0.060	0.572	**−0.402**	**<0.001**	**−0.646**	**<0.001**	**−0.205**	**0.050**	−0.202	0.054
Mid swing speed (deg/s)	−0.119	0.257	**−0.358**	**<0.001**	**−0.784**	**<0.001**	−0.175	0.095	−0.127	0.227
Left Sensor										
Propulsion duration (s)	0.094	0.370	**0.386**	**<0.001**	**0.732**	**<0.001**	**0.241**	**0.021**	0.119	0.261
Propulsion acceleration (deg/s^2)	−0.027	0.802	**−0.305**	**0.003**	**−0.676**	**<0.001**	−0.156	0.137	−0.119	0.258
Mid stance speed (deg/s)	−0.007	0.950	−0.196	0.061	**−0.568**	**<0.001**	−0.106	0.316	−0.104	0.323
Speed norm (deg/s)	−0.094	0.370	**−0.415**	**<0.001**	**−0.533**	**<0.001**	**−0.223**	**0.033**	**−0.231**	**0.027**
Toe-off speed (deg/s)	−0.033	0.754	**−0.407**	**<0.001**	**−0.567**	**<0.001**	**−0.224**	**0.032**	−0.173	0.099
Mid swing speed (deg/s)	−0.126	0.231	**−0.369**	**<0.001**	**−0.724**	**<0.001**	−0.176	0.093	−0.112	0.287

Linear correlations between the gait parameters and Fried frailty phenotypes were evaluated using Spearman's coefficient (*rho*). Statistical significance was assessed with alpha = 0.050 and are bolded in the table. The left and right sensor showed similar correlations with Fried frailty phenotypes.

3.3. Neural Network Modeling

Bootstrapping (iteration = 500) was used on the neural network to find the 95% confidence interval of the frailty assessment using the data from the left and right shin sensor separately. Using data from the sensor worn on the left shin, the lower and upper bound of the AUC ranges from 0.900–0.913 for non-frail, 0.838–0.854 for pre-frail, and 0.914–0.931 for frail group. Using only gait data from the sensor worn on the right shin, the lower and upper bound limit of the AUC were 0.893–0.905 for non-frail, 0.842–0.857 for pre-frail, and 0.945–0.958 for frail group. The smallest AUC for the classification of frailty was in the pre-frail group when using gait data from either the left or right worn sensor (Figure 4).

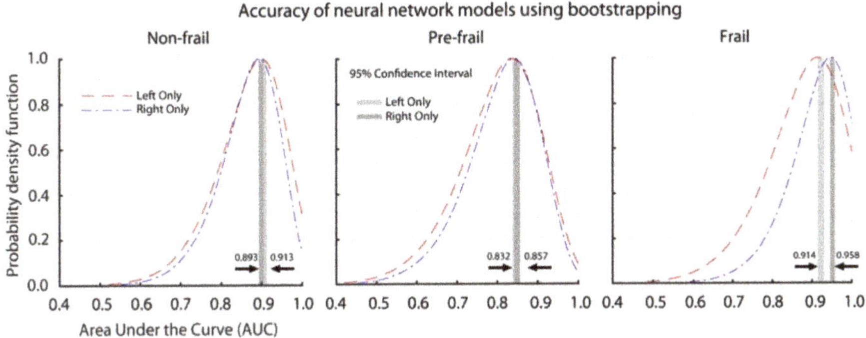

Figure 4. Probability distribution function the Area under the Curve (AUC) of two different sensor configurations. The confidence interval (shaded region) was calculated using bootstrapping (iteration = 500). The upper and lower limit of the confidence interval of the sensor configuration are also shown.

4. Discussion

Assessment of frailty status is a critical component of delivering better healthcare to the aging population [59]. Timely treatment and intervention could be prescribed or recommended if frailty could be identified early. Currently, clinical assessment of frailty is performed in a supervised setting by trained personnel. Furthermore, current assessments are limited to classification such as non-frail, pre-frail, or frail. However, with the proliferation of wearable technology, embedding sensors into daily living activities and wearables devices could provide new avenues to obtain real-time assessment of frailty and greater granularity in the classification. In this study, we demonstrated the feasibility of using a foot-worn wearable sensor to monitor and detect different frailty stages in ambulatory adults using quantifiable gait characteristics with an emphasis on the propulsion phase of walking. The results could potentially be used to evaluate frailty status in unsupervised setting; allowing for future development of a single-sensor system to assess frailty assessment at home, clinic, and even outdoor environment.

Several wearable platforms have been developed to quantify physical frailty, to distinguish presence or absence of frailty phenotypes (e.g., slowness, exhaustion, weakness, low activity, and shrinking), and/or to differentiate different frailty stages (e.g., non-frail, pre-frail, and frail) [17–28]. These studies have mainly focused on quantifying frailty by measuring functional performance during different physical tasks, such as a 20s rapid elbow flexion-extension test [17–19], balance [20,21] and gait tests [22,23], physical activity monitoring [24,25], and postural transition test, such as the Timed Up and Go Test [26–28]. However, their proposed sensor location are not always suitable for remote and continuous monitoring of frailty outside of clinical setting or under unsupervised condition. Extracting frailty related parameters from sensors during lower extremity tasks could yield new opportunities for alternative form factors, such as different types of footwear (e.g., socks, shoes, braces, etc.), to monitor frailty during daily living.

Substantial works have been done to utilize gait performance to identify frailty [60–62]. For example, Castell et al. showed that people who are at higher risk of frailty had a lower walking speed [63] and that gait speed could be used as a predictor of adverse event outcome in older adults. In this study, we also observed a reduction in the mid swing speed in the non-frail (336.9 deg/s), pre-frail (-15%, 288.3 deg/s), and frail (-32%, 230.0 deg/s) participants. However, the focus on a single speed parameter might over simplify a multifaceted syndrome such as frailty. Schwenk et al. [16] suggested that parameters beyond gait speed could provide more granularity to the frailty assessment and adopted for different diseased population. For example, Thiede et al. [39] has demonstrated that frail individual with peripheral arterial disease tends to walk slower and in shorter steps. In this study, we observed a slower and weaker propulsive performance in those who were identified as frail when compared to pre-frail and non-frail group. For instance, the propulsion duration increased by an average of 17% as the non-frail participants become pre-frail, and it substantially increased by 58% in frail population, which could be a manifestation of slowness, weakness, and exhaustion phenotype. Furthermore, the propulsion acceleration dropped by 16% and 46% for pre-frail and frail group, when compared with non-frail. Propulsion acceleration was significantly correlated with weakness and slowness phenotype when using the sensor data from the right shin (Table 4). The inability to accelerate the body forward may be explained by advancing weakness in adults who become pre-frail or frail. This may be due to muscle loss from sarcopenia [23] (manifesting the shrinking phenotype) or fat infiltration and loss of muscle quality and force production capacity in older adults [64]. While monitoring for exhaustion was not directly possible as some participants had only a few completed gait cycles (two or more) in the 4.57 m (15 ft) walking test, the decline in angular velocity may indicate the progression of exhaustion since these movement are modulated by smaller lower body muscles (e.g., popliteus) that may become exhausted much faster and more frequent than the larger muscles (e.g., soleus). This hypothesis was observed in the correlation between speed norm and exhaustion phenotype (rho $= -0.248$, $p = 0.017$). Limitation of the movement of the speed norm has been shown to restrict the ability of the knee and ankle joint to generate maximum ground reaction force [65,66], which might be indicative of weakness and exhaustion frailty phenotype.

Frailty is a geriatric syndrome with high prevalence in older adults, and, as expected, the age of the non-frail participants was younger than the pre-frail and frail group (Table 1). However, there was no statistical difference in age among the three groups. The similarity in age for the three groups emphasizes the need for development of sensor-based algorithm for the continuous and standalone monitoring of older adults. Early detection of pre-frail status might create the possibility of reversing the condition or delaying the transition to frail status through intervention. This motivates the development of a deep learning algorithm [67,68] to assess frailty while using the propulsion phase parameters, which were found to be sensitive in identifying the three groups of non-frail, pre-frail, and frail across a diverse cohort (e.g., peripheral arterial disease, HIV, diabetes mellitus, etc.).

Two different sensor configurations were analyzed in this study. Data from the left and right sensor worn on the shin were evaluated separately. Using data collected from a single sensor (left or right), we were able to achieve accuracy, as defined using the AUC, between 84% (in pre-frail population) to 96% (in frail population). This indicates that the algorithm was able to classify frail participant at 96% accuracy using the gait parameters that were proposed in the study. These results suggested that proposed gait parameters are highly associated with frailty stages, especially in frail and non-frail participants (90% accuracy). As expected, the transition toward severe stages of frailty is more difficult to assess; however, our algorithm was able to classify pre-frail participants with 84% accuracy. The selected parameters are robust in predicting frailty, regardless of whether the sensor is attached to the left or the right shin. These results could potentially encourage the integration of a single-sensor system to assess frailty by measuring gait performance, which might be more suitable for unsupervised setting. Currently, clinical assessment [13,69] are limited to the classification of non-frail, pre-frail, and frail. However, for clinicians, the knowledge gaps in the gradation of the severity of frailty could dilute the effect of targeted intervention. More gradation of frail severity could provide complementary information to clinicians in making critical health care decisions [59,70,71]. Using deep learning algorithm can help to develop a more continuous scale, which might result in a more refined stratification of frailty status.

From sensor type point of view, we have demonstrated that all the parameters of interest could be extracted from a single gyroscope attached to lower extremities. This could make it more suitable for integration into smart footwear, such as shoes, socks, and braces. Unlike accelerometers, which are sensitive to sensor location [72,73] or pressure sensors that are sensitive to wear effect, and thus need regular calibration [74,75], gyroscope is insensitive to sensor-location as long as the segment is assumed to be rigid and it does not need regular calibration [50,73], thus making it more suitable for unsupervised setting. This also facilitates the deployment of the proposed algorithm in varieties of smart footwear, including smart sock (e.g., Sensoria smart socks, Sensoria Fitness, WA, USA), pressure offloading footwear (e.g., Optima Molliter, MC, Italy), ankle braces (e.g., Smart Moore Balance Brace, Orthotics Holdings Inc., AZ, USA), smart shoes (e.g., Sensoria Walk, Sensoria Fitness, WA, USA), and enhanced their capability to remotely monitor frailty status and its progression to different frailty stages without the need of frequent calibration or assessment by trained staff or under supervised condition.

The method for deploying the proposed algorithm for the remote monitoring of frailty stages is beyond of the scope of this study. However, one potential deployment scenario of the algorithm could be to integrate a gyroscope sensor into a sock that is similar to the design that was proposed by Sensoria smart socks (Sensoria Fitness, WA, USA). Using a gyroscope, prolonged unbroken walking bouts (e.g., more than 20 consecutive steps) could be detected during the activity of daily living using the algorithm proposed by Aminian et al. [76]. Once these unbroken walking bouts are detected, the physical frailty could be quantified based on the propulsion performance using the model that is proposed in this study. The cutoff for 20 consecutive steps was selected based on a secondary analysis of the data reported by Moufawad el Achkar et al. [77]. Their study revealed that the average cadence estimated from walking bouts with more than 20 steps, measured during activities of daily living in non-frail older adults, was approximately 110 steps/minute and 90 steps/minute for walking bouts, with less than 20 consecutive steps. Schwenk et al. [22] analyzed gait data during a walking test that was performed at habitual speed and under supervised condition. Their study reported a cadence of 111 steps/minute for non-frail and 100 steps/minute for pre-frail individuals. Together, it could be speculated that daily unbroken walking bouts of greater than 20 consecutive steps might better represent the habitual walking speed than those with less than 20 consecutive steps. According to Najafi et al. [78,79], based on studies in people with diabetes, it is anticipated that over 50 bouts of walking per day with 20 steps or more could be collected in non-frail and pre-frail population. Thus, for determining progression in frailty stages (targeting non-frail and pre-frail population), the proposed scenario seems to be practical. But, this needs to be confirmed in another study. This scenario may also help to improve the accuracy by averaging the results of over 50 or more detected prolonged unbroken walking bouts during a day. To improve the autonomy and battery life, the system could be defaulted to be in sleep mode and only be activated when three consecutive steps are detected and return to sleep mode if walking is stopped before 20 steps or if it exceeds more than 30 steps. The cutoff for 30 steps was defined based on Lindemann et al. [80]. Their study suggested that after achieving steady state walking, which is often occurred before 10 consecutive steps, 20 consecutive steps and 40 consecutive steps resulted in the same average values for major gait parameters (e.g., stride length, stride time, etc.). Thus, it is speculated that walking longer than 30 consecutive steps may not influence the estimated propulsion performance. On the other hand, longer step count during prolonged walking bout may add a potential confounder that is associated with fatigue.

In this study, we analyzed over 161 participants; however, the population was more skewed toward the non-frail and pre-frail population. Even with a small sample size of frail participants, we were able to achieve significantly high effect size across the three groups. Similarly, we were limited to the number of gait cycle for each participant. A study by Lindemann et al. has suggested that steady-state walking in frail elderly does not occur until at least 2.5 m (8 ft) into walking, which is approximately six steps [80]. However, during a 4.57 m (15 ft) single task walking, the number of steady-state gait cycle was limited. Thus, the acceleration phase of the walking task might induce confounding factors during the propulsive phase of frail older adults. More importantly, these short gait cycles might not capture the exhaustion phenotype (fatigue) as suggested by Fried. Lastly, these data were collected under a structured single walking task and in a controlled laboratory environment, which might have an impact on gait performance. In a future study, we hope to apply the same model to gait data during unsupervised setting (using a single embedded sensor in footwear, offloading device, socks, etc.) to determine the efficacy of these parameters to assess frailty during daily living activities. Additionally, the engineering feasibility of integrating the proposed algorithm into wearable devices to assess frailty under unsupervised condition must be considered in future study; however it is beyond the scope of the current study. This study proposes a new algorithm to assess frailty using gait parameters with emphasis on the propulsion phase of the gait cycle. This development is an important facet in a multidisciplinary approach to develop smart footwear to monitor frailty.

5. Conclusions

This study demonstrates that a foot-worn sensor-derived gait measures during the propulsive phase of walking can be sensitive metrics in assessing frailty. Using these metrics, we have developed and validated a predictive model that could be used for unsupervised and real-time assessment using wearable sensor. These results could motivate the development and integration of single-sensor system into wearable footwear in order to assess frailty during daily living activities.

Author Contributions: H.R. contributed to the design and conception of study, data analysis, and interpretation of the results. H.N. contributed in data analysis, modeling, and interpretation of the results. H.L. contributed in design and conception of study and data gathering. B.N. contributed to the design and conception of study and interpretation of the results. All authors contributed to the draft and revision of the manuscript.

Funding: Partial support was provided by the National Institutes of Health/National Institute on Aging (award number 2R42AG032748), the National Institutes of Health/National Cancer Institute (award number 1R21CA190933-01A1), Baylor College of Medicine, and Michael E. DeBakey Department of Surgery.

Acknowledgments: The content is solely the responsibility of the authors and does not necessarily represent the official views of sponsors. We would like to thank Manuel Gardea for assistance with data analysis.

Conflicts of Interest: The proposed algorithm is protected by a provisional patent own by Baylor College of Medicine. All authors are listed as an inventor. The founding sponsors had no role in the design of the study; in the collection, analyses, or interpretation of data; in the writing of the manuscript, and in the decision to publish the results.

References

1. An Aging Nation. Available online: https://www.census.gov/library/visualizations/2017/comm/cb17-ff08_older_americans.html (accessed on 25 September 2017).
2. Kojima, G.; Kendrick, D.; Skelton, D.A.; Morris, R.W.; Gawler, S.; Iliffe, S. Frailty predicts short-term incidence of future falls among British community-dwelling older people: A prospective cohort study nested within a randomised controlled trial. *BMC Geriatr.* **2015**, *15*, 155. [CrossRef] [PubMed]
3. Schultz, M.; Rosted, E.; Sanders, S. Frailty is associated with a history with more falls in elderly hospitalised patients. *Dan. Med. J.* **2015**, *62*, A5058. [PubMed]
4. Mohler, M.J.; Wendel, C.S.; Taylor-Piliae, R.E.; Toosizadeh, N.; Najafi, B. Motor Performance and Physical Activity as Predictors of Prospective Falls in Community-Dwelling Older Adults by Frailty Level: Application of Wearable Technology. *Gerontology* **2016**, *62*, 654–664. [CrossRef] [PubMed]
5. Lin, H.S.; Peel, N.M.; Hubbard, R.E. Baseline Vulnerability and Inpatient Frailty Status in Relation to Adverse Outcomes in a Surgical Cohort. *J. Frailty Aging* **2016**, *5*, 180–182. [PubMed]
6. Arya, S.; Kim, S.I.; Duwayri, Y.; Brewster, L.P.; Veeraswamy, R.; Salam, A.; Dodson, T.F. Frailty increases the risk of 30-day mortality, morbidity, and failure to rescue after elective abdominal aortic aneurysm repair independent of age and comorbidities. *J. Vasc. Surg.* **2015**, *61*, 324–331. [CrossRef] [PubMed]
7. Karam, J.; Tsiouris, A.; Shepard, A.; Velanovich, V.; Rubinfeld, I. Simplified frailty index to predict adverse outcomes and mortality in vascular surgery patients. *Ann. Vasc. Surg.* **2013**, *27*, 904–908. [CrossRef] [PubMed]
8. Joseph, B.; Toosizadeh, N.; Orouji Jokar, T.; Heusser, M.R.; Mohler, J.; Najafi, B. Upper-Extremity Function Predicts Adverse Health Outcomes among Older Adults Hospitalized for Ground-Level Falls. *Gerontology* **2017**, *63*, 299–307. [CrossRef] [PubMed]
9. Chang, Y.-W.; Chen, W.-L.; Lin, F.-G.; Fang, W.-H.; Yen, M.-Y.; Hsieh, C.-C.; Kao, T.-W. Frailty and its impact on health-related quality of life: A cross-sectional study on elder community-dwelling preventive health service users. *PLoS ONE* **2012**, *7*, e38079. [CrossRef] [PubMed]
10. Garcia-Nogueras, I.; Aranda-Reneo, I.; Pena-Longobardo, L.M.; Oliva-Moreno, J.; Abizanda, P. Use of Health Resources and Healthcare Costs associated with Frailty: The FRADEA Study. *J. Nutr. Health Aging* **2017**, *21*, 207–214. [CrossRef] [PubMed]
11. Mohler, M.J.; Fain, M.J.; Wertheimer, A.M.; Najafi, B.; Nikolich-Zugich, J. The Frailty syndrome: Clinical measurements and basic underpinnings in humans and animals. *Exp. Gerontol.* **2014**, *54*, 6–13. [CrossRef] [PubMed]
12. Cesari, M.; Gambassi, G.; van Kan, G.A.; Vellas, B. The frailty phenotype and the frailty index: Different instruments for different purposes. *Age Ageing* **2014**, *43*, 10–12. [CrossRef] [PubMed]
13. Fried, L.P.; Tangen, C.M.; Walston, J.; Newman, A.B.; Hirsch, C.; Gottdiener, J.; Seeman, T.; Tracy, R.; Kop, W.J.; Burke, G.; et al. Frailty in older adults: Evidence for a phenotype. *J. Gerontol. Ser. A Biol. Sci. Med. Sci.* **2001**, *56*, M146–M156. [CrossRef]
14. Clegg, A.; Young, J.; Iliffe, S.; Rikkert, M.O.; Rockwood, K. Frailty in elderly people. *Lancet* **2013**, *381*, 752–762. [CrossRef]
15. Zhou, H.; Sabbagh, M.; Wyman, R.; Liebsack, C.; Kunik, M.E.; Najafi, B. Instrumented Trail-Making Task to Differentiate Persons with No Cognitive Impairment, Amnestic Mild Cognitive Impairment, and Alzheimer Disease: A Proof of Concept Study. *Gerontology* **2017**, *63*, 189–200. [CrossRef] [PubMed]
16. Schwenk, M.; Howe, C.; Saleh, A.; Mohler, J.; Grewal, G.; Armstrong, D.; Najafi, B. Frailty and technology: A systematic review of gait analysis in those with frailty. *Gerontology* **2014**, *60*, 79–89. [CrossRef] [PubMed]
17. Lee, H.; Joseph, B.; Enriquez, A.; Najafi, B. Toward Using a Smartwatch to Monitor Frailty in a Hospital Setting: Using a Single Wrist-Wearable Sensor to Assess Frailty in Bedbound Inpatients. *Gerontology* **2017**. [CrossRef] [PubMed]
18. Toosizadeh, N.; Joseph, B.; Heusser, M.R.; Orouji Jokar, T.; Mohler, J.; Phelan, H.A.; Najafi, B. Assessing Upper-Extremity Motion: An Innovative, Objective Method to Identify Frailty in Older Bed-Bound Trauma Patients. *J. Am. Coll. Surg.* **2016**, *223*, 240–248. [CrossRef] [PubMed]
19. Toosizadeh, N.; Mohler, J.; Najafi, B. Assessing Upper Extremity Motion: An Innovative Method to Identify Frailty. *J. Am. Geriatr. Soc.* **2015**, *63*, 1181–1186. [CrossRef] [PubMed]

20. Zhou, H.; Lee, H.; Lee, J.; Schwenk, M.; Najafi, B. Motor Planning Error: Toward Measuring Cognitive Frailty in Older Adults Using Wearables. *Sensors* **2018**, *18*, 926. [CrossRef] [PubMed]

21. Galan-Mercant, A.; Cuesta-Vargas, A.I. Mobile Romberg test assessment (mRomberg). *BMC Res. Notes* **2014**, *7*, 640. [CrossRef] [PubMed]

22. Schwenk, M.; Mohler, J.; Wendel, C.; D'Huyvetter, K.; Fain, M.; Taylor-Piliae, R.; Najafi, B. Wearable sensor-based in-home assessment of gait, balance, and physical activity for discrimination of frailty status: Baseline results of the Arizona frailty cohort study. *Gerontology* **2015**, *61*, 258–267. [CrossRef] [PubMed]

23. Rosenberg, I.H. Sarcopenia: Origins and clinical relevance. *J. Nutr.* **1997**, *127*, 990S–991S. [CrossRef] [PubMed]

24. Razjouyan, J.; Naik, A.D.; Horstman, M.J.; Kunik, M.E.; Amirmazaheri, M.; Zhou, H.; Sharafkhaneh, A.; Najafi, B. Wearable Sensors and the Assessment of Frailty among Vulnerable Older Adults: An Observational Cohort Study. *Sensors* **2018**, *18*, 1336. [CrossRef] [PubMed]

25. Parvaneh, S.; Mohler, J.; Toosizadeh, N.; Grewal, G.S.; Najafi, B. Postural Transitions during Activities of Daily Living Could Identify Frailty Status: Application of Wearable Technology to Identify Frailty during Unsupervised Condition. *Gerontology* **2017**, *63*, 479–487. [CrossRef] [PubMed]

26. Galan-Mercant, A.; Cuesta-Vargas, A.I. Differences in Trunk Accelerometry Between Frail and Nonfrail Elderly Persons in Sit-to-Stand and Stand-to-Sit Transitions Based on a Mobile Inertial Sensor. *JMIR Mhealth Uhealth* **2013**, *1*, e21. [CrossRef] [PubMed]

27. Greene, B.R.; Doheny, E.P.; O'Halloran, A.; Anne Kenny, R. Frailty status can be accurately assessed using inertial sensors and the TUG test. *Age Ageing* **2014**, *43*, 406–411. [CrossRef] [PubMed]

28. Galan-Mercant, A.; Cuesta-Vargas, A.I. Differences in trunk accelerometry between frail and non-frail elderly persons in functional tasks. *BMC Res Notes* **2014**, *7*, 100. [CrossRef] [PubMed]

29. Hegde, N.; Zhang, T.; Uswatte, G.; Taub, E.; Barman, J.; McKay, S.; Taylor, A.; Morris, D.M.; Griffin, A.; Sazonov, E.S. The Pediatric SmartShoe: Wearable Sensor System for Ambulatory Monitoring of Physical Activity and Gait. *IEEE Trans. Neural Syst. Rehabil. Eng.* **2018**, *26*, 477–486. [CrossRef] [PubMed]

30. Bamberg, S.J.; Benbasat, A.Y.; Scarborough, D.M.; Krebs, D.E.; Paradiso, J.A. Gait analysis using a shoe-integrated wireless sensor system. *IEEE Trans. Inf. Technol. Biomed.* **2008**, *12*, 413–423. [CrossRef] [PubMed]

31. Gonzalez, I.; Fontecha, J.; Hervas, R.; Bravo, J. An Ambulatory System for Gait Monitoring Based on Wireless Sensorized Insoles. *Sensors* **2015**, *15*, 16589–16613. [CrossRef] [PubMed]

32. Rampp, A.; Barth, J.; Schulein, S.; Gassmann, K.G.; Klucken, J.; Eskofier, B.M. Inertial sensor-based stride parameter calculation from gait sequences in geriatric patients. *IEEE Trans. Bio-Med. Eng.* **2015**, *62*, 1089–1097. [CrossRef] [PubMed]

33. Mariani, B.; Jimenez, M.C.; Vingerhoets, F.J.; Aminian, K. On-shoe wearable sensors for gait and turning assessment of patients with Parkinson's disease. *IEEE Trans. Bio-Med. Eng.* **2013**, *60*, 155–158. [CrossRef] [PubMed]

34. Nsenga Leunkeu, A.; Lelard, T.; Shephard, R.J.; Doutrellot, P.L.; Ahmaidi, S. Gait cycle and plantar pressure distribution in children with cerebral palsy: Clinically useful outcome measures for a management and rehabilitation. *NeuroRehabilitation* **2014**, *35*, 657–663. [PubMed]

35. Schlachetzki, J.C.M.; Barth, J.; Marxreiter, F.; Gossler, J.; Kohl, Z.; Reinfelder, S.; Gassner, H.; Aminian, K.; Eskofier, B.M.; Winkler, J.; et al. Wearable sensors objectively measure gait parameters in Parkinson's disease. *PLoS ONE* **2017**, *12*, e0183989. [CrossRef] [PubMed]

36. Nguyen, H.; Lebel, K.; Bogard, S.; Goubault, E.; Boissy, P.; Duval, C. Using Inertial Sensors to Automatically Detect and Segment Activities of Daily Living in People With Parkinson's Disease. *IEEE Trans. Neural Syst. Rehabil. Eng.* **2018**, *26*, 197–204. [CrossRef] [PubMed]

37. McCormick, L.; Martin, L.; Thomas, J. 1Introducing Gait Speed to Assess Frailty Outcomes In Day Hospital Patients. *Age Ageing* **2016**, *45*, i1. [CrossRef]

38. Martínez-Ramírez, A.; Martinikorena, I.; Gómez, M.; Lecumberri, P.; Millor, N.; Rodríguez-Mañas, L.; García García, F.J.; Izquierdo, M. Frailty assessment based on trunk kinematic parameters during walking. *J. Neuroeng. Rehabil.* **2015**, *12*, 48. [CrossRef] [PubMed]

39. Thiede, R.; Toosizadeh, N.; Mills, J.L.; Zaky, M.; Mohler, J.; Najafi, B. Gait and balance assessments as early indicators of frailty in patients with known peripheral artery disease. *Clin. Biomech.* **2016**, *32*, 1–7. [CrossRef] [PubMed]

40. Griffin, T.M.; Roberts, T.J.; Kram, R. Metabolic cost of generating muscular force in human walking: Insights from load-carrying and speed experiments. *J. Appl. Physiol.* **2003**, *95*, 172–183. [CrossRef] [PubMed]

41. Dudzińska-Griszek, J.; Szuster, K.; Szewieczek, J. Grip strength as a frailty diagnostic component in geriatric inpatients. *Clin. Interv. Aging* **2017**, *12*, 1151–1157. [CrossRef] [PubMed]

42. Elhadi, M.M.O.; Ma, C.Z.; Wong, D.W.C.; Wan, A.H.P.; Lee, W.C.C. Comprehensive Gait Analysis of Healthy Older Adults Who Have Undergone Long-Distance Walking. *J. Aging Phys. Act.* **2017**, *25*, 367–377. [CrossRef] [PubMed]

43. Davis, R.B.; DeLuca, P.A. Gait characterization via dynamic joint stiffness. *Gait Posture* **1996**, *4*, 224–231. [CrossRef]

44. Grewal, G.; Sayeed, R.; Yeschek, S.; Menzies, R.A.; Talal, T.K.; Lavery, L.A.; Armstrong, D.G.; Najafi, B. Virtualizing the assessment: A novel pragmatic paradigm to evaluate lower extremity joint perception in diabetes. *Gerontology* **2012**, *58*, 463–471. [CrossRef] [PubMed]

45. Reistetter, T.A.; Graham, J.E.; Deutsch, A.; Markello, S.J.; Granger, C.V.; Ottenbacher, K.J. Diabetes comorbidity and age influence rehabilitation outcomes after hip fracture. *Diabetes Care* **2011**, *34*, 1375–1377. [CrossRef] [PubMed]

46. Veeravelli, S.; Najafi, B.; Marin, I.; Blumenkron, F.; Smith, S.; Klotz, S.A. Exergaming in Older People Living with HIV Improves Balance, Mobility and Ameliorates Some Aspects of Frailty. *J. Vis. Exp.* **2016**. [CrossRef] [PubMed]

47. Tombaugh, T.N.; McIntyre, N.J. The mini-mental state examination: A comprehensive review. *J. Am. Geriatr. Soc.* **1992**, *40*, 922–935. [CrossRef] [PubMed]

48. Taylor, H.L.; Jacobs, D.R., Jr.; Schucker, B.; Knudsen, J.; Leon, A.S.; Debacker, G. A questionnaire for the assessment of leisure time physical activities. *J. Chronic Dis.* **1978**, *31*, 741–755. [CrossRef]

49. Najafi, B.; Helbostad, J.L.; Moe-Nilssen, R.; Zijlstra, W.; Aminian, K. Does walking strategy in older people change as a function of walking distance? *Gait Posture* **2009**, *29*, 261–266. [CrossRef] [PubMed]

50. Najafi, B.; Khan, T.; Wrobel, J. Laboratory in a box: Wearable sensors and its advantages for gait analysis. *Conf. Proc. IEEE Eng. Med. Biol. Soc.* **2011**, *2011*, 6507–6510. [PubMed]

51. Ayachi, F.; Nguyen, H.; Goubault, E.; Boissy, P.; Duval, C. The Use of Empirical Mode Decomposition-Based Algorithm and Inertial Measurement Units to Auto-Detect Daily Living Activities of Healthy Adults. *IEEE Trans. Neural Syst. Rehabil. Eng.* **2016**. [CrossRef] [PubMed]

52. Razjouyan, J.; Lee, H.; Parthasarathy, S.; Mohler, J.; Sharafkhaneh, A.; Najafi, B. Improving Sleep Quality Assessment Using Wearable Sensors by Including Information From Postural/Sleep Position Changes and Body Acceleration: A Comparison of Chest-Worn Sensors, Wrist Actigraphy, and Polysomnography. *J. Clin. Sleep Med.* **2017**, *13*, 1301–1310. [CrossRef] [PubMed]

53. Eng, J. Receiver Operating Characteristic Analysis: A Primer1. *Acad. Radiol.* **2005**, *12*, 909–916. [CrossRef] [PubMed]

54. Swets, J.A. Indices of discrimination or diagnostic accuracy: their ROCs and implied models. *Psychol. Bull.* **1986**, *99*, 100–117. [CrossRef] [PubMed]

55. Hanley, J.A.; McNeil, B.J. The meaning and use of the area under a receiver operating characteristic (ROC) curve. *Radiology* **1982**, *143*, 29–36. [CrossRef] [PubMed]

56. Shieh, G. Confidence intervals and sample size calculations for the weighted eta-squared effect sizes in one-way heteroscedastic ANOVA. *Behav. Res. Methods* **2013**, *45*, 25–37. [CrossRef] [PubMed]

57. Cohen, J. *Statistical Power Analysis for the Behavioral Sciences*; Lawrence Erlbaum Associates: Mahwah, NJ, USA, 1988.

58. Spearman, C. The proof and measurement of association between two things. By C. Spearman, 1904. *Am. J. Psychol.* **1987**, *100*, 441–471. [CrossRef] [PubMed]

59. Alvarez-Nebreda, M.L.; Bentov, N.; Urman, R.D.; Setia, S.; Huang, J.C.-S.; Pfeifer, K.; Bennett, K.A.; Ong, T.D.; Richman, D.; Gollapudi, D.; et al. Recommendations for preoperative management of frailty from the Society for Perioperative Assessment and Quality Improvement (SPAQI). *Perioper. Care Oper. Room Manag.* **2018**, *10*, 1–9. [CrossRef]

60. Kramer, D.B.; Tsai, T.; Natarajan, P.; Tewksbury, E.; Mitchell, S.L.; Travison, T.G. Frailty, Physical Activity, and Mobility in Patients With Cardiac Implantable Electrical Devices. *J. Am. Heart Assoc.* **2017**, *6*. [CrossRef] [PubMed]

61. Savva, G.M.; Donoghue, O.A.; Horgan, F.; O'Regan, C.; Cronin, H.; Kenny, R.A. Using timed up-and-go to identify frail members of the older population. *J. Gerontol. A Biol. Sci. Med. Sci.* **2013**, *68*, 441–446. [CrossRef] [PubMed]

62. Podsiadlo, D.; Richardson, S. The Timed "Up & Go": A Test of Basic Functional Mobility for Frail Elderly Persons. *J. Am. Geriatr. Soc.* **1991**, *39*, 142–148. [PubMed]

63. Castell, M.-V.; Sánchez, M.; Julián, R.; Queipo, R.; Martín, S.; Otero, Á. Frailty prevalence and slow walking speed in persons age 65 and older: Implications for primary care. *BMC Fam. Pract.* **2013**, *14*, 86. [CrossRef] [PubMed]

64. Rahemi, H.; Nigam, N.; Wakeling, J.M. The effect of intramuscular fat on skeletal muscle mechanics: Implications for the elderly and obese. *J. R. Soc. Interface* **2015**, *12*, 20150365. [CrossRef] [PubMed]

65. Chang, Y.H.; Kram, R. Limitations to maximum running speed on flat curves. *J. Exp. Biol.* **2007**, *210*, 971–982. [CrossRef] [PubMed]

66. Luo, G.; Stefanyshyn, D. Limb force and non-sagittal plane joint moments during maximum-effort curve sprint running in humans. *J. Exp. Biol.* **2012**, *215*, 4314–4321. [CrossRef] [PubMed]

67. Liu, W.; Zhang, C.; Ma, H.; Li, S. Learning Efficient Spatial-Temporal Gait Features with Deep Learning for Human Identification. *Neuroinformatics* **2018**. [CrossRef] [PubMed]

68. Uddin, M.Z.; Khaksar, W.; Torresen, J. A robust gait recognition system using spatiotemporal features and deep learning. In Proceedings of the IEEE International Conference on Multisensor Fusion and Integration for Intelligent Systems (MFI), Daegu, Korea, 16–18 November 2017.

69. Rockwood, K.; Blodgett, J.M.; Theou, O.; Sun, M.H.; Feridooni, H.A.; Mitnitski, A.; Rose, R.A.; Godin, J.; Gregson, E.; Howlett, S.E. A Frailty Index Based On Deficit Accumulation Quantifies Mortality Risk in Humans and in Mice. *Sci. Rep.* **2017**, *7*, 43068. [CrossRef] [PubMed]

70. Drey, M.; Pfeifer, K.; Sieber, C.C.; Bauer, J.M. The Fried frailty criteria as inclusion criteria for a randomized controlled trial: Personal experience and literature review. *Gerontology* **2011**, *57*, 11–18. [CrossRef] [PubMed]

71. Walston, J. Frailty Research Moves Beyond Risk Assessment. *J. Gerontol. A Biol. Sci. Med. Sci.* **2017**, *72*, 915–916. [CrossRef] [PubMed]

72. Tong, K.; Granat, M.H. A practical gait analysis system using gyroscopes. *Med. Eng. Phys.* **1999**, *21*, 87–94. [CrossRef]

73. Aminian, K.; Najafi, B. Capturing human motion using body-fixed sensors: Outdoor measurement and clinical applications. *Comput. Anim. Virtual Worlds* **2004**, *15*, 79–94. [CrossRef]

74. Liedtke, C.; Fokkenrood, S.A.; Menger, J.T.; van der Kooij, H.; Veltink, P.H. Evaluation of instrumented shoes for ambulatory assessment of ground reaction forces. *Gait Posture* **2007**, *26*, 39–47. [CrossRef] [PubMed]

75. Zhang, K.; Sun, M.; Lester, D.K.; Pi-Sunyer, F.X.; Boozer, C.N.; Longman, R.W. Assessment of human locomotion by using an insole measurement system and artificial neural networks. *J. Biomech.* **2005**, *38*, 2276–2287. [CrossRef] [PubMed]

76. Aminian, K.; Najafi, B.; Bula, C.; Leyvraz, P.F.; Robert, P. Spatio-temporal parameters of gait measured by an ambulatory system using miniature gyroscopes. *J. Biomech.* **2002**, *35*, 689–699. [CrossRef]

77. Moufawad El Achkar, C.; Lenoble-Hoskovec, C.; Paraschiv-Ionescu, A.; Major, K.; Bula, C.; Aminian, K. Physical Behavior in Older Persons during Daily Life: Insights from Instrumented Shoes. *Sensors* **2016**, *16*, 1225. [CrossRef] [PubMed]

78. Najafi, B.; Crews, R.T.; Wrobel, J.S. Importance of time spent standing for those at risk of diabetic foot ulceration. *Diabetes Care* **2010**, *33*, 2448–2450. [CrossRef] [PubMed]

79. Najafi, B.; Grewal, G.S.; Bharara, M.; Menzies, R.; Talal, T.K.; Armstrong, D.G. Can't Stand the Pressure: The Association Between Unprotected Standing, Walking, and Wound Healing in People With Diabetes. *J. Diabetes Sci. Technol.* **2017**, *11*, 657–667. [CrossRef] [PubMed]
80. Lindemann, U.; Najafi, B.; Zijlstra, W.; Hauer, K.; Muche, R.; Becker, C.; Aminian, K. Distance to achieve steady state walking speed in frail elderly persons. *Gait Posture* **2008**, *27*, 91–96. [CrossRef] [PubMed]

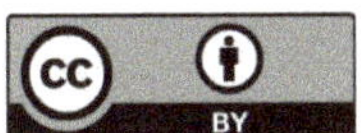

© 2018 by the authors. Licensee MDPI, Basel, Switzerland. This article is an open access article distributed under the terms and conditions of the Creative Commons Attribution (CC BY) license (http://creativecommons.org/licenses/by/4.0/).

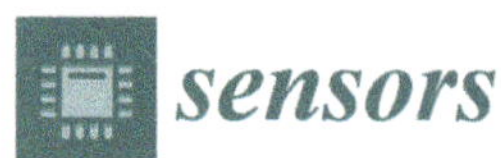

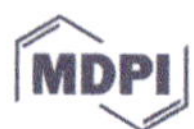

Article

Inertial Sensor-Based Variables Are Indicators of Frailty and Adverse Post-Operative Outcomes in Cardiovascular Disease Patients

Rahul Soangra [1] and Thurmon E. Lockhart [2],*

[1] Department of Physical Therapy, Crean College of Health and Behavioral Sciences, Chapman University, Orange, CA 92866, USA; soangra@chapman.edu

[2] School of Biological and Health Systems Engineering, Ira A. Fulton Schools of Engineering, Arizona State University, Tempe, AZ 85287, USA

* Correspondence: Thurmon.lockhart@asu.edu; Tel.: +1-480-965-1499

Received: 26 February 2018; Accepted: 31 May 2018; Published: 2 June 2018

Abstract: Cardiovascular disease (CVD) patients with intrinsic cardiac cause for falling have been found to be frail and submissive to morbidity and mortality as post-operative outcomes. In these older CVD patients, gait speed is conjectured by the Society of Thoracic Surgeons (STS) as an independent predictor of post-operative morbidity and mortality. However, this guideline by STS has not been studied adequately with a large sample size; rather it is based largely on expert opinions of cardiac surgeons and researchers. Although one's gait speed is not completely associated with one's risk of falls, gait speed is a quick robust measure to classify frail/non-frail CVD patients and undoubtedly frail individuals are more prone to falls. Thus, this study examines the effects of inertial sensor-based quick movement variability characteristics in identifying CVD patients likely to have an adverse post-operative outcome. This study establishes a relationship with gait and postural predictor variables with patient's post-operative adverse outcomes. Accordingly, inertial sensors embedded inside smartphones are indispensable for the assessment of elderly patients in clinical environments and may be necessary for quick objective assessment. Sixteen elderly CVD patients (Age 76.1 ± 3.6 years) who were scheduled for cardiac surgery the next day were recruited for this study. Based on STS recommendation guidelines, eight of the CVD patients were classified as frail (prone to adverse outcomes with gait speed $\leq$ 0.833 m/s) and the other eight patients as non-frail (gait speed > 0.833 m/s). Smartphone-derived walking velocity was found to be significantly lower in frail patients than that in non-frail patients ($p < 0.01$). Mean Center of Pressure (COP) radius ($p < 0.01$), COP Area ($p < 0.01$), COP path length ($p < 0.05$) and mean COP velocity ($p < 0.05$) were found to be significantly higher in frail patients than that in the non-frail patient group. Nonlinear variability measures such as sample entropy were significantly lower in frail participants in anterior-posterior ($p < 0.01$) and resultant sway direction ($p < 0.01$) than in the non-frail group. This study identified numerous postural and movement variability parameters that offer insights into predictive inertial sensor-based variables and post-operative adverse outcomes among CVD patients. In future, smartphone-based clinical measurement systems could serve as a clinical decision support system for assessing patients quickly in the perioperative period.

Keywords: frailty prediction; fall risk; smartphone based assessments; adverse post-operative outcome

---

1. Introduction

Falls [1] and frailty [2,3] in elderly patients are multifactorial [4] and are attributed to a complex interaction of intrinsic and extrinsic risk factors superimposed on normal aging process [5–8]. Patients with intrinsic cardiac cause for falling have been found to have higher mortality rate than those with non-cardiovascular or unknown causes of falls [9]. Falls in cardiovascular disease (CVD) patients are reported to be caused by underlying cardiovascular disorders or are linked to aging [10]. It remains unclear which factors are responsible for high fall risk in CVD patients, but some experts speculate that certain environments, medications, age-related changes, and diseases make a particular genotype of people vulnerable to frailty and falls in CVD patients [11,12]. This frailty phenotype is independently predictive of falls [13]. Some researchers have also linked functional limitation [14–17], poor nutritional status [14,15,18], cognitive impairment [15,19,20], depression [20,21] and loneliness [22] with cardiovascular disorders and frailty. Since both fall risk and frailty are multifactorial problems, a better understanding of the variables linked to these problems on post-operative outcomes is imperative.

Analysis of gait and postural predictor variables that describe the underlying neuromuscular function are indispensable for the diagnosis and treatment of elderly patients and may be necessary for objectively assessing CVD patients for their post-operative outcomes. Bereft of multisystem reserves, the elderly CVD patients (particularly who are frail) are increasingly vulnerable to an array of adverse health outcomes, including sarcopenia, hospitalization, negative energy balance, exhaustion, falls, and loss of independence [23] and mortality. It is evident that the elderly with cardiovascular disorders along with a history of falling have a two-thirds chance of falling over the next year [7]. In addition to inherent fall risk in older CVD patients, there exists heterogeneity of health status and this leads to increased risk of post-operative complications [16,24], and thus surgical decision-making is challenging for clinicians. Preoperative risk assessment is essential but there is a paucity of tools for predicting operative risk. Physiologic reserve in an older adult can determine his/her resilience to recover from an operation. However, there is no standardized method of measuring physiologic reserve in older surgical patients [24]. Frailty is a marker of decreased physiologic reserves and resistance to stressors [13,25–27] and predicts operative risk in older surgical patients [24]. In clinical operative settings, clinicians have tried to link postoperative adverse outcomes with various components of frailty [28].

Researchers have also reported that age remains an independent risk factor even after controlling for co-morbid illnesses and functional impairment for postoperative complications [14–16,19,28,29]. Chronological age of a patient does not reflect his/her biological age, and elderly patients have a range of biological statuses that vary from robust to frail [11,30]. Recently, the Society of Thoracic Surgeons (STS) has conjectured gait speed in CVD patients as an independent predictor of post-operative morbidity and mortality. However, this guideline by STS is based largely on expert opinion and a single walking characteristic i.e., gait speed. Although one's gait speed is not well associated with one's risk of falls, gait speed remains a quick robust measure to classify frail/non-frail CVD patients and undoubtedly frail individuals are more prone to falls [31–33]. The objective of this study is to utilize laboratory-validated tools [34,35] to assess gait and posture-related movement variability characteristics using inertial sensors (widely used in fall-risk assessment), and apply it to a clinical setting for quick assessment of post-operative adverse outcomes in cardiovascular patients. It was hypothesized that inertial sensors can help identify a subset of patients and as such their gait and posture measures have potential to identify patients with a high probability of adverse post-operative health outcome.

2. Materials and Methods

Sixteen CVD patients have been included in this study (Table 1). Patients were included in the study only if they: (i) Consented to participate and were above 70 years of age (ii), were going to be operated on the next day for cardiovascular disorder (cardiac surgery), (iii) were cognitively able to follow instructions and, (iv) were able to ambulate. The patients were categorized into a frail (F) group (walking velocity ≤ 0.833 m/s) and non-frail (NF) group (walking velocity > 0.833 m/s). The sample population had five females (ID17, ID18, and ID20–22) and 11 males.

Table 1. Means and standard deviations of patients' anthropometric and age information.

Anthropometric Variables	Frail		Non-Frail		All CVD Patients	
	Mean	**SD**	**Mean**	**SD**	**Mean**	**SD**
Age (years)	76.38	4.03	76.00	3.55	76.18	3.67
Height (cm)	172.34	12.92	171.30	6.43	171.81	9.87
Weight (kg)	87.41	20.32	77.41	15.89	82.40	18.36
BMI (kg/m^2)	29.69	7.46	26.26	4.73	27.97	6.28

Patients scheduled for cardiac surgery and present to the Cardiac Surgery Pre-Surgical Testing (PST) area of the hospital were screened by the PST nurse to determine whether all inclusion criteria were met. If the patient was found eligible for inclusion into the study, the PST nurse requested the patient if he/she were interested in talking about the study. If the patient was interested, a consenter (registered nurse specialist) discussed the study with the patient, answered all relevant questions about the study, and obtained written consent according to the IRB.

Patients who met all inclusion criteria and had consented were requested to wear a waist belt and a smartphone (inside holster) was clipped to the waist belt. All the experiments were conducted in a well-lit room with an unobstructed walking area with clear floor markings at 0 m and 5 m (Figure 1). The patients were asked to rise from the chair to a standing position and follow instruction as per the voice commands of the app (Table 2). Patients were allowed to use their walking aid (cane, walker) if they needed. A standard digital stopwatch was used; the stopwatch was started with the first footfall after the 0 m line and stopped with the first footfall after the 5 m line. The walk was repeated 3 times, with sufficient time for subject recuperation between trials. Each 5 m walk time (in seconds) was recorded on the data collection form (Figure 2). The average speed for the 3 trials was calculated and was also recorded on the data collection form. The participant's postural transition time and static postural stability was measured using the floor embedded forceplate beside the bariatric chair and smartphone-based inertial sensors. The walking speed and other gait characteristics were also determined using smartphone-based inertial sensors.

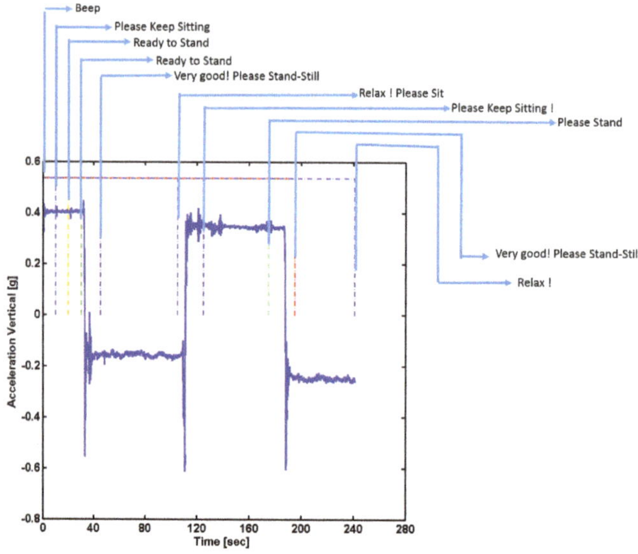

Figure 1. Truncation of smartphone IMU signals using temporal information of voice commands through the app.

Table 2. Voice commands used in app for data collection in clinical environment.

Time Interval (s)	Sound & Voice Commands	Total Elapsed Time (s)
0	Beep	0
10	Please Keep Sitting	10
10	Ready to Stand	20
10	Please stand	30
10	Very Good! Please Stand Still	40
65	Relax! Please Sit	105
60	Please Keep Sitting!	165
10	Ready to Stand	175
10	Very Good! Please Stand Still	185
65	Relax!	250

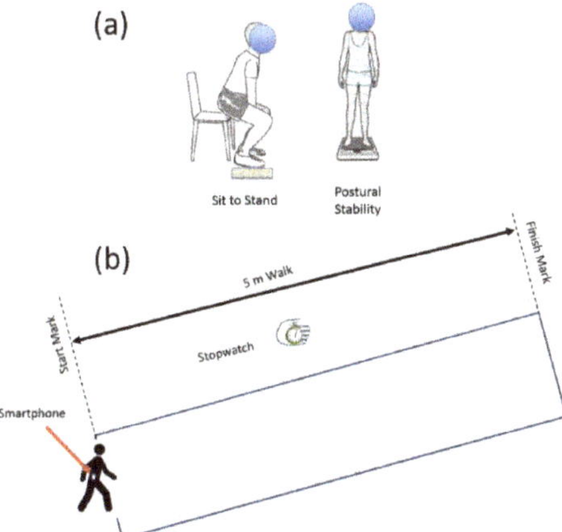

Figure 2. All patients (**a**) stand still for 60 s and perform sit-to-stand transitions; (**b**) walk a distance of 5 m.

Instrumentation: In this study, we used an Apple Iphone 5 instrument (iPhone 5, Apple Inc., Cupertino, CA, USA) which contains an ultra-compact low-power high-performance 3-axis "nano" MEMS accelerometer, LIS331DLH. The LIS331DLH has user selectable full scales of ±2 g/±4 g/±8 g and it is capable of measuring accelerations with output data rates 0.5 Hz to 1 kHz. It is capable of measuring acceleration data with a data sampling rate of 1000 Hz. It also contains a low-power 3-axis angular rate sensor, L3G4200D. The L3G4200D has a full scale of ±250/±500/±2000 degrees per second and can measure angular rates at a user-selectable bandwidth. An iOS 6-based app, named as "Lockhart Monitor" (App available freely on iOS store) was designed to collect data at a sampling frequency of 50 Hz. The app was programmed in objective C language using Xcode 4 IDE (Integrated Development Environment). The data was collected from inbuilt sensors, accelerometers and gyroscopes in the smartphone and stored in it. The collected data was either transferred using cloud service/Email or by a USB cable to the computer for data analyses. Further data processing was accomplished using custom-made Matlab (MATLAB version 6.5.1, 2003, The MathWorks Inc., Natick, MA, USA) routines. The app was designed after consultations with human factors specialists and clinical requirements from registered nurse specialists. The designed mobile app consisted of a start and stop button and recorded voice instructions were provided through the app with ample rest duration inbetween each performed activity (Table 2). The signals were truncated using the temporal information of voice commands through the app (Figure 1). A portable forceplate (Bertec Corporation, FP4060-05-PT, Columbus, OH, USA) was used to measure postural stability information.

Data Analyses: The smartphone data from each participant was collected and saved in two files: (i) The three trials of 5 m gait data (ii) and postural standing and sit-to-stand transition were collected in another data file. The data was resampled to 50 Hz, using the timestamps registered by the smartphone. The continuously collected data was then truncated at intervals and the truncated signal was used for further analysis (Figure 1). The signals were filtered using a low-pass Butterworth filter with zero lag at a cut-off frequency of 6 Hz. This cut-off frequency was selected since human movements are below 3 Hz [36,37].

To quantify the postural transition several parameters were derived from the forceplate placed below the feet of the patients while standing. Body uplift jerk [Newton/s] was defined as the rate of change of force during the sit-to-stand transition. It was calculated as the slope of the line connecting the highest force to the lowest vertical force for sit-to-stand and stand-to-sit transitions (Figure 3).

$$BUJ = \frac{dF_V}{dt},\tag{1}$$

where F_V is vertical force and Δt is the transition time for sit-to-stand or stand-to-sit transition.

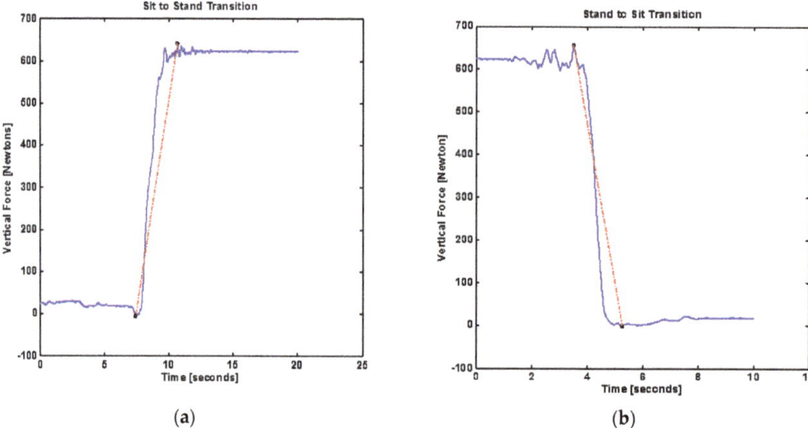

Figure 3. (**a**) Sit-to-stand vertical force (F_V), Δt is time taken from the minimum vertical force to maximum vertical force and body jerk (slope as dotted red-line); (**b**) stand-to-sit vertical force (F_V), Δt is time taken from the minimum vertical force to maximum vertical force and associated body jerk (slope as dotted red-line).

Jerk [m/s^3] was computed using accelerometer signals from steady state to maximum acceleration achieved during sit-to-stand or stand-to-sit movements. Figure 4 shows a typical signal of sit-to-stand from a smartphone accelerometer. Sway radius [mm] was calculated as the resultant of the mean of sway in AP and ML trajectories. Root Mean Square [mm] value of sway trajectory in a particular direction (AP or ML) was computed. Sway area [mm^2] was computed using mean sway radius.

Gait speed [m/s] was computed using inertial sensors of the smartphone for a 5 m long walk [34]. Acceleration signals from three directions were used to compute resultant acceleration. The resultant acceleration signals were filtered using a 4th order dual low-pass butterworth filter with a cut-off frequency as 6 Hz. One half second moving window variance was computed and the threshold was set using initial stand still data (Figure 5) as per the experimental protocol. Once start and stop time are detected, average velocity is computed over a 5 m distance walk. Root Mean Square (RMS) is a measure of dispersion of the data relative to zero, whereas standard deviation is a measure of dispersion relative to mean. This value is an indication of average magnitude of accelerations in each direction during a complete walking trial [38].

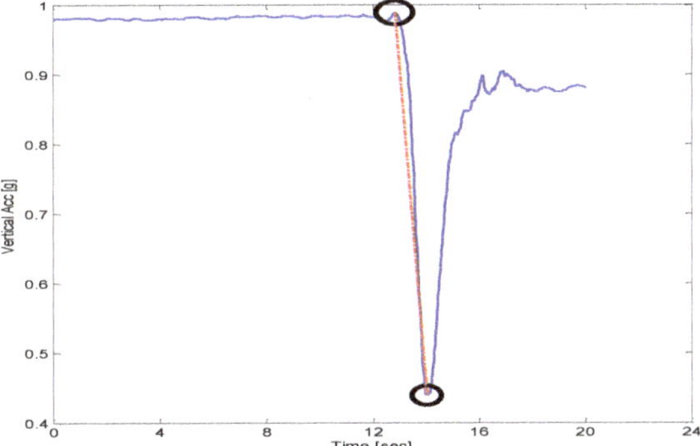

Figure 4. Peak flexion acceleration during sit-to-stand or stand-to-sit movements. Dotted red-line shows the slope as jerk.

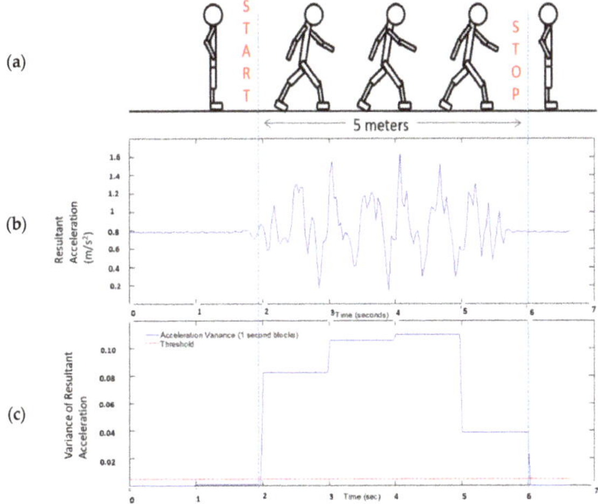

Figure 5. (**a**) The test starts from still-standing followed by 5 m walk and stops at still-standing as well; (**b**) resultant acceleration signals (in g-units); (**c**) moving window (0.5 s) variance of low-pass filtered resultant acceleration.

Where RMS_AP, RMS_ML, and RMS_V represent root mean square accelerations in anterior-posterior, medial-lateral and vertical directions, respectively (Table 3). RMS is statistical measure of magnitude of acceleration in each direction. RMSR represents the ratio between RMS in each direction and the RMS vector magnitude (RMST). RMSR is apparently the RMS normalized by the RMST. Harmonic ratio was described by Gage [39] and Smidt [40], to provide an indication of smoothness and rhythm of acceleration patterns. The harmonic ratio proposed by Gage is based on the premise that a stable rhythmic gait pattern should consist of acceleration patterns that repeat in multiples of two. Those which do not repeat in multiples of two are out of phase accelerations and therefore manifest as irregular accelerations during walking. The harmonic content of acceleration signal is evaluated in each direction using stride frequency as the fundamental frequency component. The acceleration signals that are in phase (even harmonics) are compared to components out of phase (odd harmonics) using finite Fourier series (Figure 6). The harmonic ratio is calculated by dividing the sum of amplitudes of the first 10 even harmonics by the first 10 odd harmonics for AP and Vertical direction (since both AP and vertical directions are biphasic for any stride) and its inverse for medio-lateral direction (basic ML pattern is limb dependent and only repeated once for any given stride). A higher harmonic ratio represents a smoother walking pattern.

Table 3. Six variability parameters were calculated using accelerations from three directions.

Details	Parameter Computation	Equation Number
RMS vector magnitude	$RMST = \sqrt{RMS\_AP^2 + RMS\_V^2 + RMS\_ML^2}$,	(2)
Normalized RMS in AP direction	$RMSR_{AP} = \frac{RMS_{AP}}{RMST}$,	(3)
Normalized RMS in ML direction	$RMSR_{ML} = \frac{RMS_{ML}}{RMST}$	(4)
Normalized RMS in Vertical direction	$RMSR_V = \frac{RMS_V}{RMST}$,	(5)
Harmonic Ratio in Vertical and AP direction	Harmonic Ratio = $\sum$ even harmonics / $\sum$ odd harmonics	(6)
Harmonic Ratio in ML direction	Harmonic Ratio = $\sum$ odd harmonics / $\sum$ even harmonics	(7)

Effects were considered significant when $p < 0.05$. We conducted initial analyses using a mixed-factor multivariate analysis of variance (MANOVA). Subsequent univariate repeated measures ANOVAs (mixed-factor design) were conducted separately for each dependent variable. Also, to control the familywise error rate Bonferroni corrections were adopted.

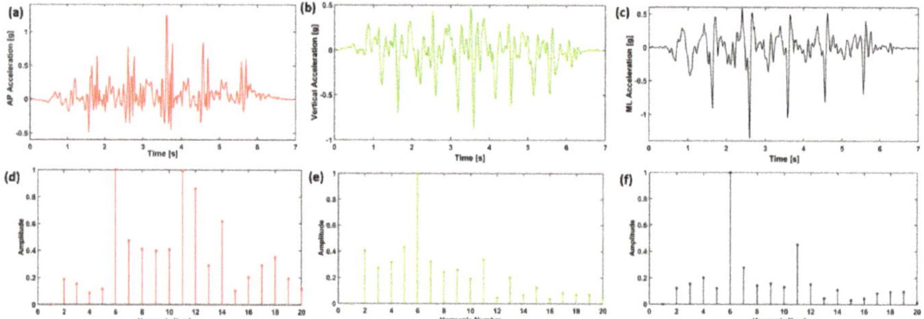

Figure 6. A representative acceleration signal of a patient with (**a**) acceleration in AP direction; (**b**) acceleration in vertical direction; (**c**) acceleration in ML direction; (**d**) harmonics of AP acceleration; (**e**) harmonics in vertical acceleration; (**f**) harmonics in ML acceleration for 5 m walk.

3. Results

Walking velocities computed using stopwatch time and smartphone time were found to be correlated with Pearson correlation coefficient = 0.8154 and spearman's rho = 0.8834 (Figure 7). Eight participants were classified as frail and eight as non-frail using the velocities from the stopwatch (with cut-off velocity = 0.833 m/s).

Table 4 lists velocities from two different systems (stopwatch vs. smartphone). Figure 8 shows an interactive dot diagram of the data of the frail and non-frail groups as displayed in dots on two vertical axes. The horizontal line indicates the cut-off point with best separation (minimal false negative and false positive results) between the two groups. The specificity = 91.3% and sensitivity = 79.2% was found for the smartphone-based velocity predictions. The mean walking velocity measured using stopwatch for frail was 0.67 m/s and that for non-frail group was 0.98 m/s. However, smartphone sensors predicted the mean walking velocity for frail group as 0.75 m/s (corrected using the regression equation in Figure 7) and for non-frail group as 0.87 m/s (Table 5). Forceplate detected a significantly higher mean COP radius ($p < 0.01$), COP area ($p < 0.01$), COP path length ($p < 0.01$), mean COP Velocity ($p < 0.01$) and higher linear variability in parameters such as SD COP-AP ($p < 0.01$), SD COP-ML ($p = 0.01$), SD COP-R ($p = 0.02$). Complexity in AP direction, as defined by approximate entropy ApEn COP-AP, was found to be significantly lower in frail patients ($p < 0.01$). In congruence to this sample, entropy was also found to be lower in AP direction ($p < 0.01$) for the frail group. Mean power frequency in anterior-posterior direction was found to be lower in the frail group than that in the non-frail group ($p < 0.01$).

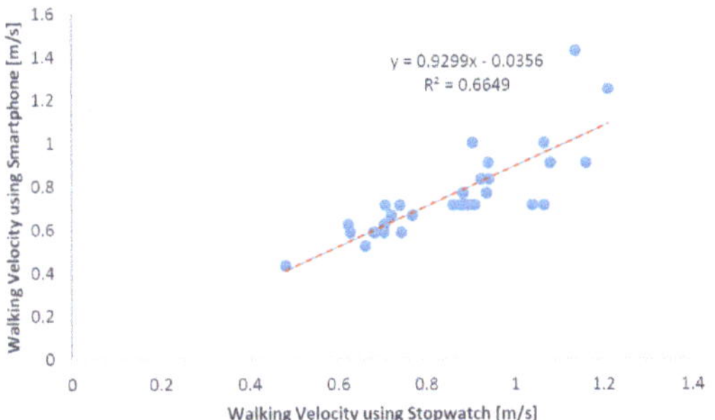

Figure 7. Relationship between the velocities of CVD patients computed from the two systems: stopwatch and smartphone. Dotted-red line shows the regression line.

Table 4. Classification of patients to frail and non-frail categories using velocities (cut-off = 0.833 m/s) from stopwatch. Velocities computed using smartphone walking signals are also listed below.

ID	Classification Frail (F), Non-Frail (NF)	Stopwatch Velocity			Smartphone Velocity			Classification Errors
		Mean	SD	CV	Mean	SD	CV	
ID04	NF	0.92	0.02	2.44	0.81	0.04	4.56	X
ID06	F	0.59	0.07	12.25	0.61	0.03	4.29	
ID08	F	0.73	0.05	6.44	0.66	0.06	9.70	
ID09	NF	1.21	0.07	5.89	1.23	0.22	17.56	
ID10	NF	1.06	0.14	12.95	0.97	0.05	5.41	
ID11	F	0.73	0.03	3.45	0.67	0.04	6.68	
ID13	F	0.83	0.09	10.27	0.75	0.07	9.11	
ID14	NF	1.06	0.02	2.34	0.81	0.16	20.38	X
ID17	F	0.67	0.01	1.51	0.58	0.05	8.60	
ID18	NF	0.91	0.03	2.97	0.70	0.07	10.36	X
ID19	F	0.58	0.09	15.04	0.59	0.14	24.14	
ID20	NF	0.97	0.10	9.92	0.88	0.04	4.95	
ID21	F	0.83	0.06	7.02	0.72	0.05	7.00	
ID22	F	0.74	0.05	6.95	0.65	0.10	16.11	
ID23	NF	0.95	0.09	9.24	0.77	0.06	7.71	
ID24	NF	1.00	0.06	6.33	1.01	0.10	10.04	

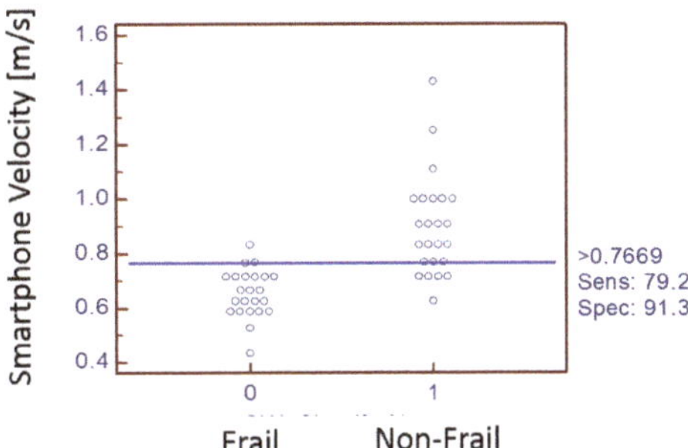

Figure 8. Integrative dot diagram suggesting specificity = 91.3% and Sensitivity = 79.2% for velocity derived from smartphone signals in classification of frail/non-frail patients.

Table 5. Linear and non-linear variability parameters from forceplate and smartphone IMU's for frail and non-frail participants.

Instrument	Variables	*p*-Value	Frail			Non-Frail		
			Mean	SD	CV	Mean	SD	CV
Stopwatch	Walking Velocity		0.67	0.08	12.03	0.98	0.13	13.10
Forceplate	Jerk [N/s]	0.83	0.01	0.00	72.96	0.01	0.00	46.55
	Peak-to-Peak Time [s]	0.09	1.81	0.86	47.33	1.38	0.69	49.71
	Mean COP Radius * [mm]	<0.01	7.38	2.02	27.30	4.88	1.59	32.60
	COP Area *	<0.01	183.37	114.36	62.36	82.44	53.97	65.46
	SD [COP-AP] *	<0.01	4.50	1.76	39.15	1.79	0.46	25.45
	SD [COP-ML] *	0.01	7.09	1.87	26.45	5.50	2.00	36.44
	SD [COP-R] *	0.02	6.63	2.20	33.17	4.98	2.33	46.87
	RMS [COP-AP]	0.92	28.61	25.42	88.87	27.62	36.61	132.51
	RMS [COP-ML]	0.08	55.13	32.29	58.57	40.29	18.68	46.36
	RMS [COP-R]	0.21	67.71	30.40	44.89	55.64	30.69	55.16
	Path Length [mm] *	<0.01	653.62	192.27	29.42	423.67	94.10	22.21
	Mean COP Velocity * [mm/s]	<0.01	21.79	6.41	29.42	14.12	3.14	22.21
	Alpha [COP-AP]	0.25	1.02	0.27	26.35	0.93	0.24	25.71
	Alpha [COP-ML]	0.13	0.93	0.20	21.40	1.03	0.24	22.85
	Alpha [COP-R]	0.20	0.92	0.21	22.31	1.01	0.24	23.47
	ApEn [COP-AP] *	<0.01	0.56	0.12	22.04	0.69	0.13	18.54
	ApEn [COP-ML]	0.25	0.74	0.15	20.58	0.69	0.14	19.83
	ApEn [COP-R]	0.28	0.71	0.17	23.49	0.66	0.12	18.56
	SampEn [COP-AP] *	<0.01	0.12	0.05	42.36	0.19	0.07	35.03
	SampEn [COP-ML]	0.30	0.19	0.09	47.49	0.16	0.07	41.49
	SampEn [COP-R]	0.34	0.18	0.09	51.19	0.16	0.05	34.15
	MPF [COP-AP] *	<0.01	0.03	0.01	35.61	0.04	0.02	35.92
	MPF [COP-ML]	0.10	0.04	0.02	44.30	0.04	0.01	32.56
Smartphone	Walk Velocity * [m/s]	<0.01	0.65	0.11	17.37	0.87	0.18	20.62
	Mean sway radius * [mm]	<0.01	14.24	3.93	27.59	8.88	3.76	42.36
	Sway Area * [mm^2]	<0.01	682.54	362.45	53.10	289.02	270.77	93.69
	Path Length * [mm]	<0.05	9217.19	2426.75	26.33	7108.34	2010.22	28.28
	Mean sway Velocity * [mm/s]	<0.05	307.19	80.80	26.30	236.94	67.01	28.28
	SD [sway-AP] *	<0.01	12.18	4.69	38.55	6.87	4.27	62.10
	SD [sway-ML] *	<0.01	10.88	3.36	30.89	7.33	2.78	37.87
	SD [sway-R] *	<0.01	8.57	2.75	32.08	5.16	2.64	51.13
	RMS [sway-AP] *	<0.01	12.17	4.69	38.55	6.87	4.27	62.10
	RMS [sway-ML] *	<0.01	10.87	3.36	30.89	7.33	2.78	37.87
	RMS [sway-R] *	<0.01	16.65	4.67	28.05	10.29	4.54	44.16
	Alpha [sway-AP]	0.30	1.03	0.32	31.11	1.15	0.28	24.45
	Alpha [sway-ML]	0.54	1.10	0.24	21.60	1.05	0.20	18.61
	Alpha [sway-R]	0.49	0.96	0.23	24.00	0.90	0.21	23.78
	ApEn [sway-AP]	0.26	1.07	0.10	8.91	1.10	0.04	3.86
	ApEn [sway-ML]	0.43	1.09	0.05	4.91	1.08	0.08	7.76
	ApEn [sway-R]	0.40	1.14	0.05	3.95	1.13	0.03	3.10
	SampEn [sway-AP] *	<0.01	1.36	0.27	20.07	1.69	0.28	16.85
	SampEn [sway-ML]	0.08	1.24	0.25	19.78	1.42	0.31	21.96
	SampEn [sway-R] *	<0.01	1.48	0.22	14.98	1.70	0.20	11.55

* significant at *p* < 0.05.

Similar to the velocities measured using the stopwatch, it was found that smartphone-based walking velocity was significantly lower in frail patients than in non-frail patients (*p* < 0.01). Mean sway radius (*p* < 0.01), sway area (*p* < 0.01), sway path length (*p* < 0.05) and mean sway velocity (*p* < 0.05) were found to be significantly higher in frail patients than in non-frail patients (Figure 9).

SD sway-AP (*p* < 0.01), SD sway-ML (*p* < 0.01), and SD sway-R (*p* < 0.01) were found to be significantly higher in frail participants. Similarly, RMS sway-AP (*p* < 0.01), RMS sway-ML (*p* < 0.01), RMS sway-R (*p* < 0.01) were also found to be significantly higher in frail participants (Figure 10).

Complexity of sway signals in anterior-posterior direction measured by sample entropy SampEn AP ($p < 0.01$) and resultant sway direction SampEn R ($p < 0.01$) were found to be significantly lower than in the non-frail group.

Post-operative outcomes in CVD patients consisted of both morbidity and mortality. Two frail patients were diagnosed with stroke (ID06 and ID21), one frail patient (ID11) with renal failure, three frail patients (ID08, ID11 and ID21) were kept for prolonged ventilation, one frail patient (ID21) had to be re-operated, 3 frail (ID06, ID11 and ID22) and 1 non-frail (ID23) were sent to a skilled nursing facility, only one frail patient (ID11) had a length of stay more than 14 days, and one frail patient had mortality (ID21) (Tables 6 and 7).

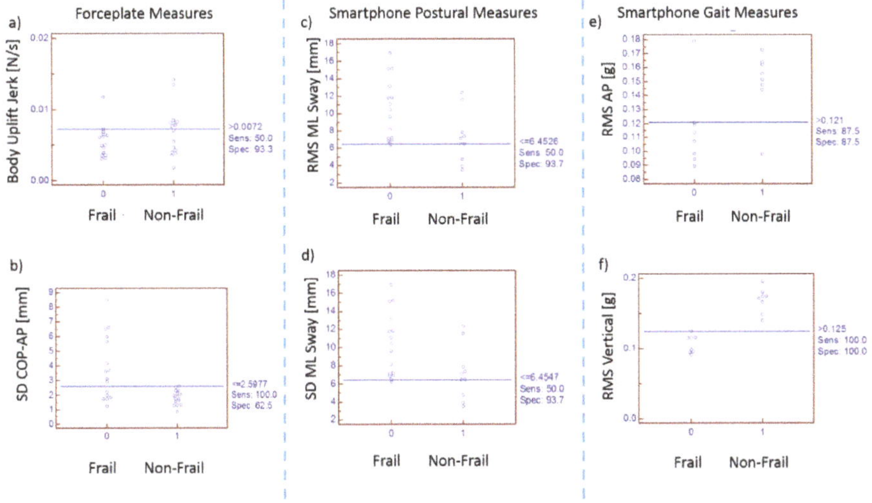

Figure 9. Interactive dot diagram of postural measures from forceplate: (**a**) Body uplift jerk; (**b**) SD of COP-AP, postural measures from smartphone; (**c**) RMS sway-ML; (**d**) SD of sway-ML and gait measures of smartphone; (**e**) RMS AP and (**f**) RMS Vertical.

Table 6. Post-operative morbidity and mortality of CVD patients.

ID	Frail/Non-Frail	Stroke	Renal Failure	Prolonged Ventilation	DSWI	Re-Operation > 24 h	Death	Skilled Nursing Facility	Length of Stay > 14 Days
ID04	NF	-	-	-	-	-	-	-	-
ID06	F	YES	-	-	-	-	-	YES	-
ID08	F	-	-	YES	-	-	-	-	-
ID09	NF	-	-	-	-	-	-	-	-
ID10	NF	-	-	-	-	-	-	-	-
ID11	F	-	YES	YES	-	-	-	YES	YES
ID13	F	-	-	-	-	-	-	-	-
ID14	NF	-	-	-	-	-	-	-	-
ID17	F	-	-	-	-	-	-	-	-
ID18	NF	-	-	-	-	-	-	-	-
ID19	F	-	-	-	-	-	-	-	-
ID20	NF	-	-	-	-	-	-	-	-
ID21	F	YES	-	YES	-	YES	YES	N/A	N/A
ID22	F	-	-	-	-	-	-	YES	-
ID23	NF	-	-	-	-	-	-	YES	-
ID24	NF	-	-	-	-	-	-	-	-

Table 7. Definitions of criteria for morbidity and mortality.

Stroke	Stroke (Central Neurological Deficit Persisting > 72 h)
RF	Renal Failure (new requirement for dialysis or increase in serum creatinine > 153 micromoles/liter [>2 mg/dL] and >2-fold the preoperative level)
Vent	Prolonged Ventilation (>24 h)
DSWI	Deep Sternal Wound Infection (requirement for operative intervention and antibiotic therapy, with positive culture)
Reop	Need for reoperation (for any reason)
SNF	Discharge to skilled Nursing Facility (health care facility) (rehabilitation, Convalescence, other hospital, nursing home) for on-going care or rehabilitation
LOS	Prolonged length of stay (>14 days postoperatively)
Death	Death (all causes)

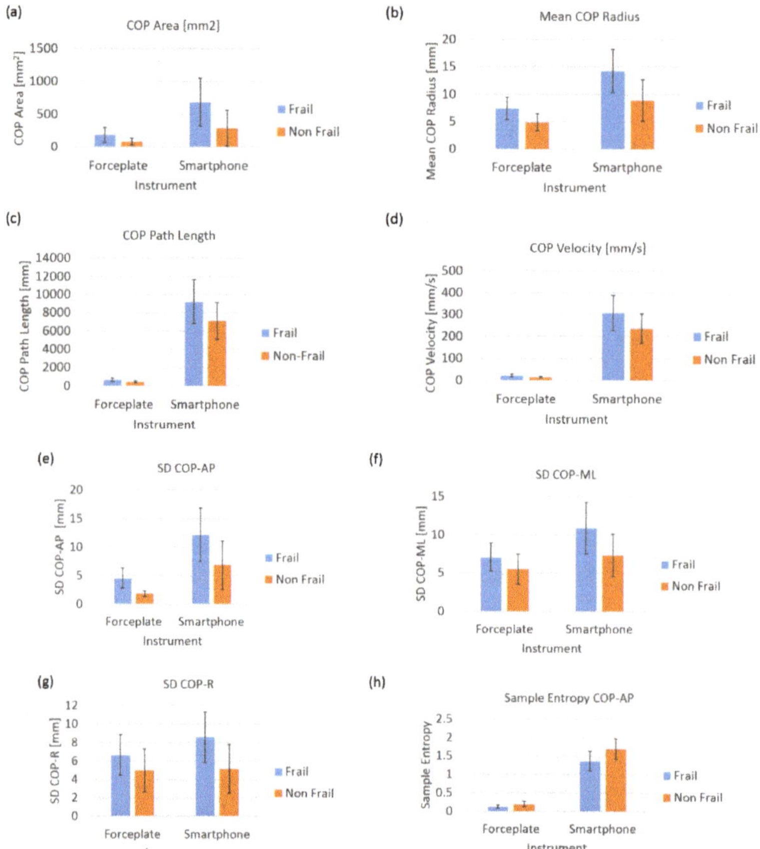

Figure 10. Postural parameters (**a**) COP Area; (**b**) Mean COP area; (**c**) COP path length; (**d**) COP Velocity; (**e**) SD of COP-AP; (**f**) SD of COP-ML; (**g**) SD of COP-R; (**h**) Sample Entropy of COP-AP from both systems i.e., forceplate and smartphone.

It was found that non-frail patients produced a higher range of accelerations while performing a sit-to-stand maneuver with lower overall variability (Table 8), whereas frail patients produced a lower range of accelerations while performing a sit-to-stand maneuver with higher variability (measured by Coefficient of variation). The variability in jerk produced during sit-to-stand was also found to be higher in frail patients than in non-frail patients. The mean time taken by frail patients in performing sit-to-stand and stand-to-sit was higher than non-frail patients (Table 8).

Table 8. Variabilities in sit-to-stand and stand-to-sit movement parameters in frail and non-frail elderly CVD patients.

Postural Transition Variables	Frail						Non-Frail					
	Sit to Stand			Stand to Sit			Sit to Stand			Stand to Sit		
	Mean	SD	CV	Mean	SD	CV	Mean	SD	CV	Mean	SD	CV
Acc Range (m/s^2)	44.6	23.8	53.4	55.3	23.0	41.6	52.4	25.0	47.7	72.6	31.3	43.0
Jerk (mm/s$^{3)}$)	15.8	13.9	87.8	17.3	12.4	71.5	15.9	9.2	58.1	21.6	11.1	51.4
Time (s)	1.6	0.6	41.8	1.5	0.7	48.0	1.4	0.4	32.4	1.3	0.3	23.1

Root mean square (RMS) in all three directions was found to be significantly different in frail and non-frail patients. Non-frail patients produced significantly higher RMS-AP ($p < 0.02$), RMS-V ($p < 0.01$) and RMS-ML ($p < 0.02$) than frail patients (Table 9).

Table 9. Harmonic ratio and root mean square (RMS-AP, ML, V) and normalized RMSR-AP, ML and V from 5 m walk smartphone signals.

Variables	Health Status					
	Frail			Non-Frail		
	Mean	SD	CV	Mean	SD	CV
Harmonic Ratio_AP	1.06	0.17	15.96	1.16	0.19	16.77
Harmonic Ratio_V	0.96	0.29	30.50	1.18	0.26	22.14
Harmonic Ratio_ML	1.09	0.37	34.36	0.98	0.25	25.19
RMS_AP *	0.12	0.03	24.50	0.15	0.02	15.23
RMS_V *	0.11	0.01	11.82	0.17	0.02	10.40
RMS_ML *	0.11	0.02	19.63	0.15	0.03	22.48
RMSR_AP	0.59	0.07	11.57	0.55	0.09	16.90
RMSR_V	0.56	0.07	12.89	0.62	0.05	8.47
RMSR_ML	0.58	0.05	9.41	0.55	0.09	15.50

* significant at $p < 0.05$.

Interactive dot diagrams indicated that RMS in a vertical direction could provide results with 100% sensitivity and 100% specificity. Variability measures such as SD and RMS from smartphone postural stability data provided specificity of 93.7% and sensitivity of 50%. The cut-off point being 6.4547 mm could classify frailty with specificity of 93.7% (Figures 9 and 10).

4. Discussion

Armed with the above-mentioned linear/nonlinear tools and inertial sensors for assessing movement variability, a trait of human movement performance, this study explored the smartphone sensor-based variables of variability in cardiovascular disease patients and their adverse post-operative outcomes. This study was conducted in a clinical environment using smartphone-based inertial sensors and found that variability of postural and gait movements in CVD patients was associated with frailty and adverse post-operative outcomes.

The Society of Thoracic Surgeons has recommended the use of quick tests such as gait speed for the assessment of frailty among cardiovascular patients. The frailty status in CVD patients is predictive of adverse health outcome, including falls, institutionalization, hospitalization and mortality [13,33,41,42].

Frail individuals are also at extremely high risk of falls, fractures and hospitalizations leading to death compared with their age-matched non-frail counterparts [13]. Gait speed suggested by the STS guideline is a robust measure in health care research, particularly among preoperative cardiac patients [43–45]. Therefore, all study patients were divided into a frail and non-frail group using the 5 m walk gait speed. This study has established a relationship between frail cardiac patients and their inherent variability and adverse post-operative outcomes after cardiac surgery. We have previously validated the use of inertial sensors in fall risk assessment in hemodialysis clinics [46,47]. Consistently, in this study, postural stability, postural transition times and gait speed (related to major health-related outcomes in frail population), are measured feasibly using smartphone inertial sensor-based methodology in clinical environments. There may be important losses of information when measurement of gait velocity is prone to human timing errors (use of stopwatch also requires experimenter's attention and reaction time to press start or stop pushbuttons after visual verification of event). In clinical practice, where gait speed is an important predictive of severe health outcomes such as mortality and a subsequent physical disability, an objective, accurate, and reliable way is required for gait speed measurement. For this study, we devised the use of a smartphone with embedded inertial sensors which capture walking characteristics of patients in clinical environments. A five meter gait speed certainly does not introduce fatigue in patients with cardiovascular impairments awaiting surgery [45]. However, some patients who are awaiting their surgery also may not be healthy enough to walk for a 5 m distance. In such scenarios, it is worthwhile to examine the effects of postural control for balance and transitioning. Although it was found that in 5 m walking trials, that stopwatch time and smartphone time were highly correlated. However, it was found that smartphone-based frail classification had classified 3 non-frails erroneously as frails. Thus, if non-frail is the desired outcome with smartphone-based gait speed, the sensitivity = 79.2% and specificity = 91.3% when the cut-off velocity is chosen as 0.766 m/s rather than the prescribed 0.833 m/s. The feasibility and agreement of this smartphone app in estimation of 5 m gait speed in a clinical environment has been reported earlier with ICC(3,k) = 0.66 for normal walking speed in healthy adults. As expected, we found frail CVD patients (0.67 ± 0.08 m/s) walked slower than non-frail (0.98 ± 0.13 m/s) counterparts.

It was also found that frail CVD patients had increased fall risk as depicted by both linear and nonlinear measures of postural sway. In support of this hypothesis, we found a significant increase in linear parameters such as mean COP radius, COP area, COP path length, mean COP Velocity for frail patients than that in non-frail patients. Coherently, it was also seen in linear variability measures that frail patients had significantly higher standard deviation (SD) in anterior-posterior, medio-lateral and resultant directions of COP. Frail patients had significantly lower complexity than the non-frail patients in COP sway in anterior posterior direction. Statistical variability such as range and SD reflect overall magnitude of COP displacement, without considering the temporal structure of the COP time series. This fundamental difference may explain that nonlinear measures of postural signals reveal subtle temporal properties of signals which are not detected through traditional linear approach [48–51]. Traditionally, higher COP displacements have been linked with less stability and consequently, pathology. However, biological systems are intrinsically complex and linear analysis does not holistically account for the time-dependent evolution of the system, eschewing patterns within the time series and an appreciable amount of information on system dynamics. Thus, an increased COP movement may not unwittingly indicate deficient postural stability, but rather an element of a healthy vigilant system able to adapt to unexpected perturbations in an attempt to maintain balance.

Entropy-based estimations of signal irregularity and concurrent organizational variability represents the adaptive capacity of frail/non-frail participants to maintain balance. Frail participants were found to have significantly lower ApEn and SaEn values during prolonged quiet standing in the AP direction, indicating greater regularity and possibly decreased complexity. The findings coincide with previous investigations [52], linked with the theory of decreased complexity attributed to pathology and aging [53]. Probably, in frail patients the bodily degrees of freedom are constrained in the AP direction compared to the ML direction, whereby coordination of the physiological system, coupled with environmental interactions, lead behavioral processes into less complex, more stable response modes (i.e., more regular sway pattern and probably closed loop short-term dependencies to restore balance). Hence, the motor system is unable to adjust to the demands inherent to frailty, therefore movements transition to a more rigid postural control behavior in the AP direction—delineated by repeated patterns (high regularity) and decreased complexity–diminishing both adaptability and stability. In this context, the decrease in complexity may be due to impaired feedback control or strength, or impaired proprioception caused due to decreased physiological reserve in frail patients leading to reduced adaptive capacity of the underlying postural system [54].

Fractal analysis of the COP time series revealed relatively marginal differences in frail versus non-frail patients in all the AP and ML and resultant directions. From a biomechanics perspective, it may also be due to inability of elderly people to control and accelerate center-of-mass (COM) over base of support, perhaps due to lack of strength and degradation of type II fibers in skeletal muscles in presence of sarcopenia or any other frailty disorder. While muscle strength was not objectively measured in this study, it has been documented that many older people have relatively weaker tibialis anterior and vastus lateralis muscle strength compared to that of healthy adults [55,56]. Frailty is also found to be related with lower level of physical activity and impaired cardiorespiratory fitness and grip strength compared to lean counterparts [13], which could possibly impair an individual's ability to correct a shift in the body's COM and effectively prevent then from falling. Probably increased postural sway could be an adaptive strategy to provide additional stability under conditions of weakness in muscles involved for postural control. Age-related deterioration of sensory and neuromuscular control mechanisms could have added to this problem [57]. Degradation of balance shows that fall risk is increased in frail CVD patients. Smartphone-based variability information was found similar to that from forceplate; in addition, root mean square acceleration in AP, ML and resultant (R) directions were found to be significantly different among the frail CVD patients than the non-frail counter parts (Table 5). Additionally, significantly higher sample entropy was found in AP direction in frail patients using the smartphone.

Most of the frail patients were met with an adverse post-operative outcome which included stroke (2 frail), renal failure (1 frail), prolonged ventilation (3 frail), reoperation (1 frail), longer length of stay (1 frail) and admissions to skilled nursing facility (3 frail and 1 non-frail); there was one mortality of a frail patient. The post-operative outcomes such as stroke, renal failure, prolonged ventilation, reoperation, longer length of stay in intensive care, and admissions to skilled nursing facility can be classified as morbidity. The one non-frail elderly participant requested discharge to a skilled nursing facility due to personal/social reasons (in absence of anyone at home to take care of them).

Walking patterns and variability may be optimal from the perspective of energy expenditure [58], temporal variability [59], spatial variability [60], and attentional demands [61]. Stability while walking is important since up to 70% of falls occur during locomotion [62,63]. Moe-Nilssen evaluated walking stability using accelerometers at the lumbar spine [64,65], and reported higher average accelerations in people with balance impairments [66]. During the course of locomotion, humans respond to multiple irregular perturbations generated by walking. The task of maintaining stability while walking primarily requires controlling the motion of COM. It has been reported that normal subjects walking with plaster casts and crutches [40], amputees walking with prosthetic limbs [67] and older people with balance problems [68] have lower harmonic ratio. But we did not find any significant differences in harmonic ratios between the frail and non-frail group for 5 m distance walk in all 3 directions.

In this study, acceleration patterns were measured at the pelvis when walking (5 m walk) to provide an indicator of whole body's stability in response to multiple unpredictable perturbations during walking. All humans have a preferable walking speed that is a combination of step length and step frequency and is an important factor in control of balance since, during walking, considerable potential for imbalance exists due to inertia of the upper body and the small contact area provided by the foot during a single limb stance [69]. This preferable or usual speed is selected to optimize the stability of the gait pattern. Hence, acceleration patterns were measured at the pelvis when walking to provide an indicator of whole body stability in response to multiple unpredictable perturbations during walking. However, we found that root mean square (RMS) in all three directions was significantly different in frail and non-frail patients. Probably, RMS acceleration is correlated with walking speed. The frail patient's comfortable walking speed selected is slower when compared to non-frail patients to minimize acceleration variability but instead RMS values were found to be significantly higher and thus were unable to provide smooth and rhythmic movements of the pelvis. The interactive dot diagram suggested that postural measures from the forceplate such as jerk, SD of COP-AP, postural measures from the smartphone such as RMS sway-ML, SD of sway-ML and gait measures of the smartphone such as RMS AP and RMS Vertical are predictive of frailty with high accuracy.

These methods build on narrative descriptions of variability by quantifying qualities of postural control, postural transition and gait could serve as an indicator of surgery outcomes in CVD patients. In combination, linear and nonlinear variability analysis quantified postural and gait control to provide a more complete understanding of the adaptive strategies used in neuromuscular control than either method could provide alone. Thus, these inertial sensor-based variables are found to have high predictive validity to identify patients with adverse post-operative outcomes through an objective method of assessment using a smartphone. These fall risk indicators of variability could be used as prescreening tools for many different kinds of surgical procedures and in turn help clinicians to identify frail patients who may need intensive rehab or to preplan their stay in hospital with specialized nursing care before they return home.

The use of smartphones as medical devices has spread pervasively worldwide in the past decade. The scope of smartphone usage has certainly exceeded that initially envisioned for only telecommunication. The performance of smartphones depends on their different model as per their processing capability and embedded sensor quality. Undoubtedly, the quality of smartphone sensors is limited by sensor inaccuracy and imprecision [70,71]. It has been found that different smartphone models have different sensor-based bias, and sensor-based noise as quantified by Allan deviation in accelerometers as velocity random-walk (VRW) and angular random-walk (ARM) [72–74]. To eliminate noise and sensor bias differences dependent on various smartphone models, we have only used one smartphone (iPhone 5, Apple, Cupertino, CA, USA) for the entire experimental study. Thus, inertial sensors embedded inside the smartphone have the potential to measure gait and posture in CVD patients, although a great deal of work is required in future research to make such research tools easy to use for clinicians. The data collection was mainly conducted by hospital staff (Registered nurse specialist) using a smartphone and forceplate in the clinical setting and experimental protocols were modified as per clinical requirements. To meet the challenges of patient safety and point of care, new technologies are needed in future such that the patient data can be acquired without hindering medical routine for patients and hospital staff.

Limitations of the Study

The strength of the conclusions of this study must be tempered by the study's limitations. The study population was limited to only 16 participants. The patients were aware that they were participating in a frailty assessment protocol. This could be a bias in the population we studied. They may be conscious of the environment and their performance may have been affected by the clinical environment (white coat syndrome). The hospital setting in which data were obtained for this study provided an unusual environment for the cardiac patients. We agree this is a special population who are battling for life and need help from physicians and researchers for their betterment. At the same time, they might be stressed to some extent for their surgery allotted for the next day and a non-laboratory setting limited the scope of this data. However, such analyses may provide insight as to the potential fall risk and chances of adverse post-operative outcomes were associated with the frail condition of patients.

Another limitation of the current study was that the smartphone-based assessments required patients to stand still before and after the 5-m walk. As automatic algorithms developed in the smartphone app determined velocity by evaluating start and stop times of movement. Automatic gait speed estimation by the smartphone required strict following of the protocol. If any other movement artifact is followed after or prior to the walking task, the movement time may get increased than the actual walking time and thus data had to be checked visually and truncated for correcting this.

5. Conclusions

The accurate measure of gait speed, as well as variability measures can improve the clinical evaluation of cardiac patients, providing an earlier detection of individuals at higher risk of major health-related events such as physical disability and mortality. This study demonstrated that a 5 m gait speed measurement using a smartphone is also a reliable objective measure; however, adhering to certain protocol is suggested for using a smartphone app. Although different methods have been used previously to measure gait speed and these have affected clinical interpretation and implementation of the gait speed [75,76]. By providing a smartphone-based clinically useful gait speed assessment method with a well-defined protocol which is simple, quick and easy to perform in clinics, it is hoped that using a smartphone for gait speed assessment will be promoted and encouraged in clinical and research settings. In addition, nonlinear postural variability measures such as complexity can be easily implemented in patients who are unable to walk but can stand still for at-least 30 s.

The study protocol and findings suggest that various variability parameters in walking and stand still posture can be easily implemented in cardiovascular clinical practice with high acceptability by the patients and clinical research staff. Patients started with standing still posture and walked at their usual pace, as if they were walking in their own home, and given no further encouragement or instructions. This data can be readily collected in non-laboratory environments and can be used to help interpret the results for future health-related events.

Author Contributions: T.E.L. conceived and designed the experiments. R.S. was majorly involved in App development, data processing and analysis. R.S. wrote the manuscript with support from T.E.L. Both authors discussed the results and contributed to the final manuscript.

Acknowledgments: This research was supported by the NSF-Information and Intelligent Systems (IIS) and Smart and Connected Health (1065442 and 1065262). We would like to thank Misha Pavel and Wendy Nilsen for their encouragement in the development of wireless health monitoring systems and fostering the support of wearable wireless health monitoring systems. Thanks also goes to tireless nurses and practitioners who have helped along the road of less traveled. We are also thankful to Saba Rezvanian for her reviews.

Conflicts of Interest: The authors declare no conflict of interest.

References

1. Bruce, J.; Ralhan, S.; Sheridan, R.; Westacott, K.; Withers, E.; Finnegan, S.; Davison, J.; Martin, F.C.; Lamb, S.E. The design and development of a complex multifactorial falls assessment intervention for falls prevention: The Prevention of Falls Injury Trial (PreFIT). *BMC Geriatr.* **2017**, *17*. [CrossRef] [PubMed]
2. Fairhall, N.; Kurrle, S.E.; Sherrington, C.; Lord, S.R.; Lockwood, K.; John, B.; Monaghan, N.; Howard, K.; Cameron, I.D. Effectiveness of a multifactorial intervention on preventing development of frailty in pre-frail older people: Study protocol for a randomised controlled trial. *BMJ Open* **2015**, *5*, e007091. [CrossRef] [PubMed]
3. Singh, M.; Stewart, R.; White, H. Importance of frailty in patients with cardiovascular disease. *Eur. Heart J.* **2014**, *35*, 1726–1731. [CrossRef] [PubMed]
4. Fleming, B.E.; Pendergast, D.R. Physical condition, activity pattern, and environment as factors in falls by adult care facility residents. *Arch. Phys. Med. Rehabil.* **1993**, *74*, 627–630. [CrossRef]
5. Tinetti, M.E.; Speechley, M.; Ginter, S.F. Risk factors for falls among elderly persons living in the community. *N. Engl. J. Med.* **1988**, *319*, 1701–1707. [CrossRef] [PubMed]
6. Campbell, A.J.; Borrie, M.J.; Spears, G.F. Risk factors for falls in a community-based prospective study of people 70 years and older. *J. Gerontol.* **1989**, *44*, M112–M117. [CrossRef] [PubMed]

7. Nevitt, M.C.; Cummings, S.R.; Kidd, S.; Black, D. Risk factors for recurrent nonsyncopal falls. A prospective study. *JAMA J. Am. Med. Assoc.* **1989**, *261*, 2663–2668. [CrossRef]

8. Tinetti, M.E.; Williams, T.F.; Mayewski, R. Fall risk index for elderly patients based on number of chronic disabilities. *Am. J. Med.* **1986**, *80*, 429–434. [CrossRef]

9. Kapoor, W.N.; Karpf, M.; Wieand, S.; Peterson, J.R.; Levey, G.S. A prospective evaluation and follow-up of patients with syncope. *N. Engl. J. Med.* **1983**, *309*, 197–204. [CrossRef] [PubMed]

10. Dey, A.B.; Stout, N.R.; Kenny, R.A. Cardiovascular syncope is the most common cause of drop attacks in the elderly. *Pac. Clin. Electrophysiol. PACE* **1997**, *20*, 818–819. [CrossRef]

11. Wilson, J.F. Frailty—And Its Dangerous Effects—Might Be Preventable. *Ann. Intern. Med.* **2004**, *141*, 489–492. [CrossRef] [PubMed]

12. Morley, J.E.; Perry, H.M., 3rd; Miller, D.K. Editorial: Something about frailty. *J. Gerontol. Ser. A Biol. Sci. Med. Sci.* **2002**, *57*, M698–M704. [CrossRef]

13. Fried, L.P.; Tangen, C.M.; Walston, J.; Newman, A.B.; Hirsch, C.; Gottdiener, J.; Seeman, T.; Tracy, R.; Kop, W.J.; Burke, G.; et al. Frailty in older adults: Evidence for a phenotype. *J. Gerontol. Ser. A Biol. Sci. Med. Sci.* **2001**, *56*, M146–M156. [CrossRef]

14. Arozullah, A.M.; Daley, J.; Henderson, W.G.; Khuri, S.F. Multifactorial risk index for predicting postoperative respiratory failure in men after major noncardiac surgery. The National Veterans Administration Surgical Quality Improvement Program. *Ann. Surg.* **2000**, *232*, 242–253. [CrossRef] [PubMed]

15. Arozullah, A.M.; Khuri, S.F.; Henderson, W.G.; Daley, J. Participants in the National Veterans Affairs Surgical Quality Improvement Program. Development and validation of a multifactorial risk index for predicting postoperative pneumonia after major noncardiac surgery. *Ann. Intern. Med.* **2001**, *135*, 847–857. [CrossRef] [PubMed]

16. Polanczyk, C.A.; Marcantonio, E.; Goldman, L.; Rohde, L.E.; Orav, J.; Mangione, C.M.; Lee, T.H. Impact of age on perioperative complications and length of stay in patients undergoing noncardiac surgery. *Ann. Intern. Med.* **2001**, *134*, 637–643. [CrossRef] [PubMed]

17. Fukuse, T.; Satoda, N.; Hijiya, K.; Fujinaga, T. Importance of a comprehensive geriatric assessment in prediction of complications following thoracic surgery in elderly patients. *Chest* **2005**, *127*, 886–891. [CrossRef] [PubMed]

18. Maurer, M.S.; Luchsinger, J.A.; Wellner, R.; Kukuy, E.; Edwards, N.M. The effect of body mass index on complications from cardiac surgery in the oldest old. *J. Am. Geriatr. Soc.* **2002**, *50*, 988–994. [CrossRef] [PubMed]

19. Marcantonio, E.R.; Goldman, L.; Mangione, C.M.; Ludwig, L.E.; Muraca, B.; Haslauer, C.M.; Donaldson, M.C.; Whittemore, A.D.; Sugarbaker, D.J.; Poss, R.; et al. A clinical prediction rule for delirium after elective noncardiac surgery. *JAMA J. Am. Med. Assoc.* **1994**, *271*, 134–139. [CrossRef]

20. Galanakis, P.; Bickel, H.; Gradinger, R.; Von Gumppenberg, S.; Forstl, H. Acute confusional state in the elderly following hip surgery: Incidence, risk factors and complications. *Int. J. Geriatr. Psychiatry* **2001**, *16*, 349–355. [CrossRef] [PubMed]

21. Berggren, D.; Gustafson, Y.; Eriksson, B.; Bucht, G.; Hansson, L.I.; Reiz, S.; Winblad, B. Postoperative confusion after anesthesia in elderly patients with femoral neck fractures. *Anesth. Analg.* **1987**, *66*, 497–504. [CrossRef] [PubMed]

22. Herlitz, J.; Wiklund, I.; Caidahl, K.; Hartford, M.; Haglid, M.; Karlsson, B.W.; Sjoland, H.; Karlsson, T. The feeling of loneliness prior to coronary artery bypass grafting might be a predictor of short-and long-term postoperative mortality. *Eur. J. Vasc. Endovasc. Surg.* **1998**, *16*, 120–125. [CrossRef]

23. Newman, A.B.; Gottdiener, J.S.; McBurnie, M.A.; Hirsch, C.H.; Kop, W.J.; Tracy, R.; Walston, J.D.; Fried, L.P. Associations of Subclinical Cardiovascular Disease With Frailty. *J. Gerontol. Ser. A Biol. Sci. Med. Sci.* **2001**, *56*, M158–M166. [CrossRef]

24. Makary, M.A.; Segev, D.L.; Pronovost, P.J.; Syin, D.; Bandeen-Roche, K.; Patel, P.; Takenaga, R.; Devgan, L.; Holzmueller, C.G.; Tian, J.; et al. Frailty as a predictor of surgical outcomes in older patients. *J. Am. Coll. Surg.* **2010**, *210*, 901–908. [CrossRef] [PubMed]

25. Boyd, C.M.; Darer, J.; Boult, C.; Fried, L.P.; Boult, L.; Wu, A.W. Clinical practice guidelines and quality of care for older patients with multiple comorbid diseases: Implications for pay for performance. *JAMA J. Am. Med. Assoc.* **2005**, *294*, 716–724. [CrossRef] [PubMed]

26. Woods, N.F.; LaCroix, A.Z.; Gray, S.L.; Aragaki, A.; Cochrane, B.B.; Brunner, R.L.; Masaki, K.; Murray, A.; Newman, A.B.; Women's Health, I. Frailty: Emergence and consequences in women aged 65 and older in the Women's Health Initiative Observational Study. *J. Am. Geriatr. Soc.* **2005**, *53*, 1321–1330. [CrossRef] [PubMed]

27. Fried, L.P.; Kronmal, R.A.; Newman, A.B.; Bild, D.E.; Mittelmark, M.B.; Polak, J.F.; Robbins, J.A.; Gardin, J.M. Risk factors for 5-year mortality in older adults: The Cardiovascular Health Study. *JAMA J. Am. Med. Assoc.* **1998**, *279*, 585–592. [CrossRef]

28. Dasgupta, M.; Rolfson, D.B.; Stolee, P.; Borrie, M.J.; Speechley, M. Frailty is associated with postoperative complications in older adults with medical problems. *Arch. Gerontol. Geriatr.* **2009**, *48*, 78–83. [CrossRef] [PubMed]

29. Alibhai, S.M.; Leach, M.; Tomlinson, G.; Krahn, M.D.; Fleshner, N.; Holowaty, E.; Naglie, G. 30-day mortality and major complications after radical prostatectomy: Influence of age and comorbidity. *J. Natl. Cancer Inst.* **2005**, *97*, 1525–1532. [CrossRef] [PubMed]

30. Mitnitski, A.B.; Graham, J.E.; Mogilner, A.J.; Rockwood, K. Frailty, fitness and late-life mortality in relation to chronological and biological age. *BMC Geriatr.* **2002**, *2*, 1. [CrossRef]

31. Millor, N.; Lecumberri, P.; Gomez, M.; Martinez, A.; Martinikorena, J.; Rodriguez-Manas, L.; Garcia-Garcia, F.J.; Izquierdo, M. Gait Velocity and Chair Sit-Stand-Sit Performance Improves Current Frailty-Status Identification. *IEEE Trans. Neural Syst. Rehabil. Eng.* **2017**, *25*, 2018–2025. [CrossRef] [PubMed]

32. Castell, M.V.; Sanchez, M.; Julian, R.; Queipo, R.; Martin, S.; Otero, A. Frailty prevalence and slow walking speed in persons age 65 and older: Implications for primary care. *BMC Fam. Pract.* **2013**, *14*, 86. [CrossRef] [PubMed]

33. Afilalo, J.; Kim, S.; O'Brien, S.; Brennan, J.M.; Edwards, F.H.; Mack, M.J.; McClurken, J.B.; Cleveland, J.C.; Smith, P.K.; Shahian, D.M.; et al. Gait Speed and Operative Mortality in Older Adults Following Cardiac Surgery. *JAMA Cardiol.* **2016**, *1*, 314. [CrossRef] [PubMed]

34. Soangra, R.; Lockhart, T.E. Agreement in gait speed from smartphone and stopwatch for five meter walk in laboratory and clinical environments. *Biomed. Sci. Instrum.* **2014**, *50*, 254–264. [PubMed]

35. Lockhart, T.E.; Soangra, R.; Chung, C.; Frames, C.; Fino, P.; Zhang, J. Development of automated gait assessment algorithm using three inertial sensors and its reliability. *Biomed. Sci. Instrum.* **2014**, *50*, 297–306. [PubMed]

36. Lockhart, T.E.; Soangra, R.; Zhang, J.; Wu, X. Wavelet based automated postural event detection and activity classification with single imu—Biomed 2013. *Biomed. Sci. Instrum.* **2013**, *49*, 224–233. [PubMed]

37. Bouten, C.V.; Koekkoek, K.T.; Verduin, M.; Kodde, R.; Janssen, J.D. A triaxial accelerometer and portable data processing unit for the assessment of daily physical activity. *IEEE Trans. Biomed. Eng.* **1997**, *44*, 136–147. [CrossRef] [PubMed]

38. Sekine, M.; Tamura, T.; Yoshida, M.; Suda, Y.; Kimura, Y.; Miyoshi, H.; Kijima, Y.; Higashi, Y.; Fujimoto, T. A gait abnormality measure based on root mean square of trunk acceleration. *J. Neuroeng. Rehabil.* **2013**, *10*, 118. [CrossRef] [PubMed]

39. Gage, H. Accelerographic analysis of human gait. *ASME Paper* **1964**, *64*, 80.

40. Smidt, G.L.; Arora, J.S.; Johnston, R.C. Accelerographic analysis of several types of walking. *Am. J. Phys. Med.* **1971**, *50*, 285–300. [PubMed]

41. Boyd, C.M.; Xue, Q.L.; Simpson, C.F.; Guralnik, J.M.; Fried, L.P. Frailty, hospitalization, and progression of disability in a cohort of disabled older women. *Am. J. Med.* **2005**, *118*, 1225–1231. [CrossRef] [PubMed]

42. Rockwood, K.; Stadnyk, K.; MacKnight, C.; McDowell, I.; Hebert, R.; Hogan, D.B. A brief clinical instrument to classify frailty in elderly people. *Lancet* **1999**, *353*, 205–206. [CrossRef]

43. Afilalo, J. Frailty in Patients with Cardiovascular Disease: Why, When, and How to Measure. *Curr. Cardiovasc. Risk Rep.* **2011**, *5*, 467–472. [CrossRef] [PubMed]

44. Afilalo, J.; Eisenberg, M.J.; Morin, J.F.; Bergman, H.; Monette, J.; Noiseux, N.; Perrault, L.P.; Alexander, K.P.; Langlois, Y.; Dendukuri, N.; et al. Gait speed as an incremental predictor of mortality and major morbidity in elderly patients undergoing cardiac surgery. *J. Am. Coll. Cardiol.* **2010**, *56*, 1668–1676. [CrossRef] [PubMed]

45. Wilson, C.M.; Kostsuca, S.R.; Boura, J.A. Utilization of a 5-Meter Walk Test in Evaluating Self-selected Gait Speed during Preoperative Screening of Patients Scheduled for Cardiac Surgery. *Cardiopul. Phys. Ther. J.* **2013**, *24*, 36–43.

46. Soangra, R.; Lockhart, T.E.; Lach, J.; Abdel-Rahman, E.M. Effects of hemodialysis therapy on sit-to-walk characteristics in end stage renal disease patients. *Ann. Biomed. Eng.* **2013**, *41*, 795–805. [CrossRef] [PubMed]

47. Lockhart, T.E.; Barth, A.T.; Zhang, X.; Songra, R.; Abdel-Rahman, E.; Lach, J. Portable, Non-Invasive Fall Risk Assessment in End Stage Renal Disease Patients on Hemodialysis. *ACM trans. Comput.-hum. Interact. A Publ. Assoc. Comput. Mach.* **2010**, 84–93. [CrossRef]

48. Handrigan, G.A.; Corbeil, P.; Simoneau, M.; Teasdale, N. Balance control is altered in obese individuals. *J. Biomech.* **2010**, *43*, 385–386. [CrossRef] [PubMed]

49. Hue, O.; Simoneau, M.; Marcotte, J.; Berrigan, F.; Dore, J.; Marceau, P.; Marceau, S.; Tremblay, A.; Teasdale, N. Body weight is a strong predictor of postural stability. *Gait Posture* **2007**, *26*, 32–38. [CrossRef] [PubMed]

50. Cavanaugh, J.T.; Guskiewicz, K.M.; Giuliani, C.; Marshall, S.; Mercer, V.; Stergiou, N. Detecting altered postural control after cerebral concussion in athletes with normal postural stability. *Br. J. Sports Med.* **2005**, *39*, 805–811. [CrossRef] [PubMed]

51. Martinez-Ramirez, A.; Lecumberri, P.; Gomez, M.; Rodriguez-Manas, L.; Garcia, F.J.; Izquierdo, M. Frailty assessment based on wavelet analysis during quiet standing balance test. *J. Biomech.* **2011**, *44*, 2213–2220. [CrossRef] [PubMed]

52. Pincus, S.M. Approximate entropy as a measure of system complexity. *Proc. Natl. Acad. Sci. USA* **1991**, *88*, 2297–2301. [CrossRef] [PubMed]

53. Lipsitz, L.A.; Goldberger, A.L. Loss of 'complexity' and aging. Potential applications of fractals and chaos theory to senescence. *JAMA* **1992**, *267*, 1806–1809. [CrossRef] [PubMed]

54. Manor, B.; Costa, M.D.; Hu, K.; Newton, E.; Starobinets, O.; Kang, H.G.; Peng, C.K.; Novak, V.; Lipsitz, L.A. Physiological complexity and system adaptability: Evidence from postural control dynamics of older adults. *J. Appl. Physiol. (1985)* **2010**, *109*, 1786–1791. [CrossRef] [PubMed]

55. Murray, M.P.; Gardner, G.M.; Mollinger, L.A.; Sepic, S.B. Strength of isometric and isokinetic contractions: Knee muscles of men aged 20 to 86. *Phys. Ther.* **1980**, *60*, 412–419. [CrossRef] [PubMed]

56. Hurley, M.V.; Rees, J.; Newham, D.J. Quadriceps function, proprioceptive acuity and functional performance in healthy young, middle-aged and elderly subjects. *Age Ageing* **1998**, *27*, 55–62. [CrossRef] [PubMed]

57. Lockhart, T.E.; Woldstad, J.C.; Smith, J.L. Effects of age-related gait changes on the biomechanics of slips and falls. *Ergonomics* **2003**, *46*, 1136–1160. [CrossRef] [PubMed]

58. Zarrugh, M.Y.; Todd, F.N.; Ralston, H.J. Optimization of energy expenditure during level walking. *Eur. J. Appl. Physiol. Occup. Physiol.* **1974**, *33*, 293–306. [CrossRef] [PubMed]

59. Maruyama, H.; Nagasaki, H. Temporal variability in the phase durations during treadmill walking. *Hum. Mov. sci.* **1992**, *11*, 335–348. [CrossRef]

60. Sekiya, N.; Nagasaki, H.; Ito, H.; Furuna, T. Optimal Walking in Terms of Variability in Step Length. *J. Orthop. Sports Phys. Ther.* **1997**, *26*, 266–272. [CrossRef] [PubMed]

61. Kurosawa, K. Effects of various walking speeds on probe reaction time during treadmill walking. *Percept. Motor Skills* **1994**, *78*, 768–770. [CrossRef] [PubMed]

62. Cali, C.M.; Kiel, D.P. An epidemiologic study of fall-related fractures among institutionalized older people. *J. Am. Geriatr. Soc.* **1995**, *43*, 1336–1340. [CrossRef] [PubMed]

63. Berg, W.P.; Alessio, H.M.; Mills, E.M.; Tong, C. Circumstances and consequences of falls in independent community-dwelling older adults. *Age Ageing* **1997**, *26*, 261–268. [CrossRef] [PubMed]

64. Moe-Nilssen, R. A new method for evaluating motor control in gait under real-life environmental conditions. Part 2: Gait analysis. *Clin. Biomech. (Bristol, Avon)* **1998**, *13*, 328–335. [CrossRef]

65. Moe-Nilssen, R. A new method for evaluating motor control in gait under real-life environmental conditions. Part 1: The instrument. *Clin. Biomech. (Bristol, Avon)* **1998**, *13*, 320–327. [CrossRef]

66. Moe-Nilssen, R. Test-retest reliability of trunk accelerometry during standing and walking. *Arch. Phys. Med. Rehabil.* **1998**, *79*, 1377–1385. [CrossRef]

67. Robinson, J.L.; Smidt, G.L.; Arora, J.S. Accelerographic, temporal, and distance gait factors in below-knee amputees. *Phys. Ther.* **1977**, *57*, 898–904. [CrossRef] [PubMed]

68. Yack, H.J.; Berger, R.C. Dynamic stability in the elderly: Identifying a possible measure. *J. Gerontol.* **1993**, *48*, M225–M230. [CrossRef] [PubMed]

69. Latt, M.D.; Menz, H.B.; Fung, V.S.; Lord, S.R. Walking speed, cadence and step length are selected to optimize the stability of head and pelvis accelerations. *Exp. Brain Res.* **2008**, *184*, 201–209. [CrossRef] [PubMed]

70. El-Sheimy, N.; Hou, H.; Niu, X. Analysis and Modeling of Inertial Sensors Using Allan Variance. *IEEE Trans. Instrum. Meas.* **2008**, *57*, 140–149. [CrossRef]
71. Grewal, M.; Andrews, A. How Good Is Your Gyro [Ask the Experts]. *IEEE Control Syst.* **2010**, *30*, 12–86. [CrossRef]
72. Aggarwal, P.; Syed, Z.; Niu, X.; El-Sheimy, N. A Standard Testing and Calibration Procedure for Low Cost MEMS Inertial Sensors and Units. *J. Navig.* **2008**, *61*. [CrossRef]
73. El-Diasty, M.; Pagiatakis, S. Calibration and Stochastic Modelling of Inertial Navigation Sensor Erros. *J. Glob. Positioning Syst.* **2008**, *7*, 170–182. [CrossRef]
74. Kos, A.; Tomazic, S.; Umek, A. Evaluation of Smartphone Inertial Sensor Performance for Cross-Platform Mobile Applications. *Sensors (Basel)* **2016**, *16*. [CrossRef] [PubMed]
75. Graham, J.E.; Ostir, G.V.; Fisher, S.R.; Ottenbacher, K.J. Assessing walking speed in clinical research: A systematic review. *J. Eval. Clin. Pract.* **2008**, *14*, 552–562. [CrossRef] [PubMed]
76. Graham, J.E.; Ostir, G.V.; Kuo, Y.F.; Fisher, S.R.; Ottenbacher, K.J. Relationship between test methodology and mean velocity in timed walk tests: A review. *Arch. Phys. Med. Rehabil.* **2008**, *89*, 865–872. [CrossRef] [PubMed]

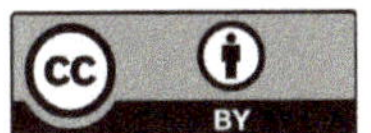

© 2018 by the authors. Licensee MDPI, Basel, Switzerland. This article is an open access article distributed under the terms and conditions of the Creative Commons Attribution (CC BY) license (http://creativecommons.org/licenses/by/4.0/).

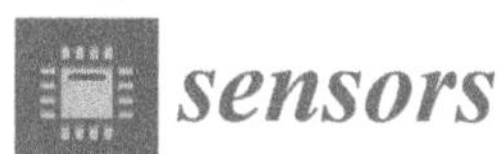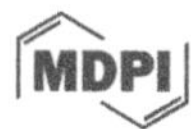

Article

Using Temporal Covariance of Motion and Geometric Features via Boosting for Human Fall Detection

Syed Farooq Ali [1], Reamsha Khan [1], Arif Mahmood [2], Malik Tahir Hassan [1] and Moongu Jeon [3,*

[1]   Department of Software Engineering, University of Management and Technology, UMT Road, C-II Johar Town, Lahore 54000, Pakistan; farooq.ali@umt.edu.pk (S.F.A.); reamshakhan1122@gmail.com (R.K.); tahir.hassan@umt.edu.pk (M.T.H.)

[2]   Department of Computer Science, Information Technology University (ITU), 346-B, Ferozepur Road, Lahore, Punjab 54000, Pakistan; arif.mahmood@itu.edu.pk

[3]   School of Electrical Engineering and Computer Science, Gwangju Institute of Science and Technology (GIST), Gwangju 61005, Korea

*   Correspondence: mgjeon@gist.ac.kr; Tel.: +82-62-715-2406

Received: 9 April 2018; Accepted: 11 June 2018; Published: 12 June 2018

Abstract: Fall induced damages are serious incidences for aged as well as young persons. A real-time automatic and accurate fall detection system can play a vital role in timely medication care which will ultimately help to decrease the damages and complications. In this paper, we propose a fast and more accurate real-time system which can detect people falling in videos captured by surveillance cameras. Novel temporal and spatial variance-based features are proposed which comprise the discriminatory motion, geometric orientation and location of the person. These features are used along with ensemble learning strategy of boosting with J48 and Adaboost classifiers. Experiments have been conducted on publicly available standard datasets including *Multiple Cameras Fall (with 2 classes and 3 classes)* and *UR Fall Detection* achieving percentage accuracies of 99.2, 99.25 and 99.0, respectively. Comparisons with nine state-of-the-art methods demonstrate the effectiveness of the proposed approach on both datasets.

Keywords: intelligent surveillance systems; human fall detection; health and well-being; safety and security

---

1. Introduction

The increasing number of aged persons has led to the uncertainty of unaided and unprovoked falls which may cause physical harm, injuries and health deterioration. These problems may become more intense if timely aid and assistance is not available. To mitigate such effects and to control the risks, there must be an accurate fall detection system. For this reason, surveillance added technology for the timely and retrospective detection of falls has become a priority for the health care industry. Therefore, the development of an intelligent surveillance system is essential, specifically, a system which has the capacity to automatically detect fall incidences using surveillance cameras.

To cope with such a crucial need, various fall detection wearable devices have been developed [1]. Some devices contain buttons and sensors that can be pressed if there is an emergency [1]. However, these devices become ineffective or even useless if the subject is unable to press the button due to unconsciousness or being far from the device. Due to the failure of wearable devices, video controlling and monitoring systems have entered the arena [1], but these systems also suffer from inaccuracy and unreliability [1]. Generic action recognition systems such as [2] may not efficiently detect falls. Due to the lack of efficiency of wearable devices and generic video systems [3], it has become necessary for customized automatic fall detection systems to be developed to cope with the challenges posed by fall detection problems. Such systems could dramatically improve the health care of older people.

In the current paper, we propose a fall detection system based on the spatial and temporal variance of different discriminative features. The proposed system is compared with nine existing algorithms on two publicly available datasets. The proposed system has exhibited excellent performance on both datasets. It may be noted that, a video surveillance system may result in a privacy issues during the continuous monitoring of older adults, and thus, has its own limitations for individual home monitoring, but it could be useful for rehabilitation centers and elderly health care houses, reformation centers [4,5], nursing homes and hospitals, electronic care environments [6], disabled care centers [7], and firearm shot damage spotting centers [8].

The remainder of this paper is organized as follows. Section 2 contains related work, Section 3 contains the proposed system, experimental evaluations are given in Section 4, conclusions and future follow in Section 5.

2. Related Work

In recent years, several vision-based techniques have been proposed for human fall detection. Some of these are based on wearable devices, such as accelerometers, while others use depth sensors, such as Microsoft Kinect. Moreover, RGB video cameras and different types of audio sensors have also been used for fall detection. Depending upon the underlying hardware, algorithms have been proposed to use one or more modalities, including accelerometer output, depth data, audio data and/or video data. Following are the broad categories of fall detection approaches and techniques.

2.1. Classification Based on Input Data Types

2.1.1. Sensor-Based

Luo et al. [9] developed a dynamic movement detection system to detect human falls. Their algorithm is based on the output of digital signals from mounted accelerometers. They filtered noisy segments using a Gaussian filter and set up a 3D body movement display which related different postures of the body to the yields of the accelerometers. Bourke et al. [10] described a procedure under supervised conditions to identify falls using tri-axial accelerometer sensors based on thresholding techniques. These sensors were mounted on the trunks and thighs of subjects. Makhlouf et al. [11] developed a multi-modal system that provided a fall detection service and an emergency service. Their system used photoelectric sensors and accelerometers to get information regarding the state of a person. If a person is in fall state, then the emergency service informs the doctor. The message sent to the specialist incorporates data about the localized area and condition of the individual. Recently, Casilari et al. [12] proposed a public repository of datasets that could be used as a common reference among the researchers to compare their algorithms. They created the UMAFall dataset that contains information about day-to-day activities and human falls. Contrary to other existing datasets that use one or two sensing points, they obtained data using five wearable sensors.

2.1.2. Audio-Based

Zigel et al. [13] presented an automatic fall discovery framework for elderly individuals particularly for when a person is unconscious or tense. The framework depends on indoor vibration and sound detection to classify human falls and other events. The classification uses features that include the shock response spectrum and Mel-frequency cepstrum coefficients. Doukas et al. [14] proposed a fall detection system based on audio and video data. Tracking of a person was done using video, and sound directionality analysis was made from audio data. Various features, including acceleration, sound proximity, average peak frequency, average signal relative amplitude, visual blob size and average movement speed were trained and tested using an SVM classifier for the detection of falls. The post-fall analysis was conducted as well to further predict if a person recovered his state or remained unconscious.

2.1.3. Image and Video-Based

Foroughi et al. [15] studied the morphological variations of silhouettes acquired from a series of videos. They concluded that the amalgamation of relative ellipse along the human body, the projection of histogram along the x-axis and y-axis and the change in the position of person's head provided beneficial cues for the determination of various behaviors of falls. Miaou et al. [16] suggested that visual detection may cause false readings as sometimes a movement appears as a fall, but, actually it may not be a fall. It could be simply a motion towards the direction of ground.

Lee et al. [17] recognized falls using image-based sensors. The data was generated by asking the subjects to randomly repeat five scenarios including lying down in a 'tucked' position, lying down in a 'stretched' position, stooping, sitting/lying down in an inactive zone and walking/standing.

Rougier et al. [18] emphasized the use of computer vision techniques to provide promising solutions for the detection of human falls. They used human shape deformation in a video sequence for human fall detection. The shape deformation from the person's silhouette was tracked along the video sequence. The fall was detected using a Gaussian mixture model. In [19], a vision-based system was proposed for human fall detection. The system used novel features of motion history for the detection of a fall. The system was run on video sequences of daily activities and simulated falls. Doulamis et al. [20] proposed a human fall detection system using cheap and low resolution cameras. Their system used adaptive background modeling using Gaussian Mixtures, and hierarchical motion estimation was used to distinguish falls from other activities, including lying, walking and sitting.

2.2. Classification Based on Classifier Types

2.2.1. Thresholding-Based

Chariff et al. [21] proposed intelligent surveillance technology to be used for the detection of dangerous events in the home environment. They tracked individuals as ellipses, and the direction of motion was utilized to recognize irregular and abnormal activities. Tao et al. [22] described the use of activity summarization in supportive homes where care is provided to aged people, but the proposed fall detection system was not capable of differentiating between a real fall incident and when the subject was just lying down.

Zaid et al. [23] used mobile robots to provide an efficient solution for fall detection in elderly people. The mobile robot system used Kinect sensor to track a target person and detect when they had fallen. Moreover, in case of a fall, an alarm was generated by sending an SMS message notification or making an emergency call.

Sumiya et al. [24] proposed a versatile robot to recognize human falls and to give details to observers. It comprised of a family portable robot with Microsoft Kinect and a PC. For simplicity, a sensor was placed on the robot which limited the blind zone by moving around with the robot. This technique improved the accuracy of fall detection compared to monitoring techniques based on fixed sensors.

2.2.2. Machine Learning-Based

Various classifiers including the Support Vector Machine (SVM), Adaboost, Multilayer Perceptron (MLP) and J48 have been used for human fall detection. Support Vector Machine, a pattern classification algorithm developed by V. Vapnik and his team at AT&T Bell Labs maps the data into higher dimensional input space and constructs an optimal plane separating the hyper-plane in this space. In [25], Foroughi et al. in 2008 implemented a Support Vector Machine to classify an event either as a fall or not a fall using feature-based approach and achieved a reliable recognition rate of 88.08%. Various other human fall detection systems use SVM for the classification of fall events (by their features) [26–28].

Debard et al. [26] proposed a feature-based approach for the detection of human falls. The proposed features included the angle of fall, aspect ratio, center velocity and head velocity. These features were trained and tested using SVM method. The drawbacks of this system include its inaccuracy to discriminate gradual fall from a person who is sitting down normally.

Ni et al. [29] developed a fall prevention framework for application in hospital wards. Their system detects if a patient gets up from the bed and generates an alarm for hospital staff to provide help. Their system used various features to detect human falls on a dataset of videos obtained from RGBD sensors of Microsoft Kinect. These included the region of interest (ROI), motion-based features, and shape-based features.

Adaboost [30], an adaptive boosting algorithm, utilizes a small number of weak classifiers that are used to construct cascades of strong classifiers. The combination of the strong classifiers into a cascade results in high accuracy and time efficiency for human fall detection. Multilayer Perceptron (MLP), a feedforward artificial neural network, is used for human fall detection systems, and achieved an accuracy of 90.15% on an ADL dataset [31].

The rule-based algorithm, J48, has also been used for the detection of human falls [32,33]. J48 is a C4.5 decision tree which is used to present different models of classification and also reveals human reasoning [34]. It has many advantages over various learning algorithms, such as its low computational cost of model generation, noise robustness and ability to handle redundant attributes and modules. It is robust even if training data contains errors or have missing attribute values [35]. Shi et al. proposed a human fall detection algorithm for classifying the human motion using the J48 decision tree classifier and achieved a sensitivity of 98.9%, a specificity of 98.5% and an overall accuracy of 98.6% [36]. In 2017, Guvensan et al. developed a system that implements the decision tree learning algorithm of J48, using five features, for detection of fall events [37]. Motivated by these algorithms, we chose the boosted J48 classifier due to its significantly higher F-measure, low computational cost and robustness to outliers and reduction of the feature space.

In the current work, we propose an algorithm under a boosting framework based on RGB video data for human fall detection. We emphasize its fast detection speed with high accuracy. We compare our work with existing state-of-the-art approaches, including Kepski et al. [38] by using KNN and SVM on the Multiple Cameras Fall Dataset [26] and the UR Fall Detection Dataset [38]. The results of our approach under an ensemble learning strategy with J48 and Adaboost outperform existing state-of-the-art approaches on both datasets in terms of percentage accuracy and execution time.

3. Proposed Fall Detection System

The first step in our proposed algorithm was to segment the foreground from the bac-ground and to identify the foreground as a person or non-person. In the second step, we computed various features from the foreground and in the third step, we trained a boosted J48 classifier for per frame classification of the foreground as a falling person or a stable moving person. In addition to the spatial information, our features also use temporal information as velocity and acceleration. Each of these steps is explained in the following sections.

3.1. Foreground Detection

A clean background image can be computed using the recently proposed background detection algorithms, such as [39–41]. The computed background image is subtracted from each frame to find the change region. Pixels with a change larger than a fixed percentage of the background image are considered to be , while the rest are considered to be the result of variation due to noise. In our experiments, we fixed this percentage at 15% of each pixel value in the background image. Then, a distance transform was computed over the changed region, followed by morphological operations, including erosion and flood filling to fill the holes in this region. To ensure that the change region contained only humans, connected components were computed and components with a size less than the minimum human size were deleted from the foreground. If a connected component had a size larger than the minimum person size threshold, it was considered to correspond to a human. Thus, a foreground mask containing only a human object was obtained. The minimum person size threshold helped to discard frames not containing a full person. Components with a size larger than the minimum person size threshold are referred to as foreground blobs in the rest of the paper.

3.2. Temporal and Spatial Variance for Falling Person Detection

In this section we discuss various types of temporal variance that we used in the proposed real-time person falling detection system. These variances include temporal variations of the aspect ratio, fall angle, speed, upper half area of bounding box and geometric center of the connected component. The temporal variance for each parameter was computed over a temporal window of size $k = 30$. This value of k was chosen after analyzing the video data and carefully conducting experiments. The value of $k = 30$ corresponded to a duration of 1 s as the frame rate of the videos was 30 frames per second. Figure 1 shows variation of the aspect ratio and other parameters with a change in person position during the process of fall.

3.2.1. Temporal Variance of the Aspect Ratio

A bounding box was computed containing the foreground blob. The aspect ratio refers to the ratio of the width to the height of this bounding box. The temporal variation of the aspect ratio is unique during the fall of a person, which was used as a feature. For a person in a stable position, the temporal variation in the aspect ratio is small, while during a fall, this variation is large. The temporal variation of the aspect ratio in a current frame was computed by taking the standard deviation of the aspect ratios of the previous k frames. After analyzing the video data and conducting experiments, the value of $k = 30$ was found to be reasonable to capture temporal variations in this parameter.

$$\sigma_{ar}^2 = \frac{1}{k} \sum_{i=1}^{k} (a_r(i) - \mu_{ar})^2 \tag{1}$$

3.2.2. Temporal Variation of the Person Angle

An ellipse was fitted in the foreground blob and a person angle was computed as the angle between the major axis of ellipse and the x-axis (horizontal axis). The person angle changed when a person fell from a standing state to a fall state. The temporal variation in the fall angle of the current frame was computed by computing the standard deviation of the fall angle of the previous $k = 30$ frames.

$$\sigma_{pa}^2 = \frac{1}{k} \sum_{i=1}^{k} (p_a(i) - \mu_{pa})^2 \tag{2}$$

3.2.3. Temporal Variation of the Motion Vector

The motion vector is the variation in the foreground blob's position between the current and the next frame. The motion magnitude increases when the body is in motion, and it reaches a high value during fall and then it becomes zero after the fall. The change in the magnitude of the body speed (B.S.) serves as an important parameter for human fall detection. The body speed is calculated by computing the motion vectors of the centroid of the foreground blob. The magnitude of motion vectors is calculated as shown in Equation (3).

$$|m_v| = \sqrt{(m_v(x))^2 + (m_v(y))^2}, \tag{3}$$

where $m_v(x)$ is the magnitude of motion vectors along the x-direction and $m_v(y)$ is the magnitude of motion vectors along the y-direction. The temporal variation in body speed gives the acceleration of the body. Figure 2 shows the body speed variation of a falling person where the number of frames and magnitude of motion vectors are plotted along x-axis and y-axis respectively. The temporal variance of m_v is computed as follows:

$$\sigma^2_{mv} = \frac{1}{k}\sum_{i=1}^{k}\left(m_v(i) - \mu_{mv}\right)^2,\tag{4}$$

where μ_{mv} is the mean motion vector over the current time window.

3.2.4. Temporal Variation of Shape Deformations

The orientation of the body shape changes significantly when a person falls. The upper half area of the foreground blob bounding box (U.H.B.B.) was used as a shape descriptor (s_d) to capture variations in the orientation of the body when fall occurs. The bounding box is divided into two equal halves. The upper half area of the upper half bounding box is high when a person is in fall state as compared to standing state. Hence, the area of the upper half of the bounding box serves as a strong feature as its value changes significantly when a person enters into a fall state from a normal state. Figure 2 shows the temporal variation of the upper half area of the bounding box of a falling person of video 1 (camera position 7) and video 3 (camera position 3), respectively. In these figures, the number of frames and number of pixels in the upper half area of bounding box are plotted along the x-axis and y-axis, respectively. The temporal variation in the upper half area of the bounding box of a current frame is computed by calculating the standard deviation in the upper half area of the bounding box from the previous $k = 30$ frames to detect if an event is a fall or not a fall.

$$\sigma^2_{sd} = \frac{1}{k}\sum_{i=1}^{k}\left(s_d(i) - \mu_{sd}\right)^2,\tag{5}$$

where μ_{sd} is the mean area of the upper-half bounding box over the current time window.

3.2.5. Temporal Variation in the Geometric Center Position

The geometric location of a foreground blob changes significantly when a person falls. This change in geometric location can be captured by taking the temporal variation of geometric center (G.C.) as a feature. The temporal variation in the x-component and y-component of the geometric center of a current frame is computed by taking the standard deviation of the x-component and y-component of the previous $k = 30$ frames. The geometric center, (x_g, y_g), is the average of the x-coordinates and y-coordinates of all boundary points (edge points) of the object

$$(x_g, y_g) = \frac{1}{n}\left(\sum_{i=1}^{n} x_i, \sum_{i=1}^{n} y_i\right),\tag{6}$$

where (x_i, y_i) represents the coordinates of the pixels in the foreground blob. Figure 2 shows the temporal variation of the geometric center of a falling person. In this figure, the number of frames and geometric center are plotted along the x-axis and y-axis, respectively.

$$\sigma^2_{gp} = \frac{1}{k}\sum_{i=1}^{k}\left(g_p(i) - \mu_{gp}\right)^2,\tag{7}$$

where μ_{gp} is the mean position of the geometric center over the current time window.

3.2.6. Temporal Variation of the Ellipse Ratio

The ellipse ratio, e_r, is defined as the ratio between the length of the major and minor axes of the ellipse containing the foreground blob. It was used as a scale invariant feature in our proposed approach for the classification of a person as fall or not a fall. Figure 1A,B shows that the ellipse ratio changes significantly when the person is moving from a standing state (A (a) & B (a)) to intermediate states (A (b), B (b) and A (c), B (c)) and then to the fall state (A (d) & B (d)). Hence, the ratio of these axes of ellipse serves as an important feature for detecting the human fall. The temporal variation of ellipse ratio is computed over the current time window

$$\sigma_{er}^2 = \frac{1}{k} \sum_{i=1}^{k} (e_r(i) - \mu_{er})^2, \tag{8}$$

where μ_{er} is the mean ellipse ratio over the current time window.

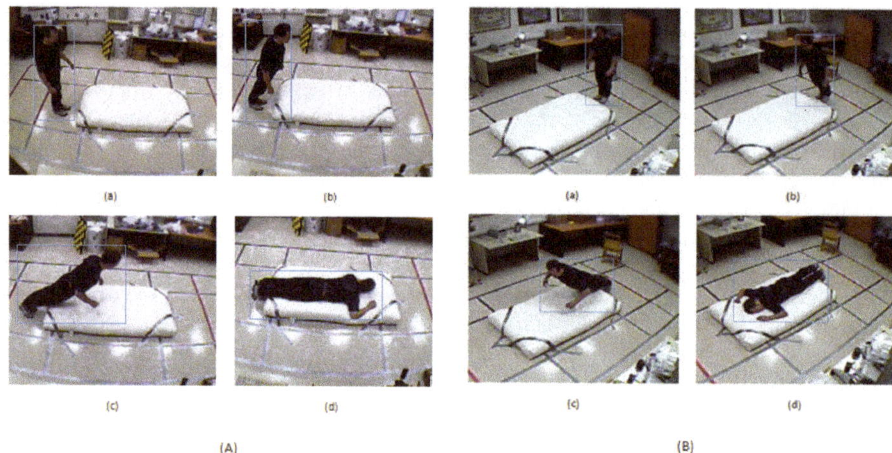

Figure 1. Temporal variation of the aspect ratio (a_r) of a falling person in the Multiple Camera Fall (MCF) dataset where a_r = width/height of bounding box of a foreground blob. The person angle (p_a), shape deformation (s_d), and ellipse ratios (e_r) are also shown for each case. (**A**) Camera 7, video 1: (**a**) $a_r = 0.45$, $p_a = 90°$, $s_d = 880.93$, $e_r = 2.02$, (**b**) $a_r = 0.48$, $p_a = 68°$, $s_d = 670.35$, $e_r = 2.17$, (**c**) $a_r = 1.45$, $p_a = 27°$, $s_d = 435.39$, $e_r = 1.85$, (**d**) $a_r = 2.85$, $p_a = 0°$, $s_d = 3252.91$, $e_r = 0.43$; (**B**) Camera 3, video 3, (**a**) $a_r = 0.44$, $p_a = 90°$, $s_d = 580.99$, $e_r = 2.12$, (**b**) $a_r = 0.52$, $p_a = 55°$, $s_d = 356.45$, $e_r = 2.05$, (**c**) $a_r = 1.46$, $p_a = 27°$, $s_d = 193$, $e_r = 1.42$, (**d**) $a_r = 2.8$, $p_a = 0°$, $s_d = 2152.48$, $e_r = 0.38$.

Figure 1 shows a comparison of different proposed feature values for two different camera views. The range of feature values despite significant view changes remained almost the same. Figure 2 shows a comparison of the temporal variation of different features in two different views. Despite significant variations in the camera viewing angle, the shape of the temporal variation remained almost the same. Both figures show that the feature values and temporal variation of values remained almost unchanged regardless of the camera viewing angle. This is the main reason for the consistent performance of the proposed algorithm across multiple camera views.

Similarly, a different camera view is shown in Figure 2. The behaviour of our features is equally good in this new figure with different camera views; this shows that our features exhibit comparable performance even with different views.

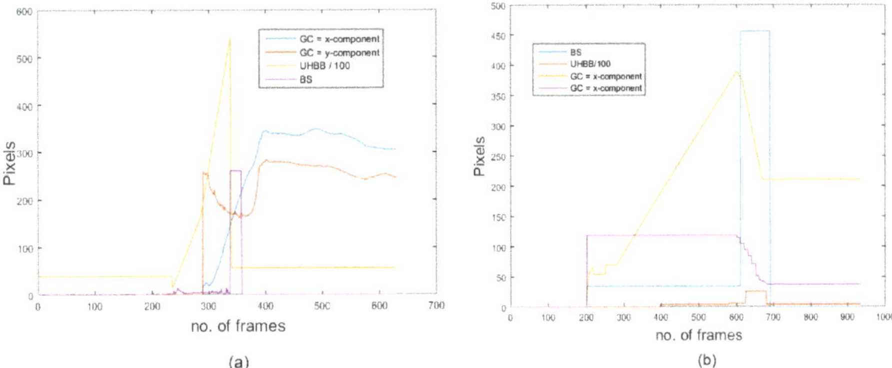

Figure 2. The temporal variation in body speed (B.S.), upper half area of the bounding box (U.H.B.B), and x-component and y-component of the geometric centre (G.C.) of a falling person on the MCF dataset: (**a**) camera 2, video 2; (**b**) camera 3, video 3.

3.3. Training Boosted J48 Classifier

Classification is the task of finding a target function that maps an attribute set to a particular class among a predefined set of classes. Various classifiers including SVM, neural networks, rule-based methods, prototype methods and exemplar-based methods exist in the literature. In the current work, we trained an ensemble of J48 classifiers, which we named 'Boosted J48'. We prefer this classification strategy over the other existing classifiers mainly because of its speed and accuracy.

Boosting is a method for combining multiple classifiers [42,43]. As the name suggests, it is a meta algorithm that is used to improve the results of the base classifier. In our case, the base classifier was J48 which is an extension of the ID3 algorithm that generates rules for the prediction of target variables [44]. The additional features of J48 include finding missing values, derivation of rules, continuous attribute value ranges, and decision tree pruning.

Boosting works sequentially, whereby the first algorithm is trained on the entire dataset, and then the rest of the algorithms are developed by fitting the residuals of the first algorithm. In this process, higher weight is given to the observations that have been poorly predicted by the previous model. Boosting is known to be sensitive to noisy data and outliers. The reason for this is that boosting overfits noisy datasets. Boosting on stable algorithms like J48 improves performance, while boosting on unstable algorithms, like MLP, may reduce performance [45].

In each iteration, the base classifier is used with a different weight over the samples of the training set. At each iteration, the computed distributions assign more weight to the incorrectly classified samples. The final classifier is obtained as a weighted average of the previous hierarchical designed classifier. We focused on the two-class classification task, where the training set is $\{(x_1, y_1), (x_2, y_2), ..., (x_N, y_N)\}$, x_i is some feature vector and $y_i \in \{-1, 1\}, i = 1, 2, ..., N$ is the label. The aim was to design an optimal classifier to predict the label of a test feature vector, x_t.

$$\hat{y} = \mathrm{sign}\{F(x_t)\} \tag{9}$$

where $\hat{y}$ is the predicted label and

$$F(x_t) = \sum_{k=1}^{K} \alpha_k \, \phi(x_t; \theta_k), \tag{10}$$

where $\phi(x_t; \theta_k)$ denotes the base classifier that returns a binary class label, $\{-1, 1\}$. The corresponding parameter vector, θ_k, describes the base classifier. An important property of boosting is its relative immunity to overfitting with an increasing K. It has been verified that even with a high number of terms, K, and consequently, a high number of parameters, the error rate on a test set does not increase but keeps decreasing and finally, reaches a low, asymptotic value.

Random Decision Forests (RDF) and J48 are both tree-based classifiers. RDF is a mixture of tree predictors, where each tree is a predicate of the values of a random vector sampled autonomously and all the trees of the forest have the same distribution [46]. As the trees in a forest become large in number, the generalization error for the forest converges to a certain limit. The votes from all trees determine the class assignments. The main limitation of RDF is its increased complexity with an increasing depth of trees when training RDF, compared to J48. That is, RDF requires more computational resources and has higher memory complexity. The learning rate of RDF is slower and its prediction process also has more computational complexity compared to an equivalent J48 classifier.

As discussed, J48 is an extension of the ID3 algorithm that generates rules for the prediction of target variables [44]. The additional features of J48 include finding missing values, the derivation of rules, continuous attribute value ranges, decision tree pruning, etc. J48 is based on the information gain ratio that is evaluated by entropy. The information gain ratio measure is used to choose the test features (attributes) at each node in the tree. The attribute with the highest information gain ratio is selected as the test feature for the current node. If we have a feature, X, and we examine the values for this feature in the training set and they are in increasing order, $A_1, A_2, ..., A_m$, then for each value, $A_j, j = 1, 2, ..., m$, the records are partitioned into 2 sets: the first set includes the X values up to and including A_j and the second set includes the X values greater than A_j [47]. For each of these m partitions, the $GainRatio(X(j), T)$ where $j = 1, 2, ..., m$ is computed, and the partition that maximizes the gain is chosen. The $GainRatio(X, T)$ is given in Equation (11):

$$GainRatio(X, T) = \frac{Gain(X, T)}{SplitInfo(X, T).}$$ (11)

Considering the information content of a message that indicates not the class to which the case belongs, but the outcome of the test on feature X, the SplitInfo is given by Equation (12):

$$SplitInfo(X, T) = -\sum_{i}^{n} \frac{|T_i|}{|T|} log_2 \frac{|T_i|}{|T|.}$$ (12)

The GainRatio(X,T) is thus the proportion of information generated by the split that is useful for the classification.

4. Experiments and Results

4.1. Datasets

We performed experiments on two publicly available datasets: the Multiple Cameras Fall (MCF) dataset (http://www.iro.umontreal.ca/~labimage/Dataset/) and the UR Fall Detection (URFD) dataset (http://fenix.univ.rzeszow.pl/~mkepski/ds/uf.html). Table 1 contains the descriptions of 20 videos from the MCF dataset captured at camera position 2. The details mentioned in Table 1 include the video number, total frames in each video, frames with falls and frames without falls. Figure 1 shows some example frames from the MCF dataset from video 1 (camera 7) and video 3 (camera 3) respectively containing various states of a falling person.

The UR Fall Detection (URFD) dataset contains frontal and overhead video sequences obtained by two Kinect sensors, with one placed at the height of 1 m from the floor and the other mounted on the ceiling with a height of 3 m. The dataset contains two kinds of falls that were performed by five people—from standing position and from sitting on the chair. The dataset was recorded at 30 frames per second. The frontal sequence contains 314 frames, in which 74 frames contain falls and 240 frames have no falls. The key frames of the URFD dataset are shown in Figure 3. The overhead sequence contains a total of 302 frames, in which 75 frames contain falls, while 227 have no falls.

Table 1. Details of the Multiple Cameras Fall (MCF) Dataset: total number of frames, number of frames containing a fall, and number of frames containing no fall in each video.

Videos	Total Frames	Fall	No Fall	Videos	Total Frames	Fall	No Fall
Video 1	1411	314	1097	Video 11	1486	608	878
Video 2	756	331	425	Video 12	1041	420	621
Video 3	883	272	611	Video 13	1240	360	880
Video 4	1033	409	624	Video 14	970	385	585
Video 5	600	266	334	Video 15	1007	367	640
Video 6	1203	513	690	Video 16	1023	320	703
Video 7	912	290	622	Video 17	992	432	560
Video 8	700	240	460	Video 18	1217	627	590
Video 9	905	360	545	Video 19	1155	390	765
Video 10	813	230	583	Video 20	2328	90	2238

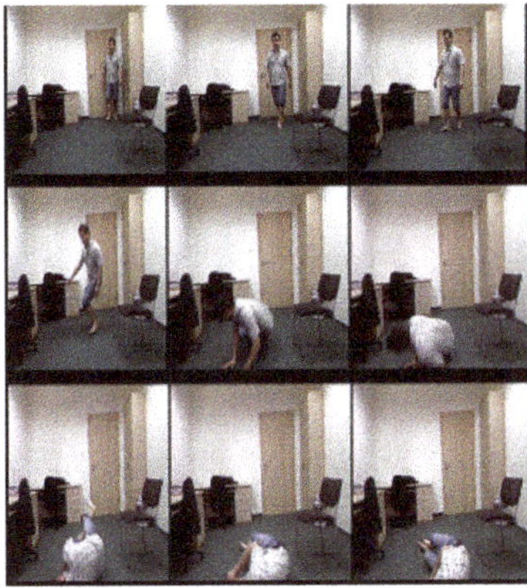

Figure 3. Selected frames from the frontal sequence of the URFD dataset.

In all experiments, 10-fold cross-validation was used. For the purpose of temporal variance computation in Equations (1)–(8), different temporal window values, k, were used. All results reported in the paper are for $k = 30$. Since the video frame rate was 30 fps, $k = 30$ corresponds to a duration of 1 s.

4.2. Comparison with Existing Approaches

The proposed algorithm was compared with existing approaches including Kepski et al. [38] using KNN and SVM, Debard (De) [26], Debard Kyrkou (DeKy) [26,30], Debard Foroughi (DeFo) [26,48], Osuna (Osu) [27], Kyrkou (Ky) [27,30] and Foroughi (Fo) [27,48].

The proposed approach, 'PA_B-J48', uses the temporal variance of motion and geometric features with an ensemble learning strategy of 'boosting with J48'. The second proposed approach, 'PA_Ada', uses the same set of features but with the Adaptive Boosting (AdaBoost) classifier. AdaBoost is an ensemble learning approach based on game theory with a main aim of combining many weak classifiers to produce a strong classifier.

Adaboost is an iterative algorithm that is used in conjunction with many other types of learning algorithms (weak learners) to improve their performance [49]. The output of weak learning algorithms is combined into a weighted sum that forms the final output of the boosted classifier. Adaboost, short for adaptive boosting, tweaks the weak learners in favor of misclassified instances by the previous classifiers. The prior knowledge of the lower bound of prediction accuracy of weak learning algorithms is not required; hence, Adaboost is suitable for many practical purposes. The algorithm is sensitive to noisy data and outliers.

The proposed algorithms work better than deep learning due to various reasons. Deep networks require very large training datasets containing millions of images to achieve good performances. Due to the limited training data being used in this study, our proposed algorithms were more suitable than the deep learning approaches.

Deep networks are computationally expensive as they require high-end GPUs to be trained on large datasets. Expensive GPUs, fast CPU, SSD storage and large RAM significantly increase the hardware cost and computational complexity of deep networks. Hence, it is not feasible to train these deep networks are not feasible on the current systems (64-bit machine with Intel core i3-3110M CPU @2.40GHz, and 4GB RAM) on which our proposed algorithm gives more than 99% percentage accuracy for various data sets.

Classical machine learning algorithms are easier to interpret and understand compared to deep learning methods. Due to thorough understanding of data and algorithms, it is easy to tune hyper-parameters and to change the design of a model. Deep learning networks have often been used like a "black box".

4.3. Performance Measures

In addition to accuracy, we used sensitivity and specificity for a comparison of our system with existing systems . These measures have also used by other fall detection systems [50].

$$Sensitivity = \frac{TP}{(TP + FN)} \tag{13}$$

$$Specificity = \frac{TP}{(TN + FP)} \tag{14}$$

where true positive (TP) is the number of falls correctly identified by the system, and false negative (FN) is the number of falls missed by the system, and true negative (TN) is the number of 'no falls' correctly identified by the system, and false positive (FP) is the number of 'no falls' missed by the system.

4.4. Experiments on the MFC Dataset

The performance of the proposed fall detection system was evaluated on the MFC dataset in three different experiments and compared with the existing state-of-the-art approaches. These experiments are discussed below.

4.4.1. Experiment 1

In the first experiment, frames of all 20 videos were combined and 10-fold cross validation was used to train and test the proposed system. All test frames were classified as fall or no fall. The resulting accuracy, sensitivity, and specificity of the existing as well as proposed methods are shown in Figure 4. The proposed PA_B-J48 has previously been shown to obtain larger accuracy than all compared methods. The proposed PA_Ada and the existing algorithms were not able to efficiently handle within class variations. A possible reason for the accuracy degradation of PA_Ada is overfitting [51]. Adaptive boosting uses a training set over and over and hence, is more prone to overfitting.

Figure 4 shows the ROC curves of the existing approaches, including De, DeKy, DeFo, Osu, Ky, Fo and proposed approaches 'PA_B-J48' and 'PA_Ada' on MCF dataset (Experiment 1). It may be observed that ROC curve of the proposed approach PA_B-J48 is better than the existing approaches.

Table 2 shows the percentage accuracy of existing approaches, including De, DeKy, DeFo, Osu, Ky, Fo, and the proposed approaches 'PA_B-J48' and 'PA_Ada' from camera position 3 and video 3 of the MCF dataset (Experiment 1). Camera 3 was placed exactly on the opposite wall from camera 2 (http://www.iro.umontreal.ca/~labimage/Dataset/). It may be observed that the proposed approach 'PA_Ada' exhibited a percentage accuracy of 99.14% with camera position 3 which is comparable with the percentage accuracy shown by camera position 2 (as can be seen in Table 3). Hence, our proposed algorithm performed robustly across different camera positions.

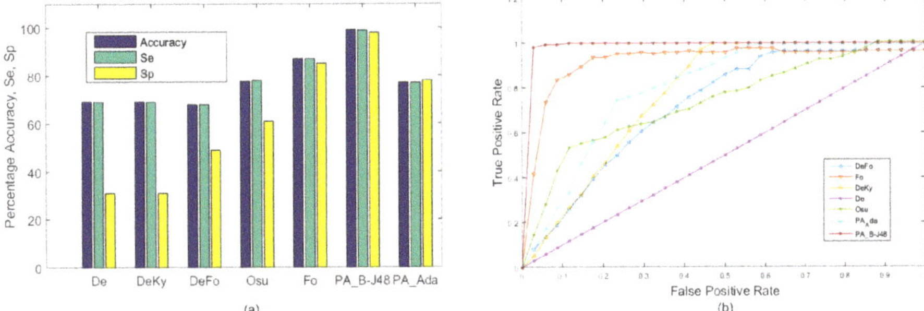

Figure 4. Experiment 1: A comparison of the existing approaches and the proposed approaches on the MCF dataset with 10-fold cross validation using two categories: 'Fall' and 'No Fall'. (**a**) Graph; (**b**) ROC curve.

Table 2. Experiment 1: Comparison of the existing approaches, De, DeKy, DeFo, Osu, Ky, and Fo, with the proposed approaches 'PA_B-J48' and 'PA_Ada' in terms of % accuracy (A) at camera position 3 of video 3 (V) of the MCF dataset with 10-fold cross validation using two categories: 'Fall' and 'No Fall'. Maximum value in each row is shown in bold.

		Existing Approaches					**Proposed Approaches**	
		De [26]	DeKy [30]	DeFo [48]	Osu [27]	Fo [48]	PA_B-J48	PA_Ada
Cam3 (V3)	A	73.23	77.09	78.37	93.47	98.39	92.4	**99.14**

Table 3. Experiment 2: Comparison of the existing approaches, De, DeKy, DeFo, Osu, Ky, and Fo, with the proposed approaches, 'PA_B-J48' and 'PA_Ada', in terms of % accuracy (A), % sensitivity (Se) and % specificity (Sp) for each Video (V) of the MCF dataset with 10-fold cross validation using two categories: 'Fall' and 'No Fall'. Maximum value in each row is shown in bold.

		Existing Approaches					**Proposed Approaches**	
Video		**De [26]**	**DeKy [30]**	**DeFo [48]**	**Osu [27]**	**Fo [48]**	**PA_B-J48**	**PA_Ada**
	A	88.65	93.76	90.50	99.23	**99.86**	99.65	98.99
V1	Se	89.00	94.00	91.00	98.00	**99.00**	**99.00**	**99.00**
	Sp	69.00	95.00	86.00	97.00	**99.00**	**99.00**	**99.00**
	A	61.83	91.76	71.24	93.03	**99.74**	99.08	99.34
V2	Se	62.00	92.00	71.00	98.00	**99.00**	**99.00**	**99.00**
	Sp	49.00	85.00	61.00	97.00	**99.00**	**99.00**	**99.00**
	A	72.79	92.86	74.94	99.88	99.89	99.89	**100.00**
V3	Se	73.00	93.00	75.00	99.00	99.00	99.00	**100.00**
	Sp	42.00	91.00	71.00	99.00	99.00	99.00	**100.00**
	A	68.41	82.95	70.45	87.40	98.35	**99.42**	88.85
V4	Se	68.00	83.00	70.00	87.00	98.00	**99.00**	89.00
	Sp	31.00	55.00	64.00	77.00	98.00	**99.00**	70.00
	A	63.42	89.38	90.12	92.03	95.72	**98.82**	94.99
V5	Se	63.00	89.00	90.00	92.00	96.00	**99.00**	95.00
	Sp	65.00	98.00	98.00	87.00	93.00	**99.00**	98.00

Table 3. *Cont.*

Video		De [26]	DeKy [30]	DeFo [48]	Osu [27]	Fo [48]	PA_B-J48	PA_Ada
	A	91.51	89.33	94.01	95.34	99.58	**99.67**	98.17
V6	Se	91.00	90.00	94.00	95.00	**100.00**	99.00	98.00
	Sp	85.00	89.00	87.00	91.00	**100.00**	99.00	98.00
	A	68.09	85.42	79.17	95.39	99.23	**99.45**	98.90
V7	Se	68.00	85.00	79.00	95.00	**99.00**	**99.00**	98.00
	Sp	32.00	62.00	76.00	89.00	**99.00**	**99.00**	98.00
	A	65.57	83.86	72.57	89.14	99.00	**99.29**	98.42
V8	Se	66.00	84.00	73.00	89.00	**99.00**	**99.00**	98.00
	Sp	32.00	61.00	78.00	72.00	98.00	**99.00**	98.00
	A	70.50	85.19	77.46	91.60	97.13	**99.45**	96.46
V9	Se	71.00	85.00	78.00	92.00	97.00	**99.00**	97.00
	Sp	52.00	90.00	74.00	97.00	95.00	**99.00**	76.00
	A	77.74	80.93	80.07	91.39	98.40	**99.02**	95.69
V10	Se	78.00	81.00	81.00	91.00	98.00	**99.00**	96.00
	Sp	65.00	52.00	52.00	84.00	94.00	**99.00**	93.00
	A	59.02	59.02	65.75	84.86	98.92	**99.53**	87.35
V11	Se	59.00	59.00	66.00	85.00	**99.00**	**99.00**	87.00
	Sp	41.00	70.00	55.00	84.00	**99.00**	**99.00**	95.00
	A	63.01	83.19	74.54	93.28	98.85	**99.33**	95.58
V12	Se	79.00	79.00	79.00	93.00	**99.00**	**99.00**	96.00
	Sp	21.00	21.00	21.00	89.00	**99.00**	**99.00**	97.00
	A	78.93	78.93	78.93	78.93	95.24	**99.11**	89.26
V13	Se	79.00	79.00	79.00	93.00	95.00	**99.00**	89.00
	Sp	21.00	21.00	21.00	6.00	84.00	**97.00**	74.00
	A	64.08	64.29	68.84	79.81	96.58	**98.96**	89.64
V14	Se	64.00	64.00	68.00	80.00	97.00	**99.00**	90.00
	Sp	36.00	39.00	51.00	57.00	95.00	**98.00**	92.00
	A	63.72	90.85	72.56	91.65	96.02	**99.50**	86.18
V15	Se	63.00	91.00	73.00	92.00	96.00	**99.00**	86.00
	Sp	40.00	70.00	72.00	96.00	95.00	**99.00**	87.00
	A	69.60	85.92	69.60	74.19	94.33	**99.41**	89.34
V16	Se	79.00	86.00	70.00	74.00	94.00	**99.00**	75.00
	Sp	30.00	67.00	30.00	42.00	90.00	**99.00**	89.00
	A	72.53	83.13	75.46	78.30	97.46	**98.83**	93.26
V17	Se	72.00	81.00	76.00	78.00	98.00	**99.00**	93.00
	Sp	27.00	70.00	47.00	49.00	93.00	**98.00**	86.00
	A	65.24	79.79	78.14	90.30	99.06	**99.18**	92.76
V18	Se	65.00	90.00	78.00	98.00	99.00	**99.00**	**99.00**
	Sp	37.00	72.00	88.00	99.00	99.00	99.00	**100.00**
	A	76.19	78.79	77.06	93.42	97.84	**99.48**	93.42
V19	Se	76.00	79.00	77.00	93.00	**99.00**	**99.00**	93.00
	Sp	48.00	52.00	56.00	88.00	55.00	**99.00**	92.00
	A	96.09	96.09	96.06	98.58	**99.87**	**99.87**	99.83
V20	Se	96.00	96.00	96.00	99.00	**100.00**	**100.00**	**100.00**
	Sp	3	3	3	65.00	96.00	**99.00**	96.00

In all experiments, the proposed algorithm performed equally well for different types of falls for various videos in the MCF dataset. We experimentally observed that the performance of our proposed algorithm was not greatly effected by the view variations in this dataset. The falls in these videos can be divided into three categories with respect to the camera angle: falling towards a side or falling towards or away from the camera. In videos 1, 3, 5, 6, 9, 10, 11, 12, 14, 15, 18, 19, and 22, the person is walking from the right to the left of the scene and falls to the side with respect to camera. In all of these videos, the person falls on his chest, while in video 6, the person falls on his back. In videos 9 and 10, the person sits on a sofa before falling. Video 11 is similar to video 9, but the person falls on a sofa rather than sitting on it. In videos 12 and 14, the person is crouching or picking up stuff from the ground before falling. In videos 15, 18, and 19, the sofa is replaced by a chair. In video 22, the person slips to the side.

The second type of fall occurs in videos 2, 4, 7, 8, and 13; the person moves from the right to the left of the scene and falls towards the camera. In video 13, the person falls on a sofa as well. In video 4, the person falls twice. The third type of fall occurs in videos 16, 17 and 20; the fall occurs away from the camera. In video 16, the person moves in a circular motion around the sofa and then falls on the sofa away from the camera. In video 20 , the person moves from the left to the right and then from the right to the left multiple times, picking up stuff from the floor, falling on a sofa multiple times and then falling on the floor in a direction away from the camera. The proposed algorithm performed almost the same on all these fall variations.

4.4.2. Experiment 2

The performance of the existing as well as the proposed algorithms on the MFC data set with 10-fold cross validation is shown in Table 3 and Figure 5. Due to relatively less with-in-class variations, performance of all algorithms increased. In this experiment, both proposed algorithms PA_B-J48 and PA_Ada performed quite well and obtained very high accuracy.

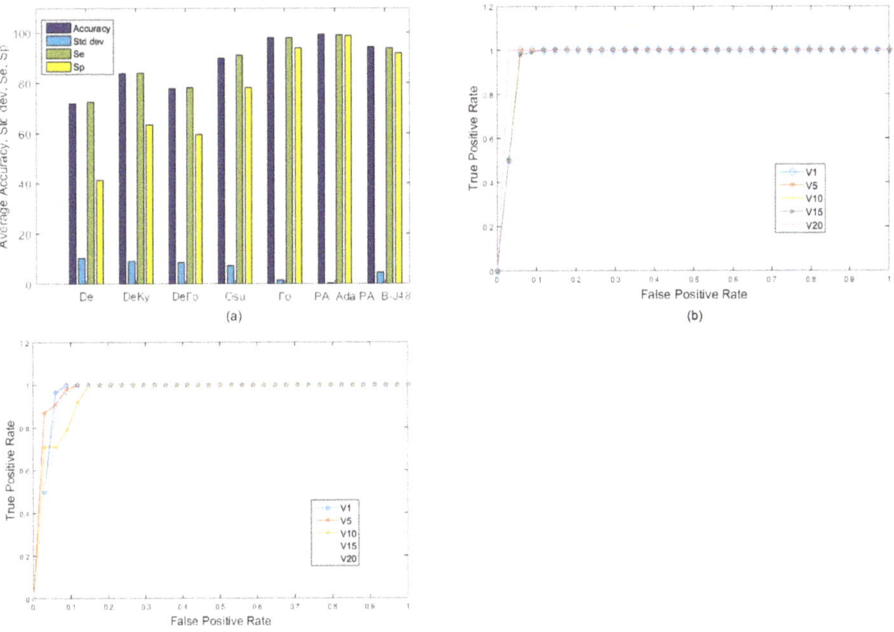

Figure 5. Experiment 2: Average comparison of the existing approaches and the proposed approaches on the MCF dataset with 10-fold cross validation using two categories: 'Fall' and 'No Fall'. (**a**) Graph; (**b,c**) ROC curve of selected videos (videos 1, 6, 10, 15, and 20) using camera 2 for the proposed approaches, PA_B-J48 and PA_Ada.

4.4.3. Experiment 3

In the third experiment, a three-class classification was performed. We added a sitting down class to evaluate the performance of the proposed algorithm in differentiating falling down from sitting down. The main difference between these two actions is the speed of performing the action. Similar to the first experiment, all 20 videos were merged together to form a single video and 10-fold cross validation was used for training and testing. Sitting down is slow and relatively gradual while falling down is rapid and relatively random. The results of this experiment are shown in Figure 6. In this experiment, the performance of PA_B-J48 remained excellent while all other methods suffered from significant accuracy degradation. This was mainly due to the similarity between the sitting and falling down classes. Moreover, adaptive boosting is more prone to overfitting large datasets and it could also serve as an important reason for the reduced performance of PA_Ada [51]. The reason for the better performance of PA_B-J48 is due to an improvement in the efficiency of the basic J48 algorithm through boosting, an ensemble learning method and more effective feature set. The J48 is a powerful decision tree method that can handle both discrete and continuous attributes. The algorithm also handles the missing values in the training data.

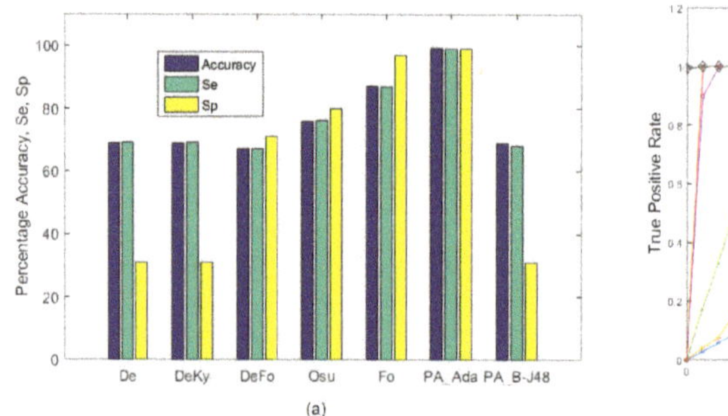
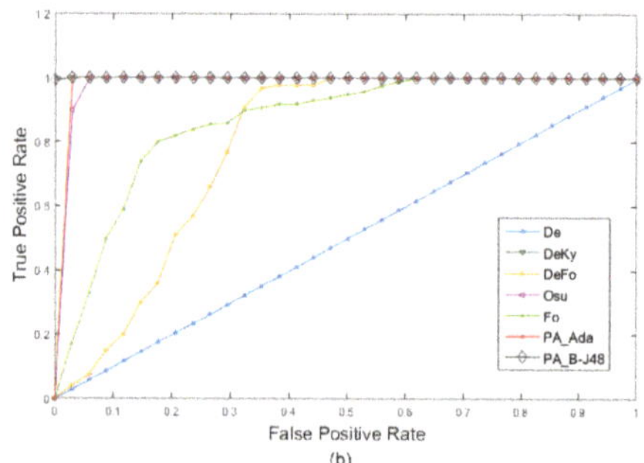

Figure 6. Experiment 3: Accuracy comparison of the existing approaches, De, DeKy, DeFo, Osu, Ky, Fo and the proposed approaches, 'PA_B-J48' and 'PA_Ada', on all videos in the MCF dataset with 10-fold cross validation using three classes i.e., 'fall', 'sitting' and 'no fall'. (**a**) Graph; (**b**) ROC curve.

4.5. Experiments on the URFD Dataset

The URFD dataset is challenging as it contains abrupt human falls and short video sequences. Moreover, the data set contains falls not only from the standing position, but also while sitting on a chair. It can be seen in the Figure 7 that our proposed approach 'PA_B-J48' outperformed the existing approaches of De, DeKy, DeFo, Osu, Fo, and Kepski et al. using KNN and SVM [38] on both frontal and overhead data sequences in terms of average accuracy, sensitivity, and specificity. Moreover, our second proposed approach also exhibited better percentage accuracy than the existing approaches of De, DeKy, DeFo, Fo, and Kepski et al. using KNN and SVM [38].

The proposed algorithm exhibited an accuracy of 99.13% on the frontal video sequence of URFD while it showed an accuracy of 99.03% of the overhead video sequence of the same dataset. This shows that accuracy degradation occurs despite significant view variation being quite minor.

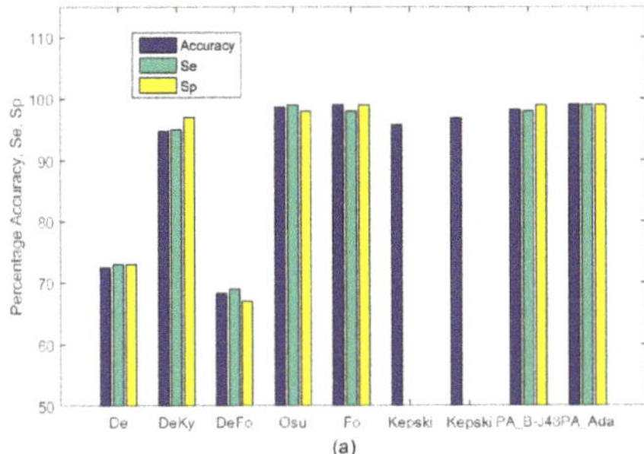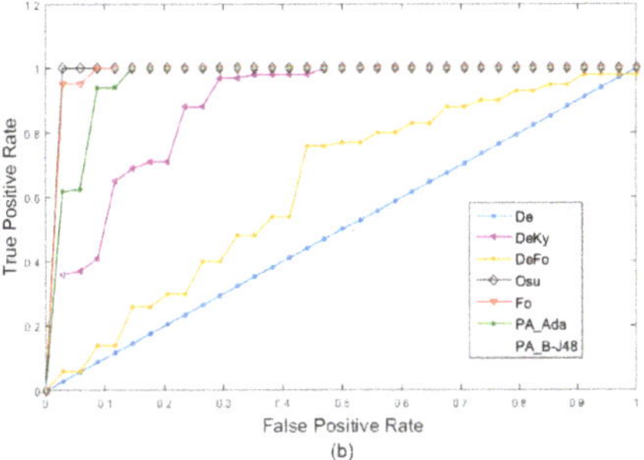

Figure 7. Experiments on the URFD dataset: comparison of accuracy, Se and Sp between the existing approaches under consideration and the proposed approach on the frontal and overhead data sequence from the URFD dataset. (**a**) Graph; (**b**) ROC curve.

4.6. Execution Time Comparison

A comparison of the execution times of the proposed approaches, PA_B-J48 and PA_Ada, with the existing approaches was performed on the MCF dataset (Experiments 1 & 3) and the URFD dataset, as shown in Table 4. All experiments were performed on a 64-bit machine with Intel Core i3-3110M CPU @2.40GHz, and 4GB RAM. In Experiment 1, the proposed PA_Ada was 9.06, 74.28, and 27.29 times faster than DeFo, Osu and Fo, respectively, while the PA_B-J48 method was 0.57, 4.72, and 1.73 times faster, respectively. In Experiment 3, the proposed PA_Ada was 4.28, 37.14, and 16.06 times faster than DeFo, Osu and Fo, respectively, while PA_B-J48 was 0.60, 5.24, and 2.27 times faster, respectively, than these methods. In both of these experiments, PA_Ada remained significantly faster than the compared algorithms. PA_B-J48 remained faster than both Osu and Fo. In both experiments, DeFo remained faster than PA_B-J48; however, its accuracy remained low. Similarly De and DeKy were faster but significantly less accurate. This shows a trade-off between accuracy and speed. The proposed algorithm uses a larger feature set than these methods to achieve a higher accuracy. By using a parallel implementation of the proposed PA_B-J48, its execution time can be significantly reduced over larger datasets. On smaller datasets such as URFD, the proposed PA_B-J48 is already among the fastest methods (Table 4).

Table 4. Comparison of execution times (seconds) of the existing approaches under consideration and the proposed approaches on the MCF dataset (Experiments 1 & 3) and on the URFD dataset. The execution time was measured on the same machine under similar operating conditions.

	Existing Approach			Proposed Approach	
Experiment	DeFo	Osu	Fo	PA_B-J48	PA_Ada
Experiment 1	16.5 s	135.19 s	49.65 s	28.63 s	1.82 s
Experiment 3	13.05 s	113.28 s	48.98 s	21.6 s	3.05 s
URFD (average)	0.12 s	0.01 s	0.32 s	0.01 s	0.025 s

5. Conclusions

An accurate and fast human fall detection system is of utmost importance for patients and aged persons for timely intervention if a fall happens, to avoid serious injuries or consequences from a fall. The work presented in this paper used the temporal variance of various discriminatory features including motion, geometric orientation and geometric location to build a fall detection system. The proposed system was trained and tested using the ensemble learning strategy and boosting with the J48 classifier as well as with the AdaBoost classifier. The proposed system was tested on two publicly available fall detection datasets and compared with eight existing algorithms. From the experiments, it was concluded that the accuracy of the proposed system was better than existing approaches for both the datasets. The proposed system was better able to differentiate between sitting down and falling down compared to existing algorithms. The proposed system also offers a faster execution time than existing methods.

This work can be extended to further improve the performance and time efficiency of human fall detection systems, specifically in more challenging datasets containing multiple people with occlusions, the same colored clothes as that of background and multisource, non-Lambertian lighting. In addition, the proposal of more novel and robust features and the development of large video repositories will play vital roles in improving the accuracy and robustness of fall detection systems. The addition of night vision functionality to a system will be an important feature of outdoor fall detection systems.

Author Contributions: Conceptualization, S.F.A.; Methodology, S.F.A. and A.M.; Software, R.K. and S.F.A.; Validation, R.K., S.F.A. and A.M.; Formal Analysis, A.M.; Investigation, S.F.A.; Resources, M.T.H. and M.J.; Data Curation, S.F.A.; Writing—Original Draft Preparation, S.F.A.; Writing—Review & Editing, A.M.; Visualization, S.F.A.; Supervision, A.M.; Project Administration, M.T.H.; Funding Acquisition, M.J.

Funding: This work was supported by the Institute for Information & Communications Technology Promotion (IITP), grant funded by the Korea government (MSIP) (No. B0101-15-0525, Development of global multi-target tracking and event prediction techniques based on real-time large-scale video analysis).

Conflicts of Interest: The authors declare no conflict of interest.

References

1. Lmberis, A.; Dittmar, A. Advanced wearable health systems and applications-research and development efforts in the European union. *IEEE Eng. Med. Biol. Mag.* **2007**, *26*, 29–33. [CrossRef]

2. Rahmani, H.; Mahmood, A.; Huynh, D.; Mian, A. Histogram of oriented principal components for cross-view action recognition. *IEEE Trans. Pattern Anal. Mach. Intell.* **2016**, *38*, 2430–2443. [CrossRef] [PubMed]

3. Tazeem, H.; Farid, M.S.; Mahmood, A. Improving security surveillance by hidden cameras. *Multimedia Tools Appl.* **2017**, *76*, 2713–2732. [CrossRef]

4. Rimmer, J.H. Health promotion for people with disabilities: The emerging paradigm shift from disability prevention to prevention of secondary conditions. *Phys. Ther.* **1999**, *79*, 495–502. [PubMed]

5. Tinetti, M.E. Preventing falls in elderly persons. *N. Engl. J. Med.* **2003**, *2003*, 42–49. [CrossRef] [PubMed]

6. Gutta, S.; Cohen-Solal, E.; Trajkovic, M. Automatic System for Monitoring Person Requiring Care and His/Her Caretaker. U.S. Patent 6,968,294, 22 November 2005.

7. Darwish, A.; Hassanien, A.E. Wearable and implantable wireless sensor network solutions for healthcare monitoring. *Sensors* **2011**, *11*, 5561–5595. [CrossRef] [PubMed]

8. Mac Donald, C.L.; Johnson, A.M.; Cooper, D.; Nelson, E.C.; Werner, N.J.; Shimony, J.S.; Snyder, A.Z.; Raichle, M.E.; Witherow, J.R.; Fang, R.; et al. Detection of blast-related traumatic brain injury in US military personnel. *N. Engl. J. Med.* **2011**, *364*, 2091–2100. [CrossRef] [PubMed]

9. Luo, S.; Hu, Q. A dynamic motion pattern analysis approach to fall detection. In Proceedings of the 2004 IEEE International Workshop on Biomedical Circuits and Systems, Singapore, 1–3 December 2004; pp. 1–5.

10. Bourke, A.; O'brien, J.; Lyons, G. Evaluation of a threshold-based tri-axial accelerometer fall detection algorithm. *Gait Posture* **2007**, *26*, 194–199. [CrossRef] [PubMed]

11. Makhlouf, A.; Nedjai, I.; Saadia, N.; Ramdane-Cherif, A. Multimodal System for Fall Detection and Location of person in an Intelligent Habitat. *Procedia Comput. Sci.* **2017**, *109*, 969–974. [CrossRef]

12. Casilari, E.; Santoyo-Ramón, J.A.; Cano-García, J.M. UMAFall: A Multisensor Dataset for the Research on Automatic Fall Detection. *Procedia Comput. Sci.* **2017**, *110*, 32–39. [CrossRef]

13. Zigel, Y.; Litvak, D.; Gannot, I. A method for automatic fall detection of elderly people using floor vibrations and sound—Proof of concept on human mimicking doll falls. *IEEE Trans. Biomed. Eng.* **2009**, *56*, 2858–2867. [CrossRef] [PubMed]

14. Doukas, C.N.; Maglogiannis, I. Emergency fall incidents detection in assisted living environments utilizing motion, sound, and visual perceptual components. *IEEE Trans. Inf. Technol. Biomed.* **2011**, *15*, 277–289. [CrossRef] [PubMed]

15. Foroughi, H.; Aski, B.S.; Pourreza, H. Intelligent video surveillance for monitoring fall detection of elderly in home environments. In Proceedings of the 11th International Conference on Computer and Information Technology (ICCIT 2008), Khulna, Bangladesh, 24–27 December 2008; pp. 219–224.
16. Miaou, S.G.; Sung, P.H.; Huang, C.Y. A customized human fall detection system using omni-camera images and personal information. In Proceedings of the 1st Transdisciplinary Conference on Distributed Diagnosis and Home Healthcare (D2H2 2006), Arlington, VA, USA, 2–4 April 2006; pp. 39–42.
17. Lee, T.; Mihailidis, A. An intelligent emergency response system: Preliminary development and testing of automated fall detection. *J. Telemed. Telecare* **2005**, *11*, 194–198. [CrossRef] [PubMed]
18. Rougier, C.; Meunier, J.; St-Arnaud, A.; Rousseau, J. Robust video surveillance for fall detection based on human shape deformation. *IEEE Trans. Circuits Syst. Video Technol.* **2011**, *21*, 611–622. [CrossRef]
19. Rougier, C.; Meunier, J.; St-Arnaud, A.; Rousseau, J. Fall detection from human shape and motion history using video surveillance. In Proceedings of the 21st International Conference on Advanced Information Networking and Applications Workshops (AINAW'07), Niagara Falls, ON, Canada, 21–23 May 2007; Volume 2, pp. 875–880.
20. Doulamis, A.; Doulamis, N.; Kalisperakis, I.; Stentoumis, C. A real-time single-camera approach for automatic fall detection. In *ISPRS Commission V, Close Range Image Measurements Techniques*; John Wiley & Sons: Hoboken, NJ, USA, 2010; Volume 38, pp. 207–212.
21. Nait-Charif, H.; McKenna, S.J. Activity summarisation and fall detection in a supportive home environment. In Proceedings of the 17th International Conference on Pattern Recognition (ICPR 2004), Cambridge, UK, 23–26 August 2004; Volume 4, pp. 323–326.
22. Tao, J.; Turjo, M.; Wong, M.F.; Wang, M.; Tan, Y.P. Fall incidents detection for intelligent video surveillance. In Proceedings of the 2005 Fifth International Conference on Information, Communications and Signal Processing, Bangkok, Thailand, 6–9 December 2005; pp. 1590–1594.
23. Mundher, Z.A.; Zhong, J. A real-time fall detection system in elderly care using mobile robot and kinect sensor. *Int. J. Mater. Mech. Manuf.* **2014**, *2*, 133–138. [CrossRef]
24. Sumiya, T.; Matsubara, Y.; Nakano, M.; Sugaya, M. A mobile robot for fall detection for elderly-care. *Procedia Comput. Sci.* **2015**, *60*, 870–880. [CrossRef]
25. Foroughi, H.; Rezvanian, A.; Paziraee, A. Robust fall detection using human shape and multi-class support vector machine. In Proceedings of the Sixth Indian Conference on Computer Vision, Graphics & Image Processing (ICVGIP'080), Bhubaneswar, India, 16–19 December 2008; pp. 413–420.
26. Debard, G.; Karsmakers, P.; Deschodt, M.; Vlaeyen, E.; Van den Bergh, J.; Dejaeger, E.; Milisen, K.; Goedemé, T.; Tuytelaars, T.; Vanrumste, B. Camera based fall detection using multiple features validated with real life video. In *Workshop Proceedings of the 7th International Conference on Intelligent Environments*; IOS Press: Amsterdam, The Netherlands, 2011; Volume 10, pp. 441–450.
27. Yu, M.; Yu, Y.; Rhuma, A.; Naqvi, S.M.R.; Wang, L.; Chambers, J.A. An online one class support vector machine-based person-specific fall detection system for monitoring an elderly individual in a room environment. *IEEE J. Biomed. Health Inform.* **2013**, *17*, 1002–1014. [PubMed]
28. Bosch-Jorge, M.; Sánchez-Salmerón, A.J.; Valera, Á.; Ricolfe-Viala, C. Fall detection based on the gravity vector using a wide-angle camera. *Expert Syst. Appl.* **2014**, *41*, 7980–7986. [CrossRef]
29. Ni, B.; Nguyen, C.D.; Moulin, P. RGBD-camera based get-up event detection for hospital fall prevention. In Proceedings of the 2012 IEEE International Conference on Acoustics, Speech and Signal Processing (ICASSP), Kyoto, Japan, 25–30 March 2012; pp. 1405–1408.
30. Kyrkou, C.; Theocharides, T. A flexible parallel hardware architecture for AdaBoost-based real-time object detection. *IEEE Trans. Very Large Scale Integr. (VLSI) Syst.* **2011**, *19*, 1034–1047. [CrossRef]
31. Kerdegari, H.; Samsudin, K.; Ramli, A.R.; Mokaram, S. Evaluation of fall detection classification approaches. In Proceedings of the 2012 4th International Conference on Intelligent and Advanced Systems (ICIAS), Kuala Lumpur, Malaysia, 12–14 June 2012; Volume 1, pp. 131–136.
32. Gjoreski, H.; Lustrek, M.; Gams, M. Accelerometer placement for posture recognition and fall detection. In Proceedings of the 2011 7th International Conference on Intelligent environments (IE), Nottingham, UK, 25–28 July 2011; pp. 47–54.
33. Kansiz, A.O.; Guvensan, M.A.; Turkmen, H.I. Selection of time-domain features for fall detection based on supervised learning. In Proceedings of the World Congress on Engineering and Computer Science, San Francisco, CA, USA, 23–25 October 2013; pp. 23–25.

34. Kaur, R.; Gangwar, R. A Review on Naive Baye's (NB), J48 and K-Means Based Mining Algorithms for Medical Data Mining. *Int. Res. J. Eng. Technol.* **2017**, *4*, 1664–1668.

35. Kapoor, P.; Rani, R.; JMIT, R. Efficient Decision Tree Algorithm Using J48 and Reduced Error Pruning. *Int. J. Eng. Res. Gen. Sci.* **2015**, *3*, 1613–1621.

36. Shi, G.; Zhang, J.; Dong, C.; Han, P.; Jin, Y.; Wang, J. Fall detection system based on inertial mems sensors: Analysis design and realization. In Proceedings of the 2015 IEEE International Conference on Cyber Technology in Automation, Control, and Intelligent Systems (CYBER), Shenyang, China, 8–12 June 2015; pp. 1834–1839.

37. Guvensan, M.A.; Kansiz, A.O.; Camgoz, N.C.; Turkmen, H.; Yavuz, A.G.; Karsligil, M.E. An Energy-Efficient Multi-Tier Architecture for Fall Detection on Smartphones. *Sensors* **2017**, *17*, 1487. [CrossRef] [PubMed]

38. Kepski, M.; Kwolek, B. Embedded system for fall detection using body-worn accelerometer and depth sensor. In Proceedings of the 2015 IEEE 8th International Conference on Intelligent Data Acquisition and Advanced Computing Systems: Technology and Applications (IDAACS), Warsaw, Poland, 24–26 September 2015; Volume 2, pp. 755–759.

39. Javed, S.; Mahmood, A.; Bouwmans, T.; Jung, S.K. Background-Foreground Modeling Based on Spatiotemporal Sparse Subspace Clustering. *IEEE Trans. Image Process.* **2017**, *26*, 5840–5854. [CrossRef] [PubMed]

40. Javed, S.; Mahmood, A.; Bouwmans, T.; Jung, S.K. Spatiotemporal Low-rank Modeling for Complex Scene Background Initialization. *IEEE Trans. Circuits Syst. Video Technol.* **2016**, *28*, 1315–1329. [CrossRef]

41. Javed, S.; Mahmood, A.; Bouwmans, T.; Jung, S.K. Superpixels-based Manifold Structured Sparse RPCA for Moving Object Detection. In Proceedings of the British Machine Vision Conference (BMVC 2017), London, UK, 4–7 September 2017.

42. Mahmood, A. Structure-less object detection using adaboost algorithm. In Proceedings of the International Conference on Machine Vision (ICMV 2007), Islamabad, Pakistan, 28–29 December 2007; pp. 85–90.

43. Mahmood, A.; Khan, S. Early terminating algorithms for Adaboost based detectors. In Proceedings of the 2009 16th IEEE International Conference on Image Processing (ICIP), Cairo, Egypt, 7–10 November 2009; pp. 1209–1212.

44. Kaur, G.; Chhabra, A. Improved J48 classification algorithm for the prediction of diabetes. *Int. J. Comput. Appl.* **2014**, *98*, 13–17. [CrossRef]

45. Tanwani, A.K.; Afridi, J.; Shafiq, M.Z.; Farooq, M. Guidelines to select machine learning scheme for classification of biomedical datasets. In Proceedings of the European Conference on Evolutionary Computation, Machine Learning and Data Mining in Bioinformatics, Tübingen, Germany, 15–17 April 2009; pp. 128–139.

46. Devasena, C.L. Comparative Analysis of Random Forest REP Tree and J48 Classifiers for Credit Risk Prediction. In Proceedings of the International Conference on Communication, Computing and Information Technology (ICCCMIT-2014), Chennai, India, 12–13 December 2015.

47. Freund, Y.; Schapire, R.; Abe, N. A short introduction to boosting. *J.-Jpn. Soc. Artif. Intell.* **1999**, *14*, 771–780.

48. Foroughi, H.; Naseri, A.; Saberi, A.; Yazdi, H.S. An eigenspace-based approach for human fall detection using integrated time motion image and neural network. In Proceedings of the 9th International Conference on Signal Processing (ICSP 2008), Beijing, China, 26–29 October 2008; pp. 1499–1503.

49. Lv, T.; Yan, J.; Xu, H. An EEG emotion recognition method based on AdaBoost classifier. In Proceedings of the Chinese Automation Congress (CAC), Jinan, China, 20–22 October 2017; pp. 6050–6054.

50. Wang, S.; Chen, L.; Zhou, Z.; Sun, X.; Dong, J. Human fall detection in surveillance video based on PCANet. *Multimedia Tools Appl.* **2016**, *75*, 11603–11613. [CrossRef]

51. Dietterich, T.; Bishop, C.; Heckerman, D.; Jordan, M.; Kearns, M. *Adaptive Computation and Machine Learning*; The MIT Press: Cambridge, MA, USA; London, UK.

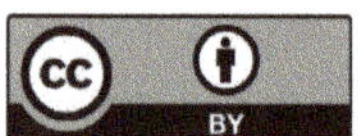
© 2018 by the authors. Licensee MDPI, Basel, Switzerland. This article is an open access article distributed under the terms and conditions of the Creative Commons Attribution (CC BY) license (http://creativecommons.org/licenses/by/4.0/).

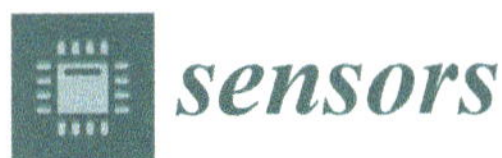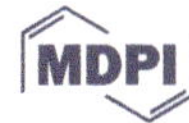

Article

A Novel and Safe Approach to Simulate Cutting Movements Using Ground Reaction Forces

Amelia S. Lanier [1,2], **Brian A. Knarr** [1,2,3], **Nicholas Stergiou** [2,4] and **Thomas S. Buchanan** [1,3,*]

[1] Biomechanics and Movement Science Program, College of Engineering, University of Delaware, Newark, DE 19716, USA; alanier@unomaha.edu (A.S.L.); bknarr@unomaha.edu (B.A.K.)

[2] Department of Biomechanics and Center for Research in Human Movement Variability, College of Education, University of Nebraska at Omaha, Omaha, NE 68182, USA; nstergiou@unomaha.edu

[3] Delaware Rehabilitation Institute, University of Delaware, Newark, DE 19716, USA

[4] Department of Environmental, Agricultural & Occupational Health, College of Public Health, University of Nebraska Medical Center, Omaha, NE 68198, USA

* Correspondence: buchanan@udel.edu; Tel.: +1-302-831-2410

Received: 1 June 2018; Accepted: 9 August 2018; Published: 11 August 2018

Abstract: Control of shear ground reaction forces (sGRF) is important in performing running and cutting tasks as poor sGRF control has implications for those with knee injuries, such as anterior cruciate ligament (ACL) ruptures. The goal of this study was to develop a novel and safe task to evaluate control or accurate modulation of shear ground reaction forces related to those generated during cutting. Our approach utilized a force control task using real-time visual feedback of a subject's force production and evaluated control capabilities through accuracy and divergence measurements. Ten healthy recreational athletes completed the force control task while force control via accuracy measures and divergence calculations was investigated. Participants were able to accurately control sGRF in multiple directions based on error measurements. Forces generated during the task were equal to or greater than those measured during a number of functional activities. We found no significant difference in the divergence of the force profiles using the Lyapunov Exponent of the sGRF trajectories. Participants using our approach produced high accuracy and low divergence force profiles and functional force magnitudes. Moving forward, we will utilize this task in at-risk populations who are unable to complete a cutting maneuver in early stages of rehabilitation, such as ACL deficient and newly reconstructed individuals, allowing insight into force control not obtainable otherwise.

Keywords: biomechanics; movement control; anterior cruciate ligament; kinetics; real-time feedback

1. Introduction

In athletic populations, the knee is a commonly injured region of the body, with younger athletes being especially at risk [1,2]. Overall, strain or sprain injuries are extremely prevalent and occur at a rate of 102 incidents per 100,000 athletes per year [3]. These types of injuries typically occur when athletes are cutting or landing from a jump [4,5]. Additionally, ankle injury models estimated that one-third of ankle injuries occur during a sharp turn or twist [6]. Medial-lateral force generation during a sharp turn or twist is additionally noted to be greater in those with functional instability of the ankle joint, emphasizing the importance of accurate shear ground reaction force (sGRF) modulation [7]. Cutting and turning tasks require modulation of sGRFs. To turn during gait, an individual first decelerates to generate a posteriorly directed GRF, and then adjusts the GRF medially or laterally to change direction [8]. In more dynamic tasks like cutting, Havens and colleagues found significant correlations between medial-lateral GRF impulse and cutting angle and performance [9,10] while Jones and colleagues found that medial/lateral GRFs significantly correlated to peak knee adduction moment during cutting and pivoting tasks [11]. sGRFs significantly dictate gait and cutting maneuvers [12–14], and so the ability to control these forces are especially important when considering their implications on other joints as the forces propagate through the body. For example, traumatic knee injuries such as anterior cruciate ligament (ACL) ruptures are often a result of simultaneous multidirectional loading involving sGRFs [15].

Many studies that aim to understand injury recovery utilize biomechanical measures (joint angle, joint translations, etc.) in conjunction with evaluation of their variability using analyses such as variance [16–19]. These analyses investigate changes among many individual features within a trial, and may focus on the amount of variation that occurs around a central point (i.e., mean and standard deviation) or singular features of the cycle (i.e., maximum or minimum). These analyses do not capture the differences in evolution of the signal over time that may occur from cycle to cycle during continuous movements. However, these subtle time varying changes that are identified through the analysis of many continuous cycles may be crucial to understand recovery, as they can indicate neuromuscular health [20]. To capture these subtle changes, a different approach can be utilized, where tools such as the Lyapunov Exponent (LyE) [21–24] can describe the temporal structure of various time series data. Larger values of the LyE indicate more divergence in the trajectories of the continuous movement cycles, while smaller values indicate less divergence. The LyE has been successfully used in numerous biomechanical applications [22,23,25]. Research focused on ACL injury and recovery indicates greater divergence (larger LyE) of knee flexion angle movement trajectories during continuous gait cycles in ACL deficient and reconstructed limbs when compared to the intact limb [21,26]. Greater kinematic divergence is present in ACL reconstructed limbs in all reconstruction types, indicating less control of the joint [21]. Alterations to divergence of knee flexion angle movement trajectories during gait post ACL injury and reconstruction may indicate functional deficits exist. However, such an evaluation was never performed with kinetic data to provide a more comprehensive picture of the changes that may occur following such an injury.

This study aims to develop and evaluate a novel and safe approach to allow participants to generate and control shear ground reaction forces similar to those generated during cutting. This study is the first but necessary step to demonstrate feasibility for a larger study that aims to understand force control via accuracy and divergence in injured populations. This study is important as it establishes the first dataset of normative/baseline force control in a healthy, uninjured population, which will allow us to better understand changes in force control as a result of injury. To understand force control of shear ground reaction forces we have developed a task using real-time visual feedback of a participant's force production. For this task to be deemed valuable, participants must be able to accurately control sGRFs (as defined by current literature), must be able to perform this task in multiple directions, must generate meaningful/functional force magnitudes, and must exhibit similar divergence of trajectories across directions and limbs. To first address force control measured via accuracy, we analyzed mean absolute error in both limbs and all directions. Based on studies utilizing a force matching task of different joints [27–29], we defined an allowable amount of absolute error to be below 10% maximum effort (MAX). To then address task performance in multiple directions, we assessed force magnitudes in both limbs and all directions. We hypothesized that task completion, as evaluated by both force magnitude and absolute error, would be similar between limbs. To determine if the force control task produced functional loads, target force magnitudes relative to subject mass were also calculated. We hypothesized that force magnitudes generated during the force control task would be greater than or equivalent to those produced during functional activities. Lastly, we wanted to be able to evaluate force control capabilities of the participants by investigating divergence of the data. Variability was analyzed by calculating the standard deviation of the absolute error of forces generated during the task for each limb and all directions. We hypothesize that the standard deviation of the absolute error will be similar across both limbs and directions during the force control task. Force control measured via divergence was also analyzed by calculating the LyE using force profiles generated during the task. We hypothesize that there will be no difference in force control measured via divergence (using the

LyE) when comparing the LyE of the right and left limb or directions of movement (anterior/posterior and medial/lateral).

2. Materials and Methods

2.1. Participants

Ten healthy individuals with no previous history of knee injuries were included: three men (age 22 ± 0.8 years, BMI 22.9 ± 0.7 kg/m^2) and seven women (age 22 ± 0.3 years, BMI 21.9 ± 2.3 kg/m^2). One subject was removed from the nonlinear analyses ($n = 9$), as they did not follow instructions to generate a smooth force pattern. This participant generated non-continuous (extreme asymptotic) force profile, which significantly impedes our ability to reliably and accurately quantify the Lyapunov Exponents. The subject was used for linear calculations ($n = 10$), as they still attempted to successfully produce the maximum forces displayed by the visual feedback. All participants were active in >50 h/yr of level I and II sports, which include running and cutting activities. This study was approved by the institutional review board at the University of Delaware and all participants provided written informed consent.

2.2. Force Control Task

All participants completed a force control task. For the force control task, participants stood on two separate force platforms (AMTI OR-6, Watertown, MA, USA) with a foot on each force plate. It should be noted that the foot morphology of each participant was not recorded, which may have affected foot placement. Throughout testing and calibration trials, the participants were in regular stance (Figure 1) facing the screen with feet positioned approximately hip width distance apart. Participants received real-time visual feedback of their force production in the leg of interest via custom written Labview code. Visual feedback of the participant's force production was presented on a screen in front of them. To visualize force production, a slider was utilized. A slider is an object that moves in response to a signal. The visual feedback format included a slider that responded to force production and two stationary indicators that identified the target force for the participants (Figure 1). The two stationary indicators represented 50% of the participant's maximum strength in that direction, based on the maximal push trials (Figure 1).

To calibrate the force control task to each participant's strength, the participants performed maximal force production trials. All participants completed the 'maximal push' trials in all shear directions (anterior, posterior, medial, and lateral) with each foot, separately. Participants were instructed to push as hard as they were able to in the four directions described above. All participants completed the 'maximal push' trials in all shear directions with each foot. After completing the 'maximal push' trials, the feedback software was calibrated, and participants began the force control testing.

Participants were instructed to control the slider and align it with the two stationary indicators. They were instructed to generate force bi-directionally (anterior/posterior or medial/lateral) and continuously to the beat of a metronome set at 60 beats per minute, and to alternatively align the slider with each stationary indicator. Participants were instructed to align the slider to each indicator alternatively and continuously and not to simply surpass the indicators. Additionally, participants were instructed to continue a cyclical and smooth trajectory if there were unable to reach the indicator. Participants were told to move to the next indicator if unable to reach the other. The force control task was two minutes in duration. Conducting the trial at 60 beats per minute for two minutes in duration was chosen to generate enough data to calculate the LyE while minimizing the duration of the trial. The force control task was conducted for both the right and left limbs and both the anterior/posterior and medial/lateral directions. This lead to a total of four conditions for each leg. Subjects were only restricted in their foot placement but were allowed to position the other joints (hip, knee, ankle) freely throughout all testing and calibration. Subjects were instructed to maintain their foot placement in the same location throughout testing. To maintain foot placement, we traced or placed tape in specific locations on the plate so subjects were able to move between trials and still maintain the same foot placement across all trials.

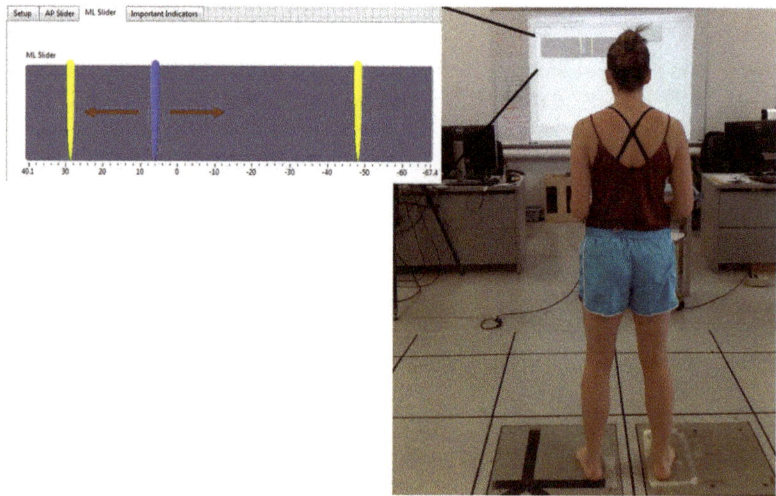

Figure 1. Experimental setup of data collection (**right**): example of visual feedback provided to study participants during the medial/lateral (ML) force control task (**left**): arrows indicate the direction the mobile cursor moves.

2.3. Data Analysis

To evaluate force control during this task, we evaluated both accuracy and divergence of the force profiles. To evaluate accuracy, we calculated a number of error measures. Using the calibration of maximal push trials and force profiles measured during the force control task, we calculated the absolute error (% Max). Absolute error was measured using custom Matlab software as the absolute value of the difference between the peak and target force for each trial. Using the maximal push trial, we recorded the maximum force production in each direction, which were then used to create the threshold levels for the indicators. From the force profiles collected during the force control trials, we compared the force generation at each peak to the 50% Max threshold. Any overshooting or undershooting of the target force was considered as an error. We calculated both the mean and standard deviation of the absolute error for both limbs (right and left) and all directions (anterior, posterior, medial, and lateral). Confidence intervals of 95% were also calculated for target force, absolute error, standard deviation of absolute error, and the LyE. In addition to our error measurements we evaluated force magnitudes per kg of body mass (N/kg) in the four directions (anterior, posterior, medial, and lateral) that were tested.

The Lyapunov exponent (LyE) was calculated using the force profiles produced during both the anterior/posterior (AP) or medial/lateral (ML) force control tasks in a manner similar to previous research [21–23,26] (Figure 2) to determine AP and ML force divergence, respectively. In all cases, unfiltered data was used to get a more accurate representation of the data, as filtering may remove subtle changes within the signal [30,31] (Figure 2). Data analysis was performed at 60 Hz. Spectral analysis revealed that the signal of interest primarily existed at 6 Hz and lower, and data was sampled at $10\times$ this frequency range (60 Hz) to ensure that sufficient points were used in the analysis without oversampling the data. We also note that a 60 Hz sampling rate is commonly used when analyzing human movement [32]. The LyE is defined as the rate of divergence of infinitesimally close trajectories [33], and is determined through a multi-step process.

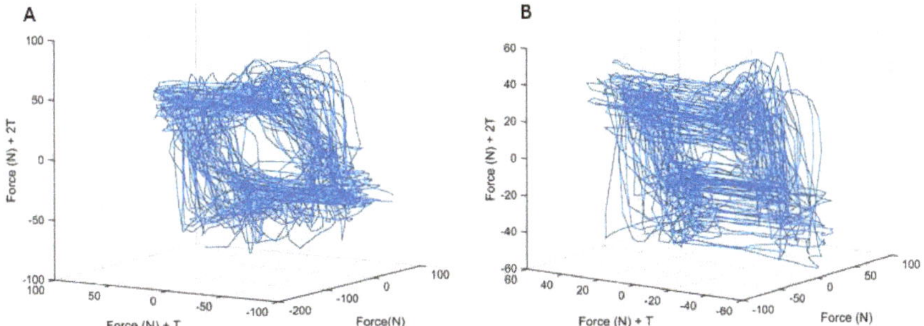

Figure 2. Depiction of trajectories of continuous movement cycles of larger and smaller Lyapunov Exponents. (**a**) Movement trajectories with a smaller Lyapunov Exponent; (**b**) Movement trajectories with a larger Lyapunov Exponent.

Calculating the LyE requires two input parameters: time lag (τ) and embedding dimension (m). Both of these parameters were used to convert our signals of interest into state space. To calculate τ, we used the Average Mutual Information (AMI) function which determines the percentage of information shared between two signals [34]. For this study, the two signals used in the AMI function were the force profile (either in the AP or ML direction) and a copy of the same force profile (Figure 3). To determine m, the Global False Nearest Neighbor (GFNN) function was used [34]. Using time delayed copies (as specified by τ) of a signal, GFNN measures the distance between trajectories in one dimension, and then increases the number of dimensions and measures again (Figure 4). A false nearest neighbor is defined by any significant changes in distance between trajectories when increasing the number of dimensions. As the dimensions are increased, the number of false neighbors is determined. The first local minima of the GFNN function was then used as m. GFNN is important to 'unfold' the data, as any folding would lead to misinterpreted LyE. Once τ and m are determined, the data are transformed in state space; in state space, the LyE can then be calculated. For this data set, each force profile was the same number of data points (3600), m was constant across trials and conditions at a value of five, while τ was calculated for each trial ($\tau = 18 \pm 0.35$). The LyE was calculated using the Wolf et al., algorithm, as this algorithm is more sensitive to changes in variability when using small data sets [32,33]. This algorithm calculates the Euclidean distance between trajectories and tracks the trajectories forward in time to determine the rate of divergence or convergence of the trajectories. It is important to note that trajectories when using LyE analysis refers to the evolution of the analyzed signal over time, which in this study is force production over time, not position data, which is sometimes used. The rate of divergence is determined for multiple trajectories and the largest, which is our value of interest, is reported. The LyE values were calculated for each subject for both the AP and ML direction providing two measures, AP LyE and ML LyE.

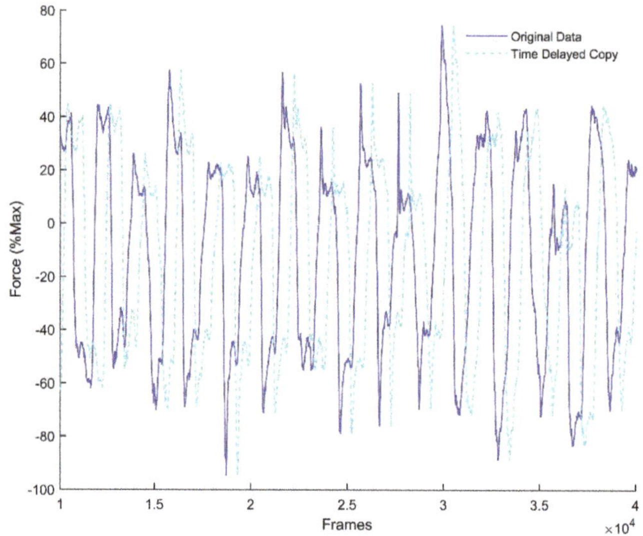

Figure 3. Original force profile (solid line) with a time delayed copy (dashed line).

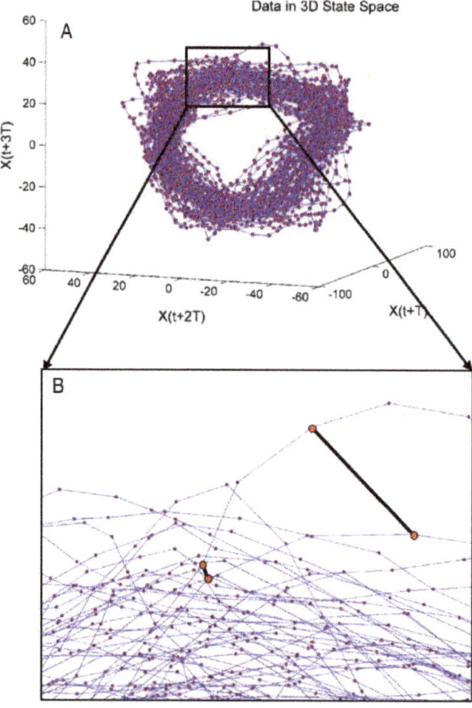

Figure 4. Force profile data X(t) transformed into 3D state space (**A**). Zoomed in view (**B**) with the distance between trajectories highlighted in black. X(t+T) represents force data shifted by the time lag, tau.

2.4. Statistical Analysis

To evaluate force control via accuracy, multiple statistical tests were performed. Descriptive statistics including minimum, maximum, and average values were also calculated for absolute error and target force. Two separate two-by-four repeated measures (limbs: right vs. left by direction: anterior vs. posterior vs. medial vs. lateral) ANOVA were conducted to determine significant differences between the group means of the target force and absolute error. For both target force and absolute error, specific pairwise comparisons within the ANOVA framework were evaluated to control for type I error inflation at a significance level of 0.05. Additionally, an upper level *t*-test was conducted to determine if the mean absolute error was greater than the allowable 10% MAX as determined by previous literature [21–23]. Lastly, a post-hoc power analysis was conducted for the absolute error values.

To further evaluate force control during the force control task via accuracy, a two-by-four repeated measures (limbs: right vs. left by direction: anterior vs. posterior vs. medial vs. lateral) ANOVA was conducted to determine significant differences for the standard deviation of the absolute error of forces generated. Lastly, a two-by-two (limbs: right vs. left by direction: AP vs. ML) fully repeated measures ANOVA was used to determine significant differences between the group means for the LyE and the standard deviation of the absolute error. One subject was removed from the LyE analysis as they were unable to generate a smooth force trajectory as they were instructed to do so. Post-hoc analysis was performed for any tests that resulted in significant interaction. The significance level was set at 0.05 and analysis was performed using SPSS (IBM Armonk, NY, USA).

3. Results

In our evaluation of both absolute error of forces generated and target force, all participants completed the force control task similarly across limbs (Tables 1 and 2). There was no significant effect of limb based on repeated measures ANOVA when comparing the means of both target force ($p = 0.117$) and absolute error ($p = 0.813$). Our analysis of target force revealed a significant effect of direction ($p < 0.001$). Target force ranged from an average of 38.53 N (left posterior) to 64.29 N (left medial). Our analysis of absolute error indicated no significant effect of either direction or interaction.

Table 1. Error calculations (mean ± standard deviation) for both the right and left limb in all directions tested during the force control task for healthy uninjured participants.

	Right Anterior	Left Anterior	Right Posterior	Left Posterior	Right Medial	Left Medial	Right Lateral	Left Lateral
Target Force (N)	41.11 ± 10.63	43.79 ± 12.88	41.72 ± 11.35	38.53 ± 9.52	54.35 ± 13.22	64.29 ± 12.05	64.07 ± 10.67	55.56 ± 12.85
Abs. Error (% Max)	6.45 ± 2.53%	5.68 ± 1.49%	7.19 ± 2.27%	8.35 ± 5.12%	6.16 ± 2.87%	5.65 ± 1.55%	5.5 ± 2.21%	5.87 ± 2.30%
St. Dev. Abs. Error (% Max)	4.86 ± 1.70%	4.50 ± 1.17%	5.62 ± 1.96%	5.77 ± 2.73%	4.31 ± 1.24%	4.28 ± 1.11%	4.09 ± 1.40%	4.59 ± 1.52%
Force (N/kg)	0.54 ± 0.21		0.60 ± 0.23		0.77 ± 0.28		0.89 ± 0.31	

Table 2. Confidence intervals of 95% for all error calculations in all directions tested during the force control task for healthy uninjured participants.

	Anterior	Posterior	Medial	Lateral
Target Force (N)	37.03–47.87	35.29–44.96	49.01–60.90	58.99–69.36
Abs. Error (%)	5.10–7.03%	5.94–9.60%	4.82–7.20%	4.71–6.45%
St. Dev. Abs. Error (%)	4.01–5.35%	4.61–6.78%	3.81–5.08%	3.61–4.76%
LyE	2.99–3.64		2.78–3.35	

Confidence intervals of 95% and average absolute error of forces generated during the force control task were below the 10% MAX allowable error (Tables 1 and 2, Figure 5). *t*-test results indicate that the average absolute error was below the 10% target ($p < 0.001$). The minimum average absolute error calculated was 5.5% MAX from the right limb in the lateral direction, while the maximum average absolute error generated was 8.35% MAX in the left limb in the posterior direction (Table 1). For each limb and direction, the average absolute error did not exceed the 10% MAX threshold, however absolute error of forces generated from the left limb in the posterior direction did exhibit large standard deviations which did exceed the 10% MAX threshold when considering standard deviations in absolute error. The post-hoc power analysis indicated sufficient power for seven out of the eight measures (seven variables $(1 - \beta) \geq 0.98$, average Cohen's d = 1.96; Absolute Error Left Limb Posterior Direction $(1 - \beta) = 0.24$, Cohen's d = 0.32).

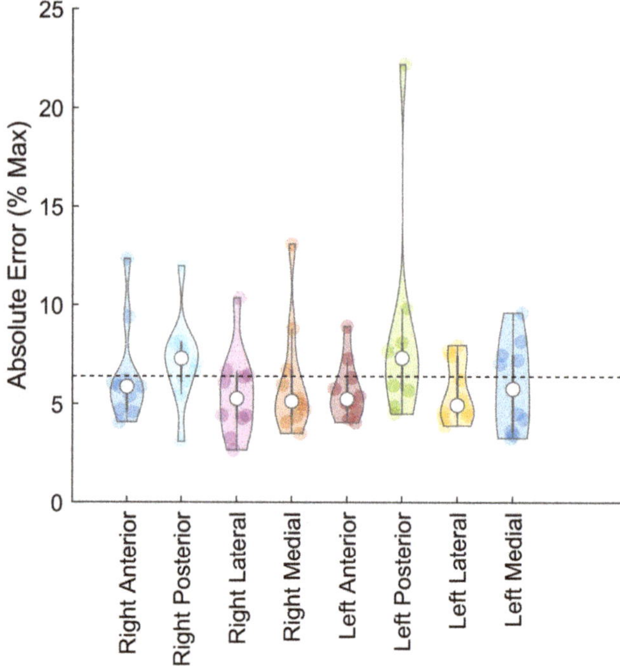

Figure 5. Violin plot of absolute error (% Max) during the force control task for each limb (right, left) and all directions (anterior, posterior, medial, lateral). Median absolute error indicated by open circle, interquartile ranges are represented by thick and thin vertical lines, and overall average is indicated by dashed line. Shaded circles represent individual subject data. * $p < 0.05$ (one-tailed t-test).

During the force control task, participants generated loads greater than that of dynamic functional tasks (Table 1). During the force control task, participants generated 0.54 N/kg, 0.60 N/kg, 0.77 N/kg, and 0.89 N/kg in the anterior, posterior, medial, and lateral directions, respectively (Table 1). Current literature reports force magnitudes ranging from 0.1–0.7 N/kg from a spectrum of activities including walking, running, and jumping [35,36].

Measures of variability indicate no differences in force control capabilities between limbs (Table 1, Figure 6). Repeated measures ANOVA comparing the standard deviation of forces generated revealed no significant effect of limb ($p = 0.783$), direction ($p = 0.132$), or interaction ($p = 0.498$, Table 1).

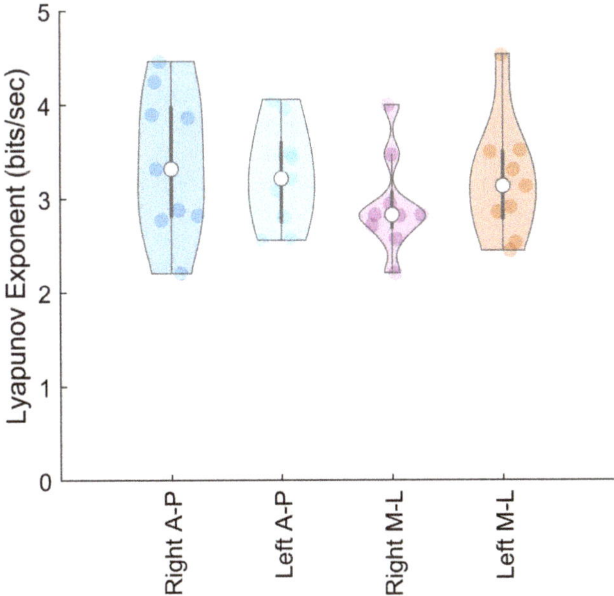

Figure 6. Violin plot of maximal Lyapunov exponent (bits/second) during the force control task. Median Lyapunov exponent indicated by open circle, interquartile ranges are represented by thick and thin vertical lines Shaded circles represent individual subject data. Data is reported for both the medial/lateral (M-L) and anterior/posterior (A-P) directions.

Based on the LyE calculated during the force control task, force control capabilities were similar across limbs for all participants (Figure 6). Our data indicate that there is no statistically significant difference in LyE values of healthy uninjured participants when comparing the right and left limb. In the right limb of healthy uninjured participants, we calculated the LyE values to be 3.39 ± 0.77 bits/s and 2.93 ± 0.52 bits/s in the AP and ML directions, respectively (Figure 6). In the left limb, we calculated the LyE to be 3.24 ± 0.55 bits/s and 3.19 ± 0.63 bits/s in the AP and ML directions (Figure 6). Additionally, our data indicate there is no statistically significant difference in the LyE values generated in the ML versus AP direction. *p*-values from the ANOVA approached significance ($p = 0.054$), but effect size calculated using Cohen's d was moderate.

4. Discussion

The aim of this study was to develop and evaluate a novel and safe approach to allow participants to generate and control shear ground reaction forces relatable to those generated during cutting. To meet this aim, we developed the force control task and evaluated it using a young, healthy and active cohort. Using real-time visual feedback of a participant's force production, we aimed to establish a task where participants are able to control ground reaction forces in multiple directions at magnitudes similar to activities of daily living. To evaluate the force control task, we measured force accuracy via absolute errors. To evaluate functional relevance, we evaluated target force and force production relative to body mass. To evaluate force control, we explored variability using standard deviation of absolute error and we explored divergence using the Lyapunov Exponent.

Our results indicate that participants were able to accurately control the multidirectional force production during the force control task. On average participants were accurate within 10% MAX with both limbs in all directions tested. Absolute error was consistent across the anterior, medial, and lateral directions with values ranging from 5.50% MAX to 6.45% MAX. Based on absolute error calculations, participants were least accurate in the posterior direction, particularly when generating force with the left limb (8.35% MAX absolute error). Larger errors generated by the left limb in the posterior direction maybe a result of strength deficits in that direction as noted by the target force which was weakest in the posterior direction (Table 1). Overall error values were below 10% MAX, across limbs and directions, indicating that participants were able to both accurately control their sGRF production in multiple directions during the force control task. This is an important and necessary finding to demonstrate that the task is achievable and feasible in a healthy population and can provide a normative baseline for evaluating performance in injured and rehabilitating populations.

A secondary goal of this task was for participants to generate forces relatable to running and cutting maneuvers. As we were unable to find literature investigating sGRF production of cutting, there are numerous studies utilizing other similar tasks which have been included. Results from this study and current research indicate that the force control task produces functionally relevant force magnitudes. Force profiles from this task reveal force generation at magnitudes larger than that of dynamic functional tasks. Participants generated forces ranging from 0.54–0.89 N/kg, with current literature reporting force magnitudes ranging from 0.1–0.7 N/kg for activities including walking, running, and jumping. AP GRF produced during gait initiation and running initiation ranges from 0.2–0.7 N/kg, while ML GRF produced gait termination ranges from 0.1–0.5 N/kg [35,36]. During a vertical jump landing, ML GRF ranges from 0.1–0.4 N/kg [35]. After analyzing calibration trials collected for this study, we found participants generate 0.54 N/kg (anterior), 0.60 N/kg (posterior), 0.77 N/kg (medial) and 0.89 N/kg (lateral) when completing the force control task. Additionally, studies utilizing a similar force control task estimated force magnitudes of ranging from 0.48 to 0.60 N/kg [36]. During the force control task, participants generate forces that are equal to or greater than that of functional tasks like walking and running. From these results, we determined that the force control task was able to be dynamically challenging and provide meaningful data on sGRF production in groups that perform high level dynamic tasks like cutting.

In our calculation of the Lyapunov Exponents, we found no statistically significant difference in force control for divergence between limbs when performing the force control task. These results were to be expected as our participants endured no major injuries to their lower limbs. Additionally, we found no statistically significant differences in force control for trajectory divergence (LyE) between directions, but participants did exhibit slightly reduced LyE values when performing the force control task in the ML direction. This may indicate better control in that direction, as a lower LyE value indicates less divergence. However, data from additional populations are needed to understand the magnitude of these differences in force control regarding divergence. These results indicate that healthy uninjured participants are able to maintain proper force control in each limb and in different directions when force control is measured via trajectory divergence.

There were some limitations in the implementation of this study. First, force control accuracy task was limited to 50% of each participant's maximum force generation, and it could be assumed that at higher levels of force production, there would be a decrease in accuracy. However, to limit the potential for injury, a lower level of force production was desired. While no participants indicated that they were unable to see the visual feedback, use of contact lenses or glasses were not recorded. In future studies, potential visual impairment will be recorded. During the force control task, no fail criteria was established to ensure participants completed the task to a certain level of accuracy. However, during data collection, the variables of interest were being monitored, and in subsequent data analysis, all trials were inspected for both the magnitude of each subject's force production and the appropriate number of cycles. By monitoring the number of cycles, we were able to ensure that the participants maintained appropriate timing.

In this study, we developed a novel task where participants accurately control sGRFs similarly with the right and left limb at functionally meaningful magnitudes in a low risk and dynamic setting. Error measured during the task was within tolerance based on related research, and divergence measures calculated during the task revealed no significant differences between limbs. We have established a standard for force control as participants generate sGRFs that can be used as a basis for comparison in other demographic and pathological populations. It is important to establish a normative baseline when using Lyapunov Exponent analysis as interpretation of the data necessitates comparisons between groups to identify trends. While a number of studies have explored the changes to the temporal structure in kinematic measures, no work has been done utilizing kinetic measures. The design of this task allows for application in at-risk populations, such as ACL deficient and newly reconstructed individuals, as the task is quasi-static but still demanding in respect to forces generated. This is important as it allows insight into the production of forces similar to functional activities, such as cutting, that would be not be obtainable otherwise. Future work will seek to understand changes to force control that may occur as a result of ACL injury and reconstruction or participation in high performance athletics, with the ultimate goal of informing both rehabilitation practices and sports training.

Author Contributions: A.S.L. and T.S.B. conceived and designed the experiments; A.S.L. performed the experiments; A.S.L., T.S.B. and N.S. analyzed the data; B.A.K. developed analysis tools; A.S.L. wrote the paper; all authors contributed to manuscript preparation.

Funding: This work was supported by the National Institutes of Health (R01-HD087459, U54-GM104941, P30-GM103333 and R01-AR046386). Nick Stergiou was supported by the Center for Research in Human Movement Variability of the University of Nebraska Omaha and the NIH (P20GM109090 and R01AG034995).

Acknowledgments: The authors would like to thank Ryan Pohlig for assistance in statistical analysis.

Conflicts of Interest: The authors declare no conflict of interest.

References

1. Nabhan, D.; Walden, T.; Street, J.; Linden, H.; Moreau, B. Sports injury and illness epidemiology during the 2014 Youth Olympic Games: United States Olympic Team Surveillance. *Br. J. Sports Med.* **2016**, *50*, 688–693. [CrossRef] [PubMed]

2. Zbrojkiewicz, D.; Vertullo, C.; Grayson, J.E. Increasing rates of anterior cruciate ligament reconstruction in young Australians, 2000-2015. *Med. J. Aust.* **2018**, *208*, 354–358. [CrossRef] [PubMed]

3. Lambers, K.; Ootes, D.; Ring, D. Incidence of patients with lower extremity injuries presenting to US emergency departments by anatomic region, disease category, and age. *Clin. Orthop. Relat. Res.* **2012**, *470*, 284–290. [CrossRef] [PubMed]

4. Boden, B.P.; Griffin, L.Y.; Garrett, W.E., Jr. Etiology and Prevention of Noncontact ACL Injury. *Phys. Sportsmed.* **2000**, *28*, 53–60. [CrossRef] [PubMed]

5. Krosshaug, T.; Nakamae, A.; Boden, B.P.; Engebretsen, L.; Smith, G.; Slauterbeck, J.R.; Hewett, T.E.; Bahr, R. Mechanisms of anterior cruciate ligament injury in basketball: Video analysis of 39 cases. *Am. J. Sports Med.* **2007**, *35*, 359–367. [CrossRef] [PubMed]

6. McKay, G.D.; Goldie, P.A.; Payne, W.R.; Oakes, B.W. Ankle injuries in basketball: Injury rate and risk factors. *Br. J. Sports Med.* **2001**, *35*, 103–108. [CrossRef] [PubMed]

7. Caulfield, B.; Garrett, M. Changes in ground reaction force during jump landing in subjects with functional instability of the ankle joint. *Clin. Biomech.* **2004**, *19*, 617–621. [CrossRef] [PubMed]

8. Glaister, B.C.; Orendurff, M.S.; Schoen, J.A.; Bernatz, G.C.; Klute, G.K. Ground reaction forces and impulses during a transient turning maneuver. *J. Biomech.* **2008**, *41*, 3090–3093. [CrossRef] [PubMed]

9. Havens, K.L.; Sigward, S.M. Whole body mechanics differ among running and cutting maneuvers in skilled athletes. *Gait Posture* **2014**, *42*, 240–245. [CrossRef] [PubMed]

10. Sigward, S.M.; Cesar, G.M.; Havens, K.L. Predictors of Frontal Plane Knee Moments During Side-Step Cutting to 45 and 110 Degrees in Men and Women: Implications for Anterior Cruciate Ligament Injury. *Clin. J. Sport Med.* **2014**, *25*, 529–534. [CrossRef] [PubMed]

11. Jones, P.A.; Herrington, L.; Graham-Smith, P. Braking characteristics during cutting and pivoting in female soccer players. *J. Electromyogr. Kinesiol.* **2016**, *30*, 46–54. [CrossRef] [PubMed]

12. Hsiao, H.; Knarr, B.A.; Higginson, J.S.; Binder-Macleod, S.A. Mechanisms to increase propulsive force for individuals poststroke. *J. Neuroeng. Rehabil.* **2012**, *12*, 40. [CrossRef] [PubMed]

13. Demes, B.; Carlson, K.J.; Franz, T.M. Cutting corners: The dynamics of turning behaviors in two primate species. *J. Exp. Biol.* **2006**, *209*, 927–937. [CrossRef] [PubMed]

14. Cloak, R.; Galloway, S.; Wyon, M. The Effect of Ankle Bracing on Peak Mediolateral Ground Reaction Force During Cutting Maneuvers in Collegiate Male Basketball Players. *J. Strength Cond. Res.* **2010**, *24*, 2429–2433. [CrossRef] [PubMed]

15. Weinhandl, J.T.; O'Connor, K.M. Influence of ground reaction force perturbations on anterior cruciate ligament loading during sidestep cutting. *Comput. Methods Biomech. Biomed. Engin.* **2017**, *20*, 1394–1402. [CrossRef] [PubMed]

16. Pollard, C.D.; Stearns, K.M.; Hayes, A.T.; Heiderscheit, B.C. Altered Lower Extremity Movement Variability in Female Soccer Players During Side-Step Cutting After Anterior Cruciate Ligament Reconstruction. *Am. J. Sports Med.* **2014**, *43*, 460–465. [CrossRef] [PubMed]

17. Goetschius, J.; Kuenze, C.M.; Hart, J.M. Knee extension torque variability after exercise in ACL reconstructed knees. *J. Orthop. Res.* **2015**, *33*, 1165–1170. [CrossRef] [PubMed]

18. Goetschius, J.; Hart, J.M. Knee-Extension Torque Variability and Subjective Knee Function in Patients with a History of Anterior Cruciate Ligament Reconstruction. *J. Athl. Train.* **2016**, *51*, 22–27. [CrossRef] [PubMed]

19. Gribbin, T.C.; Slater, L.V.; Herb, C.C.; Hart, J.M.; Chapman, R.M.; Hertel, J.; Kuenze, C.M. Differences in hip–knee joint coupling during gait after anterior cruciate ligament reconstruction. *Clin. Biomech.* **2016**, *32*, 64–71. [CrossRef] [PubMed]

20. Decker, L.M.; Moraiti, C.; Stergiou, N.; Georgoulis, A.D. New insights into anterior cruciate ligament deficiency and reconstruction through the assessment of knee kinematic variability in terms of nonlinear dynamics. *Knee Surg. Sports Traumatol. Arthrosc.* **2011**, *19*, 1620–1633. [CrossRef] [PubMed]

21. Moraiti, C.O.; Stergiou, N.; Vasiliadis, H.S.; Motsis, E.; Georgoulis, A. Anterior cruciate ligament reconstruction results in alterations in gait variability. *Gait Posture* **2010**, *32*, 169–175. [CrossRef] [PubMed]

22. Wurdeman, S.R.; Myers, S.A.; Stergiou, N. Transtibial amputee joint motion has increased attractor divergence during walking compared to non-amputee gait. *Ann. Biomed. Eng.* **2013**, *41*, 806–813. [CrossRef] [PubMed]

23. Wurdeman, S.R.; Myers, S.A.; Jacobsen, A.L.; Stergiou, N. Adaptation and Prosthesis Effects on Stride-to-Stride Fluctuations in Amputee Gait. *PLoS ONE* **2014**, *9*, e100125. [CrossRef] [PubMed]

24. Stergiou, N.; Decker, L.M. Human movement variability, nonlinear dynamics, and pathology: Is there a connection? *Hum. Mov. Sci.* **2011**, *30*, 869–888. [CrossRef] [PubMed]

25. Dingwell, J.B.; Cusumano, J.P. Nonlinear time series analysis of normal and pathological human walking. *Chaos* **2000**, *10*, 848–863. [CrossRef] [PubMed]

26. Stergiou, N.; Moraiti, C.; Giakas, G.; Ristanis, S.; Georgoulis, A.D. The effect of the walking speed on the stability of the anterior cruciate ligament deficient knee. *Clin. Biomech.* **2004**, *19*, 957–963. [CrossRef] [PubMed]

27. Baweja, H.S.; Patel, B.K.; Martinkewiz, J.D.; Vu, J.; Christou, E.A. Removal of visual feedback alters muscle activity and reduces force variability during constant isometric contractions. *Exp. Brain Res.* **2009**, *197*, 35–47. [CrossRef] [PubMed]

28. Boucher, J.-A.; Normand, M.C.; Descarreaux, M. Trunk isometric force production parameters during erector spinae muscle vibration at different frequencies. *J. Neuroeng. Rehabil.* **2013**, *10*, 89. [CrossRef] [PubMed]

29. Boucher, J.-A.; Normand, M.C.; Boisseau, É.; Descarreaux, M. Sensorimotor control during peripheral muscle vibration: An experimental study. *J. Manip. Physiol. Ther.* **2015**, *38*, 35–43. [CrossRef] [PubMed]

30. Mees, A.I.; Judd, K. Dangers of geometric filtering. *Phys. D* **1993**, *68*, 427–436. [CrossRef]

31. Rapp, P.E. A Guide to Dynamical Analysis. *Integr. Physiol. Behav. Sci.* **1994**, *29*, 311–327. [CrossRef] [PubMed]

32. Cignetti, F.; Decker, L.M.; Stergiou, N. Sensitivity of the wolf's and rosenstein's algorithms to evaluate local dynamic stability from small gait data sets. *Ann. Biomed. Eng.* **2012**, *40*, 1122–1130. [CrossRef] [PubMed]

33. Wolf, A.; Swift, J.B.; Swinney, H.L.; Vastano, J.A. Determining Lyapunov exponents from a time series. *Phys. D* **1985**, *16*, 285–317. [CrossRef]

34. Abarbanel, H.D.I.; Brown, R.; Sidorowich, J.J.; Tsminring, L.S. The analysis of observed chaotic data in physical systems. *Rev. Mod. Phys.* **1993**, *65*, 1331–1392. [CrossRef]

35. McClay, I.S.; Robinson, J.R.; Andriacchi, T.P.; Frederick, E.C.; Gross, T.; Martin, P.; Valiant, G.; Williams, K.R.; Cavanagh, P.C. A Profile of Ground Reaction Forces in Professional Basketball. *J. Appl. Biomech.* **1994**, *10*, 222–236. [CrossRef]

36. Smith, A.J.J.; Flaxman, T.E.; Speirs, A.D.; Benoit, D.L. Reliability of knee joint muscle activity during weight bearing force control. *J. Electromyogr. Kinesiol.* **2012**, *22*, 914–922. [CrossRef] [PubMed]

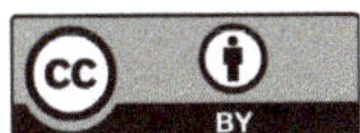

© 2018 by the authors. Licensee MDPI, Basel, Switzerland. This article is an open access article distributed under the terms and conditions of the Creative Commons Attribution (CC BY) license (http://creativecommons.org/licenses/by/4.0/).

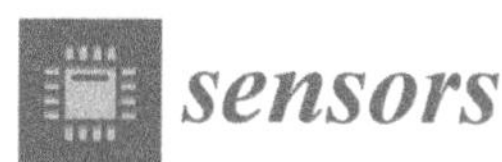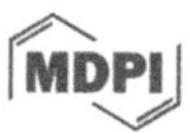

Article

Automatic Classification of Gait Impairments Using a Markerless 2D Video-Based System

Tanmay T. Verlekar [1,*], Luís D. Soares [2] and Paulo L. Correia [1]

[1]   Instituto de Telecomunicações, Instituto Superior Técnico, 1049-001 Lisbon, Portugal; plc@lx.it.pt
[2]   Instituto de Telecomunicações, Instituto Universitário de Lisboa (ISCTE-IUL), 1649-026 Lisbon, Portugal; lds@lx.it.pt
*   Correspondence: tanmay.verlekar@lx.it.pt; Tel.: +351-969-152-739

Received: 12 July 2018; Accepted: 18 August 2018; Published: 21 August 2018

Abstract: Systemic disorders affecting an individual can cause gait impairments. Successful acquisition and evaluation of features representing such impairments make it possible to estimate the severity of those disorders, which is important information for monitoring patients' health evolution. However, current state-of-the-art systems perform the acquisition and evaluation of these features in specially equipped laboratories, typically limiting the periodicity of evaluations. With the objective of making health monitoring easier and more accessible, this paper presents a system that performs automatic detection and classification of gait impairments, based on the acquisition and evaluation of biomechanical gait features using a single 2D video camera. The system relies on two different types of features to perform classification: (i) feet-related features, such as step length, step length symmetry, fraction of foot flat during stance phase, normalized step count, speed; and (ii) body-related features, such as the amount of movement while walking, center of gravity shifts and torso orientation. The proposed system uses a support vector machine to decide whether the observed gait is normal or if it belongs to one of three different impaired gait groups. Results show that the proposed system outperforms existing markerless 2D video-based systems, with a classification accuracy of 98.8%.

Keywords: gait analysis; biomechanical gait features; impaired gait classification

---

1. Introduction

Gait can be defined as a coordinated, cyclic combination of movements that results in human locomotion. Being a highly cognitive task, the manner of walking is unique to an individual [1]. However, it can be altered because of physical injuries and systemic disorders. These injuries/disorders can affect human locomotion and posture, typically resulting in reduced walking speed and step length [2]. Gait of an individual under such circumstances can be considered as impaired. By analyzing biomechanical features derived from gait, such as speed, cadence, step length, stance time, or swing time, it is possible to infer whether the observed gait is impaired, and in some cases even distinguish between different disorders that cause gait impairments, and their severity [3]. The same set of biomechanical gait features can also be used to predict fall risks in elderly populations [4] or head impacts in athletes [5].

Nowadays, the acquisition and clinical evaluation of biomechanical gait features is performed in dedicated laboratories, using a sophisticated equipment setup and with the help of specialized personnel, resulting in an expensive and time-consuming task [6]. The goal of this paper is to present a novel system that performs automatic detection and classification of gait impairments, based on the acquisition and evaluation of biomechanical gait features, using a single 2D video camera, thus making its operation possible in daily life settings, such as in clinics or even at home.

1.1. State-of-the-Art

Biomechanical features for the evaluation of an individual's gait can be acquired using several types of systems. Based on the acquisition process, they can be classified into sensor-based or vision-based systems [7]. Sensor-based systems use devices such as force sensitive resistors [8], pressure mats [9], accelerometers [10] and inertial measurement units (IMUs) [11], to acquire signals representing human motion. These sensors, which can be expensive or inaccessible to most individuals, can be setup up on the floor or attached to the body of the individual. The signals thus obtained can be processed to estimate biomechanical gait features such as velocity, cadence, step length and step time, which are effective in evaluating the individual's gait [10,11]. Setting up the selected sensors can be complex, in some cases having to be done by clinical professionals, as is often the case with body worn sensors. The processing of the resulting signals, to extract biomechanical features and perform their analysis, is also done by trained professionals.

Vision-based systems rely on the use of cameras to capture image sequences, from which biomechanical gait features can be extracted. Depending on the way the captured information is represented and processed, these systems can be classified into [1]:

- Model-based systems;
- Appearance-based systems.

Model-based systems typically rely on the use of images obtained from multiple calibrated cameras, depth sensing cameras, or a combination of both, to model the gait of an individual [12]. The use of multiple calibrated cameras allows the systems to estimate features such as the height, distance between the feet [13], or the joint angles [14]. Their performance can be further improved by using fish-eye cameras and passive markers to highlight the key joint positions [15]. A widely used model-based system for clinical evaluations is the optoelectronic motion capture system. An example of such a system is presented in [6], with the configuration of six calibrated infra-red cameras, and forty-four passive markers attached to selected body positions, for characterizing an individual's gait, while other configurations can be considered. Optoelectronic motion capture systems are considered as the gold standard for clinical evaluations, because of the accuracy of the features obtained. A drawback of this type of system is that it can only be operated in special laboratories due to the complex setup and the need for calibrations before use [7]. Thus, simpler setups have been proposed using depth sensing cameras to acquire the skeletal model of an individual, from which it is possible to estimate features [16] such as, joint positions [17], or motion history [18]. The accuracy of such systems is lower than that of the optoelectronic motion capture system, and their operation is typically limited to a range between 80 cm and 4 m.

On the other hand, appearance-based systems are typically markerless and rely on a single 2D camera, with the spatio-temporal information obtained from the captured video sequence being used to estimate biomechanical gait features. This system configuration was initially used for biometric recognition applications [19], performing well even under unconstrained conditions [20,21]. The biometric features used for recognition can be derived from representations such as the gait energy image (GEI). Such features have also been used to perform classification of gait disorders, for instance resulting from Parkinson's disease, neuropathy, hemiplegia and diplegia [22], or to detect the amount of movement and movement broadness of an individual's feet [23].

Different gait representations can be considered to better characterize an individual's health. Several appearance-based systems extract biomechanical gait features, such as step length, leg angles, gait cycle time [24,25] cadence, speed, and stride length [26], or the fraction of the stance and swing phases during a gait cycle [27], using the body silhouettes computed from a 2D video sequence. The above features are distinctive enough to classify gait as normal or impaired. Appearance-based systems can also estimate posture instabilities using biomechanical features such as lean and ramp angles [28], axial ratio and change in velocity [29]. Other appearance-based systems distinguish between normal and wavering, faltering or falling gait using features such as homeomorphisms between 2D lattices of binary silhouettes [30].

Appearance-based systems based on 2D video do not have access to depth information, which can limit their accuracy when compared to some sensor or model-based systems. However, the major body articulations are clearly visible during a gait cycle, notably if video is captured from a lateral viewpoint, often designated as the canonical view [31]. In those conditions, the features obtained from a single 2D video camera contain enough information to characterize an individual's gait, with the advantage that the system is much easier to install and operate in a daily life setting, when compared to model or sensor-based systems.

1.2. Motivation and Contribution

Most state-of-the-art markerless systems using a single 2D camera only perform a binary classification of gait as being either normal or impaired, since the classification of the type of gait impairment is a significantly more challenging task given the biomechanical gait features that are typically used. However, such classifications can provide a preliminary assessment of the type or the severity of a disorder. The automatic classification performed by the proposed system, also makes such preliminary assessments accessible to individuals in a daily life setting, where a constant presence of trained professionals is not possible.

Some systems, such as the one reported in [22], can distinguish between different types of gait disorders using biometric gait features derived from a GEI. However, their performance is poor when trying to distinguish gait disorders such as diplegia and Parkinson, as the resulting GEIs are very similar [22]. In such cases, the usage of additional biomechanical gait features, such as leg joint angles [22], or step length, foot flat ratio and speed, can lead to a significantly better performance. However, obtaining these features from a 2D video sequence can be challenging, with self-occlusions and the lack of depth information often leading to poor classification results. The self-occlusion problem can be especially difficult to handle for some gait impairments caused by disorders such as Parkinson's disease, where the short strides cause the feet to remain occluded throughout the gait cycle, as discussed in Section 2.2.

This paper presents a novel markerless appearance-based system that acquires biomechanical gait features from a single 2D camera, able to describe an individual's gait even under self-occlusions. These features include step length, foot flat ratio, speed, normalized step count, torso orientation, shift in center of gravity (COG) and the amount of movement while walking. Most state-of-the-art markerless 2D video based systems that compute step length, do not differentiate between the left and the right leg. Thus, the proposed system improves on the state-of-the-art by distinguishing the left and right step lengths, which allows identifying the limb(s) contributing to the impaired gait. Also, the proposed "amount of movement" feature helps to identify motion restricted limbs. Together, these features can be used to measure gait symmetry. The proposed system also computes a temporal feature, "foot flat ratio", that estimates the fraction of time during which the foot is in complete contact with the ground during the stance phase. This feature is significantly more descriptive than the previously considered stance/swing phase during a gait cycle [23], and along with speed and normalized step count it allows the proposed system to more reliably detect deviations from normal gait. Also, novel body related features are proposed, such as torso orientation and shift in COG, which allow estimating posture instabilities, such as a hunchback. The proposed system can therefore detect gait impairments and, in a first stage, classify an individual as having gait impairments affecting the left, the right or both sides of the body.

The rest of the paper is organized as follows: Section 2 presents the proposed system and the acquired biomechanical gait features. Section 3 presents experimental results. Section 4 provides a discussion about the quality of the features obtained, and the classification accuracy of the proposed system using a support vector machine (SVM) classifier. Section 5 presents conclusions and suggests directions for future work.

2. Methods

The architecture of the proposed system, which takes a 2D video as input, is presented in Figure 1. After an initial pre-processing step to extract binary silhouettes from the 2D video, the following two sets of biomechanical gait features are computed:

- Feet-related features—These features are obtained using the spatio-temporal information available from the individual's feet area and include: (i) left and right step lengths, and step length symmetry; (ii) normalized step count; (iii) speed; and (iv) left and right foot flat ratios;
- Body-related features—These features are obtained using information from the entire body of an individual, thus reflecting posture, and include features such as: (i) amount of movement in the left and the right side of the body, movement symmetry; (ii) shift in the COG with respect to its center of support (COS); and (iii) torso orientation.

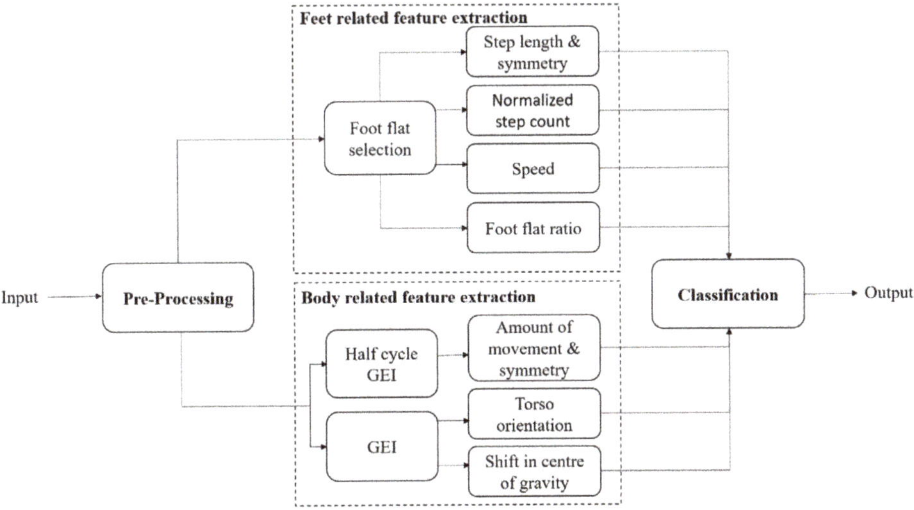

Figure 1. Proposed system architecture.

These features can then be used to decide whether the observed gait is impaired and, if it is, to classify gait impairments into different groups. The proposed system performs the classification using an SVM. Each of the main modules of the proposed architecture are detailed in the following sections.

2.1. Pre-Processing

The proposed system performs background subtraction [32] on the input 2D video, to obtain a sequence of binary silhouettes of the walking individual. The silhouettes are then normalized with respect to height, while maintaining their original aspect ratio. The normalization step, applied to each frame, makes the proposed system robust to scale changes, such as those resulting from a varying distance between an individual and the camera. The distance between the feet of the individual is then approximated as the width of a rectangular bounding box fitted onto the silhouettes [33]. Using the silhouettes and the distance between the feet, the proposed system can compute the desired biomechanical gait features.

2.2. Feet Related Feature Extraction

The gait of an individual consists of repetitions of a gait cycle. It begins and ends with an event called the "initial contact", which occurs when the heel of the foot being observed first meets the ground. The distance covered between the initial contact of the observed (left or right) foot and the initial contact of the other foot is called step length. In a healthy individual, detecting the initial contact, and thus estimating the step length can be easy since the feet are spread wide apart while walking [24]. However, in the presence of certain impairments that affect gait, the strides can be extremely short, leading to self-occlusions (i.e., the part of the body closer to the camera occludes other parts of the body), as illustrated in the right side of Figure 2a. Under such conditions, identifying the exact instant of initial contact or estimating the step length using a silhouette can be difficult.

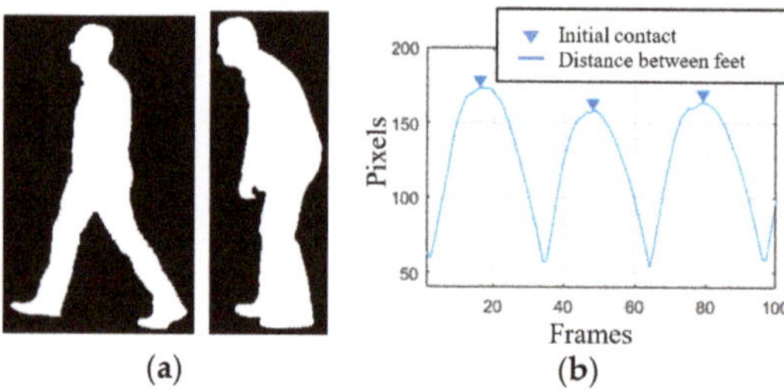

Figure 2. (**a**) Silhouettes belonging to a healthy individual (left) and an individual suffering from a systemic disorder (right); (**b**) plot representing the distance between feet along a gait sequence.

The proposed system tackles this problem by detecting the "foot flat" instants, defined as the part of the gait cycle during which the foot is in complete contact with the ground. A gait cycle includes two foot flat instants, one for each of the feet, occurring right after the initial contact. To minimize the effect of self-occlusions in the presence of very short step lengths, foot flat instances are detected by analyzing half of the gait cycle at a time, i.e., the span between two consecutive initial contact events (of opposite feet). However, since determining the exact instant of initial contact is difficult, the proposed system approximates it as the instant in time where the distance between the two feet (i.e., width of the rectangular bounding box fitted onto the silhouettes) is maximum [23], as illustrated in Figure 2b.

Moreover, to obtain foot flat positions, only the feet region of the silhouettes is of interest, so an average feet image, $AFI(x, y, t)$, can be created by keeping only the lower 10% fraction of the silhouettes, selected according to the human anatomy ratio [34]. The AFI is computed by averaging the resulting T feet silhouettes images, $I_{feet}(x, y, t)$, available between two initial contacts, according to Equation (1), and illustrated in Figure 3a,b. The averaging process makes the system more robust against any uncertainty in the estimation of the initial contact instant:

$$AFI(x, y, t) = \frac{1}{T} \sum_{t=1}^{T} I_{feet}(x, y, t) \tag{1}$$

(a)   (b)

Figure 3. *Cont.*

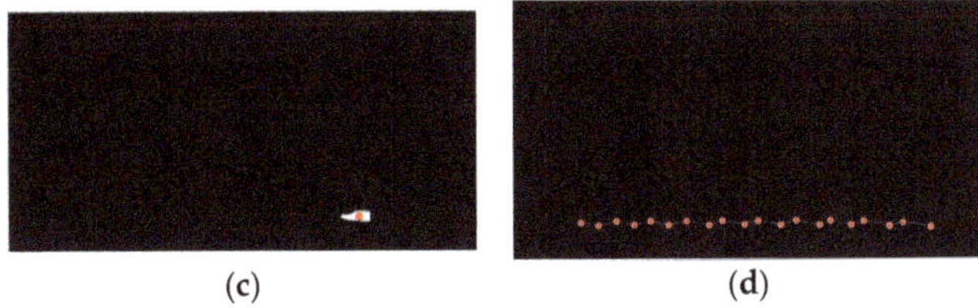

(c)   (d)

Figure 3. (**a**) Segmented feet silhouettes between two initial contacts; (**b**) AFI obtained by averaging the feet silhouettes; (**c**) position of the foot flat obtained by applying a threshold; (**d**) centroids of foot flat obtained for the entire video sequence.

Since the AFI highlights the foot when it is in complete contact with the ground, by applying the Otsu thresholding [35] to the AFI the position of the foot flat can be obtained, as illustrated in Figure 3c. The resulting foot flat positions are used for computation of feet related features as detailed in the following subsections.

2.2.1. Step Length (*SL*)

The step length can be measured using the foot flat positions obtained from the entire video sequence. However, due to the lack of depth information, there can be a significant difference between the scales of the two feet. Thus, to minimize errors, the proposed system computes the centroid of each foot flat and measures the Euclidean distance between two consecutive centroids as the step length.

Knowing the walking direction of an individual with respect to the camera, the proposed system can identify the foot closer to the camera as the right or the left foot. Thus, the proposed system can estimate both the left and right step lengths. To identify which foot is closer to the camera, since depth information is not available, the foot flat centroid positions can be used. As illustrated in Figure 3d, the centroid of the foot further away from the camera appears at a more elevated position in the image. Thus, by comparing the y-coordinate of the centroids, the step lengths can be classified as either left or the right step lengths. Since the video sequence contains multiple gait cycles and thus allow computing multiple feature values, a median is computed to increase the proposed system's robustness to outliers [23]. So, the proposed system computes the median of the left and right step lengths as SL_i^{left} and SL_j^{right}, respectively. A step length symmetry score, SL_{symm}, can then be computed as the absolute difference between the medians of left and the right step lengths, according to Equation (2). Since, the silhouettes are normalized during the pre-processing step the symmetry score remains consistent across different video sequences:

$$SL_{symm} = |median(SL_i^{left}) - median(SL_j^{right})| \tag{2}$$

2.2.2. Normalized Step Count (C) and Speed (S)

The proposed system can also compute the normalized step count and speed of an individual's movement using the foot flat information. Normalized step count, C, is computed as the total number of foot flat instances, k, divided by the total distance travelled, according to Equation (3). The distance travelled is measured as the length summation of the n observed steps, SL. The distance is measured in pixels due to the silhouette height normalization performed during pre-processing, which makes the system robust to scale changes:

$$C = \frac{k}{\sum_{i=1}^{n} SL_i} \tag{3}$$

The speed, S, of an individual's movement is computed by dividing the total distance travelled by the duration of the video sequence, according to Equation (4). The duration of the video sequence, d (in seconds), is measured between the first and last initial contacts:

$$S = \frac{1}{d} \sum_{i=1}^{n} SL_i \tag{4}$$

2.2.3. Foot Flat Ratio (*FFR*)

A walking video sequence is composed of several repetitions of a gait cycle, delimited by the initial contacts of the observed foot. It is also possible to divide each gait cycle into two phases separated by a "toe off" event, occurring when the toe of the foot being observed just leaves the ground. The phase before the toe off is called the stance phase, while the phase following the toe off is called the swing phase. Using the initial contact and the toe off, the proposed system can estimate the duration of the stance phase. As discussed in [23], the duration of the stance and swing phases are not unique enough to distinguish between different types of gait impairments. However, the amount of time the foot remains in complete contact with the ground, during the stance phase, can change significantly depending on the type of gait impairments. Thus, the proposed system computes a "foot flat ratio" feature, which can be defined as the fraction of the stance phase for which the foot remains in complete contact with the ground.

To compute the foot flat ratio, *FFR*, the proposed system measures the amount of overlap between the foot flat and the silhouettes belonging to the corresponding stance phase. It estimates the foot flat duration by counting the number of frames for which the foot flat is completely covered by the silhouettes—see Figure 4. Foot flat ratio values, for both the left and right feet, can then be computed according to Equation (5):

$$FFR = \frac{flat\ foot\ duration}{stance\ phase\ duration} \tag{5}$$

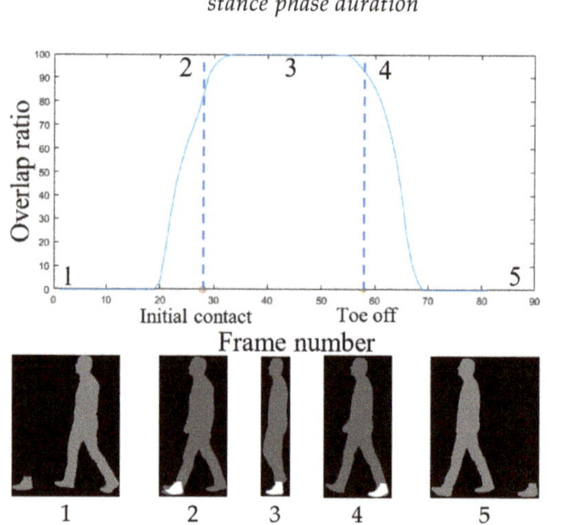

Figure 4. Plot representing the foot flat overlap ratio (**top**) and the corresponding silhouettes (**bottom**).

2.3. Body Related Feature Extraction

Apart from the feet, the body of an individual can also provide significant information about gait impairments that an individual may be suffering from. For example, an individual's movements can become severely restricted and the posture of the individual can be severely altered due to disorders such as Parkinson's disease [2]. Thus, a measurement of the amount of movement and posture instability can be useful for classifying such gait impairments. Also, in some cases, the movement of a single limb may be restricted, or more restricted than the other limb. Therefore, analyzing the movement for every half gait cycle can be useful.

2.3.1. Amount of Movement (*AOM*)

The proposed system computes the amount of movement during every half gait cycle using the entropy. However, unlike what was done for feet related features computation, here the half gait cycle is delimited by the mid-stance and mid-swing events, as it contains the part of the gait cycle where individuals shift the body weight from one side of the body to the other. The proposed system can thus capture movement restrictions while shifting weight onto the impaired side of the body. The mid-stance and mid-swing instants are approximated as the instants of the gait cycle when the distance between the two feet is minimum, corresponding to the valleys in the representation of Figure 1b. The silhouettes belonging to the considered half gait cycle, numbered from 1 to P, can then be cropped, $I_c(x, y, p)$ and averaged to obtain the half cycle GEI, $GEI_{hc}(x, y, p)$, according to Equation (6) [17]:

$$GEI_{hc}(x, y, p) = \frac{1}{P} \sum_{p=1}^{P} I_c(x, y, p) \tag{6}$$

The "amount of movement" feature, *AOM*, can then be computed over the half cycle GEI according to Equation (7), where P_i is the probability that the difference between two adjacent pixels is equal to i. As illustrated in Figure 5b,d, the restriction in movement can be effectively represented using Shannon entropy [36]:

$$AOM = -\sum_i P_i log_2 P_i \tag{7}$$

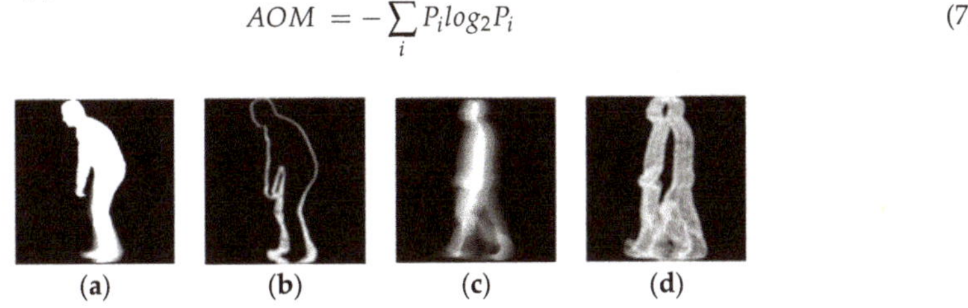

(a)   (b)   (c)   (d)

Figure 5. Half cycle GEI computed using impaired (**a**) and healthy (**c**) gait silhouettes, and the corresponding entropy representations (**b,d**).

Following the indexing of the foot flat, the amount of movement features can also be classified into left, AOM_i^{left} and right, AOM_i^{rigth}, according to the foot that enters into an initial contact during the considered half gait cycle. A symmetry measure, AOM_{symm}, can also be computed to represent the difference in movement between left and right, according to Equation (8):

$$AOM_{symm} = |median(AOM_i^{left}) - median(AOM_j^{right})| \tag{8}$$

2.3.2. Shift in COG (COG_{shift})

As illustrated in Figure 6, certain types of gait impairments caused by disorders such as Parkinson's disease, can affect the posture of an individual, being reflected as a change in the orientation of the torso and therefore as a shift in the individual's COG with respect to the COS (center of the base of support). Healthy individuals walk such that their COG and COS are always approximately vertically aligned. The proposed system computes the amount of shift using a GEI computed similarly to (6), but over the entire gait cycle. Using the GEI provides robustness to variations in the shift in COG occurring at different instants of the gait cycle. The COG is measured as a weighted centroid of the GEI, using the GEI intensity values as weights. The COS is measured as the center of the feet region of the GEI, obtained by segmenting the feet using a human anatomy ratio [34]. The shift in COG, COG_{shift}, can then be computed as the absolute difference between the horizontal coordinates of the COG and COS, according to Equation (9):

$$COG_{shift} = |COG_x - COS_x| \tag{9}$$

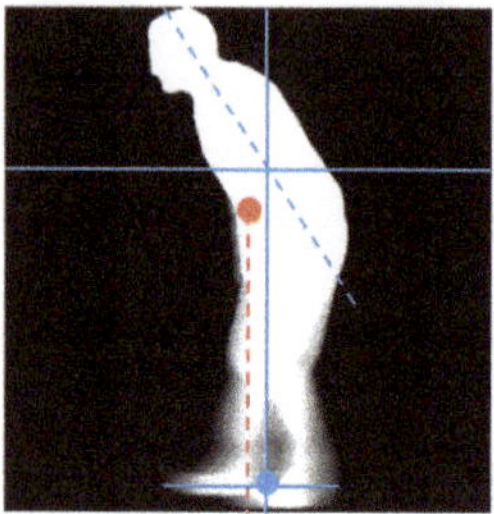

Figure 6. GEI highlighting shift in COG (middle silhouette point) with respect to the COS (lower silhouette point) and the orientation of the torso.

2.3.3. Torso Orientation (*TO*)

The last feature considered, called torso orientation, *TO*, is also computed using the complete GEI. The proposed system selects the torso using the human anatomy ratios presented in [34]. It then performs principal component analysis over the torso and measures the angle (θ) between the horizontal axis and the first principal component, $PC(PC_x, PC_y)$, according to Equation (10) [33]:

$$TO\ (\theta^\circ) = \left| tan^{-1}\left(\frac{PC_y}{PC_x} \right) \times \frac{180}{\pi} \right| \tag{10}$$

2.4. Classification

The proposed system can perform classification in two different ways. First, the system can use each feature to classify gait as either normal or impaired. The paper tests the discriminative power of each feature to classify gait as normal or impaired by using the two-sample *t*-test with unequal variances [37]. This test can be used to determine whether two samples are drawn from the same or from different population groups. Thus, the results of the test can be interpreted to identify the features that are more significant in differentiating between normal and impaired gait.

Although an individual feature can be used to classify gait as either normal or impaired, the type of impairments that can be detected may vary depending on the features used. For instance, features such as shift in COG or torso orientation can help detect posture instabilities, features such as step length or amount of movement can be used to detect asymmetric gait, while features such as foot flat ratio, normalized step count or speed can be used to detect slow moving gait and other deviations. Thus, using all the available features together can allow the proposed system to further classify gait based on the type of impairment. It can also allow identification of disorders, or even determine the severity of such disorders. For example, Parkinson's disease reduces the walking speed, alters the posture and restricts the movement of an individual, while disorders such as hemiplegia restrict the movement of a single side of the body.

The proposed system can distinguish between gait impairments caused by such disorders using the proposed biomechanical gait features. It is also possible to identify the side of the body whose movement is more affected, such as in the case of hemiplegia, as the considered features allow differentiating between left and right side impairments. The proposed system performs such classifications using a SVM, a discriminative classifier that separates data using a hyperplane [38]. To improve the classification accuracy of the proposed system, the SVM is used with a quadratic kernel.

2.5. Test Protocol

Two different tests are considered to evaluate the proposed system. The first test analyzes the discriminative power of each feature, and the second test analyzes the classification accuracy of the whole system. Thus, to successfully evaluate the proposed system, the following protocols are defined.

2.5.1. Two Sample *t*-Test

To test the ability of each feature to differentiate between normal (NM) and impaired (FB, RL, LL) gait sequences, a two-sample *t*-test with unequal variances and a significance level of 0.05 is conducted. The null hypothesis for the test states that the two samples are drawn from the same population group. Thus, given two sample sets of a feature, drawn from the available NM and one of the three impaired sequence groups, the test will return a p-value, which can be used to either accept or reject the null hypothesis. The p-value is the probability of finding the observed, or more extreme, result when the null hypothesis of a test is true. If the p-value is above the significance level of the test (in this case 0.05), the null hypothesis is accepted. Otherwise, the alternate hypothesis, that the two sample sets are drawn from two different population groups, is accepted. Accepting the alternate hypothesis also suggests that the feature being tested is discriminative enough to differentiate between the two samples.

2.5.2. Gait Type Classification Using SVM

The classification accuracy the proposed system is analyzed using a fivefold cross-validation technique. The technique divides the data into five sets, where each set contains features from two different Individuals. Thus, the training and testing set are mutually exclusive, with respect to the participating individuals. Next, the classification step is repeated 5 times such that each time, one of the five sets is used for testing and the other four sets are used for training the system. Finally, an average is computed to represent the classification accuracy of the system. The advantage of using fivefold cross-validation is that the variance of the resulting estimate is reduced as the results do not depend on a particular way of partitioning the data.

3. Results

The ability of the features to distinguish the left and right limbs, assess gait symmetry, posture instabilities, speed changes and other deviations from normal gait allows the proposed system to distinguish between different types of gait impairments. However, due to the lack of publicly available databases, the proposed system is currently tested only on the INIT gait database presented in [23]. This database contains binary silhouettes of ten individuals (nine males, one female) simulating eight different gait impairments. All the sequences are acquired in a lateral view and the type of impairment is manually annotated to create the ground truth. Each individual is recorded two different times in a LABCOM studio [23] at 30 fps, capturing multiple gait cycles per each recorded sequence. Since the first four simulated impairments correspond to restricted arm movement, testing is done considering the other four feet related impairment simulations, for which the proposed system can compute relevant feet and body related features. The tested sequences are labelled as: restricted full body movement (FB), restricted right leg movement (RL), restricted left leg movement (LL) and normal gait (NM). FB sequences simulate disorders such as Parkinson disease while, RL and LL sequences simulate disorders such as hemiplegia.

Following the protocol described in Section 2.5.1, each feature obtained from the proposed system is tested for its ability to characterize gait impairments. *t*-Test results are presented in Table 1, while the mean and the standard deviation of the features are presented in Table 2. The decision to perform the *t*-test is made considering the size of the INIT database presented in [23]. Assuming that feature samples are normally distributed, the *t*-test provides an assessment of the reliability of a given feature in in being able to differentiate between normal and impaired gait, while taking the sample size into consideration. Thus, the features resulting in lower p-values can be expected to be more significant in differentiating between normal and impaired gait.

Table 1. Two sample t-test with unequal variances and significance level of 0.05 performed between normal and impaired gait.

	FB	RL	LL
SL Left	1.56×10^{-21}	2.59×10^{-2}	4.01×10^{-9}
SL Right	1.05×10^{-23}	1.44×10^{-10}	3.88×10^{-2}
SL Symmetry	1.74×10^{-1}	5.29×10^{-10}	1.38×10^{-9}
FFR Left	4.48×10^{-7}	1.00×10^{-3}	4.89×10^{-4}
FFR Right	4.82×10^{-7}	3.25×10^{-4}	1.08×10^{-1}
S	7.02×10^{-16}	1.33×10^{-4}	1.48×10^{-4}
C	4.47×10^{-11}	2.50×10^{-5}	1.11×10^{-5}
TO	2.94×10^{-14}	6.46×10^{-1}	8.75×10^{-1}
COG_{shift}	6.87×10^{-3}	1.54×10^{-4}	4.97×10^{-2}
AOM Left	8.04×10^{-16}	3.328×10^{-1}	2.04×10^{-9}
AOM Right	1.98×10^{-19}	1.25×10^{-7}	5.97×10^{-1}
AOM Symmetry	2.46×10^{-3}	1.21×10^{-7}	1.94×10^{-9}

Table 2. Mean and standard deviation of all the observed gait features belonging to different groups.

	FB	RL	LL	NM
SL Left (pixels)	48.49 ± 12.70	115.16 ± 13.24	70.95 ± 25.26	124.19 ± 11.28
SL Right (pixels)	41.19 ± 10.24	63.24 ± 23.36	108.69 ± 21.90	120.68 ± 11.56
SL Symmetry (pixels)	7.28 ± 6.18	51.92 ± 18.61	45.90 ± 17.20	5.137 ± 3.08
FFR Left (%)	0.80 ± 0.09	0.70 ± 0.05	0.68 ± 0.09	0.64 ± 0.04
FFR Right (%)	0.75 ± 0.09	0.66 ± 0.05	0.67 ± 0.06	0.60 ± 0.06
S (pixels/s)	37.04 ± 8.86	63.11 ± 15.31	64.77 ± 13.44	81.41 ± 11.37
C (steps/pixels)	0.025 ± 0.005	0.013 ± 0.002	0.013 ± 0.001	0.010 ± 0.000
TO (°)	62.87 ± 6.25	84.97 ± 3.00	85.25 ± 3.24	85.40 ± 2.85
COG_{shift} (pixels)	12.39 ± 5.93	4.65 ± 2.25	6.40 ± 2.85	8.08 ± 2.84
AOM Left (entropy)	1.76 ± 0.31	3.12 ± 0.14	2.51 ± 0.29	3.17 ± 0.11
AOM Right (entropy)	1.58 ± 0.25	2.35 ± 0.42	3.01 ± 0.24	3.10 ± 0.11
AOM Symmetry (entropy)	0.17 ± 0.12	0.77 ± 0.39	0.55 ± 0.21	0.06 ± 0.05

The proposed system is further tested to check its ability to classify different gait impairments into different groups. The system is tested using a fivefold cross validation technique, following the protocol described in Section 2.5.2. Its classification accuracy is reported in Table 3, along with the confusion matrix in Table 4.

Table 3. Classification accuracy of the proposed and state-of-the-art systems.

Method	Classification Accuracy
Leg angle method [24]	72.5%
GEI method [22]	75.0%
Proposed system	98.8%

Table 4. Confusion matrix for the proposed system.

		Predicted Group			
		FB	RL	LL	NM
	FB	100%	0%	0%	0%
True Group	RL	0%	95%	0%	5%
	LL	0%	0%	100%	0%
	NM	0%	0%	0%	100%

4. Discussion

The proposed system can identify the left and the right leg, which allows a more complete characterization of gait impairments than was possible with the system described in [23]. This can be concluded from Table 1, where each entry presents the *p*-value of the two-sample *t*-test. The first row of the table presents the results between the NM and FB groups. The results show significantly low *p*-values for almost all the computed features. The lowest values are observed for step length, amount of movement and torso orientation, suggesting that these features are more significant when differentiating between NM and FB gait. The low *p*-values are due to shorter step lengths, restricted body movement and a hunched posture. The hunched posture also causes a significant difference in the shift in the COG feature, represented by a low *p*-value in Table 1. The speed of the individuals in the NM group is also significantly different from the FB group. This is represented by low *p*-values for the speed, normalized step count and the foot flat ratio. The only feature that accepts the null hypothesis is the step length symmetry, indicating that when differentiating between NM and FB gait the symmetry feature will perform poorly, as in these cases the steps length of both the legs are similar. However, the step length symmetry and amount of movement symmetry features are significant when differentiating between NM and RL/LL gait, as indicated by their low *p*-values in Table 1. The *p*-value for the other features, such as step length, foot flat ratio, speed, normalized step count and shift in COG, are also low suggesting that they are significant enough to distinguish between the two groups. The features that accept the null hypothesis for RL/LL gait are the torso orientation and the amount of movement for the unrestricted side of the body. However, this is expected as the torso orientation feature is only effective in severe posture instability cases, such as hunchbacks, and the amount of movement of the unrestricted side is expected to be similar to NM group.

To better illustrate the difference between the different types of gait, each entry in Table 2 presents the mean and standard deviation of each feature belonging to the respective group. Using Table 2, it can be seen that the FB gait is significantly slower than the NM gait, indicated by low speed, high normalized step count and a large fraction of time spent in foot flat during stance phase. The step lengths are also significantly shorter than the NM group. However, there is no significant difference between the left and the right foot, as indicated by low step length symmetry values and the amount of movement symmetry values. Also, the bending of torso and the shift in COG is significantly larger than the NM gait—see Table 2. For the RL/LL groups, the restricted leg/side of the body is indicated by short step length and low amount of movement (entropy values) in Table 2. However, the gait is relatively fast as indicated by the higher speed and lower normalized step count values. Finally, it should be noted that the shift in COG feature is effective in differentiating between normal and all the three types of impaired gait, as illustrated in Table 1, but it is not very precise in its measurement—see Table 2. The low precision in the measurement is caused by camera distortions, whose effect is severe, especially at the start and at the end of the gait sequence. Although its precision is not as good as that of other features, its ability to differentiate between different gait impairments allows the proposed system to successfully classify the gait as being normal or impaired.

Next, the ability of the proposed system to classify gait across different impairment groups is tested following the fivefold cross-validation technique and the resulting classification accuracy is reported in Table 3. These results indicate that the proposed system performs extremely well, being able to classify gait sequences as FB, RL, LL or NM with a correct classification accuracy of 98.8%. The results also indicate that there is a significant variation between the feature values observed for each group. Table 3 also contains a comparison of the proposed system against the state-of-the-art markerless 2D video based systems, tested using the same fivefold cross-validation technique. The leg angle method, presented in [24], can be effective when there is sufficient separation between legs. However, even in NM group, it becomes difficult to distinguish between the two legs during mid stance and mid swing phases, while in the FB sequences there is no separation between the two legs during the entire gait cycle. The work presented in [22] uses a GEI along with SVM to perform classification of gait impairments. The use of GEI allows the method to successfully differentiate between FB and NM groups, but there are significant misclassifications between the NM, RL and LL groups, reducing the overall classification accuracy to 75%—see Table 3. Even with a linear SVM, the proposed system performs better than the GEI method [22] with a correct classification accuracy of 95.0%, following the fivefold cross-validation technique. A second drawback of the GEI method [22] is that the GEIs used for the classification process do not provide any additional information about the gait impairments, while the proposed system provides measurable features that can be used to further analyze an individual's gait. Thus, it can be concluded that the biomechanical features used by the proposed system provide a better representation for gait impairment detection and classification. The performance of the proposed system can also be analyzed using the confusion matrix presented in Table 4. It shows that the proposed system performs extremely well—in fact, only a single sequence is misclassified which, due to the limited size of the available database, results in a 5% penalty to the classification accuracy of the RL group. It should also be noted that the falsely classified sequence is poorly simulated, as can be observed by the mean step length of the left and right legs, leading to its classification into the NM group. The results from the Table 4 show that the proposed system operates with an average recall of 98.75% and precision of 98.80%. The average recall and precision of the methods presented in [22] is 75% and 76.07%, and [24] is 72.5% and 72.89% respectively, suggesting that the proposed system performs significantly better than the state-of-the-art methods. Also, the goodness index of the proposed system is 0.0177 which makes it "optimal" according to [39].

5. Conclusions

The paper presents a novel markerless system that performs successful acquisition and evaluation of an individual's gait using a single 2D video camera. It evaluates individuals' gait using biomechanical gait features acquired from their binary silhouettes. These features allow the proposed system to classify an individual's gait across different gait impairments. The classification accuracy of the proposed system is significantly better than the current state-of-the-art.

The features acquired by the proposed system can be classified into two types. The first type is related to the feet of an individual. They include features such as step length, normalized step count, speed and the fraction of foot flat during a stance phase. The proposed system can distinguish among the features obtained from the left and the right foot, thus allowing the system to estimate gait symmetry. The second type of features are related to the entire body of an individual. They include features such as the amount of movement while walking, torso orientation and the shift in the COG with respect to its COS. Similarly, to feet related features, features such as the amount of movement are computed separately for either feet, to compute a symmetry score. Apart from detecting the left-right symmetry, the proposed system also detects posture instabilities using torso orientation and the shift in COG, while other features such as normalized step count and speed are used to detect the deviation from the normal gait. Using a SVM classifier, the proposed system performs almost 100% correct classification across four different types of gait on the INIT database.

Due to the lack of publicly available databases, the proposed system is currently tested on a database containing only twenty simulated sequences for each impairment type. Therefore, the future work will consider testing of the proposed system on a larger database, containing a larger variation in gait impairments, acquired from real patients. The resulting features will also be validated using the gold standard sensor or vision-based systems. The low precision of the shift in COG feature will be improved by rectifying the camera distortions in the pre-processing step. Another possible extension is to include features reflecting different arm related impairments, thus allowing the proposed system to perform an improved evaluation of an individual's health. The features can also be explored to predict fall risks in elderly populations.

Author Contributions: All authors were fully involved in the review and preparation of the manuscript.

Funding: This research was funded by Instituto de Telecomunicações under Fundação para a Ciência e Tecnologia Grant UID/EEA/50008/2013.

Conflicts of Interest: The authors declare no conflict of interest. The funders had no role in the design of the study; in the collection, analyses, or interpretation of data; in the writing of the manuscript, and in the decision to publish the results.

References

1. Makihara, Y.; Matovski, D.; Nixon, S.; Carter, J.; Yagi, Y. Gait recognition: Databases, representations, and applications. In *Wiley Encyclopedia of Electrical and Electronics Engineering*; Wiley: Hoboken, NJ, USA, 2015.
2. Azevedo Coste, C.; Sijobert, B.; Pissard-Gibollet, R.; Pasquier, M.; Espiau, B.; Geny, C. Detection of freezing of gait in Parkinson disease: Preliminary results. *Sensors* **2014**, *14*, 6819–6827. [CrossRef] [PubMed]
3. Debi, R.; Elbaz, A.; Mor, A.; Kahn, G.; Peskin, B.; Beer, Y.; Agar, G.; Morag, G.; Segal, G. Knee osteoarthritis, degenerative meniscal lesion and osteonecrosis of the knee: Can a simple gait test direct us to a better clinical diagnosis. *Orthop. Traumatol. Surg. Res.* **2017**, *103*, 603–608. [CrossRef] [PubMed]
4. Howcroft, J.; Lemaire, E.D.; Kofman, J.; McIlroy, W.E. Dual-Task Elderly Gait of Prospective Fallers and Non-Fallers: A Wearable Sensor-Based Analysis. *Sensors* **2018**, *18*, 1275. [CrossRef] [PubMed]
5. Wu, L.C.; Kuo, C.; Loza, J.; Kurt, M.; Laksari, K.; Yanez, L.Z.; Stitzel, J.D. Detection of American football head impacts using biomechanical features and support vector machine classification. *Sci. Rep.* **2017**, *8*, 855. [CrossRef] [PubMed]
6. Vanrenterghem, J.; Gormley, D.; Robinson, M.; Lees, A. Solutions for representing the whole-body centre of mass in side cutting manoeuvres based on data that is typically available for lower limb kinematics. *Gait Posture* **2010**, *31*, 517–521. [CrossRef] [PubMed]
7. Muro-De-La-Herran, A.; Garcia-Zapirain, B.; Mendez-Zorrilla, A. Gait analysis methods: An overview of wearable and non-wearable systems, highlighting clinical applications. *Sensors* **2014**, *14*, 3362–3394. [CrossRef] [PubMed]
8. Howell, A.M.; Kobayashi, T.; Hayes, H.A.; Foreman, K.B.; Bamberg, S.J.M. Kinetic gait analysis using a low-cost insole. *IEEE Trans. Biomed. Eng.* **2013**, *60*, 3284–3290. [CrossRef] [PubMed]
9. Webster, K.E.; Wittwer, J.E.; Feller, J.A. Validity of the GAITRite® walkway system for the measurement of averaged and individual step parameters of gait. *Gait Posture* **2005**, *22*, 317–321. [CrossRef] [PubMed]
10. Wang, J.S.; Lin, C.W.; Yang, Y.T.C.; Ho, Y.J. Walking pattern classification and walking distance estimation algorithms using gait phase information. *IEEE Trans. Biomed. Eng.* **2012**, *59*, 2884–2892. [CrossRef] [PubMed]
11. Anwary, A.R.; Yu, H.; Vassallo, M. An Automatic Gait Feature Extraction Method for Identifying Gait Asymmetry Using Wearable Sensors. *Sensors* **2018**, *18*, 676. [CrossRef] [PubMed]
12. Stone, E.E.; Skubic, M. Passive in-home measurement of stride-to-stride gait variability comparing vision and Kinect sensing. In Proceedings of the Annual International Conference of the IEEE Engineering in Medicine and Biology Society, Boston, MA, USA, 30 August–3 September 2011.
13. Lin, K.W.; Wang, S.T.; Chung, P.C.; Yang, C.F. A New View-Calibrated Approach for Abnormal Gait Detection. In *Advances in Intelligent Systems and Applications-Volume 2*; Springer: Berlin/Heidelberg, Germany, 2013; pp. 521–529.
14. Leu, A.; Ristić-Durrant, D.; Gräser, A. A robust markerless vision-based human gait analysis system. In Proceedings of the 6th IEEE International Symposium on Applied Computational Intelligence and Informatics, Timisoara, Romania, 19–21 May 2011.
15. Islam, A.; Asikuzzaman, M.; Garratt, M.A.; Pickering, M.R. 3D kinematic measurement of human movement using low cost fish-eye cameras. In Proceedings of the Eighth International Conference on Graphic and Image Processing, Tokyo, Japan, 29–31 October 2017.
16. Springer, S.; Yogev Seligmann, G. Validity of the kinect for gait assessment: A focused review. *Sensors* **2016**, *16*, 194. [CrossRef] [PubMed]
17. Hu, R.Z.L.; Hartfiel, A.; Tung, J.; Fakih, A.; Hoey, J.; Poupart, P. 3D Pose tracking of walker users' lower limb with a structured-light camera on a moving platform. In Proceedings of the IEEE Computer Society Conference on Computer Vision and Pattern Recognition Workshops, Colorado Springs, CO, USA, 20–25 June 2011.

18. Chaaraoui, A.A.; Padilla-López, J.R.; Flórez-Revuelta, F. Abnormal gait detection with RGB-D devices using joint motion history features. In Proceedings of the 11th IEEE International Conference and Workshops on Automatic Face and Gesture Recognition, Ljubljana, Slovenia, 4–8 May 2015.

19. Han, J.; Bhanu, B. Individual recognition using gait energy image. *IEEE Trans. Pattern Anal. Mach. Intell.* **2006**, *2*, 316–322. [CrossRef] [PubMed]

20. Verlekar, T.T.; Correia, P.L.; Soares, L.D. View-invariant gait recognition system using a gait energy image decomposition method. *IET Biom.* **2017**, *6*, 299–306. [CrossRef]

21. Verlekar, T.; Correia, P.; Soares, L. View-invariant gait recognition exploiting spatio-temporal information and a dissimilarity metric. In Proceedings of the International Conference of the Biometrics Special Interest Group, Darmstadt, Germany, 21–23 September 2016.

22. Nieto-Hidalgo, M.; García-Chamizo, J.M. Classification of Pathologies Using a Vision Based Feature Extraction. In Proceedings of the International Conference on Ubiquitous Computing and Ambient Intelligence, Philadelphia, PA, USA, 7–10 November 2017; Springer: New York, NY, USA, 2017.

23. Ortells, J.; Herrero-Ezquerro, M.T.; Mollineda, R.A. Vision-based gait impairment analysis for aided diagnosis. In *Medical & Biological Engineering & Computing*; Springer: New York, NY, USA, 2018.

24. Nieto-Hidalgo, M.; Ferrández-Pastor, F.J.; Valdivieso-Sarabia, R.J.; Mora-Pascual, J.; García-Chamizo, J.M. A vision based proposal for classification of normal and abnormal gait using RGB camera. *J. Biomed. Inform.* **2016**, *63*, 82–89. [CrossRef] [PubMed]

25. Nieto-Hidalgo, M.; Ferrández-Pastor, F.J.; Valdivieso-Sarabia, R.J.; Mora-Pascual, J.; García-Chamizo, J.M. Vision based gait analysis for frontal view gait sequences using rgb camera. In Proceedings of the International Conference on Ubiquitous Computing and Ambient Intelligence, Las Palmas Gran Canaria, Spain, 29 November–2 December 2016; Springer: Cham, Switzerland, 2016.

26. Serrano, M.M.; Chen, Y.P.; Howard, A.; Vela, P.A. Automated feet detection for clinical gait assessment. In Proceedings of the IEEE 38th Annual International Conference of the Engineering in Medicine and Biology Society, Orlando, FL, USA, 16–20 August 2016.

27. Nieto-Hidalgo, M.; Ferrández-Pastor, F.J.; Valdivieso-Sarabia, R.J.; Mora-Pascual, J.; García-Chamizo, J.M. Vision based extraction of dynamic gait features focused on feet movement using RGB camera. In *Ambient Intelligence for Health*; Springer: Cham, Switzerland, 2015.

28. Krishnan, R.; Sivarathinabala, M.; Abirami, S. Abnormal gait detection using lean and ramp angle features. In *Computational Intelligence in Data Mining—Volume 1*; Springer: New Delhi, India, 2016.

29. Nguyen, T.N.; Huynh, H.H.; Meunier, J. Extracting silhouette-based characteristics for human gait analysis using one camera. In Proceedings of the Fifth Symposium on Information and Communication Technology, Hanoi, Viet Nam, 4–5 December 2014; ACM: New York, NY, USA, 2014.

30. Bauckhage, C.; Tsotsos, J.K.; Bunn, F.E. Automatic detection of abnormal gait. *Image Vis. Comput.* **2009**, *27*, 108–115. [CrossRef]

31. Stuberg, W.A.; Colerick, V.L.; Blanke, D.J.; Bruce, W. Comparison of a clinical gait analysis method using videography and temporal-distance measures with 16-mm cinematography. *Phys. Ther.* **1988**, *68*, 1221–1225. [PubMed]

32. Zivkovic, Z.; Van Der Heijden, F. Efficient adaptive density estimation per image pixel for the task of background subtraction. *Pattern Recognit. Lett.* **2006**, *27*, 773–780. [CrossRef]

33. Verlekar, T.T.; Soares, L.D.; Correia, P.L. Gait recognition in the wild using shadow silhouettes. *Image Vis. Comput.* **2018**, *76*, 1–13. [CrossRef]

34. Choudhury, S.D.; Tjahjadi, T. Silhouette-based gait recognition using Procrustes shape analysis and elliptic Fourier descriptors. *Pattern Recognit.* **2012**, *45*, 3414–3426. [CrossRef]

35. Otsu, N. A threshold selection method from gray-level histograms. *IEEE Trans. Syst. Man Cybern.* **1979**, *9*, 62–66. [CrossRef]

36. Shannon, C.E. A mathematical theory of communication. *ACM SIGMOBILE Mob. Comput. Commun. Rev.* **2001**, *5*, 3–55. [CrossRef]

37. Chatfield, C. *The Analysis of Time Series: An Introduction*; Chapman & Hall: New York, NY, USA, 1989.

38. Allwein, E.L.; Schapire, R.E.; Singer, Y. Reducing multiclass to binary: A unifying approach for margin classifiers. *J. Mach. Learn. Res.* **2000**, *1*, 113–141.
39. Taborri, J.; Scalona, E.; Rossi, S.; Palermo, E.; Patanè, F.; Cappa, P. Real-time gait detection based on Hidden Markov Model: Is it possible to avoid training procedure? In Proceedings of the MeMeA, Turin, Italy, 7–9 May 2015; pp. 141–145.

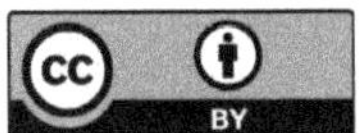

© 2018 by the authors. Licensee MDPI, Basel, Switzerland. This article is an open access article distributed under the terms and conditions of the Creative Commons Attribution (CC BY) license (http://creativecommons.org/licenses/by/4.0/).

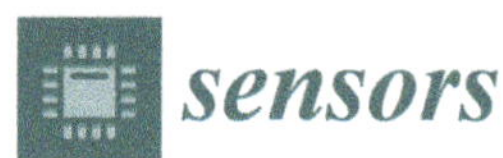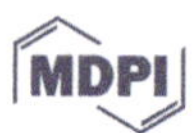

Article

Wearable Sensor Data to Track Subject-Specific Movement Patterns Related to Clinical Outcomes Using a Machine Learning Approach

Dylan Kobsar [1,*] **and Reed Ferber** [1,2,3]

1   Faculty of Kinesiology, University of Calgary, 2500 University Dr NW, Calgary, AB T2N 1N4, Canada; rferber@ucalgary.ca
2   Running Injury Clinic, Calgary, AB T2N 1N4, Canada
3   Faculty of Nursing, University of Calgary, Calgary, AB T2N 1N4, Canada
*   Correspondence: dylan.kobsar@ucalgary.ca

Received: 27 June 2018; Accepted: 23 August 2018; Published: 27 August 2018

Abstract: Wearable sensors can provide detailed information on human movement but the clinical impact of this information remains limited. We propose a machine learning approach, using wearable sensor data, to identify subject-specific changes in gait patterns related to improvements in clinical outcomes. Eight patients with knee osteoarthritis (OA) completed two gait trials before and one following an exercise intervention. Wearable sensor data (e.g., 3-dimensional (3D) linear accelerations) were collected from a sensor located near the lower back, lateral thigh and lateral shank during level treadmill walking at a preferred speed. Wearable sensor data from the 2 pre-intervention gait trials were used to define each individual's typical movement pattern using a one-class support vector machine (OCSVM). The percentage of strides defined as outliers, based on the pre-intervention gait data and the OCSVM, were used to define the overall change in an individual's movement pattern. The correlation between the change in movement patterns following the intervention (i.e., percentage of outliers) and improvement in self-reported clinical outcomes (e.g., pain and function) was assessed using a Spearman rank correlation. The number of outliers observed post-intervention exhibited a large association (ρ = 0.78) with improvements in self-reported clinical outcomes. These findings demonstrate a proof-of-concept and a novel methodological approach for integrating machine learning and wearable sensor data. This approach provides an objective and evidence-informed way to understand clinically important changes in human movement patterns in response to exercise therapy.

Keywords: accelerometer; machine learning; pattern recognition; sensors; gait; clinical; knee; osteoarthritis

---

1. Introduction

As wearable sensors become more and more ubiquitous in today's world, so does their use in human movement analysis. Given their size, affordability and ease of use, wearable inertial sensors can provide a clinically accessible alternative to more expensive conventional three-dimensional (3D) motion capture systems [1]. A further advantage of these devices is that they can be placed at variety of body locations (e.g., wrist, torso, lower limbs, etc.) and collect data continuously over many strides both in and outside of a laboratory or clinical setting [2]. However, a fundamental problem in collecting data from multiple sensors over long periods of time is that datasets quickly become exceedingly large, complex, and, most importantly, clinically uninterpretable. To counter this problem, many clinical investigations have examined simple wearable sensor outputs such as gait speed, step times and other discrete variables [3–5]. Nevertheless, there remains a vast amount of data being created by today's wearable sensors that goes unanalyzed and may itself hold the key to answering important clinical questions [6]. Therefore, there is a need to develop more sophisticated and complex methods to extract, process and present this data in clinically meaningful ways [6–9].

Perhaps the most promising way to utilize the vast amounts of data generated by modern wearable sensors is the field of machine learning [6]. Machine learning involves the integration of statistics and computer science to identify patterns in large datasets [10]. These pattern recognition tools provide the opportunity to quickly process and compare large wearable sensor datasets between or within different clinical populations or subgroups [11–15]. While group-based models can be effective in identifying clinically relevant differences in gait between individuals, there remain a number of important limitations. Most notably, group-based models require the curation of datasets that contain a large number of subjects to externally validate a model [16]. In the world of clinical gait biomechanics, even with the support of wearable sensors, recruiting and testing large numbers of patients can be difficult or impractical. Moreover, with the large amount of heterogeneity in some clinical populations (e.g., osteoarthritis; OA [17]), this becomes even more difficult.

Alternatively, subject-specific models can be used to identify gait patterns and track changes within a single patient. Used in conjunction with wearable sensors collecting data over hundreds or thousands of individual gait cycles, these subject-specific models have demonstrated the ability to outperform group-based models in identifying clinically relevant changes in gait [18,19]. A unique approach to this model is the application of a one-class classification algorithm, wherein the machine learning algorithm attempts to define the multivariate properties or boundaries for a typical observation in the dataset [20]. When applied to a gait pattern, this approach can define the current state of a subject's gait pattern and, in turn, identify changes or outliers from the original pattern. Moreover, this method can do this without the need for additional training data from conditions that may be currently unknown or yet to exist (e.g., individual data on future injury states or rehabilitation outcomes). Research has examined the ability of similar, subject-specific one-class models to identify typical gait patterns in cattle [21] and, more notably, deviations from baseline human gait patterns when perturbed by a knee brace [22]. However, to our knowledge no research has examined the opposite proposition of identifying potentially advantageous deviations from a baseline gait pattern over the course of an intervention in a clinical population.

Therefore, the objective of this research was to establish a proof-of-concept of a subject-specific one-class model's ability to identify clinically relevant changes in gait patterns over the course of rehabilitation. Specifically, our research question was: are changes in gait patterns correlated with clinical improvements following a 6-week exercise intervention in knee OA patients? It was hypothesized that patients who benefited most from the exercise intervention (i.e., improvements in self-reported pain, function, etc.) would also demonstrate the greatest changes in their gait patterns (i.e., increased percentage of outlier gait cycles) following the intervention, as assessed by a Spearman's rank correlation ($\alpha < 0.05$).

2. Methods

2.1. Subjects

A subset of 8 knee OA patients (Sex: 4F/4M, Age: 58 (5) years, Body Mass Index: 25.3 (4.8) kg/m^2, walking speed: 1.1 (0.15) m/s) were analyzed from a larger exercise intervention [11]. These patients were selected for the current analysis as they completed two baseline gait trials before the intervention, as well as one gait trial post-intervention. All participants were required to be radiographically diagnosed with knee OA and able to walk without assistive devices. For additional inclusion and exclusion criteria see Kobsar et al., 2017 [11]. This study was approved by the Conjoint Health Research Ethics Board at the University of Calgary (E-22417: Approved 14 June 2014) and all participants provided written, informed consent prior to participating.

2.2. Protocol

Participants completed two baseline gait trials on different days, within one week of beginning the exercise intervention. In each session, participants wore four wearable inertial sensors (iNEMO inertial module, STmicroelectronics, Geneva, Switzerland) securely fastened to their lower back (approximately the L3 vertebrae), lateral thigh, lateral shank and dorsum of the foot on the most affected leg. See Figure 1. In order to safeguard against potentially high impact accelerations at the foot, the highest accelerometer and gyroscope range setting (acceleration range ±16 g, gyroscope range $\pm2000°$/s, sampling rate 100 Hz) was used for the foot sensor. Further, the same range settings were selected across all remaining sensors to maintain data consistency. While all four sensors collected both linear acceleration and angular velocity data, only linear acceleration data from the three most proximal sensors (i.e., lower back, thigh and shank) were used for modeling the subject-specific gait patterns. The fourth sensor on the dorsum of the foot was used solely for gait event detection, to be discussed in the following section.

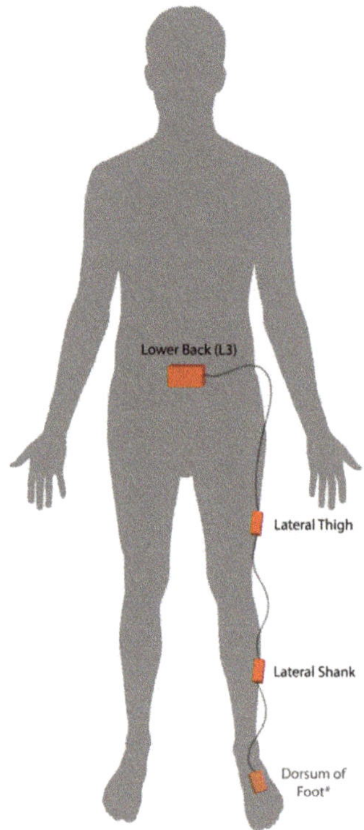

Figure 1. Placement of inertial sensors on the most affected side of knee osteoarthritis patients. * Sensor on the dorsum of the foot was only used for event detection and gait cycle segmentation.

All participants walked on a level treadmill (Bertec, Columbus, OH, USA) for a short acclimatization period at a self-selected pace, before 2.5 min of data were collected. A trial length of 2.5 min was used to obtain a minimum of 100 gait cycles per session, as this has been a recommended for similar machine learning analyses [23]. The same protocol and self-selected pace were used during the post-intervention gait trial. Participants also completed a Knee injury and Osteoarthritis Outcome Score (KOOS) before and after the intervention to assess changes, if any, in self-reported pain, symptoms, function in daily living and knee related quality of life following the intervention [24].

The exercise intervention itself was a 6-week therapist-directed, hip-focused muscle strengthening intervention detailed in Kobsar et al., 2017 [11].

2.3. Data Analysis

2.3.1. Pre-Processing

Linear acceleration data underwent a static attitude correction to align each sensor with the global vertical and horizontal planes [25,26]. Following this correction, all 3D linear acceleration and angular velocity data were filtered with a 10 Hz low-pass 4th order recursive Butterworth filter. The angular velocity data of the foot sensor was used to determine gait events (e.g., initial contact and toe-off) in a manner previously validated [26–28]. Specifically, initial contact and toe-off events were determined as the zero-crossing preceding stance and the negative peak following stance in the angular velocity signals about mediolateral axis, respectively. These gait events allowed for gait cycle segmentation and time-normalization of all sensor data (e.g., 60 points for stance; 40 points for swing). Three-dimensional linear accelerations were concatenated within each sensor (i.e., 3 axes $\times$ 100 data points combined to a 1 $\times$ 300 vector) and across all 3 sensors (i.e., 1 $\times$ 300 vectors from back, thigh and shank sensors combined) to form a 1 $\times$ 900 vector which defined the overall movement pattern for each individual gait cycle. Finally, the linear acceleration data from each gait trial were stored in an m $\times$ 900 matrix, where "m" equals the number of gait cycles recorded during the 2.5 min of data collection. The average number of gait cycles per session was 135 (10).

2.3.2. Data Reduction and Feature Selection

Prior to computing the boundaries of the subject-specific one-class model, the 900 point vectors defining each gait cycle were reduced to a set of principal components (PCs). To do so, data from both baseline gait trials were combined, resulting in an average of 270 gait cycles collected over 5 min of walking data. These data were then standardized to a mean of 0 and a standard deviation of 1, before being transformed into linearly uncorrelated PCs using a principal component analysis [11,29]. The PCs that explained at least 95% of the total variance in the original data were selected as features for the algorithm [30]. Therefore, the scores on these PCs across all baseline gait cycles were used as the features to define the overall gait pattern of a subject. Given that this was a subject-specific model, a total of 8 principal component analyses were conducted on baseline data (i.e., one for each subject). Therefore, each patient had their own unique set of gait features to be used in modeling their gait pattern. Post-intervention data were reduced and features (i.e., PC scores) were computed in the same manner as the baseline. This procedure involved utilizing the data reduction outputs generated from the baseline data (i.e., mean, standard deviation and PC loading coefficients) to ensure the post-intervention PC scores were appropriately aligned with their corresponding baseline data.

2.3.3. Defining Subject-Specific One-Class Models

Subject-specific, one-class models were defined using baseline gait features (i.e., reduced PC scores) in conjunction with a one-class support vector machine (OCSVM). The OCSVM requires only one example, or class of data (i.e., positive cases), which are used to maximize the space between these data and the origin in high-dimensional feature space [31,32]. In essence, this approach attempts to define and minimize a hypersphere wherein most of the data are found and thereby define a "typical" observation or gait cycle data set. This decision boundary can then be used as a classifier to determine if new data fits within this hypersphere (i.e., positive case or "typical" gait cycle) or outside of this hypersphere (i.e., negative case, "atypical," or outlier gait cycle) [33]. This method has been shown to be successful in detecting outlier cases across a number of different machine learning applications [20,33–35]. In the current investigation, we used "fitcsvm," available from Matlab (The MathWorks Inc., Natick, MA, USA), which utilizes the algorithm defined by Schölkopf et al. [31,32]. The boundary definition for this classifier was trained using the baseline features retained following the above-mentioned data reduction technique (i.e., PC scores depicting 95% of total variance). The training of this boundary was done using a Gaussian kernel function, in combination with a "ν" parameter for regularization. This parameter was chosen based on the value that achieved less than 1% outliers in a randomly selected 20% cross-validation set from baseline data. In other words, the OCSVM decision boundary was set wide enough to include 99% of the baseline gait cycles and thereby define a "typical" gait cycle data set. It should also be noted that to ensure the method was entirely subject-specific, this regularization parameter definition was conducted separately within each individual. Finally, post-intervention data were tested to determine the percentage of gait cycles that were defined as outliers given the baseline-derived multivariate boundary threshold.

Two simplified visualizations of this boundary definition, using only 2 PCs, are shown in Figure 2. Figure 2A shows an example where no post-intervention gait cycles fell outside the baseline-defined OCSVM boundary (i.e., 0% outliers), suggesting no change in gait patterns following the intervention. Alternatively, in Figure 2B, a large number of post-intervention gait cycles fell outside the baseline-defined OCSVM boundary (i.e., approximately 30% outliers), suggesting the patient's gait pattern has changed in response to the intervention. However, it should again be noted that the OCSVM boundary and subsequent results were based on a high-dimensional PC space for each subject. Alternatively, these examples in Figure 2 represent only a 2-dimensional sub-space for ease of visualization and understanding.

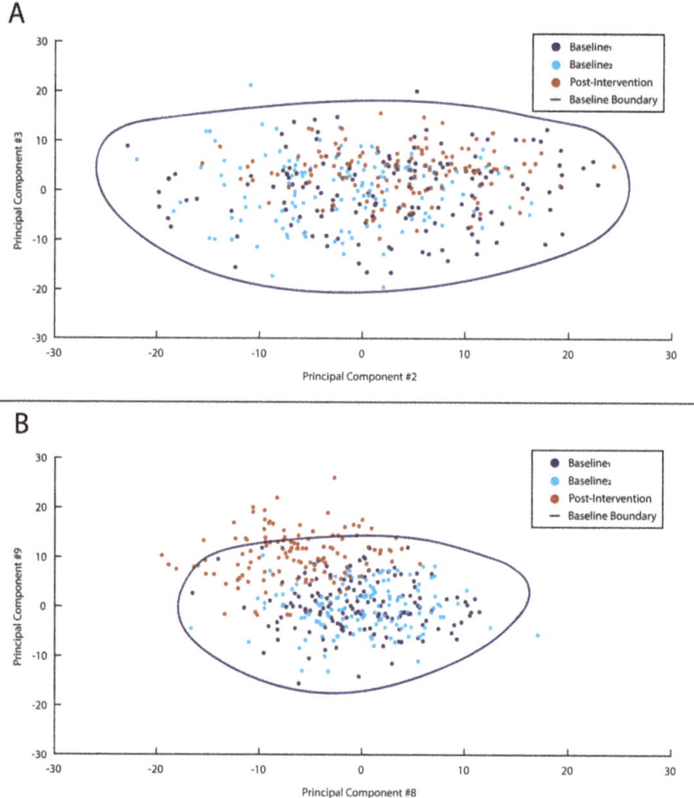

Figure 2. Simplified visualizations of boundary definitions (blue line) defined by baseline data (dark blue and light blue circles) and tested on post-intervention data (red circles). In example (**A**), no post-intervention gait cycles are defined as outliers, while in example (**B**) approximately 30% are viewed as outliers.

2.3.4. Statistical Analysis

The primary variables of interest were: (i) percentage of gait cycles defined as outliers in the post-intervention gait trial; and (ii) average improvement in self-reported subscales of pain, symptoms, function in daily living and knee related quality of life (i.e., post-intervention scores—baseline scores). A non-parametric correlation, Spearman's rank correlation (ρ), was used to assess the association between these two variables. A correlation of 0.10–0.29, 0.30–0.49 and 0.5+ were interpreted as small, medium and large, respectively [36]. Any subjects that reported no change or negative change were assessed as a zero-net change, based on the purpose of identifying the relationship of gait pattern deviation to clinical improvements.

3. Results

The average number of PCs retained to describe 95% of the total variance in each subject was 84 (5). The average percentage of gait cycles defined as outliers in the 20% cross-validated baseline data and post-intervention gait trial data were 0.5 (0.4)% and 17.7 (17.1)%, respectively. The best regularization parameters (v) selected for the single-subject boundary thresholds were found to range between 0.1–0.8, with an average value of 0.4 (0.3). The percentage of outlier gait cycles in the post-intervention gait session achieved a large association ($\rho = 0.78$; $p = 0.02$) with the improvement in self-reported clinical outcomes following the intervention. This association, with non-parametric (Spearman rank correlation; ρ) and parametric coefficients (Pearson's correlation; r), is visualized using a scatter plot in Figure 3.

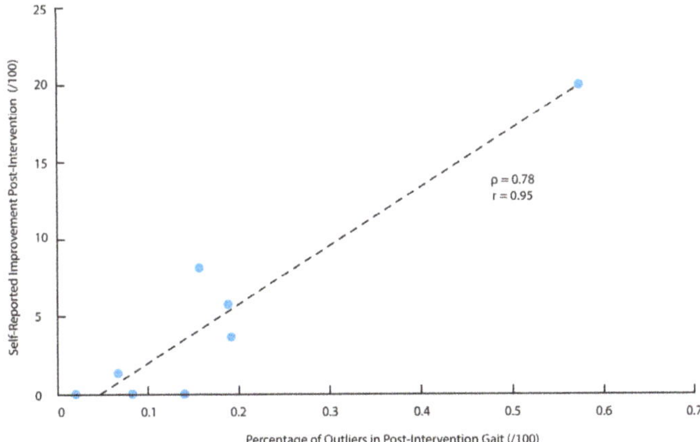

Figure 3. The percentage of outlier in post-intervention data displayed a large association with the self-reported improvement in post-intervention (i.e., change in Knee Injury Osteoarthritis Outcome Scores subscales): Spearman rank correlation (ρ) = 0.78 and Pearson correlation coefficient (r) = 0.95.

4. Discussion

The purpose of this study was to establish a proof-of-concept for the use of a machine learning approach for assessing patient-specific changes in gait following an exercise therapy intervention. In support of our hypothesis, patients who benefited most from the exercise intervention also demonstrated the greatest overall change in gait patterns, as defined by the single-subject OCSVM models. This finding was demonstrated by the significant association ($\rho = 0.78$; $p = 0.02$) between the percentage of outlier gait cycles observed in post-intervention gait and clinical outcome improvement. In the context of previous univariate models examining the association of changes in muscle strength ($r^2 = 0.28$–0.31; [37]) or pain sensitization ($\rho = 0.28$–0.35; [38]) to changes in self-reported outcomes in knee OA patients following exercise, the current association is comparatively large. To our knowledge, this is the first study to integrate pattern recognition algorithms with wearable technology to define objective, subject-specific biomechanical outcomes related to clinical improvements. Moreover, the current findings support the recent recommendation of utilizing subject-specific models in wearable sensor research [19].

In general, these findings are in accordance with a similar subject-specific one-class model approach used by Cola et al. [22], however there are a number of important distinctions. First, Cola et al. [22] examined artificially prescribed gait perturbations in healthy subjects to identify negative deviations from their "typical" gait patterns. In contrast, the current study introduced a 6-week exercise intervention to identify presumably positive deviations from a knee OA patient's "typical" pattern. In addition to the contrasting clinical application, there remain a number of differences in the method itself, such as; (i) the number of sensors used (3 vs. 1), (ii) the number of days used to train baseline patterns (2 vs. 1) and (iii) the algorithm to define typical patterns (SVM vs. k-means). However, perhaps the most important distinction between the current study and that of Cola et al. [22] is the manner in which the features and threshold parameters were selected. Specifically, the work by Cole et al. [22] introduced gait perturbations in a controlled and standardized manner, which afforded the authors the ability to deliberately select the best features (i.e., 11 gait variables out of 43 total) and threshold parameters for identifying these perturbations in future gait data collections. While this a priori knowledge of the gait perturbations may be appropriate for identifying a known or consistent gait perturbation, it is not possible in clinical practice where the potential change is unknown. Alternatively, the current study uses a completely unsupervised approach, with no a priori feature selection or information of how a patient's gait may or may not change. In doing so, we were able to define a holistic and objective measure of subject-specific changes in gait mechanics following an exercise intervention, something rarely seen in previous OA research.

While exercise interventions have consistently demonstrated improvements in the pain and function of knee OA patients, identifying concomitant changes in gait patterns has been rarely reported using conventional group-based methods [39–42]. Given that much of this research has examined single, discrete variables (e.g., knee adduction moment), the sensitivity of this type of univariate statistical approaches is questionable [17]. In contrast, the current study supports previous research suggesting examining multivariate and/or multi-segment changes may better quantify the overall biomechanical changes that occur after an exercise intervention [43,44]. Nevertheless, these multivariate changes often remain limited when assessed in conventional group-based analyses [44]. This further suggests that exercise interventions may not elicit any consistent change in gait patterns, univariate or multivariate, across heterogeneous diseases such as knee OA [39–42]. Therefore, a significant strength of the current study is the introduction of an alternative, single-subject model to track multivariate, multi-segment changes in gait biomechanics. Further, this approach is directly aligned with the ongoing shift towards precision medicine and personalized treatment approaches [45,46].

Given the complex nature of the proposed analysis, it becomes increasingly important to concentrate on ways to translate this information to the clinician and patient in a relevant and meaningful manner. The first and most simplistic way to translate this information is in the form of a percentage score from 0% to 100%, with 0% being no change in gait pattern and 100% being a complete change in overall gait pattern. In this instance, the output becomes easily interpretable but a somewhat black box assessment of the overall change. Alternatively, these holistic changes in gait patterns could be further stratified into sensors/segments and planes of movement to identify which sensors and axes were most important in driving the overall change, similar to Phinyomark et al. [47]. Finally, a more conventional waveform analysis could be used to examine the specific changes that may have occurred in relation to the baseline boundary. A brief representative example of this analysis is presented in Figure 4. In this example, while the thigh sensor appears to contain the most important changes for this individual, it is evident that there are a number of multi-segment changes occurring as well. Although many of these changes appear subtle, it remains unclear whether such changes accumulating over thousands of gait cycles per day may relate to a clinically important change in the mechanical loading of the knee joint. Therefore, the current study remains a proof-of-concept approach assessing this novel evidence-informed approach.

Further work is required to develop highly specific and clinically relevant data visualizations and outcomes, as well as relating these biomechanical outcomes to long-term disease progression.

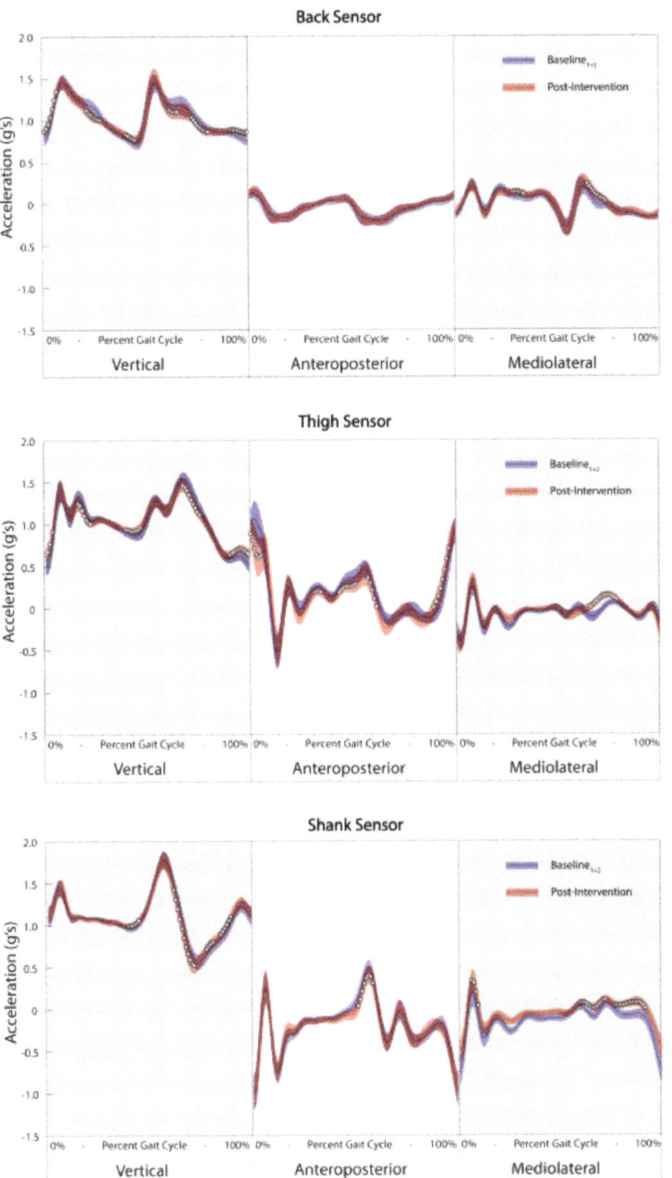

Figure 4. Example of waveform analysis of three-dimensional linear accelerations from the back (**top**), thigh (**middle**) and shank (**bottom**) visualizing changes in post-intervention data (red line) compared to baseline data (blue line). Data is presented from the patient who demonstrated the greatest number of gait cycle outliers post-intervention. White circles represent areas of the waveform where differences between baseline and post-intervention data are statistically significant (Holm-Bonferroni corrected *p*-value of less than 0.05) and have a large effect size (Cohen's d > 0.8).

Limitations and Future Directions

As is with any proof-of-concept study, there are a number of important limitations that must be discussed and addressed in future research. First, the sample size for this study was relatively small. Nevertheless, given the subject-specific model utilized the analysis, the limited sample size would only have affected strength of the relationship between gait cycle outliers and clinical improvements across the patients. However, it would not influence the fit of any individual models themselves and thus there is no increased risk of overfitting related to the sample size. To this point, additional subjects would be beneficial in filling out the space in Figure 3 but would not change the current position of any data points in the space. Second, two baseline trials, amassing a total of 5 min of walking data with an average of 270 gait cycles, were used to train each subject's typical pattern. Given the highly controlled data collection environment, gait cycles collected over two separate days were thought to be sufficient in order to account for any potential between-day errors or variability. Nevertheless, future research should examine the impact of including more than 2 days of gait data as this will likely become more important in less controlled gait assessment protocols. Another potential limitation is the amount of data collected and utilized for the analysis (i.e., continuous waveform data from three sensors). While on-board preprocessing would likely provide the most efficient management of data, based on our previous research the limiting factor in this may be the event detection itself [48]. Nevertheless, this topic remains outside the scope of the current proof-of-concept study and future work may look to examine the most efficient ways preprocess and package the data for analysis. Lastly, our data was filtered with a 10 Hz low-pass filter as we were primarily interested in the overall pattern of gait, rather than high frequency impact accelerations or vibrations. Future research may look to include additional frequency-based parameters in their analysis to further define potential changes in gait.

5. Conclusions

The current study demonstrates a successful proof-of-concept for the use of a subject-specific one-class model for identifying individualized changes in gait patterns in response to an exercise intervention. The changes in gait patterns observed with this method were found to be associated with improvements in self-reported clinical measures, following the 6-week rehabilitation protocol. Therefore, this novel method effectively integrates machine learning and wearable technology to provide an objective and evidence-informed way to understand clinically important changes in human movement patterns.

Author Contributions: Conceptualization, D.K. and R.F.; Data curation, D.K.; Formal analysis, D.K.; Methodology, D.K.; Supervision, R.F.; Writing-original draft, D.K.; Writing-review & editing, D.K. and R.F.

Funding: We would like to thank Alberta Innovates—Health Solutions (20140433) and the Canadian Institutes of Health Research (GSD-128743) for their funding support.

Acknowledgments: The authors would like to thank our research coordinators Karen Pulsifer and Jill Baxter, as well as all participants who so generously gave their time to be involved in this study.

Conflicts of Interest: The authors declare no conflict of interest. The funding sponsors had no role in the design of the study; in the collection, analyses, or interpretation of data; in the writing of the manuscript and in the decision to publish the results.

References

1. Tao, W.; Liu, T.; Zheng, R.; Feng, H. Gait analysis using wearable sensors. *Sensors* **2012**, *12*, 2255–2283. [CrossRef] [PubMed]
2. Shull, P.B.; Jirattigalachote, W.; Hunt, M.A.; Cutkosky, M.R.; Delp, S.L. Quantified self and human movement: A review on the clinical impact of wearable sensing and feedback for gait analysis and intervention. *Gait Posture* **2014**, *40*, 11–19. [CrossRef] [PubMed]
3. Zhang, H.; Yan, S.; Fang, C.; Guo, X.; Zhang, K. Clinical evaluation and gait characteristics before and after yotal knee arthroplasty based on a portable gait analyzer. *Orthop. Surg.* **2016**, *8*, 360–366. [CrossRef] [PubMed]

4. Barrois, R.; Gregory, T.; Oudre, L.; Moreau, T.; Truong, C.; Pulini, A.A.; Vienne, A.; Labourdette, C.; Vayatis, N.; Buffat, S.; et al. An automated recording method in clinical consultation to rate the limp in lower limb osteoarthritis. *PLoS ONE* **2016**, *11*, e0164975. [CrossRef] [PubMed]

5. Pau, M.; Caggiari, S.; Mura, A.; Corona, F.; Leban, B.; Coghe, G.; Lorefice, L.; Marrosu, M.G.; Cocco, E. Clinical assessment of gait in individuals with multiple sclerosis using wearable inertial sensors: Comparison with patient-based measure. *Mult. Scler. Relat. Disord.* **2016**, *10*, 187–191. [CrossRef] [PubMed]

6. Ferber, R.; Osis, S.T.; Hicks, J.L.; Delp, S.L. Gait biomechanics in the era of data science. *J. Biomech.* **2016**, *49*, 3759–3761. [CrossRef] [PubMed]

7. Gregory, C.M.; Embry, A.; Perry, L.; Bowden, M.G. Quantifying human movement across the continuum of care: From lab to clinic to community. *J. Neurosci. Methods* **2014**, *231*, 18–21. [CrossRef] [PubMed]

8. Cohen, S.; Bataille, L.R.; Martig, A.K. Enabling breakthroughs in Parkinson's disease with wearable technologies and big data analytics. *Mhealth* **2016**, *2*, 20. [CrossRef] [PubMed]

9. Chen, S.; Lach, J.; Lo, B.; Yang, G.Z. Toward pervasive gait analysis with wearable sensors: A systematic review. *IEEE J. Biomed. Health Inform.* **2016**, *20*, 1521–1537. [CrossRef] [PubMed]

10. Deo, R.C. Machine learning in medicine. *Circulation* **2015**, *132*, 1920–1930. [CrossRef] [PubMed]

11. Kobsar, D.; Osis, S.T.; Boyd, J.E.; Hettinga, B.A.; Ferber, R. Wearable sensors to predict improvement following an exercise intervention in patients with knee osteoarthritis. *J. Neuroeng. Rehabil.* **2017**, *14*, 94. [CrossRef] [PubMed]

12. Mannini, A.; Trojaniello, D.; Cereatti, A.; Sabatini, A.M. A machine learning framework for gait classification using inertial sensors: Application to elderly, post-stroke and huntington's disease patients. *Sensors* **2016**, *16*, 134. [CrossRef] [PubMed]

13. Palmerini, L.; Rocchi, L.; Mazilu, S.; Gazit, E.; Hausdorff, J.M.; Chiari, L. Identification of characteristic motor patterns preceding freezing of gait in Parkinson's disease using wearable sensors. *Front. Neurol.* **2017**, *8*, 1–12. [CrossRef] [PubMed]

14. Drover, D.; Howcroft, J.; Kofman, J.; Lemaire, E.D. Faller classification in older adults using wearable sensors based on turn and straight-walking accelerometer-based features. *Sensors* **2017**, *17*, 321. [CrossRef] [PubMed]

15. Riaz, Q.; Vögele, A.; Krüger, B.; Weber, A. One small step for a man: Estimation of gender, age and height from recordings of one step by a single inertial sensor. *Sensors* **2015**, *15*, 31999–32019. [CrossRef] [PubMed]

16. Lubetzky-Vilnai, A.; Ciol, M.; McCoy, S.W. Statistical analysis of clinical prediction rules for rehabilitation interventions: Current state of the literature. *Arch. Phys. Med. Rehabil.* **2014**, *95*, 188–196. [CrossRef] [PubMed]

17. Mills, K.; Hunt, M.A.; Ferber, R. Biomechanical deviations during level walking associated with knee osteoarthritis: A systematic review and meta-analysis. *Arthritis Care Res. (Hoboken)* **2013**, *65*, 1643–1665. [CrossRef] [PubMed]

18. Rodríguez-Martín, D.; Samà, A.; Pérez-López, C.; Català, A.; Arostegui, J.M.M.; Cabestany, J.; Bayés, À.; Alcaine, S.; Mestre, B.; Prats, A.; et al. Home detection of freezing of gait using Support Vector Machines through a single waist-worn triaxial accelerometer. *PLoS ONE* **2017**, *12*, e0171764. [CrossRef] [PubMed]

19. Benson, L.C.; Clermont, C.A.; Bošnjak, E.; Ferber, R. The use of wearable devices for walking and running gait analysis outside of the lab: A systematic review. *Gait Posture* **2018**, *63*, 124–138. [CrossRef] [PubMed]

20. Mourão-Miranda, J.; Hardoon, D.R.; Hahn, T.; Marquand, A.F.; Williams, S.C.R.; Shawe-Taylor, J.; Brammer, M. Patient classification as an outlier detection problem: An application of the One-Class Support Vector Machine. *Neuroimage* **2011**, *58*, 793–804. [CrossRef] [PubMed]

21. Haladjian, J.; Haug, J.; Nüske, S.; Bruegge, B. A wearable sensor system for lameness detection in dairy cattle. *Multimodal Technol. Interact.* **2018**, *2*, 27. [CrossRef]

22. Cola, G.; Avvenuti, M.; Vecchio, A.; Yang, G.Z.; Lo, B. An on-node processing approach for anomaly detection in gait. *IEEE Sens. J.* **2015**, *15*, 6640–6649. [CrossRef]

23. Mundfrom, D.J.; Shaw, D.G.; Ke, T.L. Minimum Sample Size Recommendations for Conducting Factor Analyses. *Int. J. Test.* **2005**, *5*, 159–168. [CrossRef]

24. Roos, E.M.; Roos, H.P.; Lohmander, L.S.; Ekdahl, C.; Beynnon, B.D. Knee Injury and Osteoarthritis Outcome Score (KOOS)—Development of a self-administered outcome measure. *J. Orthop. Sports Phys. Ther.* **1998**, *28*, 88–96. [CrossRef] [PubMed]

25. Tundo, M.D.; Lemaire, E.; Baddour, N. Correcting Smartphone orientation for accelerometer-based analysis. In Proceedings of the 2013 IEEE International Symposium on Medical Measurements and Applications (MeMeA), Gatineau, QC, Canada, 4–5 May 2013; pp. 58–62. [CrossRef]

26. Kobsar, D.; Osis, S.T.; Phinyomark, A.; Boyd, J.E.; Ferber, R. Reliability of gait analysis using wearable sensors in patients with knee osteoarthritis. *J. Biomech.* **2016**, *49*, 3977–3982. [CrossRef] [PubMed]

27. Fraccaro, P.; Walsh, L.; Doyle, J.; O'Sullivan, D. Real-world gyroscope-based gait event detection and gait feature extraction. In Proceedings of the eTELEMED—The Sixth International Conference on eHealth, Telemedicine, and Social Medicine, Barcelona, Spain, 24–27 March 2014.

28. Rampp, A.; Barth, J.; Schuelein, S.; Gassmann, K.-G.; Klucken, J.; Eskofier, B.M. Inertial Sensor-Based Stride Parameter Calculation From Gait Sequences in Geriatric Patients. *IEEE Trans. Biomed. Eng.* **2015**, *62*, 1089–1097. [CrossRef] [PubMed]

29. Deluzio, K.J.; Astephen, J.L. Biomechanical features of gait waveform data associated with knee osteoarthritis: An application of principal component analysis. *Gait Posture* **2007**, *25*, 86–93. [CrossRef] [PubMed]

30. Nigg, B.M.; Baltich, J.; Maurer, C.; Federolf, P. Shoe midsole hardness, sex and age effects on lower extremity kinematics during running. *J. Biomech.* **2012**, *45*, 1692–1697. [CrossRef] [PubMed]

31. Schölkopf, B.; Platt, J.C.; Shawe-Taylor, J.; Smola, A.J.; Williamson, R.C. Estimating the Support of a High-Dimensional Distribution. *Neural Comput.* **2001**, *13*, 1443–1471. [CrossRef] [PubMed]

32. Schölkopf, B.; Williamson, R.; Smola, A.; Shawe-Taylor, J.; Platt, J. Support vector method for novelty detection. In Proceedings of the 12th International Conference on Neural Information Processing Systems (NIPS'99), Cambridge, MA, USA, 29 November–4 December 1999.

33. Zhang, X.; Gu, C.; Lin, J. Support vector machines for anomaly detection. In Proceedings of the 2006 6th World Congress on Intelligent Control and Automation, Dalian, China, 21–23 June 2006.

34. Lukashevich, H.; Nowak, S.; Dunker, P. Using one-class SVM outliers detection for verification of collaboratively tagged image training sets. In Proceedings of the 2009 IEEE International Conference on Multimedia and Expo, New York, NY, USA, 28 June–3 July 2009.

35. Guerbai, Y.; Chibani, Y.; Hadjadji, B. The effective use of the one-class SVM classifier for handwritten signature verification based on writer-independent parameters. *Pattern Recognit.* **2015**, *48*, 103–113. [CrossRef]

36. Cohen, J. *Statistical Power Analysis for the Behavioral Sciences*; Lawrence Erlbaum: New Jersey, NJ, USA, 1988; ISBN 978-0-12-179060-8.

37. Bokaeian, H.R.; Bakhtiary, A.H.; Mirmohammadkhani, M.; Moghimi, J. Quadriceps strengthening exercises may not change pain and function in knee osteoarthritis. *J. Bodyw. Mov. Ther.* **2018**, *22*, 528–533. [CrossRef] [PubMed]

38. Henriksen, M.; Klokker, L.; Graven-Nielsen, T.; Bartholdy, C.; Schjødt Jørgensen, T.; Bandak, E.; Danneskiold-Samsøe, B.; Christensen, R.; Bliddal, H. Association of exercise therapy and reduction of pain sensitivity in patients with knee osteoarthritis: A randomized controlled trial. *Arthritis Care Res. (Hoboken)* **2014**, *66*, 1836–1843. [CrossRef] [PubMed]

39. Henriksen, M.; Klokker, L.; Bartholdy, C.; Schjoedt-Jorgensen, T.; Bandak, E.; Bliddal, H. No effects of functional exercise therapy on walking biomechanics in patients with knee osteoarthritis: Exploratory outcome analyses from a randomised trial. *BMJ Open Sport Exerc. Med.* **2017**, *2*. [CrossRef] [PubMed]

40. Bennell, K.L.; Kyriakides, M.; Metcalf, B.; Egerton, T.; Wrigley, T.V.; Hodges, P.W.; Hunt, M.A.; Roos, E.M.; Forbes, A.; Ageberg, E.; et al. Neuromuscular versus quadriceps strengthening exercise in patients with medial knee osteoarthritis and varus malalignment: A randomized controlled trial. *Arthritis Rheumatol.* **2014**, *66*, 950–959. [CrossRef] [PubMed]

41. Bennell, K.L.; Hunt, M.A.; Wrigley, T.V.; Hunter, D.J.; McManus, F.J.; Hodges, P.W.; Li, L.; Hinman, R.S. Hip strengthening reduces symptoms but not knee load in people with medial knee osteoarthritis and varus malalignment: A randomised controlled trial. *Osteoarthr. Cartil.* **2010**, *18*, 621–628. [CrossRef] [PubMed]

42. Sled, E.A.; Khoja, L.; Deluzio, K.J.; Olney, S.J.; Culham, E.G. Effect of a home program of hip abductor exercises on knee joint loading, strength, function, and pain in people with knee osteoarthritis: A clinical trial. *Phys. Ther.* **2010**, *90*, 895–904. [CrossRef] [PubMed]

43. Gaudreault, N.; Mezghani, N.; Turcot, K.; Hagemeister, N.; Boivin, K.; De Guise, J.A. Effects of physiotherapy treatment on knee osteoarthritis gait data using principal component analysis. *Clin. Biomech.* **2011**, *26*, 284–291. [CrossRef] [PubMed]

44. Brenneman, E.C.; Maly, M.R. Identifying changes in gait waveforms following a strengthening intervention for women with knee osteoarthritis using principal components analysis. *Gait Posture* **2018**, *59*, 286–291. [CrossRef] [PubMed]
45. Buford, T.W.; Pahor, M. Making preventive medicine more personalized: Implications for exercise-related research. *Prev. Med.* **2012**, *55*, 34–6. [CrossRef] [PubMed]
46. Karsdal, M.A.; Christiansen, C.; Ladel, C.; Henriksen, K.; Kraus, V.B.; Bay-Jensen, A.C. Osteoarthritis—A case for personalized health care? *Osteoarthr. Cartil.* **2014**, *22*, 7–16. [CrossRef] [PubMed]
47. Phinyomark, A.; Hettinga, B.A.; Osis, S.; Ferber, R. Do intermediate- and higher-order principal components contain useful information to detect subtle changes in lower extremity biomechanics during running? *Hum. Mov. Sci.* **2015**, *44*, 91–101. [CrossRef] [PubMed]
48. Benson, L.C.; Clermont, C.A.; Osis, S.T.; Kobsar, D.; Ferber, R. Classifying running speed conditions using a single wearable sensor: Optimal segmentation and feature extraction methods. *J. Biomech.* **2018**, *71*, 94–99. [CrossRef] [PubMed]

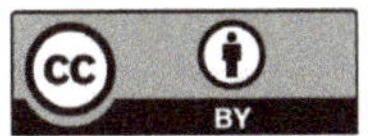

© 2018 by the authors. Licensee MDPI, Basel, Switzerland. This article is an open access article distributed under the terms and conditions of the Creative Commons Attribution (CC BY) license (http://creativecommons.org/licenses/by/4.0/).

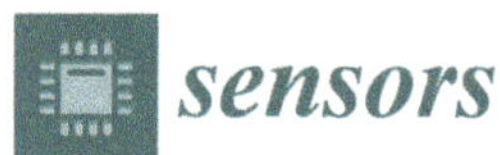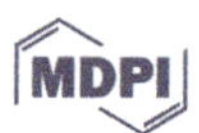

Article

Examination of the Effect of Suitable Size of Shoes under the Second Metatarsal Head and Width of Shoes under the Fifth Metatarsal Head for the Prevention of Callus Formation in Healthy Young Women

Ryutaro Kase [1], Ayumi Amemiya [1,*], Rena Okonogi [2], Hiroki Yamakawa [3], Hisayoshi Sugawara [1], Yuji L. Tanaka [1], Masatoshi Komiyama [1] and Taketoshi Mori [4]

[1]   Department of Nursing Physiology, Graduate School of Nursing, Chiba University, 1-8-1 Inohana, Chuo-ku, Chiba-shi, Chiba 260-8672, Japan; rkase@chiba-u.jp (R.K.); h.sugawara@chiba-u.jp (H.S.); yuji@faculty.chiba-u.jp (Y.L.T.); mkomi@faculty.chiba-u.jp (M.K.)

[2]   Department of Nursing, Hospital of Jichi Medical University Saitama Medical Center, 1-847 Amanuma-cho, Oomiya-ku, Saitama-shi, Saitama 330-8503, Japan; leana-viking2013@ezweb.ne.jp

[3]   Nature's Walk Ltd., 3-2-3 Honcyou, Chuo-ku, Chiba-shi, Chiba 260-0012, Japan; yamakawa@natureswalk.co.jp

[4]   Department of Life Support Technology (Molten), Graduate School of Medicine, The University of Tokyo, 7-3-1 Hongo, Bunkyo-ku, Tokyo 113-0033, Japan; tmoriics-tky@umin.ac.jp

*   Correspondence: amemiya-a@chiba-u.jp; Tel.: +81-43-226-2402

Received: 22 August 2018; Accepted: 27 September 2018; Published: 28 September 2018

Abstract: Excessive pressure and shear stress while walking cause a risk of callus formation, which eventually causes foot ulcers in patients with diabetes mellitus. Callus under the second metatarsal head (MTH) has been associated with increased shear stress/pressure ratios (SPR). Callus under the fifth MTH has been associated with increased peak shear stress (PSS). The purpose of this study is to examine whether the effect of the suitable size and width of shoes prevents diabetic foot ulcers under the second and fifth MTH. We measured the pressure and shear stress by testing three kinds of sizes and two types of width of shoes. Significant difference was not observed in the SPR under the second MTH among different sizes of shoes. However, the pressure and shear stress were significantly lower when putting on shoes of fit size compared with larger sizes. The PSS under the fifth MTH was significantly smaller when putting on shoes of fit width compared with those of narrow width. Wearing shoes of fit size and width has the potential to prevent callus formation by reducing the pressure and shear stress constituting SPR under the second MTH and PSS under the fifth MTH.

Keywords: shear stress; shoe; callus; walking; woman

---

1. Introduction

From 1980 to 2014, the number of patients with diabetes mellitus has increased from 108 million to 422 million [1]. The global prevalence of diabetes among adults over 18 years has also increased from 4.7% to 8.5% in the same period [1]. According to a projection by the World Health Organization (WHO), diabetes will be the seventh leading cause of mortality by 2030 [2]. Diabetes is associated with several complications, including neuropathy, retinopathy, and diabetic kidney disease, of which diabetic foot ulcer constitutes one that develops in 4–10% of patients with diabetes [3]. Reportedly, 25% of patients with diabetes experience diabetic foot ulcers within their lifetime [3]. Moreover, diabetic foot ulcers show frequent recurrence, and 7–20% of patients with diabetic foot ulcers have to undergo leg amputations, accounting for a 15–40 times higher ratio of leg amputation in patients with diabetes compared with healthy people [4]. Foot ulcers not only lead to amputation of the lower limb, they also adversely affect individuals' quality of life (QOL), reduce physical activity, and aggravate psychological stress [5]. A study has estimated that diabetic ulcer-related costs averaged over $13,000 per episode, excluding costs associated with psychosocial issues, decline in the QOL, and lost productivity [6]. Thus, the prevention of diabetic foot ulcers is imperative not only for patients, but also both socially and economically.

Callus is one of the leading causes of diabetic foot ulcers. Callus occurs by the thickening of the stratum corneum by repeated pressure and overloading [7]. Reportedly, callus formation precedes ulcer formation in over 82% of patients with diabetic foot ulcers [7]. In addition, the relative risk for ulceration in a callused region is 11.0 compared with that without callus [8,9]. Therefore, the prevention of callus leads to the prevention of diabetic foot ulcers.

It has been reported that 42% of lower limb amputations are estimated to be shoe-related, 8% of which could have been avoided by wearing appropriate footwear [10]. A report has mentioned that the pressure on the plantar during walking is not significantly different between the patient group using a custom-made insole and that using prefabbed insoles [11], suggesting that changing merely the insole has no effect on reducing the pressure on the plantar. Presently, custom footwear with confirmed efficacy in preventing callus formation is available [12,13]. However, in the clinical setting, it has been reported that only 22% patients with diabetes have worn custom footwear [14]. This is possible because patients with diabetes do not recognize the importance of callus formation prevention, and custom footwear is expensive as well. In addition, it is not feasible to wear customized footwear to merely prevent callus formation. In this study, it was hypothesized that pressure and shear stress decreased if prefabric footwear was suitable in width and size, which is effective in preventing callus formation.

Several studies have measured the pressure on the plantar of patients with diabetes during walking. Repeated pressure and shear stress during walking contribute to callus formation on the plantar region [15,16]. In fact, patients with callus, even after removing the callus, exhibit significantly higher peak pressure (PP) during walking than patients without callus [17]. A report has stated that both plantar shear stress and shear stress–time integral values are elevated in diabetic patients with peripheral neuropathy, suggesting the potential clinical significance of these factors in ulceration [18]. Despite the potential significance of shear stress, few researches have measured shear stress because of technical difficulty, especially during walking.

However, ShokacChip^{TM} (Touchence Inc., Tokyo, Japan), a newly developed sensor, has facilitated the measurement of pressure and shear stress applied to an insole of footwear. Since the measurement method was new, this study was measured for young healthy subjects. Using ShokacChip^{TM}, a study has revealed that callus is associated with an increased shear stress/normal stress (pressure) ratios (SPR) under the second metatarsal head (MTH) and with higher peak shear stress (PSS) under the fifth MTH [19]. In addition, it has been suggested that callus formation under the second MTH is caused by wearing large shoes, and that callus formation under the fifth MTH is associated with wearing narrow shoes [20]. Thus, it was hypothesized that wearing shoes of suitable size and width is effective to reduce pressure and shear stress under the second and fifth MTH. In other words, it was hypothesized that it leads to the prevention of callus formation. To the best of our knowledge, no study has yet investigated differences in the pressure and shear stress among various sizes and widths of shoes.

Thus, the present study aimed to examine the pressure and shear stress under the second and fifth MTH during walking and confirm whether there is a difference between suitable shoes and large shoes that can lead to the prevention of callus formation. In addition, the present study aimed to confirm whether there is a difference between suitable shoes and narrow shoes that can lead to the prevention of callus formation.

2. Materials and Methods

2.1. Research Design and Procedure

In this study, variables were compared with crossover design. This study was conducted and reported according to a part of a Consolidated Standards of Reporting Trials (CONSORT) checklist [21].

2.2. Participants Recruitment and Ethics

In this study, 49 healthy adults without diabetes who could walk without support were enrolled as study participants using a snowball sampling method. This study focused on women, since they tended to wear incorrectly sized shoes [22,23]. This study was conducted in accordance with the Declaration of Helsinki, and the protocol was approved by the Ethical Committee of the Graduate School of Nursing, Chiba University (28-65: November/22/2016) (Chiba, Japan). In addition, written informed consent was obtained from each participant before enrollment.

2.3. Footwear Type

In this study, a skilled prosthetist and orthotist measured participants' feet sizes and selected a pair of fit shoes for each participant. The experimental shoes that were used prepared different sizes of the same product. These shoes were made from leather and were brand shoes called gute wahl. These shoes were recommended by Shoes Meister for diabetic foot ulcers. Three sizes of experimental shoes—fit size, 1-cm larger size and 2-cm larger size—were tested to measure the pressure and shear stress under the second MTH. For the fifth MTH, the following two types of experimental shoes were tested: fit width and narrow width. Experimental shoes of narrow width were prepared by inserting a cork insole of 6-mm thickness in the fit shoes. The cork insole was prepared by the prosthetist and an orthotist by cutting a cork sheet. The cork insole was thinned only at the heel for preventing the shoes from coming off during walking.

2.4. Pressure and Shear Stress under the Second MTH

Participants put on unified socks during the test. If there was a callus, at certain locations on the plantar surface, eventually sensors read higher values as calluses increase the tissue rigidity. In the case of calluses on the plantar region, all of the calluses were removed prior to data collection in this study. First, the prosthetist and orthotist obtained participants' footprints. Next, the foot length and width of standing participants were measured, and a fit size of shoes was selected. Second, the researcher directly attached sensors of ShokacChip™ (Touchence Inc.) on the plantar region of participants. Then, converters were put on the front shin portion and wirelessly connected to a personal computer. All of the participants tested the three sizes of shoes. The prosthetist and orthotist assisted participants with putting on the shoes in order to avoid any difference in the manner of shoe wearing. The order of testing the three sizes of shoes was randomly selected. Third, participants walked approximately 15 m as practice for confirming that they did not experience any pain or interference on walking with the attached sensors. Lastly, external force (pressure and shear stress) was measured (details in "Data Collection"). All of the participants walked approximately 15 m twice as the measurement walk, and the researcher recorded all of the sensor data, ensuring that the sensors were operating during the study. In addition, an assistant measured 15 m of walking time using a stopwatch. After obtaining the measurements for one size of shoes, measurements were obtained for the other two types of shoes in the same manner.

2.5. Measurement of Pressure and Shear Stress under the Fifth MTH

Measurements were obtained for the fifth MTH via the same procedure that was used for the second MTH. However, in this case, only two types of shoes, fit width and narrower than fit width, were tested.

2.6. Data Collection

The pressure and shear stress were measured using ShokacChip^{TM}. The high sensitivity was realized for three-dimensional axes by processing three piezoelectric elements and locating them at three-dimensional axes on the 2-mm^2 chip. Notably, the sensor size was $\varphi 10.0 \times 1.3$ mm (t); as it was very small and thin, it could measure the in-shoe pressure and shear stress of the plantar under each MTH region. The reliability and validity of the system for measuring the in-shoe plantar pressure and shear stress have been previously established [24]. In this study, coefficients of variation (CV) and intraclass correlation coefficients (ICC) were confirmed. The mean CV was 9.7%. The mean ICC was 0.943 [24]. Even though this sensor does not require any calibration before each measurement, calibration was performed before measuring with shoes.

In this study, the external force variables, including PP, pressure time integral (PI), PSS, and shear stress integral (SSI) of each walking cycle were calculated from the data of external force recorded by the sensor. These variables have been frequently used in previous studies [18–20,24]. In addition, the SPR, which is considered to be associated with callus formation, was calculated by dividing the shear stress by the normal stress (pressure), concretely, using peak value (SPR-p) and time-integral value (SPR-i, calculated by dividing the SSI by the PI value). Furthermore, data regarding age, sex, height, weight, body mass index (BMI), the number of callus under the second MTH and fifth MTH, foot length, and foot width were obtained.

2.7. Data Analysis

The variables of the external force were obtained by averaging 12 steps after removing the first and last three steps. Data analysis was performed for each second and fifth MTH by using MATLAB R2012a (The Math Works, Inc., Natick, MA, USA). Statistical analyses were performed using IBM SPSS Statistics ver.23.0 (Chicago, IL, USA). The Cohen's d effect size was 0.45, and sample size was 41 when calculated based on the previous study [25]. Normality analyses were conducted before data analysis. A paired *t*-test was conducted to compare the external force value due to shoe differences. In this study, p = 0.05 two-tailed was considered statistically significant. In addition, the calculated Cohen's d effect size was described in the results. Descriptive data were expressed as the mean ± standard deviation of continuous variables and n (%) for categorical variables. The external force values were represented as bar graphs in these figures. These bar graphs in the figure contained standard errors. Further, Pearson's test was used whether there was a correlation between the difference of width (shoes versus feet) and the PSS.

3. Results

In this study, 49 participants were enrolled, and 54 and 44 feet were used for obtaining measurements of variables for the second and fifth MTH, respectively. Table 1 summarizes the characteristics of all of the participants. Calluses under the second MTH were observed in 29 of 54 feet, whereas those under the fifth MTH were observed in nine of 44 feet.

When putting on shoes of fit size, the PSS under the second MTH was significantly smaller than those putting on larger sizes [1-cm large size: p < 0.001, d = 0.40 (Figure 1a); 2-cm large size: p = 0.01, d = 0.53 (Figure 2a)]. In addition, the PP under the second MTH was significantly smaller (p = 0.001, d = 0.33) when testing shoes of fit size compared with shoes of 1-cm large size (Figure 1a). The PI under the second MTH in cases of fit-sized shoes was significantly smaller than those in cases of larger sizes [1-cm large size: p = 0.002, d = 0.36 (Figure 1b); 2-cm large size: p = 0.012, d = 0.35 (Figure 2b)]. In addition, the SSI under the second MTH was significantly smaller (p = 0.034, d = 0.28) when putting on the fit size than when putting on the 1-cm large size (Figure 1b). Furthermore, the SSI under the second MTH was significantly smaller (p = 0.023, d = 0.38) when testing the fit size than when testing the 2-cm large size (Figure 2b). Thus, the SSI significantly increased when participants put on larger shoes. However, even when different sizes of shoes were tested, significant difference was not observed in the SPR-p and SPR-i, which were associated with the callus formation under the second MTH.

Table 1. Patient characteristics.

	Measurement of Second MTH	Measurement of Fifth MTH
Number of patients	27	22
Number of feet	54	44
Age (y)	26.9 ± 7.2	26.7 ± 7.3
Sex (n)		
Man	0	0
Woman	27 (55%)	22 (45%)
Height (cm)	156.0 ± 5.0	157.2 ± 4.6
Weight (kg)	56.9 ± 10.0	55.4 ± 9.3
BMI	23.1 ± 3.7	22.4 ± 3.5
Number of feet with callus under the second MTH	29 (53.7%)	-
Number of feet with callus under the fifth MTH	-	9 (20.5%)
Feet length (cm)	23.0 ± 0.9	22.9 ± 1.0
Feet width (cm)	22.1 ± 2.0	22.6 ± 1.3

n (%); mean $\pm$ SD, BMI; body mass index, MTH; metatarsal head.

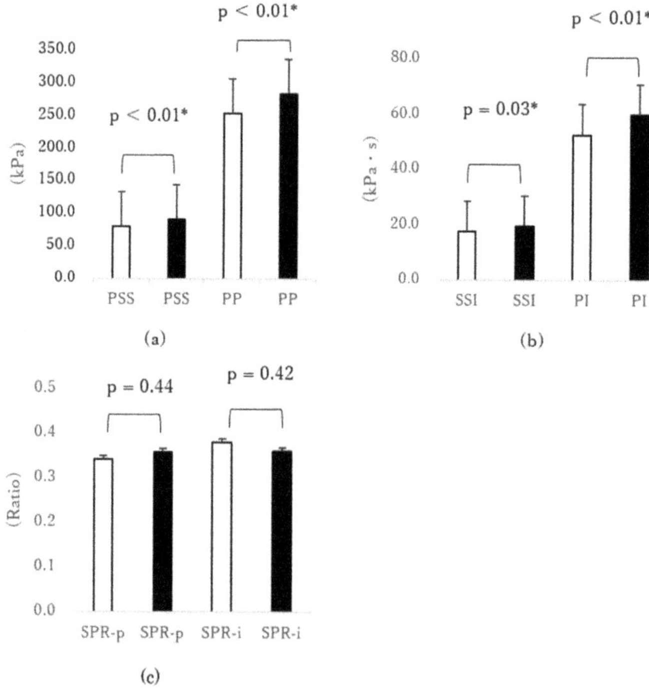

Figure 1. Comparison of external force under the second MTH due to differences in shoe size (□ fit size vs. ■ 1-cm larger size). (**a**) Peak normal stress (pressure) (PP) and peak shear stress (PSS), (**b**) normal stress (pressure) time integral (PI) and shear stress time integral (SSI), and (**c**) shear stress/normal stress (pressure) ratio of peak value (SPR-p) and shear stress/normal stress (pressure) ratio of time integral value (SPR-i). * $p < 0.05$ paired *t*-test. Error bar was standard error (SEM). MTH: metatarsal head.

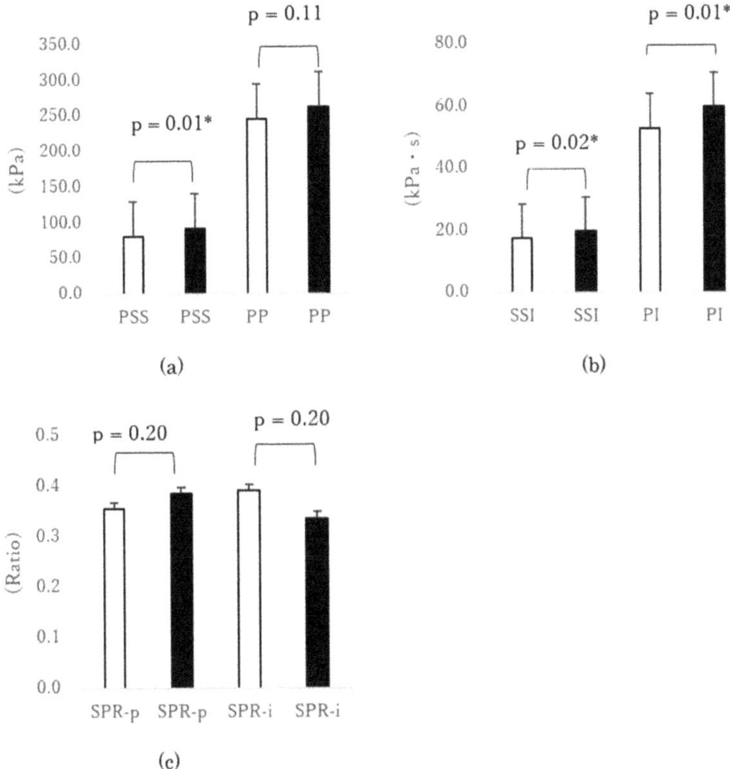

Figure 2. Comparison of external force under the second MTH due to differences in shoe size (□ fit size vs ■ 2-cm larger size). (**a**) Peak normal stress (pressure) (PP) and peak shear stress (PSS), (**b**) normal stress (pressure) time integral (PI) and shear stress time integral (SSI), and (**c**) shear stress/normal stress (pressure) ratio of peak value (SPR-p) and shear stress/normal stress (pressure) ratio of time integral value (SPR-i). * p < 0.05 paired *t*-test. Error bar was standard error (SEM). MTH: metatarsal head.

The PSS under the fifth MTH was significantly smaller (p < 0.01, d = 0.42) when putting on shoes of fit width than when putting on shoes of narrower width (Figure 3a). However, significant differences were not observed in the others under the fifth MTH.

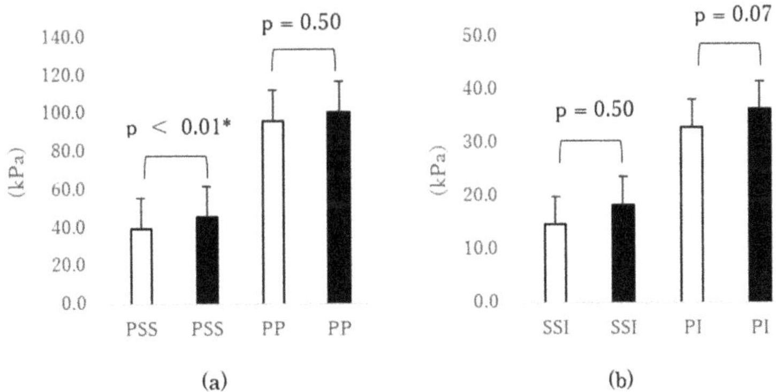

Figure 3. *Cont.*

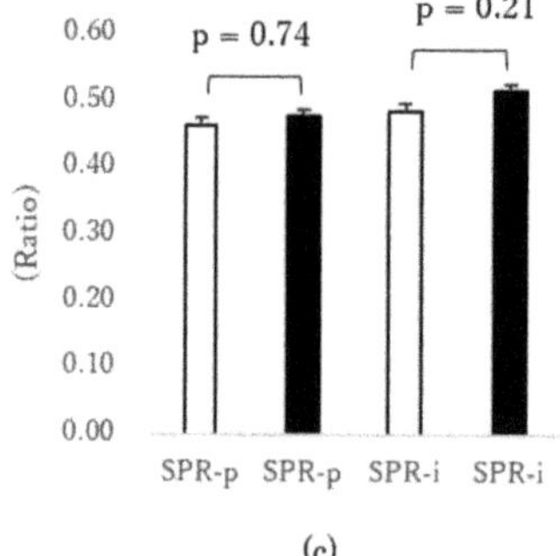

(c)

Figure 3. Comparison of external force under the fifth MTH due to differences in shoe width (□ fit width vs. ■ narrow width). (**a**) Peak normal stress (pressure) (PP) and peak shear stress (PSS), (**b**) normal stress (pressure) time integral (PI) and shear stress time integral (SSI), and (**c**) shear stress/normal stress (pressure) ratio of peak value (SPR-p) and shear stress/normal stress (pressure) ratio of time integral value (SPR-i). * $p < 0.05$ paired *t*-test. Error bar was standard error (SEM). MTH: metatarsal head.

The difference between the participants' foot width and shoe width was seven mm on average in case of shoes of fit width, in which shoes were wider than feet. In contrast, the average of the difference was −3 mm for narrow shoes, in which shoes were narrower than feet. The correlation coefficient between the difference of width (shoes versus feet) and the PSS was −0.26, which was only a weak negative correlation (Figure 4).

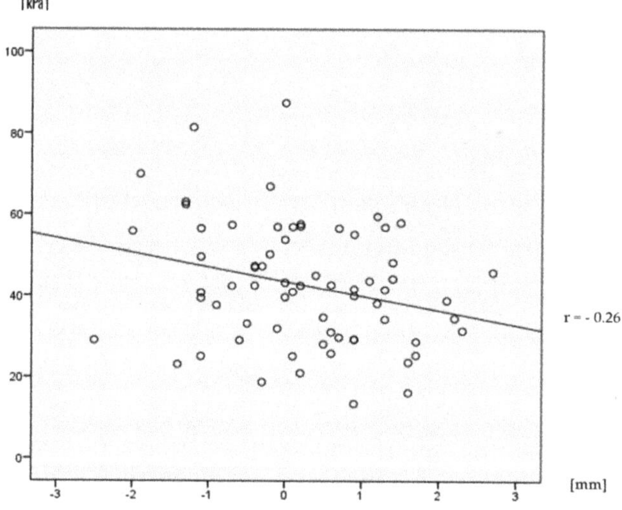

Figure 4. Relationship between the difference of width (shoes vs. feet) and PSS. The straight line is the correlation line. Dots are samples.

4. Discussion

This is the first study to reveal the pressure and shear stress under the second and fifth MTH when young healthy participants put on shoes of different sizes or widths for preventing callus formation. For the second MTH, the findings of this study revealed that the PI and SSI decreased by wearing suitably sized footwear compared with larger sized footwear; these valuables comprised the SPR that is associated with the prevention of the callus formation. In addition, the findings also revealed that the PSS associated with the callus formation at the fifth MTH decreased by wearing footwear of suitable width.

Regarding the shoe size, the PI, SSI, and PSS under the second MTH were significantly smaller when putting on fit-sized shoes compared to larger-sized shoes. The PI and SSI comprise SPR, which is associated with the prevention of callus formation [19]. However, significant difference was not observed in the SPR-i that is associated with the callus formation under the second MTH, because in this study, both SSI and PI decreased by putting on fit shoes. Assumedly, as the large sliding of the plantar occurs when walking, wearing larger-size shoes results in an increase in the PI, SSI, and PSS under the second MTH. Thus, it has been clear that unsuitable shoes augment pressure and shear stress. Wearing suitably sized shoes is effective at reducing pressure and shear stress and leading to the prevention of callus formation under the second MTH.

Regarding the width of shoes, the PSS under the fifth MTH was smaller when putting on shoes of fit width compared with those of a narrow width. In addition, the correlation coefficient between the difference between the foot width and shoes width and the PSS was −0.26, which was a weak negative correlation in the range between narrow shoes and shoes that fit (Figure 4). The results of this study support that the width of the outdoor shoes was narrow, which is related to the callus formation [26]. The relative risk for callus formation is 2.03 when comparing wearing narrow shoes with suitable shoes, and the relative risk for corn formation is 6.18, respectively [26]. Further, callus formation has been shown to be associated with higher PSS under the fifth MTH [19]. The present data proved a previous suggestion that callus formation under the fifth MTH is associated with wearing narrow shoes [20]. As the fifth MTH has a thinner subcutaneous tissue than the first and second MTH regions, the mechanical load may not be absorbed by the subcutaneous tissue. From the results of this study, it is considered that if a person wears narrow shoes, the shear stress increases, because the foot is pressed against both sides of the shoes. On the other hand, when wearing fit shoes that are somewhat wider than feet, the foot spread by the load is not pressed against the sides of the shoes, and the shear stress is decreased. Thus, it is suggested that wearing footwear of suitable width has been effective at reducing pressure and shear stress, and thus preventing callus formation under the fifth MTH.

A previous study on shoe selection has reported that the use of incorrectly sized shoes significantly correlates with pain and ulceration [27]. Another study that is based on data from 227 women has reported that 48.5% were wearing incorrectly sized shoes, of which 12.8% were wearing shoes that were at least 1 cm larger than their feet [23]. A study that examined 65 older adults verified that 72% participants were, in fact, wearing incorrectly sized shoes (65% were wearing shoes larger than their feet) [27]. On the contrary, a study evaluating 356 women (age 20–60 years) has reported that 88% of patients were wearing shoes that were narrower than their feet [22]. As the proportion of older adults is high among patients with diabetes [28], they are more likely to wear larger-size shoes. Moreover, it has been revealed that an incorrect width of shoes has been worn by people who selected incorrect shoes [23]. Therefore, it is possible that patients with diabetes tend to frequently wear unsuitable shoes. Perhaps, it is difficult for people to select suitable shoes because it is difficult to find shoes with all applicable sizes, widths, and shoe fittings in everyday life. This might be why patients with diabetes frequently wear unsuitable shoes. It would very be important for patients with diabetes to find suitable shoes at least regarding the points of size and width in order to reduce the pressure and shear stress that lead to callus formation.

This study has some limitations. First, all of the participants were healthy people without diabetes. Compared with healthy participants, patients with diabetes or diabetic neuropathy have abnormal plantar pressure distribution as follows: elevated plantar pressure because of the motion of small rolling during the mid-stance [29], an impaired ability to stabilize their body when walking on irregular surfaces [30], foot deformity [31], limitation of the joint range of motion, and muscle weakness [32,33]. Second, patients with diabetes are often older than the participants of this study. Thus, it is quite likely that these characteristics of patients with diabetes affect the results in the clinical setting. In future, it is necessary to assess the effect of wearing shoes of suitable size and width in patients with diabetes.

Third, since only women were included in this study, the findings of this study are limited to woman. Finally, an insufficient sample size due to a lack of shoe size has affected the results. Data collection was finished before reaching the target sample size, since the shoe size could not have been sufficiently collected, and data collection time was limited. In future study, it will be important to increase the sample size and include males, a diabetic cohort, and a higher body mass index cohort.

5. Conclusions

This is the first study to compare the pressure and shear stress under the second and fifth MTH from wearing different sizes of shoe in young healthy participants. Apparently, the PI and SSI under the second MTH decrease by wearing suitably sized shoes compared with larger shoes. Furthermore, the PSS under the fifth MTH decreases by wearing shoes of a suitable width rather than narrow shoes. Therefore, there is a possibility that wearing shoes of suitable width and size can reduce pressure and shear stress and thus lead to the prevention of callus formation and diabetic foot ulcers.

Author Contributions: Conceptualization, A.A.; Data curation, R.K. and A.A.; Formal analysis, R.K., A.A. and R.O.; Funding acquisition, A.A.; Investigation, R.K., A.A., R.O., H.Y. and H.S.; Methodology, A.A.; Project administration, A.A.; Supervision, T.M.; Writing—original draft, R.K. and A.A.; Writing—review & editing, A.A., Y.L.T. and M.K.

Funding: Research supported by MEXT KAKENHI Grant Numbers (JP16H06675, JP16K12949) and NAKANISHI MUTSUKO NURSUING PRACTICE RESEARCH FUND.

Acknowledgments: We wish to express my appreciation to our participants. We would especially like to express my gratitude to German orthopedic shoe technician Meister Karsten Rieche and Yukie Oonuma for their professional advice.

Conflicts of Interest: The authors report no relevant conflict of interests.

References

1. World Health Organization. Available online: http://www.who.int/mediacentre/factsheets/fs312/en/ (accessed on 20 February 2018).

2. Mathers, C.D. Projections of Global Mortality and Burden of Disease from 2002 to 2030. *PLoS Med.* **2006**, *3*, e442. [CrossRef] [PubMed]

3. Singh, N. Preventing foot ulcers in patients with diabetes. *J. Am. Med. Assoc.* **2005**, *293*, 217–228. [CrossRef] [PubMed]

4. Frykberg, R.G. Diabetic foot disorders. A clinical practice guideline (2006 revision). *J. Foot Ankl. Surg.* **2006**, *45*, S1–S66. [CrossRef]

5. Brod, M. Quality of life issues in patients with diabetes and lower extremity ulcers: Patients and care givers. *Qual. Life Res.* **1998**, *7*, 365–372. [CrossRef] [PubMed]

6. Stockl, K. Costs of lower-extremity ulcers among patients with diabetes. *Diabetes Care* **2004**, *27*, 2129–2134. [CrossRef] [PubMed]

7. Sage, R.A. Outpatient care and morbidity reduction in diabetic foot ulcers associated with chronic pressure callus. *J. Am. Podiatr. Med. Assoc.* **2001**, *91*, 275–279. [CrossRef] [PubMed]

8. Murray, H.J. The association between callus formation, high pressures and neuropathy in diabetic foot ulceration. *Diabet. Med.* **1996**, *13*, 979–982. [CrossRef]

9. Waaijman, R. Risk factors for plantar foot ulcer recurrence in neuropathic diabetic patients. *Diabetes Care* **2014**, *37*, 1697–1705. [CrossRef] [PubMed]

10. Reiber, G.E. Who is at risk of limb loss and what to do about it? *J. Rehabil. Res. Dev.* **1994**, *31*, 357–362. [PubMed]

11. Paton, J.S. A comparison of customised and prefabricated insoles to reduce risk factors for neuropathic diabetic foot ulceration: A participant-blinded randomised controlled trial. *J. Foot Ankl. Res.* **2012**, *5*, 31. [CrossRef] [PubMed]

12. Janisse, D. Pedorthic management of the diabetic foot. *Prosthet. Orthot. Int.* **2015**, *39*, 40–47. [CrossRef] [PubMed]

13. Mayfield, J.A.; Reiber, G.E.; Sanders, L.J.; Janisse, D.; Pogach, L.M. Preventive Foot Care in People With Diabetes. *Diabetes Care* **2003**, *26*, S78. [CrossRef] [PubMed]

14. Knowles, E.A. Do people with diabetes wear their prescribed footwear? *Diabet. Med.* **1996**, *13*, 1064–1068. [CrossRef]

15. Singh, D. Callosities, corns and calluses. *BMJ. Br. Med. J.* **1996**, *312*, 1403–1406. [CrossRef]

16. Freeman, D.B. Corns and calluses resulting from mechanical hyperkeratosis. *Am. Fam. Physician* **2002**, *65*, 2277–2285. [PubMed]

17. Pataky, Z. The impact of callosities on the magnitude and duration of plantar pressure in patients with diabetes mellitus. A callus may cause 18,600 kilograms of excess plantar pressure per day. *Diabetes Metab.* **2002**, *28*, 356–361. [PubMed]

18. Yavuz, M. American Society of Biomechanics Clinical Biomechanics Award 2012: Plantar shear stress distributions in diabetic patients with and without neuropathy. *Clin. Biomech.* **2014**, *29*, 223–229. [CrossRef] [PubMed]

19. Amemiya, A. Shear Stress-Normal Stress (Pressure) Ratio Decides Forming Callus in Patients with Diabetic Neuropathy. *J. Diabet. Res.* **2016**, *2016*, 3157123. [CrossRef] [PubMed]

20. Amemiya, A. Investigation of External Force on Plantar Associated with Callus in Diabetic Neuropathy Patients and Its Relationship with their Leg Motions for Foot Ulcer Prevention. Ph.D. Thesis, The University of Tokyo, Tokyo, Japan, 2016.

21. Moher, D. CONSORT 2010 Explanation and Elaboration: Updated guidelines for reporting parallel group randomised trials. *Int. J. Surg.* **2012**, *10*, 28–55. [CrossRef] [PubMed]

22. Frey, C. American Orthopaedic Foot and Ankle Society women's shoe survey. *Foot Ankl.* **1993**, *14*, 78–81. [CrossRef]

23. De Castro, A.P. The Relationship Between Wearing Incorrectly Sized Shoes and Foot Dimensions, Foot Pain, and Diabetes. *J. Sport Rehabil.* **2010**, *19*, 214–225. [CrossRef]

24. Amemiya, A. Establishment of a measurement method for in-shoe pressure and shear stress in specific regions for diabetic ulcer prevention. In Proceedings of the 2016 38th Annual International Conference of the IEEE Engineering in Medicine and Biology Society (EMBC), Orlando, FL, USA, 16–20 August 2016; pp. 2291–2294.

25. Menz, H.B. Plantar pressures are higher under callused regions of the foot in older people. *Clin. Exp. Dermatol.* **2007**, *32*, 375–380. [CrossRef] [PubMed]

26. Menz, H.B. Footwear characteristics and foot problems in older people. *Gerontology* **2005**, *51*, 346–351. [CrossRef] [PubMed]

27. Burns, S.L. Older people and ill fitting shoes. *Postgrad. Med. J.* **2002**, *78*, 344–346. [CrossRef] [PubMed]

28. World Health Organization. Global report on diabetes. Available online: http://apps.who.int/iris/bitstream/10665/204871/1/9789241565257_eng.pdf?ua=1 (accessed on 20 February 2018).

29. Amemiya, A. Elevated plantar pressure in diabetic patients and its relationship with their gait features. *Gait Posture* **2014**, *40*, 408–414. [CrossRef] [PubMed]

30. Menz, H.B. Walking stability and sensorimotor function in older people with diabetic peripheral neuropathy. *Arch. Phys. Med. Rehabil.* **2004**, *85*, 245–252. [CrossRef] [PubMed]

31. Ledoux, W.R. Biomechanical differences among pes cavus, neutrally aligned, and pes planus feet in subjects with diabetes. *Foot* **2003**, *24*, 845–850. [CrossRef] [PubMed]

32. Andersen, H. Muscle strength in type 2 diabetes. *Diabetes* **2004**, *53*, 1543–1548. [CrossRef] [PubMed]

33. Sacco, I.C. Abnormalities of plantar pressure distribution in early, intermediate, and late stages of diabetic neuropathy. *Gait Posture* **2014**, *40*, 570–574. [CrossRef] [PubMed]

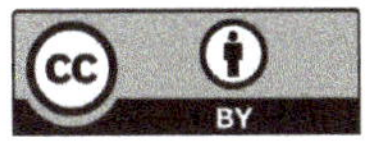 © 2018 by the authors. Licensee MDPI, Basel, Switzerland. This article is an open access article distributed under the terms and conditions of the Creative Commons Attribution (CC BY) license (http://creativecommons.org/licenses/by/4.0/).

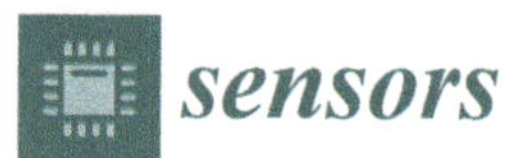 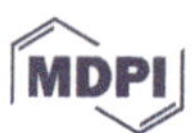

Article

Towards an Automated Unsupervised Mobility Assessment for Older People Based on Inertial TUG Measurements

Sandra Hellmers [1],*
, Babak Izadpanah [1], Lena Dasenbrock [2], Rebecca Diekmann [1], Jürgen M. Bauer [3], Andreas Hein [1] and Sebastian Fudickar [1]

[1] Carl von Ossietzky University Oldenburg, 26129 Oldenburg, Germany; babak_izadpanah83@yahoo.com (B.I.); rebecca.diekmann@uni-oldenburg.de (R.D.); andreas.hein@uni-oldenburg.de (A.H.); sebastian.fudickar@uni-oldenburg.de (S.F.)
[2] Peter L. Reichertz Institute for Medical Informatics, 30625 Hannover, Germany; lena.dasenbrock@plri.de
[3] Center for Geriatric Medicine, University Heidelberg, 69117 Heidelberg, Germany; Juergen.Bauer@bethanien-heidelberg.de
* Correspondence: sandra.hellmers@uni-oldenburg.de

Received: 30 July 2018; Accepted: 29 September 2018; Published: 2 October 2018

Abstract: One of the most common assessments for the mobility of older people is the Timed Up and Go test (TUG). Due to its sensitivity regarding the indication of Parkinson's disease (PD) or increased fall risk in elderly people, this assessment test becomes increasingly relevant, should be automated and should become applicable for unsupervised self-assessments to enable regular examinations of the functional status. With Inertial Measurement Units (IMU) being well suited for automated analyses, we evaluate an IMU-based analysis-system, which automatically detects the TUG execution via machine learning and calculates the test duration. as well as the duration of its single components. The complete TUG was classified with an accuracy of 96% via a rule-based model in a study with 157 participants aged over 70 years. A comparison between the TUG durations determined by IMU and criterion standard measurements (stopwatch and automated/ambient TUG (aTUG) system) showed significant correlations of 0.97 and 0.99, respectively. The classification of the instrumented TUG (iTUG)-components achieved accuracies over 96%, as well. Additionally, the system's suitability for self-assessments was investigated within a semi-unsupervised situation where a similar movement sequence to the TUG was executed. This preliminary analysis confirmed that the self-selected speed correlates moderately with the speed in the test situation, but differed significantly from each other.

Keywords: TUG; IMU; frailty; geriatric assessment; machine learning; wearable sensors; semi-unsupervised; self-assessment; domestic environment; functional decline

---

1. Introduction

The early detection of functional decline, which occurs with age and results, among others, in an increased fall risk, is important to initiate timely preventive measures, slow down the progress of decline and maintain older peoples' independent living. The Timed Up and Go test (TUG), developed by Podsiadlo and Richardson [1], is a well-established assessment and one of the most frequently-used tests for mobility. This test assesses the basic mobility skills, which make up important abilities for independent living. Besides balance and strength, mobility is one of the essential components of physical function [2]. The TUG consists of several components of everyday movements (see Figure 1). At the beginning of the test, the patient is sitting on a chair leaning against the backrest. Then, she or he gets up from the chair, walks 3 m, turns around, walks back and sits down again. The test starts with the request and stops when the participant is seated again correctly in the chair with his/her back resting at the back of the chair. According to the necessary duration, the patient's mobility is categorized into four groups: <10 s freely mobile, 11–19 s mostly independent, 20–29 s variable mobility, >30 s impaired mobility. Therefore, a faster time indicates a better functional performance. The TUG test is an established and widely-used test as part of geriatric assessments, and the intra-rater, inter-rater and test-retest reliability of the individual components of the instrumented TUG (iTUG) have been shown to be excellent to good for total duration in patients with Parkinson's disease [3]. Therefore, the TUG test is a suitable test to investigate temporal progressions. For example, van Iersel et al. [4] pointed out that the TUG test is sensitive to clinically-relevant changes in functional mobility in frail elderly patients within a period of two weeks. Over time, the TUG test was enhanced several times: Wall et al. [5] introduced the Expanded Timed Get-up-and-Go (ETGUG) test, in which the length was increased to 10 m, and times for each of the components tasks were measured separately using a multi-memory stopwatch.

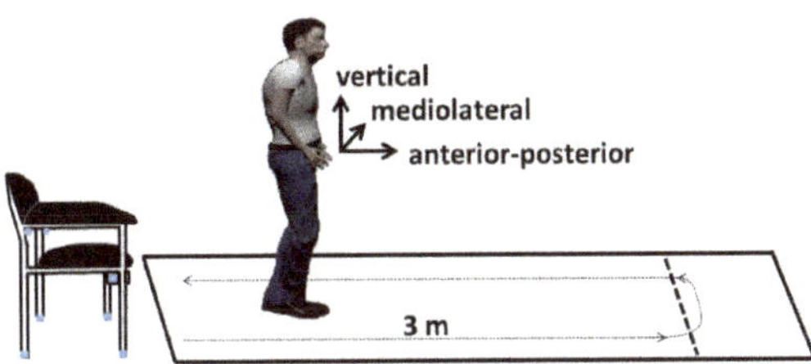

Figure 1. Setting of the Timed up and Go (TUG) test in our study. The test is measured by an IMU integrated into a belt. Additionally, a stopwatch and the automated/ambient TUG (aTUG) system are reference measures. The coordinate orientation of the Inertial Measurement Unit (IMU) is illustrated in the figure.

The advantage of the TUG test is its simplicity: the short test duration, the low required equipment and the possibility to perform the test even for patients with functional impairments. However, because of the importance of detecting early changes in functional decline, these assessment should be performed regularly and in a high frequency to initiate early interventions and slow down the functional decline. To relieve clinicians and reduce the stress for the patients, these assessments should take place in the daily life of the patients in the form of unsupervised self-assessments. Inertial Measurement Units (IMU) are well suited for automated analyses and can be easy to use, flexible and inexpensive, thus suitable for self-guided assessments.

Sprint et al. [6] provided in their survey an overview of the TUG test and technologies utilized for TUG instrumentation. Besides video-based measurements, ambient technologies and wearable or smartphone-based technologies have been already used for studies. The automated/ambient TUG (aTUG) [7] uses ambient sensors attached to a chair and provides a fully-automated TUG test execution. The aTUG consists of a laser range scanner for gait analysis, force sensors in the chair legs to analyze the components of rising from the chair or sitting down and a laser barrier to measure the test duration, which shows a high correlation with stop-watch measurements [8].

The suitability of the aTUG system in diverse health care environments was already shown in [9].

Wearable sensors have become quite popular, and therefore, IMU were used in several studies. Table 1 shows a selection of studies, which used inertial measurement units or smartphones for TUG analyses.

Table 1. Selection of studies that used inertial sensors for TUG analyses. The study population, as well as the placement of the IMU and the analyses method are listed in detail. Parkinson's disease is abbreviated as PD; Accelerometer (Acc); Gyroscope (Gyro); Magnetometer (Magn); instrumented TUG (iTUG).

Article	Year	Population n (Years) (Average Age $\pm$ SD)	Technology, Placement	Methods, Analyses
Higashi et al. [10]	2008	10 healthy (21.0 $\pm$ 2), 20 hemiplegic (68.3 $\pm$ 11)	2 IMU (3D-Acc/Gyro), waist, upper thigh, video camera	duration of TUG phases, rule-based
Salarin et al. [11]	2010	12 PD (60.4 $\pm$ 8.5), 10 control (60.2 $\pm$ 8.2)	7 IMU forearms, shanks, thighs, sternum	automatic detection of TUG components, rule-based
Chiari [12]	2011	20 early-mild PD, 20 healthy	1 Acc lumbar segment L5	Feature selection, discrimination of PD and non-PD with accuracy of 92.5%
Jallon et al. [13]	2011	19 subjects	1 IMU (3D-Acc), 3D-Magn, chest	Bayesian classifier, Accuracy TUG phases detection near 85%
Adame et al. [14]	2012	10 healthy (63.2 $\pm$ 10.1), 10 early stage PD (58.8 $\pm$ 9.5), 10 advanced stage PD (66.2 $\pm$ 4.8)	1 IMU, lower back	Estimation of TUG phases duration: small mean error, dynamic time warping
Milosevic et al. [15]	2013	3 PD, 4 healthy	Android Smartphone 3D-Acc, 3D-Gyro, 3D-Magn, chest	self-administered and automated TUG, rule-based
Reinfelder et al. [16]	2015	16 PD	2 IMU, SHIMMER 2R, 3D-Acc, 3D-Gyro, lateral side of both shoes	TUG phases recognition, Support Vector Machine, sensitivity: 81.80%
Nguyen et al. [17]	2017	4 females (67.8 $\pm$ 10.4) 8 males (66.6 $\pm$ 3.6) early stages PD	motion capture suit 17 IMU (3D-Acc/Gyro), 3D-Magn, each body segment	TUG activities recognition sensitivity: 97.6%, specificity: 92.7% modifications 100% accur. rule-based

Already in 2008, Higashi et al. [10] developed the TUG-T and measured the duration of the six single components of the test (standing up, walking forward, turn one, walking back, turn two and sitting down) with two inertial sensors. An instrumented version of the TUG (iTUG) was proposed to measure the duration of four components (sit-to-stand, steady-state gait, turning, turn-to-sit) and a set of balance and gait parameters [11], but required seven inertial sensors. Reinfelder et al. [16] developed a TUG phase segmentation system with two IMU and reached a mean sensitivity of 81.80% over all phases by using a support vector machine. A smartphone application called sTUG was developed by Milosevic et al. [15], which completely automates the iTUG test, determines the beginning and the end of the test and quantifies its individual phases. With a system of 17 IMU and a rule-based algorithm, accuracies of 100% could be achieved for TUG phases' recognition [17].

Many studies in the literature focus on the discrimination between different diseases or phenotypes such as Parkinson's disease or fallers like for example [12,18]. Although there are good results for combined use of multiple IMU, the recognition accuracy of the TUG phases with a single IMU can be improved and should be confirmed for larger study populations. Many studies used rule-based algorithms, while some others used logistic regression models for fall prediction [19], dynamic time warping [14] or for example feature selection [12]. Until now, only a rather small minority use machine learning for the TUG classification like [16]. However, in order to support a higher motion variety and motion anomalies, machine learning might be more suitable regarding different study populations, which differ for example in age, functional status or diseases, which affect the locomotor system. Additionally, these studies do not focus on settings beyond the laboratory, as well as automated self-assessments, except Milosevic et al. [15]. However, Milosevic's system needs the interaction of the user (start and stop record) since it cannot identify phases of the TUG execution automatically in a longer sequence.

Thus, we develop an activity recognition via machine learning and a rule-based algorithm, which detects both standardized TUG-sequences and similar sequences, which may occur in daily life and is more naturalistic than the standard TUG setup. We used one single IMU integrated into a belt to enable an easy use and an unobtrusive sensor placement, especially regarding future self-assessments at home. After the validation of our system under standardized conditions in a laboratory environment, we evaluate the suitability for future self-assessments by a non-standardized situation with similar movement patterns to the TUG test.

In contrast to the previous studies, we conducted a study with a larger sample size to cover common age-related varieties of motion patterns and corresponding anomalies. As the ground truth, we applied both clinical caregivers (stopwatch measurements) and the aTUG system. In comparison to Milosevic's system, we chose a more unobtrusive and easier sensor placement than the chest. Our system can be used without assistance and interactions. Another major difference lies in the application of a machine learning algorithm instead of a rule-based algorithm. Since a high variance in movement patterns or strategies can occur, especially for transitions, in older adults, machine learning algorithms might be more robust than rule-based algorithms. If large datasets are available, which cover a majority of these variances, it is preferable to use machine learning. Rule-based algorithms need to be very complex to take different study populations into account, which differing in functional status or diseases. With increasing complexity, reading and adjusting a rule-based system becomes often cumbersome.

In summary, we want to develop an accurate system for automated mobility assessments for older people based on inertial TUG measurements, which is able to be used in clinical environments, as well as in future unsupervised self-assessments at home for a high variety of patients.

2. Materials and Methods

In order to evaluate an approach for automated measurement and analysis of the TUG test based on 3D accelerometer and 3D gyroscope data via machine learning, we included 157 participants in our study (87 female (59%), 60 male (41%)), aged 70 years and above. Table 2 lists the characteristics of our study population. The data of 10 participants were excluded in this analysis, due to a low signal-to-noise ratio or a wrong positioning of the sensor (cf. also Figure 2).

Table 2. Characteristics of our included study population ($n = 148$) with minimum (min), maximum (max) and mean-value (mean), as well as the standard deviation (SD) of age in years, body weight in kg and body height in cm.

	Min	Max	Mean	SD
age (years)	70	87	75.22	3.83
weight (kg)	46.85	110.80	76.01	13.94
height (cm)	145.80	188.70	167.43	9.50

Besides the TUG test, the screening study consists of other different geriatric tests such as the Short Physical Performance Battery (SPPB), the Stair Climb Power Test (SCPT), the 6-min walk test, frailty criteria and counter movement lump. These tests were measured in a conventional way by medical professionals and additionally with ambient and wearable technology. More details are described in [20]. The study has been approved by the appropriate ethics committees (ethical vote: Hannover

Medical School, No. 6948; ethical vote: Carl von Ossietzky University, Drs.33/2016) and conducted in accordance with the Declaration of Helsinki.

We used a five-fold cross-validation. Therefore, our dataset was randomly divided into 5 equally-sized subsamples. One subsample (20% of the data) was retained as the validation data for testing the model, and the remaining 4 subsamples (80%) were used as training data. The cross-validation process was then repeated 5 times, with each of the 5 subsamples used once as the validation data. Figure 2 illustrates the data used for our machine learning model. Due to optimization steps and to enable an increased sensitivity, we added additional data of a younger study population (n = 39, 23–38 years) for left and right turnings, as well as sit-to-stand and stand-to-sit transitions, which were underrepresented in our dataset. Imbalanced data refer often to classification problems because standard classifiers tend to be overwhelmed by the large classes and ignore the small ones [21]. Before this optimization step, data of these activities were underrepresented in comparison to walking and sitting.

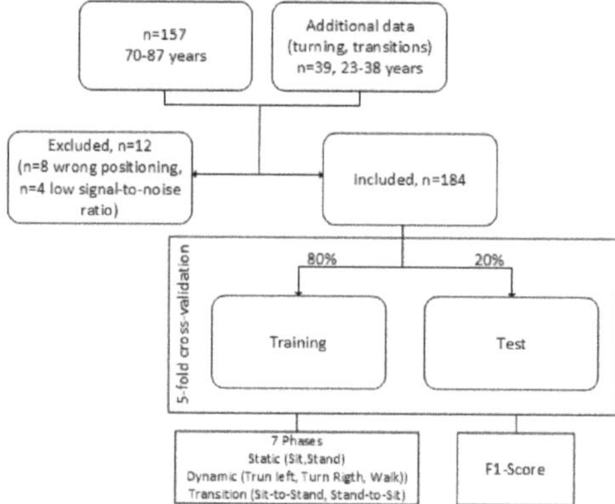

Figure 2. Used data for the machine learning model. Additional data of a younger study population (n = 20, aged 23–37 years) was included for optimization of the recognition of turnings and transitions.

The geriatric tests in our study were supported by technology. Thereby, the TUG was technically measured via the aTUG system and the sensor belt, which are described in the following.

2.1. aTUG System

The aTUG system is illustrated in Figure 3. It includes four force sensors (FS) in each chair leg, a laser range scanner (LRS) and a light barrier (LB). The force sensors (rated force: 1 kN, accuracy class: 1%) measure the force distribution on the chair. Especially the transitions (sit-to-stand, stand-to-sit) can be analyzed by these sensors. The TUG duration analysis by force sensors achieved a root mean square error (RMSE) of 0.90 s after calibration [8]. The laser range scanner (Hokuyo UTM-30LX, Hokuyo Automatic Co., Ltd., Osaka, Japan) was used for gait analyses during the walking phases and the turning. Additionally, a light barrier (OSRAM LD271, OSRAM Opto Semiconductors GmbH, Regensburg, Germany) was mounted at the backrest of the chair to detect the beginning and end of the TUG test. All sensors are commercially available. The aTUG system is able to detect the duration of the TUG test with a mean error of 0.05 s and a standard deviation of 0.59 s [22].

Due to its valid and precise measurements, the aTUG system is used as the reference system.

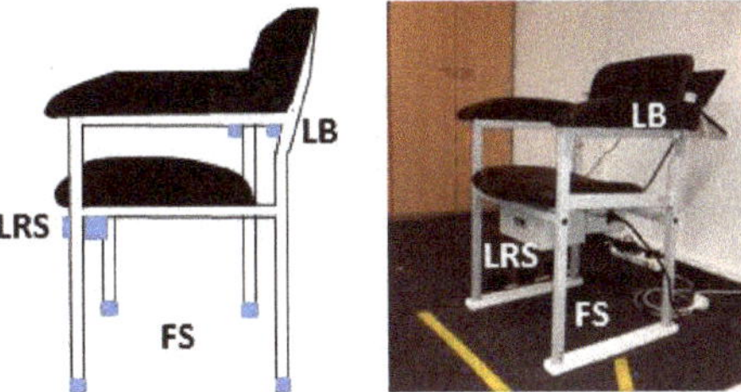

Figure 3. The aTUG system is used for automated TUG tests and includes force sensors (FS) in each chair leg, a laser range scanner (LRS) and a light barrier (LB).

2.2. Sensor-Belt

Besides the aTUG system, a wearable system was utilized, which is also commercially available. Figure 4 shows the sensor system, which is integrated into a belt and worn at the hip. The dimension of the sensor unit is about 11 cm × 2.5 cm (battery included), and the overall weight of the belt is 140 g. This compact and light system enables an easy, unobtrusive and comfortable measurement. The sensor unit consists of a triaxial accelerometer (Bosch BMA180, Bosch Sensortec GmbH, Reutlingen, Germany), gyroscope (STMicroelectronics L3GD20H, STMicroelectronics, Geneva, Switzerland) and magnetometer, as well as a barometer. The sensitivity of the accelerometer is ±16G and the resolution 12 bit, while the sensitivity of the gyroscope lies at $\pm 2000 \text{ deg} \cdot \text{s}^{-1}$. We used a general sampling rate of 100 Hz in our study. The orientation of the sensors is illustrated in Figure 1. The correct placement of the sensor belt, as well as the position of the sensor unit inside the belt were checked for each participant of our study by our physical therapists or study nurses and was adapted individually to ensure a correct alignment between the L3 and L5 lumbar vertebral body. Especially regarding our machine learning approach, a correct alignment is important for a good classification performance.

In our study, we used only the inertial sensors (accelerometer and gyroscope) to avoid over-fitting, because the magnetometer is highly influenced by environmental noise (metal chair). The barometer can be used to detect changes in height. However, since the accuracy lies about ±10 cm, the air pressure data were excluded due to their low additional information content.

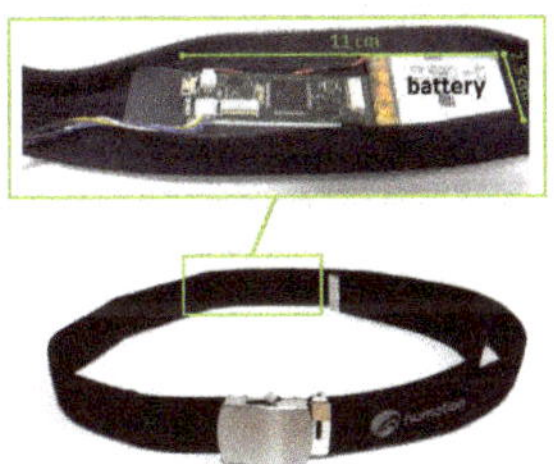

Figure 4. The sensor belt includes a 3D accelerometer, gyroscope and magnetometer, as well as a barometer.

2.3. Machine Learning and Algorithm

2.3.1. Pattern of TUG Test and Labeling

Figure 5 shows exemplarily the acceleration and gyroscope data of one person in three axes (vertical, mediolateral and anterior-posterior) during the TUG test. The coordinate orientation of the sensors is illustrated in Figure 1. The different phases of the TUG are marked in Figure 5. The static activity of sitting at the beginning and the end of the TUG can be easily recognized based on its nearly constant values of acceleration and angular velocity. Especially for the phases of turning, the gyroscope data in y-direction show significant peaks. The walking phases are characterized by peaks, which can be used for step detection. In the shown example are three steps before the participants starts the turning. The overall duration of this tests is about 12 s ($14-2$ s). The decision between turning and stand-to-sit at the end of the TUG test can be difficult, because of a possible overlay of these movements.

Supervised learning is a type of machine learning algorithm that uses a known dataset to make predictions for a new dataset. To create this training set, the TUG-phases are manually labeled by experts regarding their acceleration and gyroscope signals via a rule-based method. After labeling, features are derived for classification for each movement. In order to describe our algorithm, we will focus on the derived features, the sliding window and the classifier in the next subsection.

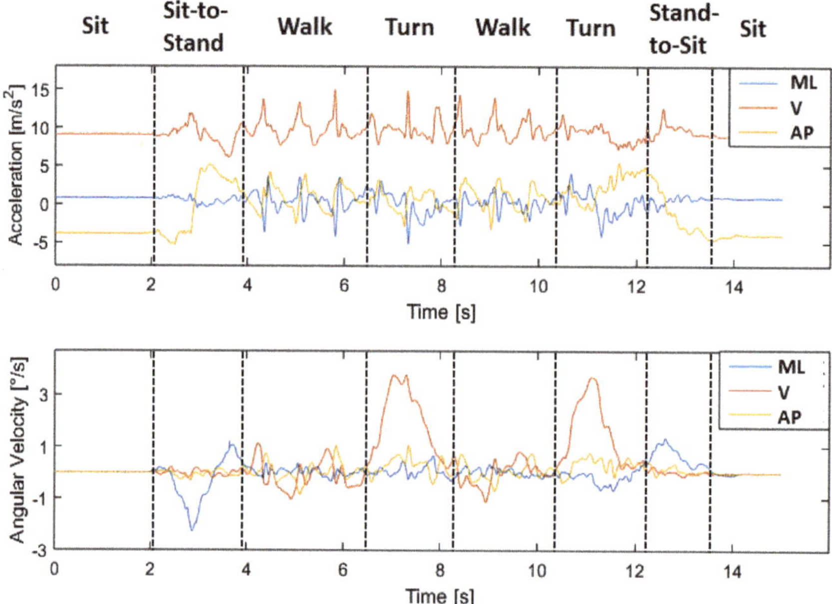

Figure 5. Example of the acceleration and gyroscope data during a TUG test. The TUG test consists of several components of everyday movements, which are marked in the graph. Each component is characterized by specific features, which are derived for machine learning classification. Medio-Lateral (ML); Vertical (V); Anterior-Posterior (AP).

2.3.2. Hierarchical Classification Model

We developed a hierarchical model for classification (see Figure 6). Therefore, four classifiers were trained. After a low pass filtering of the raw data, the first classifier (1) distinguished between static and dynamic activities, as well as transitions. If the state was classified, the other classifiers (2)–(4) characterized the activities in detail after filtering the raw data with the mentioned filters in Table 3.

The features of the specific phases are extracted to characterize the movements. The used features are:

- Auto Correlation (AC)
- Pitch (P)
- Root Mean Square (RMS)
- Signal Magnitude Area (SMA)
- Spectral Entropy (SE)

- Mean (M)
- Standard Deviation (SD)
- Signal Energy (SE)
- Signal Vector Magnitude (SVM)
- Correlation (C)

A detailed description of each feature and its calculation can be found in [23].

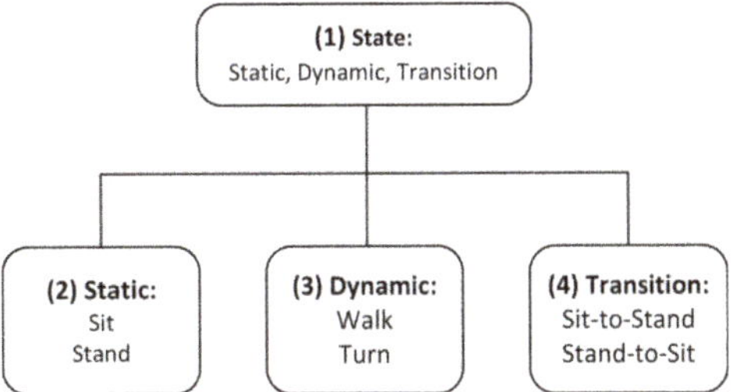

Figure 6. Hierarchical classification model. The first classifier distinguished between the state, and the others classify the possible activities of each state.

Since activity recognition requires a careful selection of feature combinations for classification, the number of features used is limited, so that only these are used, which significantly improves the classification model. This is done because, on the one hand, not every feature combination is suitable for each classification and, on the other hand, the computation time must remain efficient.

We used four different classification models to optimize our activity recognition: Boosted Decision Trees (BDT) [24,25], Boosted Decision Stump (BDS) [26], Multilayer Perceptrons (MLP) [27] and Adaptive Multi-Hyperplane Machine (AMM) [28]. The *F1*-score,recall, precision and accuracy are used for validations: the *F1*-score is the harmonic mean of precision, and recall and is defined by:

$$F1 = 2 \cdot \frac{precision \cdot recall}{precision + recall}, \tag{1}$$

where precision and recall are defined by:

$$precision = \frac{tp}{tp + fp} \tag{2}$$

and:

$$recall = \frac{tp}{tp + fn}, \tag{3}$$

with *tp* as true positive, *fp* as false positive and *fn* as false negative. The accuracy is defined by:

$$accuracy = \frac{tp + tn}{tp + tn + fp + fn}, \tag{4}$$

with *tn* as true negative.

Table 3 sums up the parameters for our classifiers, which were determined after optimization analyses.

The methods, as well as the sliding window parameters and the feature sets are different for each classifier. The combinations with the best results are presented here (cf. Table 4). Thereby, the features were calculated in each case for all components of Acceleration (Acc), Gyroscope (Gyro) or for both (Acc + Gyro).

Table 3. Parameters for our classifiers: method, size and step-width of the sliding window, as well as the noise reduction filter and feature set. The abbreviations of the features are listed in the text. The used data for each feature are specified in brackets at the end of the line: Acceleration data (Acc), Gyroscope data (Gyro). The abbreviations HL and HN stand for hidden layer and hidden nodes. The cut-off frequency of the specific filters is f_c. AC, Auto Correlation; C, Correlation; SMA, Signal Magnitude Area.

	Classifier	Method	Window Size (s)	Step Width (s)	Filter	Feature-Set
(1)	State	Boosted Decision Trees	1.405	0.072	Low pass ($f_c = 6.1\,\text{Hz}$)	AC, C, Mean (Acc), RMS, SD, SE (Acc + Gyro)
(2)	Static	Multilayer Perceptrons (5 HL, 7 HN)	2.511	0.427	-	Mean, SMA (Acc), Pitch, AC, C (Acc + Gyro)
(3)	Dynamic	Multilayer Perceptrons (3 HL, 44 HN)	1.853	0.249	Gaussian $\sigma = 0.23$	RMS (Acc), Pitch, AC, C, SMA, SD (Acc + Gyro)
(4)	Transition	Multilayer (4 HL, 40 HN) Perceptrons (4 HL, 40 HN)	1.135	0.073	Low pass ($f_c = 4.5\,\text{Hz}$)	RMS (Acc), Mean, SE (Gyro), AC, C, SMA, SD (Acc + Gyro), Pitch

Table 4. *F1*-scores of the classification methods for the different classifiers: Boosted Decision Trees (BDT), Multilayer Perceptrons (MLP).

Classifier	*F1*-Score (%)	Method (%)
State	96.6	BDT
Static	97.3	MLP
Dynamic	97.5	MLP
Transition	94.8	MLP

2.4. TUG Analyses Algorithm

The raw data are classified via our hierarchical classification model as described in Section 2.3.2. Since we want to detect complete TUG sequences, we used a rule-based model to identify the TUG test via its specific phases and their order. For this, the order of the automatically generated labels of the classified sub-activities will be checked. A valid TUG sequence consists of the following phases (see Figures 1 and 5):

Sit-to-stand → walk → turn → walk → turn → stand-to-sit.

Since the sub-activities can be expected to include some classification errors, due to the false-positive rates of the trained classifiers (see Table 4), and to take the variations of performing the TUG test into account, we included the following approach to increase the robustness of the algorithm. Nine models were specified as valid TUG sequences. Especially, doubled activities such as turn-turn were accepted as valid and were combined as one turn. Another valid model consisted of the combination sit-to-stand → stand-to-sit → walk, which is implausible and indicates a misclassification. Therefore, our model allows minor illogical classification errors. For example:

- Sit-to-stand → stand-to-sit → walk → turn → turn → walk → turn → stand-to-sit
- Sit-to-stand → walk → turn → turn → walk → turn → stand-to-sit
- ...

Especially regarding the aim to analyze further unsupervised-assessments in non-standardized settings, this more robust approach might be more applicable. A list of all models and their accuracies is presented in the Results Section 3.3. The duration of each phase can be determined by these motion labels, as well as the overall duration of the TUG test. In the evaluationsection, we compare our results with stopwatch measurements by medical experts and the aTUG system.

3. Results

After the description of the study design, sensors used and the algorithms, we want to focus on our results in the following.

3.1. Results of the Hierarchical Classification Model

Table 4 shows the results of the F1-scores for the best combination of each method. While boosted decision trees achieved the highest F1-score for the state-classification, multilayer perceptrons were most suitable for the classification of static and dynamic activities, as well as transitions.

3.2. Results of TUG-Phases' Classification

The results for recall, precision, accuracy and F1-score for our classification of each TUG component are listed in Table 5. We achieved F1-scores >0.94 for the static activities standing and sitting, as well as for the dynamic activity walking. However, especially for the short movements such as the transitions and turnings, we only achieved F1-scores between 0.70 and 0.81. For further optimization, more data of these activities are needed, because these movements are still underrepresented, even though we used additional data. However, accuracies above 0.96 could be achieved for all TUG components.

Table 5. Results of our classification model for static (sit, stand) and dynamic (walk, turn around) activities, as well as transitions (sit-to-stand, stand-to-sit).

Classifier	Activity	Recall	Precision	Accuracy	F1-Score
Static	Sit	0.93	0.96	0.96	0.95
	Stand	0.96	0.91	0.97	0.94
Dynamic	Turn around	0.78	0.83	0.99	0.81
	Walk	0.98	0.98	0.98	0.97
Transition	Sit-to-Stand	0.84	0.66	0.99	0.74
	Stand-to-Sit	0.94	0.56	0.99	0.70

3.3. Results of TUG Classification

The TUG classification followed a rule-based model. The detected activities had to be in a specific order to be recognized as a valid TUG test. Since one of the valid models could be found in the data, the duration of the whole activity was calculated based on the durations of the single phases. The resulting duration had to be below 30 s to be accepted as TUG-test since durations over 30 s were not realistic because they failed our inclusion criteria.

As already mentioned in Section 2.4, nine models were accepted as valid TUG tests, to increase the robustness of our algorithm. The accuracy was estimated in accordance with Equation (4). The cumulative accuracy A_i was calculated by the sum of the accuracies of the nine valid models A_j:

$$A_i = \sum_{i=1}^{j} A_j \tag{5}$$

Table 6 lists the included models and the accuracies of TUG test detection.

Table 6. Included models and the resulting recognition accuracy, as well as the cumulative accuracy. The order of the activities for each model is listed in following terms: sit-to-stand (↑), Walk (W), Turn (T), stand-to-sit (↓).

#	Model	Accuracy A_j (%)	Cum.Accuracy A_i (%)
1	↑ *W T W T* ↓	15.37	15.37
2	↑↓ *W T W T* ↓	52.15	67.52
3	↑↓ *T W T* ↓	12.35	79.87
4	↑↓ *T* ↓	5.67	85.54
5	↑↓ *W T* ↓	4.34	89.88
6	↑ *T W T* ↓	2.34	92.22
7	↑↓ *W T W T W* ↓	1.67	93.89
8	↑ *W T W T W* ↓	1.33	95.22
9	↑ *W T* ↓	1.33	96.55

The model in the first line corresponds to the standard sequence of TUG phases. With these nine considered models, we reach a recognition accuracy of 96.55%, which corresponds to the cumulative accuracy. Of course, more models can be created to achieve higher accuracies, but this would also lead to a higher false-positive rate.

3.4. Comparison with Stopwatch Measurement

In order to validate our system regarding the measurement of the total time, we compared our results with two reference measurements, assumed as the gold standard. Besides the automated, technical measures, medical professionals measured the test duration by stopwatch. The histogram in Figure 7 shows the needed test duration for our study population (stopwatch measurements). Due to the left-skewed distribution, we estimated a gamma distribution (red line).

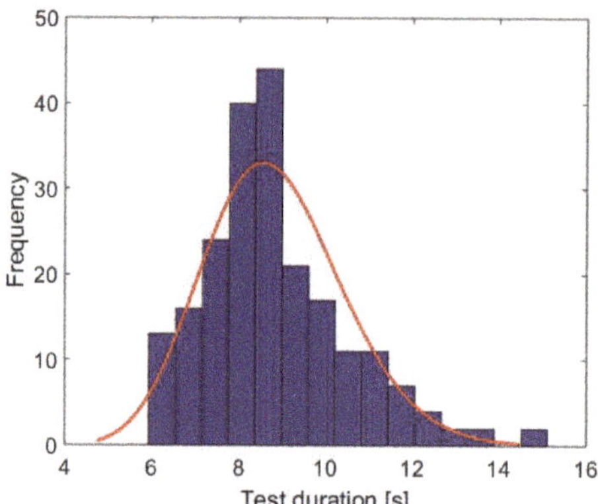

Figure 7. Distribution of the TUG test duration (stopwatch measurements) and the estimated gamma distribution (red line).

A correlation analysis between the stopwatch and automated measurements showed a significant correlation with an excellent correlation coefficient of $r = 0.97$ and a p-value of <0.001. Figure 8 refers to the comparison between the measured test duration by stopwatch and our IMU system. As expected, there was a linear relationship. A regression analysis results in the following relation:

$$TUG\_Duration_{IMU} = 0.90 \cdot TUG\_Duration_{stopwatch} + 0.766 \tag{6}$$

Additionally, a Bland–Altman plot was used to analyze the agreement between both systems (see Figure 8b). Since the mean value was near zero, our IMU-based system had no fixed bias.

The minimal detectable change differed in the literature between 1.14 s [29] and 3.4 s [30]. Therefore, differences within the mean ±1.96 SD were not clinically important, and the two methods may be used interchangeably.

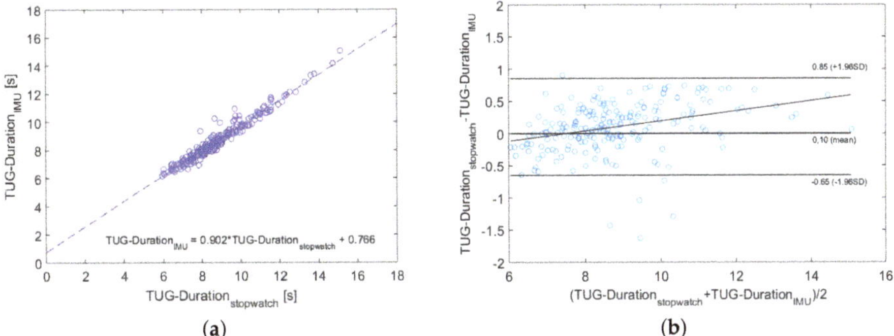

Figure 8. Comparison between stopwatch and IMU measurements. The dashed line represents the linear regression line and corresponds to the stated equation in (**a**). The Bland–Altman plot and its characteristic values are shown in (**b**). (**a**) Correlation analysis; (**b**) Bland–Altman plot.

3.5. Comparison with the aTUG System

As already mentioned, we used the aTUG as an additional reference system. The correlation analysis has shown an excellent correlation coefficient of $r = 0.99$ and a p-value of <0.001. Figure 9 shows the comparison between the aTUG and the IMU results. Again, there is a linear relationship:

$$TUG\_Duration_{IMU} = 1.01 \cdot TUG\_Duration_{aTUG} + 0.954 \tag{7}$$

This was in good agreement with our previous findings. The marginally better correlation between aTUG and IMU than the stopwatch and IMU might be due to the inter-tester reliability, which influences the stopwatch measurements. Even though, these influences have been shown to be minimal [20].

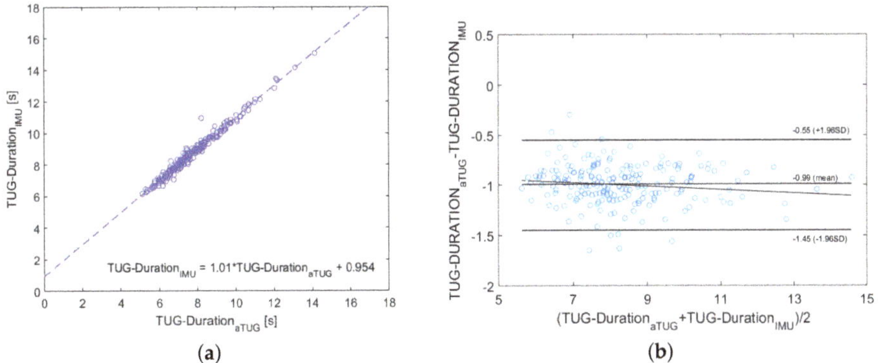

Figure 9. Comparison between aTUG and IMU measurements. The dashed line represents the linear regression line and corresponds to the stated equation in (**a**). The Bland–Altman plot and its characteristic values are shown in (**b**). (**a**) Correlation analysis; (**b**) Bland–Altman plot.

The Bland–Altman plot indicated a consistent bias, which can be adjusted by subtracting the mean difference from the biased method. The differences within the mean 1.96 SD were not clinically important either. Therefore, these two methods can be also used interchangeably.

3.6. Suitability for Self-Assessments

In order to evaluate the suitability of the sensor-belt for self-assessments, we asked the participants to wear the belt after the assessment for one week during the day. Since the battery runtime was about two days, the participants were instructed to load the battery every night, which worked well for most participants. Due to the individual positioning of the sensor-unit in the belt between the L3 and L5 lumbar vertebral body by the medical experts in the assessments, the sensor could also be positioned with a sufficient precision by the participants themselves. To confirm the suitability of our TUG classification for self-assessments, we classified the complete recordings of the test battery within the assessment, which consisted of several tests such as for example the short physical performance battery, the frailty criteria or the stair climb power test. Figure 10 shows our assessment room. To make an intermediate step to future home-assessments, we analyzed a semi-unsupervised situation. Within this test battery, the participants were asked to change seats (from Chair 1 to the aTUG-system (Chair 2)) as a preparation for the TUG-test (see Figure 10).

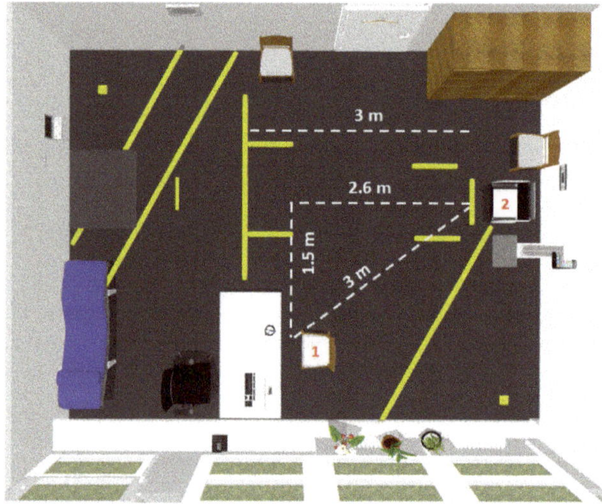

Figure 10. Sketch of our laboratory. Within a semi-unsupervised situation, the participants change from Chair 1 to Chair 2.

In this semi-unsupervised situation, the participants stood up from Chair 1 and walked with one turning to Chair 2 and sat down. This sequence was similar to a TUG sequence. The walking distances (white lines in Figure 10) varied between 3 m and about 4.1 m. Therefore, the mean distance was assumed to be 3.55 m.

Due to our set of valid TUG models, our system had the ability to recognize also these modified TUG sequences. Besides the already analyzed supervised TUG-tests, we identified 190 additional sequences in our data, which had a similar series of movements to the TUG test. In order to analyze this semi-unsupervised situation, we compared these results of 78 participants with the TUG-test duration. For better comparability, we normalized the data to the assumed walking distance (TUG-test: 6 m, change seats: 3.55 m). This approach had the limitation that the duration of the transfer movements (sit-to-stand, stand-to-sit) were supposed to be approximately the same, as well as the participants chose a mean distance of 3.55 m for changing seats. However, this first approximation showed a moderate correlation ($r = 0.51$, $p < 0.01$) between these parameters. Figure 11 shows the normalized test durations.

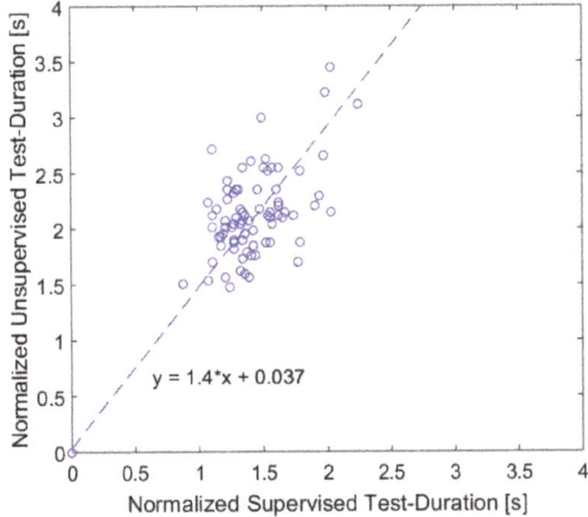

Figure 11. Comparison of the normalized durations of the TUG-test and the semi-unsupervised test situation.

The results show that the self-selected speed was significantly slower than the speed in the test situation regarding the Wilcoxon test ($p < 0.01$), which was applied due to the not normally distributed TUG test duration (see Figure 7). By assuming that the transfer movements and turnings were approximately the same, the differences in speed lied in the self-selected gait speed.

In order to investigate the correlation of the TUG test with the other battery of assessments, Pearson's linear correlation coefficient was computed between the Standard TUG duration (STUG) and Unsupervised TUG duration (UTUG) with different geriatric tests. The results are listed in Table 7. The standardized TUG test had a higher correlation coefficient in all test than the semi-unsupervised TUG test.

Table 7. Correlation coefficients of the Standard TUG duration (STUG) and Unsupervised TUG duration (UTUG) with other geriatric tests like for example the chair rising and gait speed of the Short Physical Performance Battery (SPPB). Significant results are marked with an asterisk (*).

	STUG		UTUG	
	r	p	r	p
Stair Climb Power Test	0.85	<0.01 *	0.52	<0.01 *
SPPB-Chair Rising Test	0.67	<0.01 *	0.28	<0.01 *
SPPB-Gait Speed	0.75	<0.01 *	0.36	<0.05 *
6-min Walk Test	−0.82	<0.01 **	−0.44	<0.01 *

4. Discussion

The main purpose of the present study was to develop an automated mobility assessments for older people based on inertial TUG measurements, which is able to be used in clinical environments, as well as in future unsupervised self-assessments at home. Therefore, we conducted a prospective study with 157 participants aged 70 and above and used the data to identify a suitable machine learning classifier for TUG-phases' recognition. We achieved accuracies over 96% in the classification of the specific TUG components and for the complete TUG sequence recognition via a rule-based approach. In comparison to other studies, these results are satisfactory, especially regarding our minimalistic sensor system of one IMU, which was positioned in a belt at the hip. To validate our results, we compared the IMU-based data with two reference systems as the criterion standard, which showed significant correlations of 0.97 (stopwatch) and 0.99 (aTUG), respectively. This underlines the suitability of our system for clinical investigations. Thus, the system is a powerful, low-cost and accurate tool for automated TUG test analyses. Further analyses of the accuracy of our system to determine each TUG phase in terms of time, related to the reference system, should be done. This might be a valuable addition, especially for clinical issues, which addresses diseases with the influences of only specific phases of the TUG test.

Since we want to detect both standardized TUG-sequences and similar sequences, which may occur in daily life and are more naturalistic than the standard TUG setup, we focused as an intermediate step to unsupervised home-assessments on a semi-unsupervised situation with similar sequences to the TUG test within the assessment. The most important limitation and simultaneously a great opportunity lie in our set of valid TUG models. On the one hand, this could lead to misclassifications in laboratory settings, but on the other hand, it allows detecting movement sequences that are similar to the TUG test. The comparison of the durations confirmed the expected result that the self-selected speed is lower in non-test situations, but there is a moderate correlation between these tests. Maybe the self-selected speed can be more sensitive to functional changes than assessments in a test situation, when a participant tries to perform particularly well. However, in our first analyses, we could not confirm this hypothesis. Correlation analyses between different geriatric tests and the TUG variations show a stronger correlation between the standard TUG test and the other tests than for the semi-unsupervised TUG. This had been expected, since a stronger correlation was expected between the test situations.

The attraction and the novelty of our approach lies in the combination of a high accuracy in TUG classification with only one single inertial measurement unit, the large study population, the automated analyses, the simplicity of our the system (no interaction required, easy to use) and the suitability of the investigation of unsupervised or rather unstandardized assessments.

The general suitability of our sensor system was investigated during a home-assessment following the clinical assessments, in which the participants wore the sensor-belt during the day for one week and wrote an activity diary. Most participants were able to load the battery and wear the belt in the correct position by themselves.

Further analyses of the home-assessment data are planed to analyze the significance regarding the detection of functional decline. Especially, the investigation of the single TUG phases in unsupervised situations might be worthwhile. In summary, our system is applicable for flexible measurement of the Timed Up and Go test performance in clinical settings, as well as in semi-unsupervised situations. The determined IMU-based test durations are in good agreement with the stopwatch measurements by medical experts and the aTUG-system. Assessments of non-standardized variations of TUG sequences might be a worthwhile enhancement for the identification of changes in the functional status, but need further investigations.

Author Contributions: Conceptualization, J.M.B., A.H. and S.F. Data curation, S.H., L.D., R.D. and S.F. Formal analysis, S.H. and B.I. Funding acquisition, J.M.B., A.H. and S.F. Investigation, S.H., L.D. and S.F. Methodology, S.H., B.I., L.D., A.H. and S.F. Project administration, R.D. and S.F. Resources, J.M.B. and A.H. Software, S.H., B.I. and S.F. Supervision, J.M.B., A.H. and S.F. Validation, S.H. and B.I. Visualization, S.H. and B.I. Writing, original draft, S.H. Writing, review and editing, S.H., B.I., L.D., R.D., A.H. and S.F.

Funding: The study is funded by the German Federal Ministry of Education and Research (Project No. 01EL1822D).

Conflicts of Interest: The authors declare no conflict of interest.

References

1.   Podsiadlo, D.; Richardson, S. The Timed Up & Go: A test of basic functional mobility for frail elderly persons. *J. Am. Geriat. Soc.* **1991**, *39*, 142–148, doi:10.1111/j.1532-5415.1991.tb01616.x. [CrossRef] [PubMed]

2. Hellmers, S.; Steen, E.E.; Dasenbrock, L.; Heinks, A.; Bauer, J.M.; Fudickar, S.; Hein, A. Towards a minimized unsupervised technical assessment of physical performance in domestic environments. In Proceedings of the 11th EAI International Conference on Pervasive Computing Technologies for Healthcare, Barcelona, Spain, 23–26 May 2017; pp. 207–216.

3. Van Lummel, R.C.; Walgaard, S.; Hobert, M.A.; Maetzler, W.; Van Dieën, J.H.; Galindo-Garre, F.; Terwee, C.B. Intra-Rater, inter-rater and test-retest reliability of an instrumented timed up and go (iTUG) Test in patients with Parkinson's disease. *PLoS ONE* **2016**, *11*, e0151881, doi:10.1371/journal.pone.0151881. [CrossRef] [PubMed]

4. Van Iersel, M.B.; Munneke, M.; Esselink, R.A.; Benraad, C.E.; Rikkert, M.G.O. Gait velocity and the Timed-Up-and-Go test were sensitive to changes in mobility in frail elderly patients. *J. Clin. Epidemiol.* **2008**, *61*, 186–191, doi:10.1016/j.jclinepi.2007.04.016. [CrossRef] [PubMed]

5. Wall, J.C.; Bell, C.; Campbell, S.; Davis, J. The Timed Get-up-and-Go test revisited: Measurement of the component tasks. *J. Rehabil. Res. Dev.* **2000**, *37*, 109. [PubMed]

6. Sprint, G.; Cook, D.J.; Weeks, D.L. Toward automating clinical assessments: A survey of the timed Up and Go. *IEEE Rev. Biomed. Eng.* **2015**, *8*, 64–77, doi:10.1109/RBME.2015.2390646. [CrossRef] [PubMed]

7. Frenken, T.; Lipprandt, M.; Brell, M.; Gövercin, M.; Wegel, S.; Steinhagen-Thiessen, E.; Hein, A. Novel approach to unsupervised mobility assessment tests: Field trial for aTUG. In Proceedings of the 2012 6th International Conference on Pervasive Computing Technologies for Healthcare (PervasiveHealth), San Diego, CA, USA, 21–24 May 2012; pp. 131–138.

8. Fudickar, S.; Kiselev, J.; Frenken, T.; Wegel, S.; Dimitrowska, S.; Steinhagen-Thiessen, E.; Hein, A. Validation of the ambient TUG chair with light barriers and force sensors in a clinical trial. *Assist. Technol.* **2018**, 1–8, doi:10.1080/10400435.2018.1446195. [CrossRef] [PubMed]

9. Frenken, T.; Frenken, M.; Gövercin, M.; Kiselev, J.; Meyer, J.; Wegel, S.; Hein, A. A novel ICT approach to the assessment of mobility in diverse health care environments. In Proceedings of the CEWIT-TZI-acatech Workshop "ICT Meets Medicine and Health"(ICTMH 2013), Bremen, Germany, 19–20 March 2013.

10. Higashi, Y.; Yamakoshi, K.; Fujimoto, T.; Sekine, M.; Tamura, T. Quantitative evaluation of movement using the timed up-and-go test. *IEEE Eng. Med. Biol. Mag.* **2008**, *27*, 38–46, doi:10.1109/MEMB.2008.919494. [CrossRef]

11. Salarian, A.; Horak, F.B.; Zampieri, C.; Carlson-Kuhta, P.; Nutt, J.G.; Aminian, K. iTUG, a sensitive and reliable measure of mobility. *IEEE Trans. Neural Syst. Rehabil. Eng.* **2010**, *18*, 303–310, doi:10.1109/TNSRE.2010.2047606. [CrossRef] [PubMed]

12. Chiari, L. Wearable systems with minimal set-up for monitoring and training of balance and mobility. In Proceedings of the 2011 Annual International Conference of the IEEE Engineering in Medicine and Biology Society (EMBC), Boston, MA, USA, 30 August–3 September 2011; pp. 5828–5832.

13. Jallon, P.; Dupre, B.; Antonakios, M. A graph based method for timed up & go test qualification using inertial sensors. In Proceedings of the 2011 IEEE International Conference on Acoustics, Speech and Signal Processing (ICASSP), Prague, Czech Republic, 22–27 May 2011; pp. 689–692.

14. Adame, M.R.; Al-Jawad, A.; Romanovas, M.; Hobert, M.; Maetzler, W.; Möller, K.; Manoli, Y. TUG test instrumentation for Parkinson's disease patients using inertial sensors and dynamic time warping. *Biomed. Eng./Biomed. Tech.* **2012**, *57*, 1071–1074, doi:10.1515/bmt-2012-4426. [CrossRef]

15. Milosevic, M.; Jovanov, E.; Milenković, A. Quantifying Timed-Up-and-Go test: A smartphone implementation. In Proceedings of the 2013 IEEE International Conference on Body Sensor Networks (BSN), Cambridge, MA, USA, 6–9 May 2013, pp. 1–6.

16. Reinfelder, S.; Hauer, R.; Barth, J.; Klucken, J.; Eskofier, B.M. Timed Up-and-Go phase segmentation in Parkinson's disease patients using unobtrusive inertial sensors. In Proceedings of the 37th Annual International Conference of the IEEE Engineering in Medicine and Biology Society (EMBC), Milan, Italy, 25–29 August 2015; pp. 5171–5174.

17. Nguyen, H.; Lebel, K.; Boissy, P.; Bogard, S.; Goubault, E.; Duval, C. Auto detection and segmentation of daily living activities during a Timed Up and Go task in people with Parkinson's disease using multiple inertial sensors. *J. Neuroeng. Rehabil.* **2017**, *14*, 26. [CrossRef] [PubMed]

18. Marschollek, M.; Nemitz, G.; Gietzelt, M.; Wolf, K.; Zu Schwabedissen, H.M.; Haux, R. Predicting in-patient falls in a geriatric clinic. *Z. Gerontol. Geriatr.* **2009**, *42*, 317–322, doi:10.1007/s00391-009-0035-7. [CrossRef] [PubMed]

19. Greene, B.R.; O'Donovan, A.; Romero-Ortuno, R.; Cogan, L.; Scanaill, C.N.; Kenny, R.A. Quantitative falls risk assessment using the timed up and go test. *IEEE Trans. Biomed. Eng.* **2010**, *57*, 2918–2926, doi:10.1109/TBME.2010.2083659. [CrossRef] [PubMed]

20. Hellmers, S.; Fudickar, S.; Büse, C.; Dasenbrock, L.; Heinks, A.; Bauer, J.M.; Hein, A. Technology supported geriatric assessment. In *Ambient Assisted Living*; Springer: Cham, Switzerland, 2017; pp. 85–100.

21. Chawla, N.V.; Japkowicz, N.; Kotcz, A. Special issue on learning from imbalanced datasets. *ACM Sigkdd Explor. Newsl.* **2004**, *6*, 1–6, doi:10.1145/1007730.1007733. [CrossRef]

22. Frenken, T.; Vester, B.; Brell, M.; Hein, A. aTUG: Fully-automated timed up and go assessment using ambient sensor technologies. In Proceedings of the 2011 5th International Conference on Pervasive Computing Technologies for Healthcare (PervasiveHealth), Dublin, Ireland, 23–26 May 2011; pp. 55–62.

23. Figo, D.; Diniz, P.C.; Ferreira, D.R.; Cardoso, J.M. Preprocessing techniques for context recognition from accelerometer data. *Pers. Ubiquitous Comput.* **2010**, *14*, 645–662, doi:10.1007/s00779-010-0293-9. [CrossRef]

24. Rokach, L.; Maimon, O. *Data Mining with Decision Trees*; World Scientific: Singapore, 2007.

25. Schapire, R.E. The boosting approach to machine learning: An overview. In *Nonlinear Estimation and Classification*; Springer: New York, NY, USA, 2003; pp. 149–171.

26. Iba, W.; Langley, P. Induction of one-level decision trees. In *Machine Learning Proceedings 1992*; Morgan Kaufmann Publishers Inc.: San Francisco, CA, USA, 1992; pp. 233–240.

27. Beale, R.; Jackson, T. *Neural Computing—An introduction*; CRC Press: Boca Raton, FL, USA, 1990.

28. Wang, Z.; Djuric, N.; Crammer, K.; Vucetic, S. Trading representability for scalability: Adaptive multi-hyperplane machine for nonlinear classification. In Proceedings of the 17th ACM SIGKDD International Conference on Knowledge Discovery and Data Mining, San Diego, CA, USA, 21–24 August 2011; pp. 24–32.

29. Alghadir, A.; Anwer, S.; Brismée, J.M. The reliability and minimal detectable change of Timed Up and Go test in individuals with grade 1–3 knee osteoarthritis. *BMC Musculoskelet. Disord.* **2015**, *16*, 174, doi:10.1186/s12891-015-0637-8. [CrossRef] [PubMed]

30. Gautschi, O.P.; Stienen, M.N.; Corniola, M.V.; Joswig, H.; Schaller, K.; Hildebrandt, G.; Smoll, N.R. Assessment of the minimum clinically important difference in the timed up and go test after surgery for lumbar degenerative disc disease. *Neurosurgery* **2017**, *80*, 380–385, doi:10.1227/NEU.0000000000001320. [CrossRef] [PubMed]

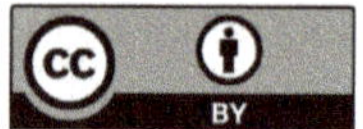

© 2018 by the authors. Licensee MDPI, Basel, Switzerland. This article is an open access article distributed under the terms and conditions of the Creative Commons Attribution (CC BY) license (http://creativecommons.org/licenses/by/4.0/).

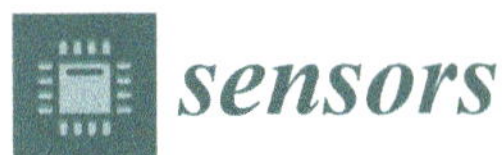 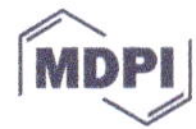

Article

Gait Symmetry Assessment with a Low Back 3D Accelerometer in Post-Stroke Patients

Wei Zhang [1],*, Matthew Smuck [2,3], Catherine Legault [4], Ma A. Ith [2,3], Amir Muaremi [5] and Kamiar Aminian [1]

1   Laboratory of Movement Analysis and Measurement Ecole Polytechnique Fédérale de Lausanne (EPFL), 1015 Lausanne, Switzerland; kamiar.aminian@epfl.ch
2   Wearable Health Lab, Department of Orthopaedic Surgery, Stanford University, Redwood City, CA 94063, USA; msmuck@stanford.edu (M.S.); mith@stanford.edu (M.A.I.)
3   Division of Physical Medicine & Rehabilitation, Stanford University, Palo Alto, CA 94304, USA
4   Stanford Stroke Center, Stanford University, Palo Alto, CA 94304, USA; clegault@stanford.edu
5   Novartis Institutes for BioMedical Research, 4056 Basel, Switzerland; amir.muaremi@novartis.com
*   Correspondence: w.zhang@epfl.ch; Tel.: +41-21-693-7606

Received: 14 August 2018; Accepted: 29 September 2018; Published: 3 October 2018

Abstract: Gait asymmetry is an important marker of mobility impairment post stroke. This study proposes a new gait symmetry index (GSI) to quantify gait symmetry with one 3D accelerometer at L3 (GSI_{L3}). GSI_{L3} was evaluated with 16 post stroke patients and nine healthy controls in the Six-Minute-Walk-Test (6-MWT). Discriminative power was evaluated with Wilcoxon test and the effect size (ES) was computed with Cliff's Delta. GSI_{L3} estimated during the entire 6-MWT and during a short segment straight walk ($GSI_{L3straight}$) have comparable effect size to one another (ES = 0.89, $p < 0.001$) and to the symmetry indices derived from feet sensors ($|ES| = [0.22, 0.89]$). Furthermore, while none of the indices derived from feet sensors showed significant differences between post stroke patients walking with a cane compared to those able to walk without, GSI_{L3} was able to discriminate between these two groups with a significantly lower value in the group using a cane (ES = 0.70, $p = 0.02$). In addition, GSI_{L3} was strongly associated with several symmetry indices measured by feet sensors during the straight walking cycles (Spearman correlation: $|\rho| = [0.82, 0.88]$, $p < 0.05$). The proposed index can be a reliable and cost-efficient post stroke gait symmetry assessment with implications for research and clinical practice.

Keywords: symmetry; trunk movement; autocorrelation; gait rehabilitation

---

1. Introduction

Stroke is the fifth leading cause of death in the United States [1]. About 80% of stroke survivors are affected by hemiparesis [1], characterized by muscle weakness and extensor spasticity in the lower extremities that can severely influence mobility in post-stroke patients. One of the typical impairments caused by this hemiparesis is gait asymmetry. In post-stroke rehabilitation programs, considerable focus is placed on the equalization of weight bearing through the lower extremities and the capacity to shift weight between the lower extremities during gait [2]. Symmetry is a target gait function to restore and is an useful outcome measure of the rehabilitation [2–6]. Despite its clinical interest and importance, there is currently no standardized method to measure gait symmetry [6,7]. Camera-based motion capture system, and pressure mats and insoles are used to analyze kinetics and kinematics of gait [4,6,8–10], and fewer studies reported different methods for gait symmetry assessment using inertial sensors [10–12]. Regardless of the tool used to measure gait, the assessment of symmetry remains a simple comparison of different spatiotemporal gait parameters between left and right sides (such as stance and swing phase, step length, etc.). To our knowledge, only one study has reported an alternative method other than aforementioned studies based on spatiotemporal gait parameters to analyze symmetry [13]. Using inertial sensors fixed on each shank, the method first applied quantization of raw sensor signals with a symbolic segmentation, then symmetry is determined by the difference ratio between the symbols of left and right side. However, a user-defined threshold on the mean squared error to determine the quantization resolution a priori limits this method's accuracy. In a recent study, we developed two simple gait symmetry indices estimated by the linear correlation coefficient and the normalized sample distance between the left and right foot pitch angular velocity [14]. The developed indices demonstrated high and comparable discriminative power than gait symmetry estimated with spatiotemporal gait parameters. Importantly, these novel methods assess gait symmetry based on signal profiles corresponding to step alternation from two sides without estimation of specific spatiotemporal gait parameters, which usually requires sophisticated signal processing and a gait model. Such a gait model is usually developed for healthy gait patterns and its reliability becomes questionable in applications with pathological gait.

Analyzing step alternation from sensor signal profile might be applicable to other sensor configurations as well. For example, one study [12] reported that asymmetry estimated by the trunk movement showed significant difference between chronic stroke patients and healthy controls, whereas comparison of side-to-side symmetry in spatiotemporal parameters did not differ between groups. However, the study reported a comparison of symmetry outcomes with only two spatiotemporal gait patterns. It is not fully clear whether the trunk movement is superior to feet kinematics for gait asymmetry estimation in post stroke patients.

In this study, we proposed and evaluated a gait symmetry index derived from a single 3D accelerometer worn at the midline of the lower back (approximately at the level of L3). The primary outcome of this study was the discriminative power of the single low back accelerometry based gait symmetry index in post-stroke patients. We compared the discriminative power to the gait symmetry indices estimated using two feet sensors that have been validated in previous studies, namely the method based on the difference ratio of various spatiotemporal gait parameters and the method based on the pitch angular velocity signal profile. The secondary outcome was the association between gait symmetry estimated by one low back accelerometer and the symmetry measured with two feet sensors.

2. Materials and Methods

2.1. Data Acquisition

Sixteen consecutively consenting post-stroke patients (nine males and seven females, average age 54 years with range 23–74, 6 using a cane) and nine healthy controls (five males and four females, average age 35 years with range 25–48) participated this study at the Physical Medicine & Rehabilitations Section and in the Department of Neurology & Neurological Sciences, at Stanford University. Six patients suffered from subcortical stroke and 10 suffered from cortical stroke. The stroke etiology was hemorrhagic in one patient and ischemic in the others. The time after stroke varied from 5 months to 11 years with a median of 20 months. Patient self-reported outcome of stroke impact scale (SIS) [15] was between 190 to 288 points with a median of 219.5 (the higher the point, the higher the impact). The ethical committee for Human Subjects Research at Stanford University approved this study. Written informed consents were obtained from the patients in the study.

Participants performed gait assessment in Six-Minute-Walk-test (6-MWT) with their comfortable walking speed under the supervision of an experienced clinical researcher. The 6-MWT is a reliable and easy to administer assessment widely used for walking function assessment following stroke [16]. At our location, the 6-MWT was conducted in a rectangular set of corridors between 15 to 25 m long linked together by 90-degree turns. During the test, patients wore a wireless inertial sensor (MTw Awinda, Xsens, Enschede, The Netherlands [17]) on top of each shoe and in the midline of the low back (approximately at the level of L3). Each sensor was held in position with an elastic band. Study participants were provided instruction before the walking assessment. When ready at the starting position (standing straight in front of the starting line), data recording started with the countdown 5 seconds prior to the command 'Start' from the clinical researcher. Recording stopped when the participant completed the 6-MWT and stood quietly at the end of the trial. Raw sensor data were transmitted to a Windows laptop via Bluetooth during the assessment. To assure good connection, a researcher walked with the laptop behind the participants during the entire 6-MWT. Meanwhile, the researcher marked down the time when the participants reached the first 90-degree turn at the end of the corridor (ca. 14 m). The sensor data collection application running on the laptop synchronized the data and exported a data file for each assessment containing 3D acceleration and 3D gyroscope data sampled at 100 Hz.

2.2. Gait Symmetry Assessment with Two Feet Sensors

2.2.1. Symmetry of Spatiotemporal Gait Parameters

We used validated algorithms [18–21] to extract spatiotemporal gait parameters from the feet sensors. Prior to processing, data were resampled to 200 Hz using linear interpolation to be consistent with the validated algorithms. In specific, gait cycles were detected based on the timing of two consecutive foot-flats [19]. Velocity and position of the foot were estimated by the numerical integration of the gravity-free acceleration data in the global frame and drift removal technique using the zero velocity update during the foot-flat period [22]. Subsequently, path length, ratio between the actual 3D path and the stride length, were estimated [22]. Heel strike and lift off angles were estimated based on the de-drifted angular velocity data [21]. Maximum angular velocity of the foot and various temporal parameters were extracted from the angular velocity signals [19]. Cycles with a turning angle between two foot-flats less than 20 degrees were considered as straight walking cycles [18]. Symmetry index (SI) was estimated using the difference ratio of the spatiotemporal parameters (listed in Table 1) of each gait cycle n according to Equation (1):

$$\text{SI}(n) = \frac{Param_{left}(n) - Param_{right}(n)}{0.5 * \left[Param_{left}(n) + Param_{right}(n) \right]} * 100\% \tag{1}$$

Table 1. Spatiotemporal parameters analyzed for each foot in one gait cycle.

Parameter [Unit]	Description
Spatial	
PathLength [% stride length]	Ratio between the length of the real path of the foot in 3D space (including both stride length and width) and stride length of one cycle.
StrikeAng [deg]	Angle between the foot and the ground at heel strike in sagittal plane.
LiftOffAng [deg]	Angle between the foot and the ground at toe off in sagittal plane.
MaxAngVel [deg/s]	Maximum pitch foot angular velocity during swing phase.
Temporal	
StanceRatio [%]	Percentage of the gait cycle during which the foot is in stance phase.
LoadRatio [%]	Percentage of the stance corresponding to loading phase defined as the time between heel strike and toe strike
FootFlatRatio [%]	Percentage of the stance corresponding to the foot-flat phase
PushRatio [%]	Percentage of the stance corresponding to push phase defined as the time between heel off and toe off.

2.2.2. Symmetry of Foot Pitch Angular Velocity

Gait symmetry was computed using the recently published algorithms [14]. The algorithms assessed symmetry using the foot pitch angular velocity signals of each gait cycle. The pitch angular velocity signal was smoothed with a 2nd order Butterworth low-pass filter (cut-off frequency of 10 Hz). The maximum lag between the signals from both feet was estimated based on cross correlation, and one signal was shifted to align left and right gait cycles. The aligned signals were segmented to individual gait cycles based on detected gait cycle of the right foot leading to two signals $\omega_{left}(n)$ and $\omega_{right}(n)$ of cycle n [19]. The gait symmetry between the left and the right signals was assessed for each cycle based on (a) Pearson correlation coefficient (denoted by GSI_{corr}) and (b) the normalized sample distance (denoted by GSI_{dist}). GSI_{dist} was the mean absolute difference between each left and right signal sample of cycle n divided by the mean range of the signals in the cycle (Equation (2)). Mean values of GSI_{corr} and GSI_{dist} of all straight walking cycles in the entire 6-MWT were calculated. The detection of gait cycle and the selection of straight walking cycles were based on the same algorithms mentioned in Section 2.2.1:

$$GSI_{dist}(n) = \frac{mean\left(\left|\omega_{left}(n) - \omega_{right}(n)\right|\right)}{0.5 * \left[range\left(\omega_{left}(n)\right) + range\left(\omega_{right}(n)\right)\right]} * 100\% \tag{2}$$

2.3. Gait Symmetry Assessment with a Single 3D Accelerometer at the Low Back

Gait cycles can be measured by analyzing the repetitive movement pattern of the center of mass (CoM) [23]. Low back (approximately L3) accelerations, which are assumed to correspond to CoM during walking, were first smoothed with a 2nd order Butterworth low-pass filter with the cut-off frequency of 10 Hz. Autocorrelation coefficients of vertical (AR_v), frontal (AR_f) and lateral (AR_l) accelerations at the low back were computed as the function of time lag (t), respectively. The biased form of autocorrelation was used to suppress the amplitude of the coefficients while t increased [23]. The maximum time lag was 4 s (400 samples), which is about 2.5 times a single stride duration in post hemiplegic stroke patients [24]. This window length was chosen to capture the repetition of stride cycles in very slow walking. Coefficient of stride cycle repetition (C_{stride}) was the sum of positive autocorrelation coefficients of the three axes as a function of t (Equation (3)). Coefficient of step repetition (C_{step}) was the norm of autocorrelation coefficients as a function of t (Equation (4)). One stride time (T_{stride}) equals to t, when C_{stride} had the maximum value. The hypothesis was that, in a perfect symmetric gait pattern, two consecutive steps have the same step duration of $0.5 * T_{stride}$. The maximum value of C_{step} was $\sqrt{3}$ when autocorrelation coefficient of each acceleration axis was 1 at zero-lag ($t = 0$). The gait symmetry index (GSI_{L3}) was C_{step} ($0.5 * T_{stride}$) normalized to its value at zero-lag (Equation (5)), so that the maximum value of GSI_{L3} was 1 in a perfect symmetric gait pattern:

$$C_{stride}(t) = AR_v(t) + AR_f(t) + AR_l(t); \; if \; AR(t) < 0, \; AR(t) = 0 \tag{3}$$

$$C_{step}(t) = \sqrt[2]{AR_v(t) + AR_f(t) + AR_l(t)} \tag{4}$$

$$GSI_{L3} = C_{step} \; (0.5 * T_{stride}) / \sqrt{3} \tag{5}$$

2.4. Statistical Analysis

Symmetry indices (SI) of each spatiotemporal gait parameter estimated by the feet sensors listed in Table 1, GSI_{corr}, GSI_{dist} and GSI_{L3} (estimated by the low back accelerometer) were computed for each post-stroke patient and each healthy control. For SI, GSI_{corr} and GSI_{dist}, mean values over all gait cycles during straight walking in the entire 6-MWT assessment period were computed. GSI_{L3} was computed for the entire 6-MWT assessment period and for the first straight course of the assessment ($GSI_{L3straight}$). Given the small sample size in this study, non-parametric statistics were applied for the analyses. Wilcoxon rank sum test was used to test whether there are significant differences in various sensor-derived gait symmetry indices between post-stroke patients and control group. In addition, effect size (ES) calculator Cliff's Delta was used to determine the discriminating power of various symmetry indices [25]. Cliff's Delta calculates the proportion of non-overlapped samples in the groups. ES = 1 or -1 indicates the two groups have no overlap. Whereas, ES = 0 means the two groups are not separable. According to a study by Romano et al., ES less than 0.147 is negligible, between 0.147 and 0.33 is small, between 0.33 and 0.474 is medium, and more than 0.474 is a large effect [26].

The correlations between the low back sensor derived symmetry indices (GSI$_{L3}$ and GSI$_{L3straight}$) and the feet sensor based symmetry indices (SI, GSI_{corr} and GSI_{dist}) were analyzed with Spearman rank correlation coefficient (ρ).

3. Results

3.1. Discriminative Power of Gait Symmetry as Measured by Various Indices

Comparison between the synchronized feet pitch angular velocity signals and the low back acceleration signals revealed that the CoM movement repeated with the gait cycles. Figure 1a shows the sensor signals of a healthy control. The vertical acceleration showed stronger repetitive patterns than frontal and lateral accelerations at each step corresponding to the foot pitch angular velocity of left and right steps, which had high similarity in this healthy control. Whereas, the lateral acceleration shows a strong repetitive pattern with each stride (two steps).

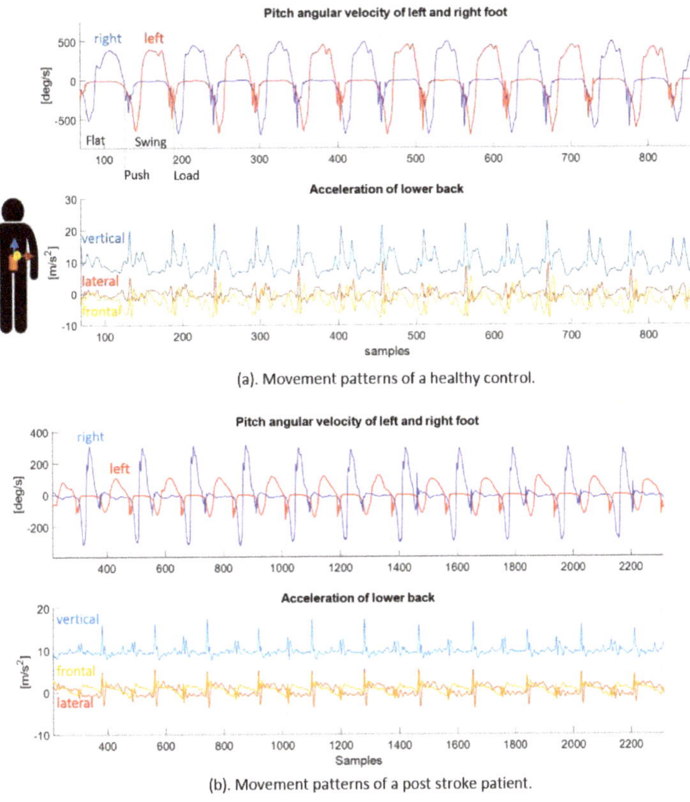

(a). Movement patterns of a healthy control.

(b). Movement patterns of a post stroke patient.

Figure 1. Synchronized pitch angular velocity signals from feet sensors and 3D acceleration signals from low back sensor. (**a**) Synchronized signals from a healthy control. (**b**) Synchronized signals from a post-stroke patient. Upper plot shows foot pitch angular velocity on the left (red) and right (blue) side during walking. Lower plot shows lower back acceleration on the vertical (blue), frontal (yellow) and lateral (red) axis. The dotted vertical lines indicate of each gait cycles detected by the feet sensors. In (**a**), time phases of foot-flat, push-up, swing and loading in one cycle of the left foot are indicated in the pitch angular velocity signal. Axes of the accelerometer at the low back are illustrated next to the acceleration signals.

Figure 1b shows sensor signals of a post-stroke patient. The foot pitch angular velocity profiles between the left and right steps had visible differences, which were reflected in the movement of the CoM as well. The vertical acceleration at the low back had poor similarity between the successive steps, but was visible between successive stride cycles. The aforementioned signal patterns were captured by the autocorrelation coefficients, C_{stride} and C_{step} as illustrated in Figure 2. The healthy control (a) had a shorter stride duration (ca. 1.05 s at maximum C_{stride}) compared to the post-stroke patient (b) (ca. 1.90 s). The coefficient of step repetition (C_{step}) of the healthy control at half stride time was higher than that in the post-stroke patient, which indicated a higher gait symmetry.

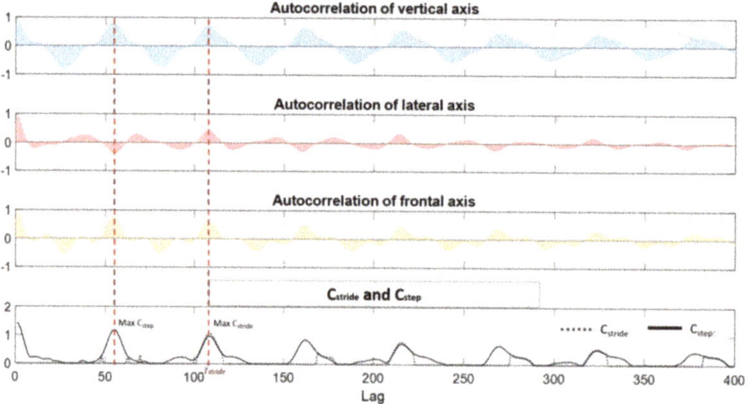

(a). 3D autocorrelation coefficients of low back acceleration of a healthy control.

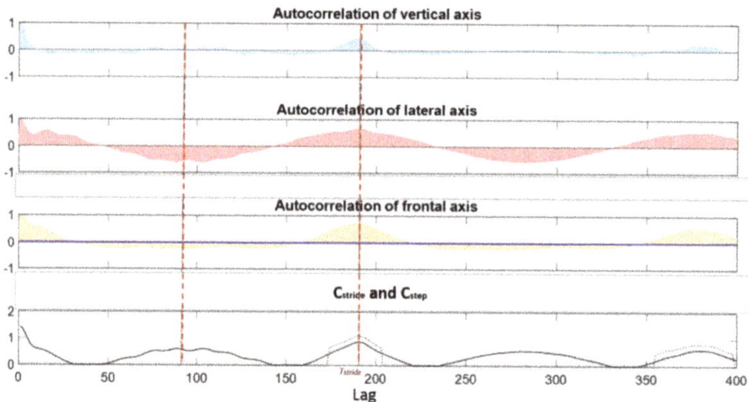

(b). 3D autocorrelation coefficients of low back acceleration in a post stroke patient.

Figure 2. Autocorrelation coefficients of 3D acceleration of lower back. (**a**) Coefficients of a healthy control. (**b**) Coefficients of a post-stroke patient. Autocorrelation coefficients in vertical (blue), lateral (red) and frontal (yellow) axis are computed with increased lag from 0 to 400 samples (4 s). C_{stride} (dotted black line) and C_{step} (solid black line) in the bottom plot are computed as a function of time lag.

Table 2 summaries the discriminative power of various gait symmetry indices. Gait symmetry measured with two feet sensors demonstrated a significant difference between healthy controls and post-stroke patients (except for symmetry of foot loading and flat ratios), among which, GSI_{dist} had the largest effect size. Gait symmetry measured with the low back accelerometer was significantly lower in post-stroke patients during the entire 6-MWT and during the shorter straight walk of the assessment.

The effect size was the same as GSI_{dist}, the best spatiotemporal parameter derived from the feet angular velocity signals. Boxplots in Figure 3 show the differences in various symmetry indices between post-stroke patients walking with and without a cane. Interestingly, GSI_{L3} was significantly lower in post-stroke patients walking with a cane compared to those able to walk without. There were no significant differences between $GSI_{L3straight}$ and any symmetry estimates provided by the feet sensors.

Table 2. Mean ± standard deviation and effect size (ES) as estimated by Cliff's Delta of various symmetry indices.

Symmetry Index (SI)	Control Group	Post-stroke	ES
Gait symmetry based on spatiotemporal gait parameter			
PathLength	0.54 ± 0.07	4.30 ± 5.69	−0.85 ***
StrikeAng	8.50 ± 4.53	35.78 ± 30.85	−0.79 **
LiftOffAng	3.78 ± 1.33	42.80 ± 37.27	−0.88 ***
MaxAngVel	6.31 ± 3.78	44.86 ± 39.23	−0.81 **
StanceRatio	3.06 ± 2.27	12.19 ± 8.06	−0.79 **
LoadRatio	22.36 ± 9.42	32.36 ± 22.06	−0.22
FootFlatRatio	5.99 ± 2.28	7.18 ± 4.98	−0.13
PushRatio	6.88 ± 3.67	25.76 ± 25.57	−0.71 **
Gait symmetry based on feet angular velocity signal profile			
GSI_{corr}	0.97 ± 0.01	0.76 ± 0.24	0.85 ***
GSI_{dist}	6.84 ± 1.23	16.87 ± 7.70	−0.89 ***
Gait symmetry based on low back accelerometry			
GSI_{L3}	0.74 ± 0.06	0.35 ± 0.22	0.89 ***
$GSI_{L3straight}$	0.69 ± 0.09	0.36 ± 0.19	0.89 ***

*** indicates $p < 0.001$, ** indicates $p < 0.01$.

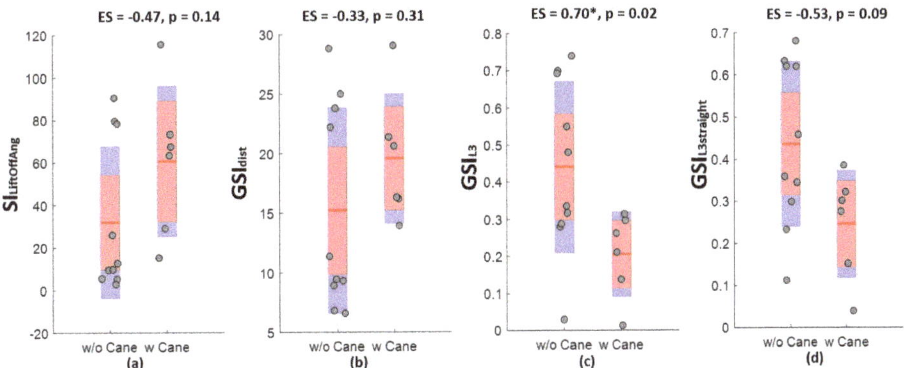

Figure 3. Boxplots of various gait symmetry indices measured in post-stroke patients with (w Cane) or without (w/o Cane) using cane. Effect size (ES) is measured with Cliff's Delta and p value is determined by Wilcoxon rank sum test. * indicates $p < 0.05$. (**a**) Comparison and effect size of $SI_{LiftOffAng}$. (**b**) Comparison and effect size of GSI_{dist}. (**c**) Comparison and effect size of GSI_{L3}. (**d**) Comparison and effect size of $GSI_{L3straight}$.

3.2. Correlations between Gait Symmetry Measured with Low Back Accelerometry and That Measured with Two Feet Sensors

Correlation analysis shown in Figure 4 indicated good consistency between gait symmetry measured with single 3D accelerometer at the low back and those measured with two feet sensors during the straight walking cycles of entire 6-MWT ($\rho = -0.88$ with $SI_{LiftOffAng}$, $\rho = 0.87$ with SI_{corr} and $\rho = -0.82$ with GSI_{dist}). Gait symmetry derived from the low back accelerometer when the participants walked through a short straight path ($GSI_{L3straight}$) were significantly correlated with feet sensor based symmetry measures as well ($\rho = -0.84$ with $SI_{LiftOffAng}$, $\rho = 0.80$ with GSI_{corr} and $\rho = -0.79$ with GSI_{dist}).

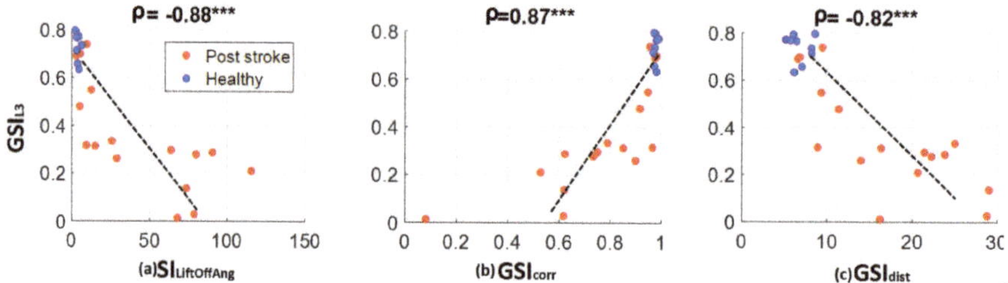

Figure 4. Correlation between gait symmetry measured with the low back accelerometer and symmetry measured with two feet sensors. Association is estimated with Spearman correlation. *** indicates $p < 0.0001$.

4. Discussion

This study developed a gait symmetry assessment with a single 3D accelerometer placed at the low back. Symmetry index estimated with the low back accelerometer, GSI_{L3}, is a measure of the repetitiveness of the gait cycles. Thus, the more symmetric the gait is, the higher the index value. On the contrary, the symmetry indices based on the spatiotemporal gait parameters with the feet sensors, SI, are measures of the degree of difference in the bilateral movement. The value decreases when the difference decreases as in symmetric gaits. Thus, SI has a negative correlation with GSI_{L3}. This is also the case for the gait symmetry measured with angular velocity signal profile GSI_{dist} using the feet sensors, as GSI_{dist} measures the difference between the bilateral foot angular velocity signals. GSI_{corr} with the feet sensors measures the correlation between the bilateral foot angular velocity signals. Its value increase when signals have higher correlation as in symmetric gaits. Hence, GSI_{corr} has a positive correlation with GSI_{L3}. More importantly, GSI_{L3} has good discriminative power comparable to symmetry indices based on spatiotemporal parameters derived from two feet sensors. GSI_{L3} has several advantages in technical implementation and clinical practice.

4.1. Advantages in Technical Implementation

A quantitative measure of the degree of asymmetry is useful for post-stroke gait rehabilitation assessment. Computing difference ratio of left and right steps based on spatiotemporal foot characteristics processes accelerometer, gyroscope, and in some cases magnetometer, barometer and foot pressure data [27], to derive gait parameters, which are high-level descriptions of information contained in the raw sensor signals. Gait modeling, advanced signal processing and complex 3D computation are required to find accurate spatiotemporal measures [18–21]. However, the challenge of accurate gait parameter estimation rises when applying the model to different pathologies, which can deviate largely from normal gait patterns. Often observed in post-stroke patients, lower limb movement is impaired by stiffness and slowness, which imposes difficulty to estimates of displacement, speed or rotation in periodic movement based on integration of inertial sensor signals [28]. Thus, the reliability of spatiotemporal-derived parameters may become questionable. To avoid this, computing symmetry (GSI_{L3}) is based on analysis of acceleration signals' repetitiveness quantified by autocorrelation coefficients. In addition, the computation is both easier and more robust than the morphology-based signal processing provided by the spatiotemporal gait parameter estimations. Compared to symmetry indices estimated with two feet sensors, GSI_{L3} is easier for technical implementation as only a single sensor is required. The computation of GSI_{L3} is based on the norm of autocorrelation coefficients rather than analysis of individual axis as presented in two studies [12,23]. Different from these studies, the proposed estimation of GSI_{L3} does not rely on detection of step alternation, which can be unreliable in people with poorly symmetric gaits as shown in Figure 2b. The biased autocorrelation coefficients decreases while time lag increases, which allows the reliable detection of the immediate next stride. In addition, estimation of GSI_{L3} during the entire 6-MWT as presented in this study has comparable discriminative power as those estimations using cleaned data (only straight walking cycles) with two feet sensors as shown in the results summarized in Table 2. Ultimately, GSI_{L3} requires less computation and it may be more feasible and robust than feet sensor based gait symmetry measures in semi- or unsupervised assessment.

4.2. Advantages in Clinical Practice

Gait symmetry is a biomarker of post-stroke rehabilitation [4]. Compared to assessment with two feet sensors, use of a single sensor worn at the low back is easier to set up in an office setting and less prone to disruption. Our results show that the low back sensor symmetry index estimated with a short straight walk is similar to that estimated with a complete 6-MWT. This implies that further simplification of the current clinical assessment procedure, to a brief walking assessment is possible. Asymmetry in spatiotemporal gait characteristics of post-stroke population, such as stance ratio, has been confirmed in other studies [3,29]. In this study, we demonstrate that asymmetry measure with a single low back accelerometer can significantly differentiate post-stroke gait from healthy gait, and can do so with an effect size that is larger than the difference in stance ratio and comparable to the best performing spatiotemporal characteristics (path length, maximum angular velocity and angle at toe lift off). This finding is confirmed by other studies of stroke survivors, where repetitiveness of the trunk accelerometry performed better than similarity between left and right step length and stride duration [12]. Furthermore, the developed symmetry index can discriminate severity of gait disturbance in the post-stroke population. In our study, the low back symmetry index could discriminate between gaits of post-stroke patients that required a cane from those who ambulating without an assistive device, comparing to the symmetry indices derived from two feet sensors that did not show significant difference between these two groups. These results suggest that the CoM accelerometry from the single low back sensor might be more sensitive to disability severity than feet kinematics within post-stroke patients. Accordingly, we suggest that gait symmetry assessment with one sensor on the low back is preferred over assessments with two feet sensors, both for in-clinic assessments and for long-term unsupervised assessments outside the clinic setting.

4.3. Limitations

The presented analyses have some limitations. We did not calibrate the low back accelerometer before gait symmetry estimation. Removal of static offset in acceleration signals and accurate alignment of axes with trunk frame may improve reproducibility of the symmetry index estimation. This is particularly important for gait symmetry assessment in individual patients during rehabilitation. In addition, test-retest reliability of the presented GSI_{L3} should be evaluated to determine the minimum detectable change using the developed index. Another limitation is with the selection of the maximum time lag for autocorrelation analysis. Four-second lag was chosen based on reported data in previous stroke study. A longer window is unlikely to affect the stride time detection. However, a shorter window may not accurately detect the stride repetition in extremely impaired stroke patients with very slow walking. A systematic examination using different window length will be required to determine the optimized configuration for computation with a patient group exhibiting large functional variations. In addition, the sample size in this study was small, yet our findings did reach statistical significance with effect sizes that suggest the sample was sufficient to support our conclusion. Still, it must be noted that age differences between the post-stroke and the control group may introduce some bias into the effect sizes of the various symmetry indices.

4.4. Future Studies

In the on-going study, we will address the clinical relevance of the developed gait symmetry assessment. Associations between clinical stroke diagnosis (including stroke etiology, SIS, self-reported recovery assessment) and the developed gait symmetry index will be analyzed. The analysis outcome will be compared to that measured by other more traditional gait markers, such as gait speed. The test-retest reliability of the developed gait symmetry index will be studied to determine the minimum detectable change that is relevant for longitudinal gait rehabilitation assessment. Future studies will also test the proposed symmetry index with large sample size to confirm the results of this study.

5. Conclusions

The proposed gait symmetry assessment with one 3D accelerometer placed on the midline of the low back shows high discriminative power in differentiating post-stroke patients from healthy controls. The outcome is comparable to the gait symmetry with spatiotemporal gait analysis using two feet sensors. The proposed method can be a cost-effective and reliable solution for post-stroke gait symmetry assessment in clinic. Assessment reproducibility and feasibility for unsupervised assessment is an important next step in our investigation to enable future studies using this method to monitor gait recovery after stroke, and to guide post-stroke gait rehabilitation.

Author Contributions: Conceptualization, W.Z. and M.S.; Methodology, W.Z. and K.A.; Software, W.Z.; Formal Analysis, W.Z. and C.L.; Data Curation, W.Z., M.A.I., and C.L.; Writing-Original Draft Preparation, W.Z.; Writing-Review & Editing, all authors.

Funding: This research is funded by Firmenich for EPFL-Stanford Exchange Program.

Acknowledgments: Authors thank all participants in the study.

Conflicts of Interest: The authors declare no conflict of interest.

References

1. Mobility after Stroke. Available online: http://www.stroke.org/stroke-resources/library/mobility-after-stroke (accessed on 7 February 2018).
2. Patterson, K.K.; Parafianowicz, I.; Danells, C.J.; Closson, V.; Verrier, M.C.; Staines, W.R.; Black, S.E.; McIlroy, W.E. Gait asymmetry in community-ambulating stroke survivors. *Arch. Phys. Med. Rehabil.* **2008**, *89*, 304–310. [CrossRef] [PubMed]
3. Olney, S.J.; Richards, C. Hemiparetic gait following stroke. Part I: Characteristics. *Gait Posture* **1996**, *4*, 136–148. [CrossRef]
4. Hsu, A.-L.; Tang, P.-F.; Jan, M.-H. Analysis of impairments influencing gait velocity and asymmetry of hemiplegic patients after mild to moderate stroke. *Arch. Phys. Med. Rehabil.* **2003**, *84*, 1185–1193. [CrossRef]
5. Yang, S.; Zhang, J.-T.; Novak, A.C.; Brouwer, B.; Li, Q. Estimation of spatio-temporal parameters for post-stroke hemiparetic gait using inertial sensors. *Gait Posture* **2013**, *37*, 354–358. [CrossRef] [PubMed]
6. Patterson, K.K.; Gage, W.H.; Brooks, D.; Black, S.E.; McIlroy, W.E. Evaluation of gait symmetry after stroke: A comparison of current methods and recommendations for standardization. *Gait Posture* **2010**, *31*, 241–246. [CrossRef] [PubMed]
7. Anna, A.S.; Wickström, N.; Eklund, H.; Zügner, R.; Tranberg, R. Assessment of Gait Symmetry and Gait Normality Using Inertial Sensors: In-Lab and In-Situ Evaluation. In *Biomedical Engineering Systems and Technologies*; Communications in Computer and Information Science; Springer: Berlin/Heidelberg, Germany, 2012; pp. 239–254. Available online: https://link.springer.com/chapter/10.1007/978-3-642-38256-7_16 (accessed on 15 November 2017).
8. Sung, P.S.; Danial, P. A Kinematic Symmetry Index of Gait Pattern Between Older Adults with and without Low Back Pain. Spine. 10 November 2017. Publish Ahead of Print. Available online: http://journals.lww.com/spinejournal/Abstract/publishahead/A_Kinematic_Symmetry_Index_of_Gait_Pattern_Between.95621.aspx (accessed on 15 November 2017).

9.   Moevus, A.; Mignotte, M.; de Guise, J.A.; Meunier, J. A perceptual map for gait symmetry quantification and pathology detection. *Biomed. Eng. OnLine* **2015**, *14*, 99. [CrossRef] [PubMed]

10.   Dewar, M.E.; Judge, G. Temporal asymmetry as a gait quality indicator. *Med. Biol. Eng. Comput.* **1980**, *18*, 689–693. [CrossRef] [PubMed]

11.   Wüest, S.; Massé, F.; Aminian, K.; Gonzenbach, R.; de Bruin, E.D. Reliability and validity of the inertial sensor-based Timed "Up and Go" test in individuals affected by stroke. *J. Rehabil. Res. Dev.* **2016**, *53*, 599–610. [CrossRef] [PubMed]

12.   Hodt-Billington, C.; Helbostad, J.L.; Moe-Nilssen, R. Should trunk movement or footfall parameters quantify gait asymmetry in chronic stroke patients? *Gait Posture* **2008**, *27*, 552–558. [CrossRef] [PubMed]

13.   Sant'Anna, A.; Wickström, N. A Symbol-Based Approach to Gait Analysis from Acceleration Signals: Identification and Detection of Gait Events and a New Measure of Gait Symmetry. *IEEE Trans. Inf. Technol. Biomed.* **2010**, *14*, 1180–1187. [CrossRef] [PubMed]

14.   Zhang, W.; Smuck, M.; Legault, C.; Ith, M.A.; Muaremi, A.; Aminian, K. Simple Gait Symmetry Measures Based on Foot Angular Velocity: Analysis in Post Stroke Patients. Honolulu, HI, USA, 2018. Available online: http://embc.embs.org/2018/wp-content/uploads/sites/35/2018/08/99118-EMBC-Final-Program.pdf (accessed on 2 September 2018).

15.   Stroke Impact Scale (SIS). Stroke Engine. Available online: https://www.strokengine.ca/en/assess/sis/ (accessed on 2 September 2018).

16.   Kosak, M.; Smith, T. Comparison of the 2-, 6-, and 12-minute walk tests in patients with stroke. *J. Rehabil. Res. Dev.* **2005**, *42*, 103–107. [CrossRef] [PubMed]

17.   MTw Awinda—Products. Xsens 3D Motion Tracking. Available online: https://www.xsens.com/products/mtw-awinda/ (accessed on 2 September 2018).

18.   Mariani, B.; Hoskovec, C.; Rochat, S.; Büla, C.; Penders, J.; Aminian, K. 3D gait assessment in young and elderly subjects using foot-worn inertial sensors. *J. Biomech.* **2010**, *43*, 2999–3006. [CrossRef] [PubMed]

19.   Mariani, B.; Rouhani, H.; Crevoisier, X.; Aminian, K. Quantitative estimation of foot-flat and stance phase of gait using foot-worn inertial sensors. *Gait Posture* **2013**, *37*, 229–234. [CrossRef] [PubMed]

20.   Mariani, B.; Jiménez, M.C.; Vingerhoets, F.J.G.; Aminian, K. On-Shoe Wearable Sensors for Gait and Turning Assessment of Patients with Parkinson's Disease. *IEEE Trans. Biomed. Eng.* **2013**, *60*, 155–158. [CrossRef] [PubMed]

21.   Mariani, B.; Rochat, S.; Büla, C.J.; Aminian, K. Heel and Toe Clearance Estimation for Gait Analysis Using Wireless Inertial Sensors. *IEEE Trans. Biomed. Eng.* **2012**, *59*, 3162–3168. [CrossRef] [PubMed]

22.   Dadashi, F.; Mariani, B.; Rochat, S.; Büla, C.J.; Santos-Eggimann, B.; Aminian, K. Gait and Foot Clearance Parameters Obtained Using Shoe-Worn Inertial Sensors in a Large-Population Sample of Older Adults. *Sensors* **2013**, *14*, 443–457. [CrossRef] [PubMed]

23.   Moe-Nilssen, R.; Helbostad, J.L. Estimation of gait cycle characteristics by trunk accelerometry. *J. Biomech.* **2004**, *37*, 121–126. [CrossRef]

24.   Von Schroeder, H.P.; Coutts, R.D.; Lyden, P.D.; Billings, E.; Nickel, V.L. Gait parameters following stroke: A practical assessment. *J. Rehabil. Res. Dev.* **1995**, *32*, 25–31. [PubMed]

25.   Macbeth, G.; Razumiejczyk, E.; Ledesma, R.D. Cliff's Delta Calculator: A non-parametric effect size program for two groups of observations. *Univ. Psychol.* **2011**, *10*, 545–555.

26.   Romano, J.; Kromrey, J.D.; Coraggio, J.; Skowronek, J.; Devine, L. Appropriate Statistics for Ordinal Level Data: Should We Really Be Using *t*-Test and Cohen'sd for Evaluating Group Differences on the NSSE and Other Surveys? BibSonomy: Arlington, Virginia, 2006. Available online: http://citeseerx.ist.psu.edu/viewdoc/download?doi=10.1.1.595.6157&rep=rep1&type=pdf (accessed on 2 September 2018).

27.   Moufawad el Achkar, C.; Lenoble-Hoskovec, C.; Paraschiv-Ionescu, A.; Major, K.; Büla, C.; Aminian, K. Physical Behavior in Older Persons during Daily Life: Insights from Instrumented Shoes. *Sensors* **2016**, *16*, 1225. [CrossRef] [PubMed]

28. Tan, U.-X.; Veluvolu, K.C.; Latt, W.T.; Shee, C.Y.; Riviere, C.N.; Ang, W.T. Estimating Displacement of Periodic Motion with Inertial Sensors. *IEEE Sens. J.* **2009**, *8*, 1385–1388. [PubMed]

29. Hesse, S.; Jahnke, M.; Schreiner, C.; Mauritz, K.-H. Gait symmetry and functional walking performance in hemiparetic patients prior to and after a 4-week rehabilitation programme. *Gait Posture* **1993**, *1*, 166–171. [CrossRef]

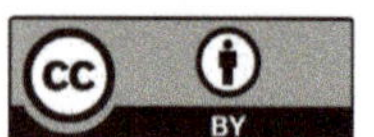

© 2018 by the authors. Licensee MDPI, Basel, Switzerland. This article is an open access article distributed under the terms and conditions of the Creative Commons Attribution (CC BY) license (http://creativecommons.org/licenses/by/4.0/).

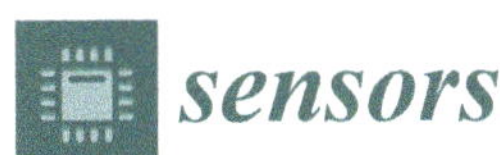 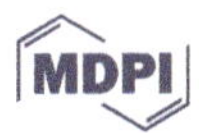

Article

Multiple-Wearable-Sensor-Based Gait Classification and Analysis in Patients with Neurological Disorders

Wei-Chun Hsu [1,2,3,]*, Tommy Sugiarto [1,2,4], Yi-Jia Lin [1], Fu-Chi Yang [5], Zheng-Yi Lin [6], Chi-Tien Sun [4], Chun-Lung Hsu [4] and Kuan-Nien Chou [7,]*

[1] Graduate Institute of Biomedical Engineering, National Taiwan University of Science and Technology, Taipei 10607, Taiwan; d10622817@mail.ntust.edu.tw (T.S.); jiajia527@gmail.com (Y.-J.L.)
[2] Graduate Institute of Applied Science and Technology, National Taiwan University of Science and Technology, Taipei 10607, Taiwan
[3] Department of Biomedical Engineering, National Defense Medical Center, Taipei 11490, Taiwan
[4] Division of Embedded System and SoC Technology, System Integration and Application Department, Information and Communication Research Laboratory, Industrial Technology Research Institute, Hsinchu 31057, Taiwan; ctsun@itri.org.tw (C.-T.S.); clh@itri.org.tw (C.-L.H.)
[5] Department of Neurology, Tri-Service General Hospital, National Defense Medical Center, Taipei 11490, Taiwan; Fuji-yang@yahoo.com.tw
[6] Department of Physical Medicine and Rehabilitation, Taipei City Hospital Zhongxing Branch, Datong District, Taipei 10341, Taiwan; DAP52@tpech.gov.tw
[7] Neurosurgery Department, Tri-Service General Hospital, Taipei 11490, Taiwan
* Correspondence: wchsu@mail.ntust.edu.tw (W.-C.H.); choukuannien@gmail.com (K.-N.C.); Tel.: +886-2730-3741 (W.-C.H.); +886-28792-3311 (K.-N.C.)

Received: 23 August 2018; Accepted: 6 October 2018; Published: 11 October 2018

Abstract: The aim of this study was to conduct a comprehensive analysis of the placement of multiple wearable sensors for the purpose of analyzing and classifying the gaits of patients with neurological disorders. Seven inertial measurement unit (IMU) sensors were placed at seven locations: the lower back (L5) and both sides of the thigh, distal tibia (shank), and foot. The 20 subjects selected to participate in this study were separated into two groups: stroke patients (11) and patients with neurological disorders other than stroke (brain concussion, spinal injury, or brain hemorrhage) (9). The temporal parameters of gait were calculated using a wearable device, and various features and sensor configurations were examined to establish the ideal accuracy for classifying different groups. A comparison of the various methods and features for classifying the three groups revealed that a combination of time domain and gait temporal feature-based classification with the Multilayer Perceptron (MLP) algorithm outperformed the other methods of feature-based classification. The classification results of different sensor placements revealed that the sensor placed on the shank achieved higher accuracy than the other sensor placements (L5, foot, and thigh). The placement-based classification of the shank sensor achieved 89.13% testing accuracy with the Decision Tree (DT) classifier algorithm. The results of this study indicate that the wearable IMU device is capable of differentiating between the gait patterns of healthy patients, patients with stroke, and patients with other neurological disorders. Moreover, the most favorable results were reported for the classification that used the combination of time domain and gait temporal features as the model input and the shank location for sensor placement.

Keywords: wearable device; gait analysis; IMU sensors; gait classification; stroke patients; neurological disorders

1. Introduction

Wearable devices, such as accelerometers, gyroscopes, or a combination of the two to form inertial measurement unit (IMU) sensors, have been widely used in gait analysis and the monitoring of physical activity. The validation of algorithms and sensor configurations has been performed in some studies, including the validation of gait event detection in systems such as the motion capture system, force platform, and gait mat system by using the golden standard [1–5]. A. Godfrey et al. in 2014 [3] validated low-cost body-worn sensors for assessing gait in healthy young and older people. Their study used an accelerometer placed on the lower back (L5) and their algorithm was validated against the golden standard from the *GaitRite* mat system. Spatiotemporal gait parameters including step time, step length, step velocity, stride time, variability, and asymmetry were calculated and compared with the result from the gait mat. Their result showed that the sensor arrangement and algorithm were valid and reliable for quantifying gait during continuous walking in both younger and older adults. Using the same sensor placement and algorithm, S. Del Din et al. in 2016 [1] applied wearable sensors for Parkinson Disease's (PD) subjects and healthy older adults. Their study found an excellent agreement for mean step time, stance time, step length, and step velocity for the older adults group, while for PD groups, agreement was found for step time, stance time, and step velocity. The efficacy of using an accelerometer placed on the distal tibia to determine the Initial Contact and Final Contact gait event was examined by J. Sinclair et al. in 2013 [4]. Compared with the golden standard from the Kitsler Force platform, they found a strong correlation in the duration of stance phase between the two methods and suggest that a shank-mounted accelerometer can be used to accurately and reliably detect gait events.

The application of a wearable device in gait analysis is not limited to gait event detection and the calculation of spatiotemporal parameters, but can be extended to investigate gait stability and variability between normal and pathological gaits [6–9] and classify various types of gait patterns [10–13]. Gait stability and harmony in children with Cerebral Palsy (CP) was examined with IMU sensors placed on the lower back (L3–L4) by M. Iosa et al. in 2012 [7,14]. Gait stability can be defined as the ability of the body segment to displace with proper speed so that the upper body oscillation can be minimized by moving the body segment in a coordinated fashion. This parameter can be quantified by measuring the upper body acceleration's dispersion and smoothness. Meanwhile, gait harmony is the ability of our body to synchronize the symmetric and rhythmic movement by means of inter-limb, intra-limb, and lower–upper coordination. This parameter also can be quantified by upper body acceleration data, in terms of their ratio between odd and even harmonics and the ratio between the gait parameters of two steps from different sides. Those parameters are important in gait analysis because they are related to the stabilization of the body center of mass in order to avoid falls and also of the head in order to steady the optical and vestibular informational flow [15].

Their study used a 10 m walking test with self-selected speed and then calculated the gait stability and gait harmony using the data from the accelerometer and gyroscope; they found a general reduction of gait stability indicated by higher Root Mean Square (RMS) acceleration, acceleration minimal value, and peak-to-peak angular velocity in children with CP [7]. Gait stability in Down syndrome (DS) and Prader–Willi syndrome (PWS) was examined using four IMU sensors placed on the pelvis, trunk, and both shanks by G. Salatino et al. in 2016 [8]. A 10 m walking test with self-selected speed was also used in this study and spatiotemporal gait parameters with RMS acceleration were calculated from the IMU sensors. They found that there were no significance differences among DS, PWS, and normal children for all calculated spatiotemporal parameters; however, acceleration RMS on the pelvic sensors was found to be greater in DS and PWS with respect to normal children.

To classify various types of gait patterns, E. Sejdic et al. in 2016 [10] examined gait signals from accelerometers placed on the lower back to extract time, frequency, and time–frequency domain features in order to differentiate gaits between healthy and clinical populations (PD and peripheral neuropathy subjects). Discriminating gaits related to neurodegenerative diseases such as PD and Huntington's disease was done in a study by Mannini et al. [12] using different machine learning techniques and

IMU sensors placed on both the shank and lower back (between L4 and S2). Both of those studies used the subject's self-preferred speed for walking trials on a treadmill and walkway, respectively.

Moreover, various types of physical activity have been examined with the use of wearable devices [16–22]. In 2004, A. V. Rowlands et al. [20] used a triaxial accelerometer placed on the hip to measure the intensity of different activities (moderate and vigorous) in young children and young adults. Meanwhile, in 2009, five different activities (walking, running, cycling, driving, and sports) were classified with a triaxial accelerometer placed on the subject's waist and different classifiers (Decision Tree and Naïve Bayes) [17].

While also still minimizing the subject's discomfort, the classification of gait patterns with a wearable device provides more mobility than does the conventional method, which uses complex and expensive motion analysis system equipment. Gait analysis using IMU sensors provides portability, low cost, and flexibility in terms of free-living data collection. Furthermore, gait classification with a wearable device can provide long-term gait assessment, especially in people with disease, by enabling the early detection of gait alteration and by the easiness of gait assessment.

Therefore, to achieve ideal results in gait pattern classification, various sensor placements and algorithms have been adopted and tested in normal people and people with disease [23–26]. A. Salarian et al. in 2013 [25] proposed a novel approach to reducing the number of sensing units for wearable gait analysis by continuing to use the double-pendulum model but with a lower number of sensors (only two gyroscope units placed on both sides of the shank). Their approach concluded that it is feasible to reduce the number of sensors needed from four to two to estimate the movement of the thigh from the movement of the shank, which will be useful for ambulatory gait analysis. While a study by A. Salarian et al. was done on PD subjects, L. Carcreff in 2018 [26] conducted a study which compared the spatiotemporal measurement performance of three wearable sensor configurations: shank and thigh, shanks, and the feet. Their placement configuration selection was based on potential applications in children with CP and their result showed that the shank-and-thigh-based sensor configuration was more robust in children with higher levels of disability.

Vienne et al. (2017) [27] published a review on the use of IMU sensors to assess gait quality in patients with neurological disorders. Their study concluded that too many protocols are being adopted in the assessment of gait using IMU sensors, including those for algorithms and sensor placement. From the total of 78 studies examined in that literature review, 16% of them were using more than one sensor with a maximum of seven sensors; half of them (39 studies) were neurological studies; more than 50 studies used the subject's self-selected speed; and 67 studies were done only in a gait laboratory or hospital, while 9 of them were done in the subject's home. Consequently, a comparison of a multitude of studies is difficult to conduct, and ascertainment of the optimal sensor placement configuration and classification algorithm is crucial.

However, no study has ever examined IMU sensor placement configuration with different classification algorithms in patients with neurological disorders. Thus, this study aimed to conduct a comprehensive analysis of the placement of multiple wearable sensors (including seven different sensors placements and five different algorithms) for gait analysis and classification in patients with neurological disorders. Features of time domain, gait temporal parameters, and a combination of both were also examined to determine which feature yielded the most favorable classification result. A comparison of the classification of sensors at multiple placements was crucial for reducing the number of sensors used and, hence, the computational load in order to increase the speed of the classification process. Our hypothesis was that sensor placement on the shank would have a better classification result since the gait event detection would be based on sensors placed on the shank.

2. Materials and Methods

2.1. Subjects

Twenty subjects participated in this study and were divided into two groups: patients with stroke and patients with other neurological disorders. The stroke patients group comprised 11 subjects (mean age = 65.2 ± 13.7 years, height = 162.1 ± 9.66 cm, and weight = 61.8 ± 6.5 kg), while the group of patients with neurological disorders other than stroke comprised the remaining 9 subjects (mean age = 66.4 ± 9.16 years, height = 167.3 ± 9.16 cm, and weight = 63.5 ± 11.1 kg) and consisted of subjects who had undergone surgery for brain tumors and had a spinal injury, brain concussion, or brain hemorrhage. Participants who met the following inclusion criteria were enrolled in this study: age ≥ 18 years; ability to understand simple instructions; ability to walk without any assistive device for at least 15 m. Participants with unstable neurological and functional status were excluded, along with those with comorbidities that would affect gait.

2.2. Equipment

Seven wireless IMU sensors from Delsys Trigno^{TM} (Delsys Inc., Boston, MA, USA) were used in this study. The IMU sensors consisted of a triaxial accelerometer, gyroscope, and magnetometer. However, this study only used data from the accelerometer and gyroscope. The triaxial accelerometer can measure acceleration up to ±16 g, and the triaxial gyroscope can measure angular velocity up to 2000°/s. The sampling rate of both the accelerometer and gyroscope was 148 Hz, and the resolution of the analog-to-digital converter was 16 bit. All IMU sensors were connected through wireless communication to the Delsys Sensor Base, which used a USB interface to transfer the data in real time to the PC. All data acquisition procedures were performed using EMGWorks 4.3.1 Acquisition software (Delsys Inc., Boston, MA, USA), and data processing and analysis was performed using Python 3.6 with an Anaconda environment.

2.3. Experimental Protocol

The IMU sensors were placed at seven locations on the subject. The first sensor was placed on the subject's lower back (L5), and the second and third sensors were placed on the subject's left and right foot, respectively. Both sides of the subject's thigh and distal tibia were used for the placement of sensors 4–7. The orientation of the sensor's axis was set to a mediolateral direction for the x axis, a vertical direction for the y axis, and an anteroposterior direction for the z axis. All of the sensors were secured with tight medical-grade tape to minimize movement artifacts. An illustration of sensor placement is shown in Figure 1.

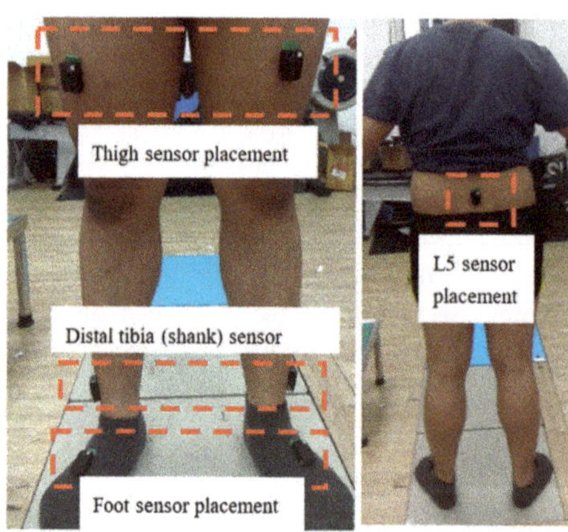

Figure 1. Illustration of the placement of the seven sensors on the subject.

After all the sensors had been placed, the subject was asked to participate in a level walking trial at their selected speed. One level walking trial included the forward and return directions of a distance of approximately 12 m. Each subject was required to complete six successful trials. All IMU sensor data were collected and saved on the PC for further analysis. In order to avoid the effect of the turn-around period, the return direction walk was excluded and only the first two strides in the forward direction (one right stride and one left stride) were used for data analysis.

Data for the stroke group and the group with other neurological disorders were collected at a hospital, whereas data for the healthy adult group were collected in the gait laboratory.

2.4. Data Processing

The triaxial accelerometer and gyroscope data from all seven sensors were extracted and exported to a .csv format file for further processing. Triaxial accelerometer data were filtered with a fourth-order bi-directional Butterworth bandpass filter with a cutoff frequency of 1–20 Hz [28] and triaxial gyroscope data were subjected to the same bandpass filter with a different cutoff frequency (0.25–30 Hz) [29]. The data collected from the distal tibia (shank) IMU sensor in this study were used to define the left and right gait cycle independently for each side.

After being filtered with the bandpass filter with the cutoff frequency at 0.25–30 Hz, the mediolateral axis of the gyroscope data was used to detect initial contact (IC) and final contact (FC) of the left and right gait cycle [5,29]. The local maximum of the filtered shank angular velocity was selected as the mid-swing area, and additional criteria were defined for peaks larger than $50°/s$ to prevent false peak selection. After the mid-swing area had been defined, other local minima before and after the mid-swing event were selected to be the FC and IC events, respectively. Specified minimal peak distance and minimal peak height were also applied to IC and FC peak detection to prevent the system from detecting the wrong peak.

The resulting IC and FC event times formed a complete gait cycle with the following sequence: IC right foot → FC left foot → IC left foot → FC right foot → IC right foot → FC left foot → IC left foot. This gait cycle comprised two complete stride cycles of the right and left feet (IC to the next ipsilateral IC gait event). Gait temporal parameters were calculated from this complete gait cycle.

Stride time:
$$Stride\ Time = IC_{(k+1)} - IC_k. \tag{1}$$

Stance time:
$$Stance\ Time = FC_{(k)} - IC_k. \tag{2}$$

Stance time:
$$Swing\ Time = IC_{(k+1)} - FC_k. \tag{3}$$

First double-limb support:
$$1st\ DLS = FC_{(k)contralateral} - IC_{(k)ipsilateral}. \tag{4}$$

Second double-limb support:
$$2nd\ DLS = FC_{(k)ipsilateral} - IC_{(k)contralateral}. \tag{5}$$

where k is the kth-order gait event.

The percentage of each gait temporal parameter was also calculated by dividing it by the stride time of its side of the gait cycle. The symmetry ratio between the left and right sides was also calculated for stride, stance, and swing parameters [30].

$$Symmetry\ Ratio = \frac{Right\ temporal\ gait\ parameter}{Left\ temporal\ gait\ parameter} \tag{6}$$

In addition to calculating gait temporal parameters, the IC and FC event times were also used to separate the accelerometer and gyroscope data into each left and right gait cycle. Data from both the triaxial accelerometer and gyroscope were segmented into the left and right strides (IC to the next ipsilateral IC gait event) and then normalized into 101 points so that all segmented data would be the same size. After the time normalization process, time domain features were extracted from the normalized data and saved for further classification purposes.

The following time domain features were extracted from the accelerometer and gyroscope data: mean, variance, kurtosis, and deviation from the normalized segmented data. Although the time domain features were extracted from all seven sensors, cycle cutting was only applied to the corresponding side (for example, the left thigh sensor was applied to the cycle from the left stride and vice versa). Therefore, a total of 192 time domain features were extracted from all seven sensors for each trial on each subject. All trials for every subject could then be combined for use in further classification processing.

2.5. Gait Event Detection

The gait event consisting of IC and FC times was extracted from the shank angular velocity data using the described method. The result of IC and FC event time detection on the right side of the gait cycle is presented in Figure 2. The local minimum before the mid-swing event was the FC event time, and the local minimum after the mid-swing was the IC event time.

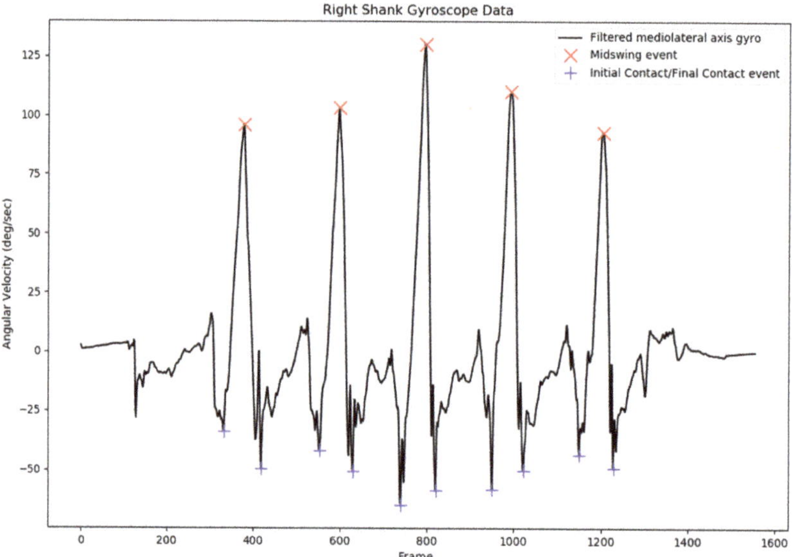

Figure 2. Initial contact (IC) and final contact (FC) event time detection from the filtered right-shank angular velocity signal.

After several configurations, specified values of minimal peak distance and minimal peak height were set at 30 data points and 100°/s for the mid-swing event, respectively. For local minima point detection, minimal peak distance and minimal peak height were set to be 50 data points and 30°/s, respectively. These values were selected to prevent detection of the wrong IC and FC event times.

The defined IC and FC event times were used to segment the filtered accelerometer and gyroscope signals into one gait cycle, for which the defined starting and end points were the IC event time and the next ipsilateral IC event time, respectively. Data for the normalized segmented acceleration and angular velocity are displayed in Figure 3.

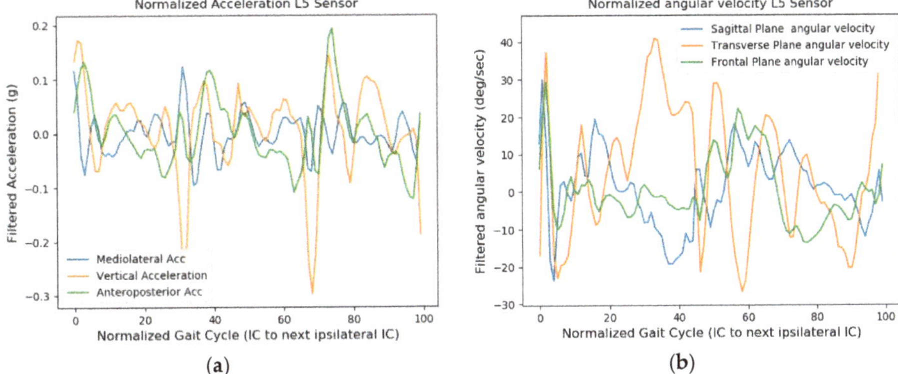

Figure 3. Normalized segmented acceleration (**a**) and angular velocity (**b**) obtained from the L5 IMU sensor data for feature extraction purposes.

2.6. Classification

Binary classification to differentiate stroke and other neurological disorders was performed using time domain features of the segmented accelerometer, gyroscope, and gait temporal features. Seven classification methods were used in this study, and the different configurations of sensors were also used to examine the most favorable sensor placement for distinguishing between the different groups. The five algorithms used in this study were as follows:

- Random forest (RF) classifier: A random forest is a supervised learning algorithm that combines decision trees and generally involves training with the bagging method. The number of trees used in this study was 1000.

- Adaboost classifier: This method was first introduced by Freund and Schapire [31]. The core principle of Adaboost is to fit a sequence of weak learners on repeatedly modified versions of data. In this study, the maximum number of estimators—at which boosting was terminated—was set to 150.

- Decision tree (DT): A decision tree is a tree-like graph that illustrates all possible decision alternatives and corresponding outcomes. It is composed of nodes where tests on specific attributes have been performed as well as leaf nodes indicating the value of the target attribute.

- Gaussian naïve Bayes (GNB): GNB is a supervised learning method that is based on applying the Bayes theorem with the *naïve* assumption of independence between each pair of features [32].

- Neural network with multilayer perceptron (MLP): MLP is a neural network capable of understanding a rich variety of nonlinear problems and uses backpropagation to classify instances [33]. The size of the hidden layer used in this study was 2000, with the *Adam* solver and an adaptive learning rate.

Hidden Markov Model (HMM)-based features and SVM classifiers were excluded in this study since these two algorithms have already been explored in many studies which classify either different types of gait patterns or different types of physical activity with wearable accelerometer/IMU sensors [12,22,34,35].

The time domain features of all subjects were combined with their corresponding true label to shape the whole subject dataset. The whole subject dataset was then split randomly with a 6:4 ratio into the training and testing datasets, respectively. The training dataset was then split 5-fold to perform *k*-fold cross-validation. The training dataset was trained with those five different algorithms and the mean accuracy of the 5-fold cross-validation method was calculated for each model. The trained model was tested with the unseen testing dataset, and the confusion matrix and accuracy were calculated and compared for each model.

In addition to the feature classification of all sensors, another classification was performed in which only the separate locations of each sensor were used as the feature with the five algorithms. The results from the classification of each sensor were then compared to identify the sensor with the best placement configuration for differentiating between the three groups.

Another classification method with calculated gait temporal parameters as the feature was used with the five algorithms. All 17 gait temporal parameters were used as the feature for the five algorithms, and the cross-validation and testing accuracies were reported and compared for each algorithm.

The next classification method combined the time domain features from the accelerometer and gyroscope with the calculated gait temporal parameters to acquire a new feature set. The new feature set then trained various algorithms to obtain the cross-validation and testing accuracy for each algorithm.

The last classification method used time domain and gait temporal features from each sensor location group separately for each independent classification. For example, the time domain features from the accelerometer and gyroscope on the left and right feet were combined to produce an independent classification result for the foot sensor. The same rule was also applied for the thigh, shank, and L5 sensors to produce four classification results for the foot, shank, thigh, and L5 sensor locations. A chart illustrating the combination of classification methods used in this study is shown in Figure 4.

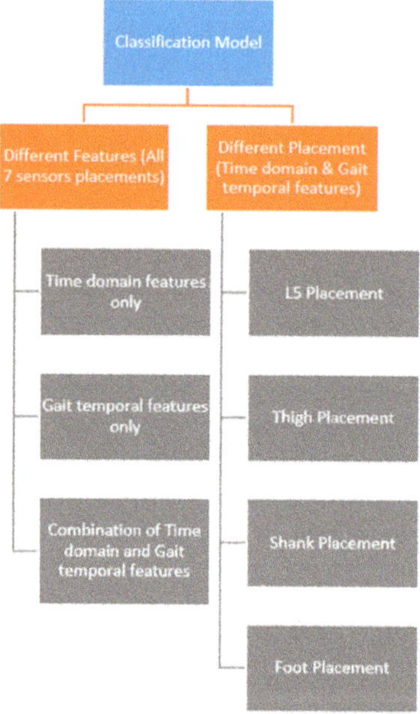

Figure 4. Chart of the seven different classification methods used in this study; the left part shows the three classification methods that used all sensor placements while the right part shows the four classification methods that used each sensor placement independently.

To eliminate redundancy and reduce the number of features, feature selection was performed according to the highest score. In this study, the feature selection method employed was a calculation of the ANOVA F-value between the label and feature, and we selected only the highest-scoring 20% of features. The new feature set resulting from reduction through the feature selection process was used in the same classification method. All feature selection processes and classifications were performed with the *scikit-learn 0.19.1* module of Python 3.6.

3. Results

Time domain features were extracted from the normalized segmented data for the triaxial accelerometer and gyroscope at the seven sensor locations. The features were then used as the input for the five classifiers, the results of which are presented in Table 1.

Table 1. Validation and testing accuracy results for the five classification methods that used time domain features of normalized segmented acceleration and angular velocity from the data from the seven sensor positions.

Seven Sensor Placements (Time Domain Features)					
Model Name	5-Fold Cross-Validation		Testing Accuracy (%)	Average Precision	Average Recall
	Mean Accuracy (%)	Standard Deviation			
Random Forest	81.08425	10.78727	82.6087	0.83	0.83
Multilayer Perceptron	78.41758	11.86194	84.78261	0.86	0.85
Naïve Bayes	86.90842	5.415183	84.78261	0.85	0.85
Adaboost	83.84615	10.60653	76.08696	0.81	0.80
Decision Tree	79.64103	10.87058	76.08696	0.76	0.76

The results obtained after the feature selection process are listed in Table 1. These results were derived from the reduced number of features, specifically only the 20% highest-scoring features according to the ANOVA F-values. The result of selected features from all the classification method used on this study showed on Appendix A.

A second classification experiment was conducted using the features for calculating gait temporal parameters. All 17 gait temporal parameters were used as features. The mean accuracy of the 5-fold cross-validation and the testing accuracy are presented in Table 2.

Table 2. Validation and testing accuracy results for the five classification methods that used features from gait temporal parameters.

Seven Sensor Placements (Gait Temporal Features)					
Model Name	5-Fold Cross-Validation		Testing Accuracy (%)	Average Precision	Average Recall
	Mean Accuracy (%)	Standard Deviation			
Random Forest	58.95238	11.24712	76.08696	0.76	0.76
Multilayer Perceptron	68.15385	11.58815	63.04348	0.68	0.63
Naïve Bayes	68.98168	11.92694	71.73913	0.76	0.72
Adaboost	55.98535	11.97776	65.21739	0.68	0.67
Decision Tree	51.49451	14.74979	60.86957	0.61	0.61

Table 3 presents the results from the classification experiment that used a combination of temporal gait parameters and time domain features with all seven sensor placements. The results from the previous classification experiment, which produced four results from four different sensor locations (L5, foot, shank, and thigh), are listed in Tables 4–7. Cross-validation mean accuracy and testing accuracy after the feature selection process are also indicated in the results.

Table 3. Validation and testing accuracy results for the five classification methods that used a combination of gait temporal parameters and time domain features.

Seven Sensor Placements (Combination of Time Domain & Gait Temporal Features)					
Model Name	5-Fold Cross-Validation		Testing Accuracy (%)	Average Precision	Average Recall
	Mean Accuracy (%)	Standard Deviation			
Random Forest	80.87912	11.62656	84.78261	0.83	0.83
Multilayer Perceptron	71.05495	13.12726	84.78261	0.88	0.85
Naïve Bayes	88.22711	3.997853	84.78261	0.85	0.85
Adaboost	79.75092	8.194112	82.6087	0.85	0.85
Decision Tree	78.1978	4.665143	80.43478	0.84	0.80

Table 4. Validation and testing accuracy for the classification method that used time domain and gait temporal features of the accelerometer and gyroscope at the L5 sensor location.

L5 Sensor Placement (Combination of Time Domain & Gait Temporal Features)					
Model Name	5-Fold Cross-Validation		Testing Accuracy (%)	Average Precision	Average Recall
	Mean Accuracy (%)	Standard Deviation			
Random Forest	66.43956	10.10788	80.43478	0.81	0.80
Multilayer Perceptron	65.68498	19.98486	50	0.68	0.61
Naïve Bayes	75.02564	10.49391	73.91304	0.81	0.78
Adaboost	66.21978	10.95326	80.43478	0.80	0.80
Decision Tree	63.56777	5.392539	65.21739	0.78	0.78

Table 5. Validation and testing accuracy for the classification method that used the time domain and gait temporal features of the accelerometer and gyroscope at the foot sensor location.

Foot Sensor Placement (Combination of Time Domain & Gait Temporal Features)					
Model Name	5-Fold Cross-Validation		Testing Accuracy (%)	Average Precision	Average Recall
	Mean Accuracy (%)	Standard Deviation			
Random Forest	70.31502	17.46668	82.6087	0.83	0.83
Multilayer Perceptron	56.60073	5.390239	60.86957	0.68	0.61
Naïve Bayes	79.01099	13.31621	78.26087	0.81	0.78
Adaboost	67.53846	12.53356	80.43478	0.80	0.80
Decision Tree	67.45788	15.14377	78.26087	0.78	0.78

Table 6. Validation and testing accuracy for the classification method that used the time domain and gait temporal features of the accelerometer and gyroscope at the shank (distal tibia) sensor location.

Shank Sensor Placement (Combination of Time Domain & Gait Temporal Features)					
Model Name	5-Fold Cross-Validation		Testing Accuracy (%)	Average Precision	Average Recall
	Mean Accuracy (%)	Standard Deviation			
Random Forest	81.0696	5.926482	82.6087	0.83	0.83
Multilayer Perceptron	81.27473	7.196452	80.43478	0.86	0.80
Naïve Bayes	83.94139	7.054515	82.6087	0.83	0.83
Adaboost	75.23077	4.176749	76.08696	0.76	0.76
Decision Tree	72.37363	5.568556	89.13043	0.90	0.89

Table 7. Validation and testing accuracy for the classification method that used the time domain and gait temporal features of the accelerometer and gyroscope at the thigh sensor location.

Thigh Sensor Placement (Combination of Time Domain & Gait Temporal Features)					
Model Name	5-Fold Cross-Validation		Testing Accuracy (%)	Average Precision	Average Recall
	Mean Accuracy (%)	Standard Deviation			
Random Forest	77.91209	13.57666	80.43478	0.83	0.83
Multilayer Perceptron	52.20513	1.810191	54.34783	0.30	0.54
Naïve Bayes	79.64103	5.478678	82.6087	0.85	0.83
Adaboost	69.39194	6.124936	80.43478	0.79	0.78
Decision Tree	64.08791	7.802167	69.56522	0.70	0.70

4. Discussion and Future Works

4.1. Discussion

This study aimed to perform a comprehensive analysis of multiple placements of wearable sensors for gait analysis and classification in patients with neurological disorders. Seven IMU sensors were placed at different locations, and gait-cycle-segmented data were used to create time domain features for classification purposes. The IC and FC gait event times were determined using filtered mediolateral acceleration data from the shank sensor. This algorithm has been commonly applied in studies using IMU sensors to define IC and FC gait event times, both in healthy individuals and in those with pathological disorders [5], including application for patients with knee arthroplasty [36], spinal cord injuries [37], and Parkinson's disease [29]. All of these studies have been in agreement and confirmed the validity of using the shank angular velocity to define gait events with the golden standard, such as motion capture systems or foot switches. De Vroey et al. (2018) [36] reported adequate to excellent intra-class correlation values overall for temporal gait parameters calculated using shank angular velocity and a camera system, also suggesting that IMU sensors can be used outside of laboratory assessments to examine the temporal gait parameters in the knee arthroplasty population.

Because this event detection method was crucial for separating the accelerometer and gyroscope data for classification purposes in the present study, the use of IMU sensors to define the IC and FC events in the study that validated the method was therefore imperative. Thus, the study conducted by K. Aminian et al. [5] was significant for the conduction of the present study because it validated the algorithm for defining IC and FC events using shank angular velocity in healthy young and elderly subjects. The results also revealed high acceptability in elderly subjects and the method was recommended for use in clinical applications, such as the monitoring of rehabilitation progress, gait analysis in patients with neurological disorders, and fall risk assessment in elderly patients.

The results from the IC and FC event detection revealed that false peak detection, which can lead to false IC and FC event detection, can be prevented with the current additional parameters applied for peak detection. The pattern in the shank angular velocity of the nonaffected side of stroke subjects was similar to that of the shank angular velocity of healthy subjects, with a less abrupt signal, as indicated in Figure 5. Although the shank angular velocity pattern of the affected side of stroke patients exhibited a more abrupt signal, the peak was still detected without any false peak detection. This phenomenon was also observed in another study involving a patient with a spinal cord injury; however, the study concluded that the gait event from the shank angular velocity could be used to detect the IC and FC events as accurately as a foot switch for both healthy subjects and those with pathological disorders [37]. An example of the shank angular velocity of a stroke subject's affected side is presented in Figure 6.

The IC and FC event detections were used to separate the acceleration and angular velocity data from the seven sensor positions for gait classification. This study performed several classification experiments using features from the time domain, gait temporal parameters, and a combination of time domain and gait temporal parameters. Classifications using only independent sensor locations with time domain and gait temporal features were also performed to examine the most accurate sensor placements for gait classification.

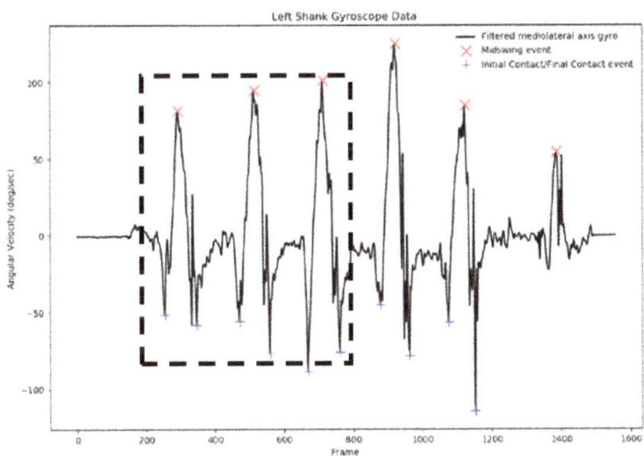
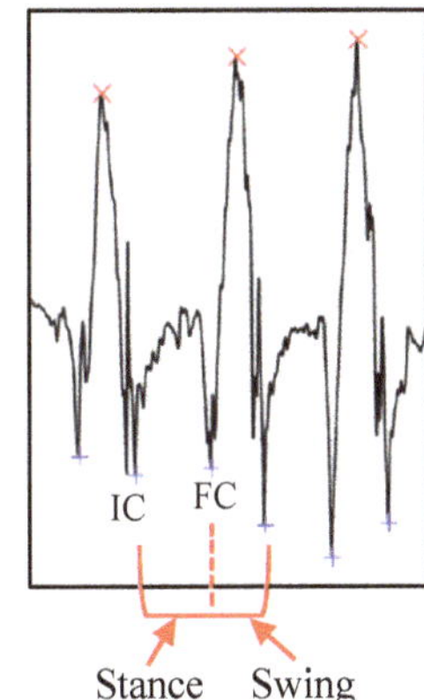

Figure 5. Typical shank angular velocity data from the nonaffected side of a stroke subject and the detailed IC and FC event times (right side).

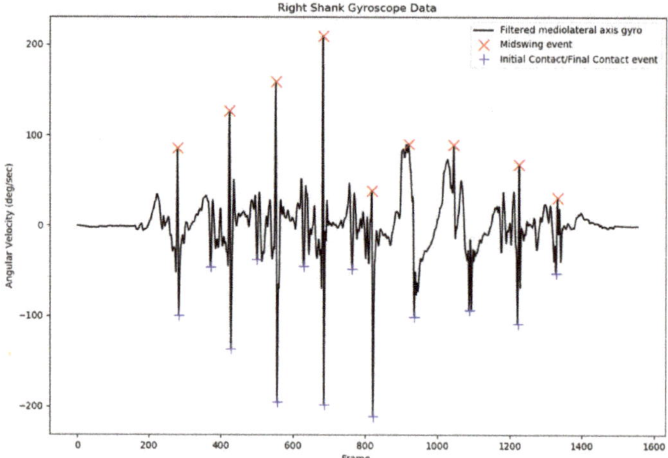

Figure 6. Typical shank angular velocity data from the affected side of stroke subjects. The figure indicates more abrupt and noisy signals in comparison with the nonaffected side.

The cross-validation accuracy and testing accuracy after feature selection were compared between the classification experiment and within-classification experiment (for different classification algorithms). The results revealed that for classifications involving only time domain features, the Naïve Bayes and MLP classifier outperformed other algorithms with 84.78% testing accuracy; however, MLP had better average precision at 0.86. Moreover, when the features changed from time domain to gait temporal parameters, the RF classifier achieved the highest testing accuracy (76.08%).

The third classification experiment combined time domain features and gait temporal parameters, and the results revealed that the MLP classifier outperformed other algorithms with 84.78% testing accuracy; MLP also had better average precision at 0.88. The results from the first three classification experiments, which used different types of features on the same sensor placement configuration, revealed that the classification with a combination of time domain and gait temporal features showed the best result with 84.78% testing accuracy and average precision and recall of 0.88 and 0.85, respectively. This testing accuracy was achieved with the MLP algorithm.

Classification with only gait temporal parameters demonstrated the lowest testing accuracy (76.08%) (with the RF method), in comparison with a combination of time domain and gait temporal features (84.78% testing accuracy with the MLP algorithm) or even with only time domain feature classification. Other studies have also reported that time domain and frequency domain features achieved higher accuracy than other classification methods using group-specific features based on the Hidden Markov Model (HMM) [12]. Although these studies used a classification algorithm (SVM) not used in the present study, the comparison of classification algorithms used in this study indicated that even using the same algorithm, the classification methods based on time domain features still outperformed those using gait temporal features and a combination of features (such as the RF method in this study). Moreover, an SVM classifier was already explored in a study classifying healthy young and older gaits [34] and in another classifying gaits between normal, hemiplegia, and PD patients [35] with both of them showing good results. Combined with HMM-based features, an SVM classifier was also explored in two previous studies by Mannini et al. which classified gaits between elderly, post-stroke, and Huntington's disease subjects [12] and classified human physical activity [22]. However, these results are in agreement with those reported in the present study because the classification results from a combination of features were more favorable than the results from using only gait temporal parameters.

Another study also used time domain features and gait temporal parameters and discovered that their method was capable of classifying three types of neurodegenerative diseases (Parkinson's disease, Huntington's disease, and amyotrophic lateral sclerosis) with up to 90.63% accuracy [38]. In contrast with our results, this study reported relatively higher accuracy for the features extracted from gait temporal parameters. The fact that both the method utilized for defining the IC and FC events and the classification algorithm differed from those used in the present study may be a reason as to why their study achieved higher accuracy. Moreover, their study extracted the time domain features from gait temporal parameters, which also influenced their results. This study also found that among the set of all features, the gait temporal parameters feature was shown to have the worst classification performance with the lowest testing accuracy (60.8%). That means that the classification which only used gait temporal parameters was able to differentiate those groups but the performance was far worse than those of other classifications which utilized the other feature sets like time domain features from the acceleration and gyroscope.

The second part of the classification experiment was a comparison of classification using different sensor placements using the same type of features (combination of time domain and gait temporal features). In this part, four sensor placement groups (L5, foot, shank, and thigh) were used for different independent classification experiments. For the foot, shank, and thigh, the features used were derived from sensors on the left and right side. The results revealed that the shank-based placement achieved the highest result with 89.13% testing accuracy with the Decision Tree algorithm. This result was in agreement with the authors' hypothesis which stated that shank-based placement might have better accuracy since the gait event definition was based on the shank sensor. Moreover, shank-based placement also outperformed all of the classification experiments which used all sensors.

These results could be attributable to the fact that all of the definitions of gait event were based on the angular velocity of the shank sensor, leading to the classification results based on the shank and thigh sensors demonstrating the highest accuracy. The results from the highest accuracy, precision, and recall from each classification method and sensor placement are shown in Table 8.

Table 8. Result from the highest accuracy, precision, and recall from each classification method and sensor placement.

Classification Method (Algorithm Used):	Testing Accuracy (%)	Average Precision	Average Recall
Shank-placement-feature-based model (DT)	89.13	0.90	0.89
Thigh-placement-feature-based model (RF)	80.43	0.83	0.83
Time-domain-feature-based model (MLP)	84.78	0.86	0.85
Model based on gait temporal parameter features (RF)	76.08	0.76	0.76
Combination-feature-based model (MLP)	84.78	0.88	0.85

Another study that also used the same algorithm to define the IC and FC gait events compared the configuration of various sensor placements for detecting IC and FC events and calculated the spatiotemporal parameters of gait in children with cerebral palsy (CP). Their results revealed that a shank-and-thigh sensor configuration yielded more robust results in children with CP and a higher level of disability [26]. This result is in agreement with our results, which revealed that the shank and thigh sensor placement group achieved the highest accuracy among the sensor placements; moreover, other results proved that the algorithm using shank angular velocity to define IC and FC gait event times is more robust than other sensor placement configurations.

4.2. Study Limitations and Future Works

The features used in this study did not include frequency domain features which may also be useful features for classifying between normal and abnormal gait. However, the current result which used a combination of time domain and gait temporal parameters already showed good results with 89.13% testing accuracy. Therefore, future study will examine the effect of adding frequency domain features for gait impairment classification. The limited sample size was also a limitation of this study, in addition to the individual differences that might exist among stroke patients and other neurological disease patients.

Future works arising from this study will be clinical applications that use the best sensor placement method showed in this study's results in order to reduce the number of sensors used and increase the subject's convenience.

5. Conclusions

The results of IC and FC gait event detection using shank angular velocity demonstrated robust detection in all three groups. False peak detection, which can lead to false gait event detection, could be prevented by using this algorithm in combination with the correct additional parameters, such as specified minimal peak distance and minimal peak height.

The comparison of various methods and features for classification among the three groups demonstrated that the classification which used features from a combination of time domain and gait temporal parameters outperformed the classification which only used features from gait temporal parameters. The best result from combination-based feature classification was achieved by the MLP algorithm with 84.78% testing accuracy.

Classification results from different sensor placements revealed that the shank-based sensor gives the best result among the sensor placements with a testing accuracy with 89.13%. The results of the present study demonstrated that the wearable IMU device is capable of differentiating between the gait patterns of healthy patients, patients with stroke, and patients with other neurological disorders.

In summary, the best classification model result among all features and sensor placement combinations was achieved by using all placements with a combination of time domain and gait temporal parameters, while the best sensor placement was shank-based sensors with a combination of time domain and gait temporal parameters and the DT algorithm. Meanwhile, the worst sensor placement resulted from the RF algorithm using L5-based sensor placement.

Author Contributions: Conceptualization, W.-C.H. and T.S.; Methodology, W.-C.H., T.S., and Y.-J.L.; Software, T.S., C.-T.S., C.-L.H.; Validation, W.-C.H. and T.S.; Formal Analysis, T.S.; Investigation, W.-C.H., T.S., and Y.-J.L.; Resources, W.-C.H., F.-C.Y., Z.-Y.L., and K.-N.C.; Data Curation, T.S., F.-C.Y., Z.-Y.L., and K.-N.C.; Writing-Original Draft Preparation, T.S.; Writing-Review & Editing, W.-C.H., T.S., Y.-J.L., C.-T.S., C.-L.H., F.-C.Y., Z.-Y.L., and K.-N.C.; Visualization, T.S.; Supervision, W.-C.H., C.-T.S., and C.-L.H.; Project Administration, W.-C.H., and K.-N.C.; Funding Acquisition, W.-C.H., and K.-N.C.

Funding: The authors gratefully acknowledge financial support from the grant from the Ministry of Science and Technology, Taiwan (MOST104-2628-E-011-006-MY3 to W.-C.H., the corresponding author Wei-Chun Hsu), the National Taiwan University of Science and Technology (TSGH-NTUST-104-05), the Tri-Service General Hospital (TSGH-NTUST-107-04), and Industrial Technology Research Institute (107A02104).

Acknowledgments: The authors would like to thank for all the subjects who participated on this study. The authors would like also to thank Dueng-Yuan Hueng from Neurosurgery Department, Tri-Service General Hospital-Taiwan for the supervision during this study.

Conflicts of Interest: The authors declare there is no conflict of interest on this study.

Appendix

In this section, the selected features from the feature selection process are shown for each classification model (Table A1).

Table A1. Result of selected features from each classification model.

Model Name	Result of Selected Features
Time domain features only	Variance of left foot acceleration Z, Mean of left foot acceleration Y, Mean of left shank acceleration X, Mean and kurtosis of left thigh acceleration X, Skewness of left shank acceleration Z, Skewness of left thigh acceleration X, Variance of right foot acceleration X, Mean of right foot acceleration Z, Kurtosis of L5 acceleration X, Kurtosis of right thigh acceleration X, Skewness of right foot acceleration X, Skewness of right thigh acceleration X, Variance of left foot gyroscope X, Y, and Z, Variance of left shank gyroscope X and Y, Variance of left thigh gyroscope Y, Kurtosis of L5 gyroscope Z, Kurtosis of left shank gyroscope X, Skewness of left foot gyroscope Y, Skewness of left thigh gyroscope Y and Z, Variance of right shank gyroscope X, Y, and Z, Variance of right thigh gyroscope X and Y, Mean of right foot gyroscope Y, Mean of right shank gyroscope Y, Kurtosis of right foot gyroscope X and Y, Kurtosis of right shank gyroscope X, Kurtosis of right thigh gyroscope Z, Skewness of right foot gyro X and Z, Skewness of right shank gyroscope X and Y.
Gait temporal features only	Right stance percentage, Right swing time, Right swing percentage, Swing ratio
Combination features (gait temporal and time domain frequency)	Right stance percentage, Right swing time, Right swing percentage, Swing ratio, Variance of left foot acceleration Z, Mean of left foot acceleration Y, Mean of left shank acceleration X, Mean and kurtosis of left thigh acceleration X, Skewness of left shank acceleration Z, Skewness of left thigh acceleration X, Variance of right foot acceleration X, Mean of right foot acceleration Z, Kurtosis of L5 acceleration X, Kurtosis of right thigh acceleration X, Skewness of right foot acceleration X, Skewness of right thigh acceleration X, Variance of left foot gyroscope X, Y, and Z, Variance of left shank gyroscope X and Y, Variance of left thigh gyroscope Y, Kurtosis of L5 gyroscope Z, Kurtosis of left shank gyroscope X, Skewness of left foot gyroscope Y, Skewness of left thigh gyroscope Y and Z, Variance of right shank gyroscope X, Y, and Z, Variance of right thigh gyroscope X and Y, Mean of right foot gyroscope Y, Mean of right shank gyroscope Y, Kurtosis of right foot gyroscope X and Y, Kurtosis of right shank gyroscope X, Kurtosis of right thigh gyroscope Z, Skewness of right foot gyro X and Z, Skewness of right shank gyroscope X and Y.
L5 sensor placement	Variance of gyroscope X and Z, Kurtosis of gyroscope Z, Mean of acceleration Z, Kurtosis of acceleration X, Right stride time, Right stance time, Right swing time and percentage, First Double Limb Support time and percentage, Stride and Swing ratio.
Foot sensor placement	Variance of left foot gyroscope Y, Skewness of left foot gyroscope Y, Variance of right foot acceleration X, Mean of right foot acceleration Z, Skewness of right foot acceleration X, Kurtosis of right foot gyroscope X, Mean of right foot gyroscope Y, Skewness of right foot gyroscope Z, Right stance percentage, Right swing time and percentage, Stride and Swing ratio.
Shank sensor placement	Skewness of left shank acceleration Z, Variance of left shank gyroscope X, Variance of right shank gyroscope X and Y Mean of right shank gyroscope Y, Kurtosis of right shank gyroscope X, Skewness of right shank gyroscope X and Y, Right stance percentage, Right swing time and percentage, Stride and Swing ratio.
Thigh sensor placement	Variance of left thigh gyroscope Y, Skewness of left thigh gyroscope Y, Skewness of right thigh acceleration X, Variance of right thigh gyroscope X and Y, Kurtosis of right thigh gyroscope Z, Right stance percentage, Right swing time and percentage, Stride and Swing ratio.

References

1. Din, S.D.; Godfrey, A.; Rochester, L. Validation of an accelerometer to quantify a comprehensive battery of gait characteristics in healthy older adults and Parkinson's disease: Toward clinical and at home use. *IEEE J. Biomed. Health Inform.* **2016**, *20*, 838–847. [CrossRef] [PubMed]
2. Trojaniello, D.; Cereatti, A.; Della Croce, U. Accuracy, sensitivity and robustness of five different methods for the estimation of gait temporal parameters using a single inertial sensor mounted on the lower trunk. *Gait Posture* **2014**, *40*, 487–492. [CrossRef] [PubMed]
3. Godfrey, A.; Del Din, S.; Barry, G.; Mathers, J.C.; Rochester, L. Within trial validation and reliability of a single tri-axial accelerometer for gait assessment. In Proceedings of the 2014 36th Annual International Conference of the IEEE Engineering in Medicine and Biology Society (EMBC), Chicago, IL, USA, 26–30 August 2014; pp. 5892–5895.
4. Sinclair, J.; Hobbs, S.J.; Protheroe, L.; Edmundson, C.J.; Greenhalgh, A. Determination of gait events using an externally mounted shank accelerometer. *J. Appl. Biomech.* **2013**, *29*, 118–122. [CrossRef] [PubMed]
5. Aminian, K.; Najafi, B.; Büla, C.; Leyvraz, P.-F.; Robert, P. Spatio-temporal parameters of gait measured by an ambulatory system using miniature gyroscopes. *J. Biomech.* **2002**, *35*, 689–699. [CrossRef]
6. Brunelli, S.; Paolucci, S.; Traballesi, M. Assessment of gait stability, harmony, and symmetry in subjects with lower-limb amputation evaluated by trunk accelerations. *J. Rehab. Res. Dev.* **2014**, *51*, 623–634.
7. Iosa, M.; Marro, T.; Paolucci, S.; Morelli, D. Stability and harmony of gait in children with cerebral palsy. *Rese. Dev. Disabil.* **2012**, *33*, 129–135. [CrossRef] [PubMed]
8. Salatino, G.; Bergamini, E.; Marro, T.; Gentili, P.; Iosa, M.; Morelli, D.; Vannozzi, G. Gait stability assessment in down and prader-willi syndrome children using inertial sensors. *Gait Posture* **2016**, *49*, S16. [CrossRef]
9. Weiss, A.; Herman, T.; Giladi, N.; Hausdorff, J.M. Objective assessment of fall risk in Parkinson's disease using a body-fixed sensor worn for 3 days. *PLoS ONE* **2014**, *9*, e96675. [CrossRef] [PubMed]
10. Sejdic, E.; Lowry, K.A.; Bellanca, J.; Redfern, M.S.; Brach, J.S. A comprehensive assessment of gait accelerometry signals in time, frequency and time-frequency domains. *IEEE Trans. Neural Syst. Rehab. Eng.* **2014**, *22*, 603–612. [CrossRef] [PubMed]
11. Zheng, H.; Yang, M.; Wang, H.; McClean, S. Machine learning and statistical approaches to support the discrimination of neuro-degenerative diseases based on gait analysis. In *Intelligent Patient Management*; Springer: Berlin/Heidelbersg, Germany, 2009; pp. 57–70.
12. Mannini, A.; Trojaniello, D.; Cereatti, A.; Sabatini, A.M. A machine learning framework for gait classification using inertial sensors: Application to elderly, post-stroke and huntington's disease patients. *Sensors* **2016**, *16*, 134. [CrossRef] [PubMed]
13. Zhang, J.; Lockhart, T.E.; Soangra, R. Classifying lower extremity muscle fatigue during walking using machine learning and inertial sensors. *Ann. Biomed. Eng.* **2014**, *42*, 600–612. [CrossRef] [PubMed]
14. Iosa, M.; Bini, F.; Marinozzi, F.; Fusco, A.; Morone, G.; Koch, G.; Martino Cinnera, A.; Bonnì, S.; Paolucci, S. Stability and harmony of gait in patients with subacute stroke. *J. Med. Biol. Eng.* **2016**, *36*, 635–643. [CrossRef] [PubMed]
15. Iosa, M.; Picerno, P.; Paolucci, S.; Morone, G. Wearable inertial sensors for human movement analysis. *Exp. Rev. Med. Dev.* **2016**, *13*, 641–659. [CrossRef] [PubMed]
16. Steele, B.G.; Holt, L.; Belza, B.; Ferris, S.; Lakshminaryan, S.; Buchner, D.M. Quantitating physical activity in copd using a triaxial accelerometer. *CHEST J.* **2000**, *117*, 1359–1367. [CrossRef]
17. Long, X.; Yin, B.; Aarts, R.M. Single-accelerometer-based daily physical activity classification. In Proceedings of the 2009 Annual International Conference of the IEEE Engineering in Medicine and Biology Society, Minneapolis, MN, USA, 3–6 September 2009; pp. 6107–6110.
18. Coley, B.; Najafi, B.; Paraschiv-Ionescu, A.; Aminian, K. Stair climbing detection during daily physical activity using a miniature gyroscope. *Gait Posture* **2005**, *22*, 287–294. [CrossRef] [PubMed]
19. Taraldsen, K.; Chastin, S.F.M.; Riphagen, I.I.; Vereijken, B.; Helbostad, J.L. Physical activity monitoring by use of accelerometer-based body-worn sensors in older adults: A systematic literature review of current knowledge and applications. *Maturitas* **2012**, *71*, 13–19. [CrossRef] [PubMed]
20. Rowlands, A.V.; Thomas, P.W.; Eston, R.G.; Topping, R. Validation of the RT3 triaxial accelerometer for the assessment of physical activity. *Med. Sci. Sport. Exer.* **2004**, *36*, 518–524. [CrossRef]

21. Plasqui, G.; Westerterp, K.R. Physical activity assessment with accelerometers: An evaluation against doubly labeled water. *Obesity* **2007**, *15*, 2371–2379. [CrossRef] [PubMed]

22. Mannini, A.; Sabatini, A.M. Machine learning methods for classifying human physical activity from on-body accelerometers. *Sensors* **2010**, *10*, 1154–1175. [CrossRef] [PubMed]

23. Khandelwal, S.; Wickström, N. Novel methodology for estimating initial contact events from accelerometers positioned at different body locations. *Gait Posture* **2018**, *59*, 278–285. [CrossRef] [PubMed]

24. Anwary, A.R.; Yu, H.; Vassallo, M. Optimal foot location for placing wearable imu sensors and automatic feature extraction for gait analysis. *IEEE Sens. J.* **2018**, *18*, 2555–2567. [CrossRef]

25. Salarian, A.; Burkhard, P.R.; Vingerhoets, F.J.G.; Jolles, B.M.; Aminian, K. A novel approach to reducing number of sensing units for wearable gait analysis systems. *IEEE Trans. Biomed. Eng.* **2013**, *60*, 72–77. [CrossRef] [PubMed]

26. Carcreff, L.; Gerber, C.N.; Paraschiv-Ionescu, A.; De Coulon, G.; Newman, C.J.; Armand, S.; Aminian, K. What is the best configuration of wearable sensors to measure spatiotemporal gait parameters in children with cerebral palsy? *Sensors* **2018**, *18*, 394. [CrossRef] [PubMed]

27. Vienne, A.; Barrois, R.P.; Buffat, S.; Ricard, D.; Vidal, P.-P. Inertial sensors to assess gait quality in patients with neurological disorders: A systematic review of technical and analytical challenges. *Front. Psychol.* **2017**, *8*, 817. [CrossRef] [PubMed]

28. Kavanagh, J.J.; Morrison, S.; James, D.A.; Barrett, R. Reliability of segmental accelerations measured using a new wireless gait analysis system. *J. Biomech.* **2006**, *39*, 2863–2872. [CrossRef] [PubMed]

29. Salarian, A.; Russmann, H.; Vingerhoets, F.J.; Dehollain, C.; Blanc, Y.; Burkhard, P.R.; Aminian, K. Gait assessment in parkinson's disease: Toward an ambulatory system for long-term monitoring. *IEEE Trans. Biomed. Eng.* **2004**, *51*, 1434–1443. [CrossRef] [PubMed]

30. Patterson, K.K.; Gage, W.H.; Brooks, D.; Black, S.E.; McIlroy, W.E. Evaluation of gait symmetry after stroke: A comparison of current methods and recommendations for standardization. *Gait Posture* **2010**, *31*, 241–246. [CrossRef] [PubMed]

31. Freund, Y.; Schapire, R.E. A decision-theoretic generalization of on-line learning and an application to boosting. *J. Comput. Syst. Sci.* **1997**, *55*, 119–139. [CrossRef]

32. Zhang, H. The optimality of naive bayes. In Proceedings of the Seventeenth International Florida Artificial Intelligence Research Society Conference, Miami Beach, FL, USA, 12–14 May 2004.

33. Bishop, C.; Bishop, C.M. *Neural Networks for Pattern Recognition*; Oxford University Press: Oxford, UK, 1995.

34. Begg, R.K.; Palaniswami, M.; Owen, B. Support vector machines for automated gait classification. *IEEE Trans. Biomed. Eng.* **2005**, *52*, 828–838. [CrossRef] [PubMed]

35. Pogorelc, B.; Bosnić, Z.; Gams, M. Automatic recognition of gait-related health problems in the elderly using machine learning. *Multimedia Tools Appl.* **2012**, *58*, 333–354. [CrossRef]

36. De Vroey, H.; Staes, F.; Weygers, I.; Vereecke, E.; Vanrenterghem, J.; Deklerck, J.; Van Damme, G.; Hallez, H.; Claeys, K. The implementation of inertial sensors for the assessment of temporal parameters of gait in the knee arthroplasty population. *Clin. Biomech.* **2018**, *54*, 22–27. [CrossRef] [PubMed]

37. Jasiewicz, J.M.; Allum, J.H.J.; Middleton, J.W.; Barriskill, A.; Condie, P.; Purcell, B.; Li, R.C.T. Gait event detection using linear accelerometers or angular velocity transducers in able-bodied and spinal-cord injured individuals. *Gait Posture* **2006**, *24*, 502–509. [CrossRef] [PubMed]

38. Daliri, M.R. Automatic diagnosis of neuro-degenerative diseases using gait dynamics. *Measurement* **2012**, *45*, 1729–1734. [CrossRef]

 © 2018 by the authors. Licensee MDPI, Basel, Switzerland. This article is an open access article distributed under the terms and conditions of the Creative Commons Attribution (CC BY) license (http://creativecommons.org/licenses/by/4.0/).

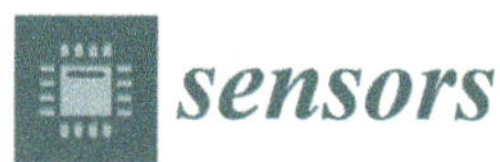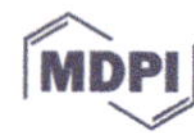

Article

Scanning Laser Rangefinders for the Unobtrusive Monitoring of Gait Parameters in Unsupervised Settings

Sebastian Fudickar [1,*], Christian Stolle [1], Nils Volkening [2] and Andreas Hein [2]

[1] Department of Health Services Research, CvO University Oldenburg, School of Medicine and Health Science, 26111 Oldenburg, Germany; christian.stolle1@uni-oldenburg.de
[2] OFFIS e.V., 26121 Oldenburg, Germany; nils.volkening@offis.de (N.V.); andreas.hein@offis.de (A.H.)
* Correspondence: sebastian.fudickar@uol.de; Tel.: +49-441-798-2849

Received: 9 August 2018; Accepted: 10 October 2018; Published: 12 October 2018

Abstract: Since variations in common gait parameters (such as cadence, velocity and stride-length) of elderly people are a reliable indicator of functional and cognitive decline in aging and increased fall risks, such gait parameters have to be monitored continuously to enable preventive interventions as early as possible. With scanning laser rangefinders (SLR) having been shown to be suitable for standardised (frontal) gait assessments, this article introduces an unobtrusive gait monitoring (UGMO) system for lateral gait monitoring in homes for the elderly. The system has been evaluated in comparison to a GAITRite (as reference system) with 86 participants (ranging from 21 to 82 years) passing the 6-min walk test twice. Within the considered 56,351 steps within an overall 7877 walks and approximately 34 km distance travelled, it has been shown that the SLR Hokuyo UST10-LX is more sensitive than the cheaper URG-04LX version in regard to the correct (automatic) detection of lateral steps (98% compared to 77%) and walks (97% compared to 66%). Furthermore, it has been confirmed that the UGMO (with the SLR UST10-LX) can measure gait parameters such as gait velocity and stride length with sufficient sensitivity to determine age- and disease-related functional (and cognitive) decline.

Keywords: gait recognition; scanning laser rangefinders (SLR), GAITRite; cadence; velocity and stride-length

---

1. Introduction

The prolongation of elderly people's ability to remain independent in their common environments is an essential necessity to assure both a high quality of living for elderly people and well-functioning health-care systems. Thus, the early detection of functional decline and a deep understanding of elderly people's locomotion processes are both essential aspects for the prevention of falls, which are the leading cause of fatal injury and the most common cause of non-fatal trauma-related hospital admissions among older adults causing over \$50 billion total medical costs in 2015 [1] and being critical for losing the ability for independent living due to the resulting potentially severe effects on patients' physical and mental health [2–6]. Thus, the reliable identification of at-risk patients at the earliest possible stage is a critical foundation to initiate appropriate preventive interventions [7] and thereby prolong functional and cognitive decline. The human gait (e.g., quantified as gait speed) has been confirmed to be a comprehensive measure and indicator for both, functional and cognitive decline [8,9]. For example, Savica et al. have investigated GAITRite measures of dementia patients and found an association between reduced gait velocity, cadence and stride length, and both global and domain-specific cognitive decline [10]. Similarly, Bridenbaugh proposed that stride speed and variability may be sensitive enough to track cognitive impairments [11].

A gait can be characterised via the following events and parameters. As shown in Figure 1, a gait cycle or stride is defined as the phases during movement of both, the left and the right feet once. In contrast, a step considers the movement of either the left or the right foot (starting with toe off/last contact and lasting till initial contact of the same foot). Thus, a stride consists of two steps. Common parameters to characterise a gait typically consider a walk, which consists of multiple sequential steps. Common parameters (listed in Table 1) such as the cadence, velocity, stride length (L/R), L/R stance phases, L/R swing phase, L/R step length and step width are calculated from the durations and distances of the stance and swing phases and the foot positions, in accordance with the following equations. Among these parameters, the latter five parameters can be derived separately for each foot.

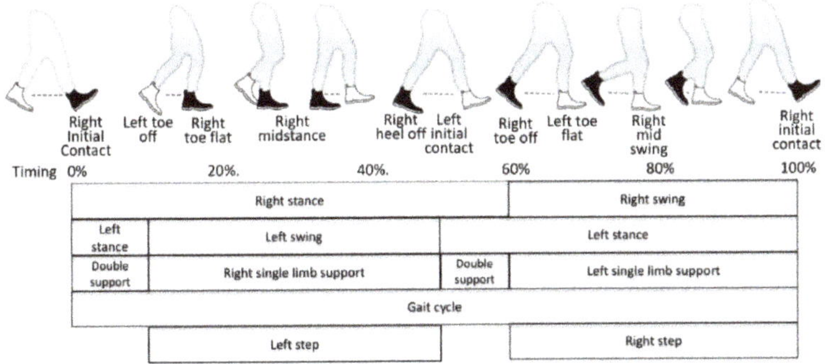

Figure 1. Gait cycle with the corresponding events (along with a typical ratio-timing based on occurrence within a gait cycle), the corresponding phases; black shoe represents right foot.

Table 1. Common gait parameters and corresponding algorithms.

Gait Parameter	Description	Algorithm	Separately per Foot
Step length [m]	Distance between the heel of one foot to the heel of the next one along walking direction (see left and right step in Figure 1)	Distance passed from toe off to initial contact.	x
Cadence [1/min]	Step frequency	Number of steps/time [min]	
Walking velocity [m/min]	Gait speed	Distance [m]/time [min] = stride_length [m] × cadence [1/min]/2	
Stance time [s]	Time each foot has contact with the ground per step (see left and right stance in Figure 1.)	Last_contact_time − first_contact_time	x
Swing time [s]	Time each foot has no contact with the ground per step (see left and right swing in Figure 1)	Step[i + 1]. first_contact_time − step[i]. last_contact_time	x
Stride length [m]	Distance from one foot hitting the ground to its next ground contact (see full gait cycle shown in Figure 1 as example for right stride).	Step_length$_{Left}$ + step_length$_{Right}$	x

A study indicated a standard deviation of 7% among for normal indoor gait velocities (as shown in Table 2) ranging (in mean) between 80–91 m/min for men and 73–81 m/min for women [12,13].

In contrast, age-related variability of the gait (e.g., due to corresponding disabilities such as arthritis) was shown for gait velocity to be ranging from 14% [14] to 29% for the transition to frailty and even 51% in case of fearful fallers. This decrease of velocity has been shown to be mainly related to a decreased stride length of approximately 10% [15,16] and even 21% for transition to frailty and 41% for fearful fallers. In contrast, the cadence shows rather minor variations among these age-related phenomena.To summarise, aging in gait can be expected to manifest in smaller rather than in less steps.

However, functional decline in terms of variations in the gait initially occur during daily activities and not during phases of peak performance within clinical assessments, for the following reasons: While being conducted in rather standardised settings and thereby assuring performance comparability among elderly people, well-accepted clinical assessments are typically not applied in a preventive manner. Furthermore, elderly people's performance within clinical assessments has been shown to be affected by the physicians' presence. In addition, due to the incomparability of clinical walkways with rather complex home environments, elderly people's performance within clinical tests is less representative of their common performance [17]. Consequently, clinical tests have been shown to result on average in 21% higher walking speeds and a mean 6% higher step-length than experienced in everyday living scenario tests and thereby have been shown to allow only limited insights into the elderly people's everyday performance [17].

Consequently, with gait being a suitable early indicator of functional and cognitive decline and being specifically sensitive in unsupervised everyday living conditions, corresponding sensitive measurement technology is required [17] that supports a frequent sufficiently sensitive unsupervised technical monitoring (and assessment) of physical performance in domestic environments, as argued by Hellmers et al. [18]. In order to be accepted for continuous monitoring of the elderly people's activities within their homes, these sensors have to preserve the participants' privacy and have to consider users' low technological readiness [19], while being sufficiently robust in regard to context variations.

Table 2. Measures for common gait parameters as an indication of clinical meaningfulness ranges as mean ([+] The selected columns as well specify standard deviation as ±SD and mean variation from the normal gender independent value in % in parenthesis).

Parameter	Men Normal [20]	Women Normal [20]	Normal (Gender Independent) [21]	Transition to Frailty[+] [16]	Fearful Fallers [+] [22]
Velocity [m/min]	86 (80–91)	77 (73–81)	82	58.2 ± 13.8 (29%)	39.6 ± 11.4 (51%)
Cadence [1/min]	111	117	113	105.7 ± 12.7 (6%)	95.4 ± 11.2 (15%)
Stride length [m]	1.46	1.28	1.41	1.11 ± 0.18 (21%)	0.83 ± 0.16 (41%)

While accurate gait analytic-systems such as the GAITRite [23] and the Vicon [24] system are commonly accepted as gold standards, they are rather unsuitable for long-term monitoring especially within domestic environments due to the associated costs and installation efforts. In regard to the unobtrusive monitoring of the gait in domestic environments, various senor types have been considered. The sensitivity of passive infrared (PIR) presence-sensors or light-barriers, due to the low granularity of the gathered information, still has to be confirmed [19,25]; and body-worn inertial measurement units (IMU) [26,27] require users' willingness and habituality of use. The following ambient sensing techniques fulfill the aforementioned criteria much better. For fine-grained insights of the gait, scanning laser rangefinders (SLR) achieve sufficient sensitivity to characterise the gait (see Table 3). SLRs send radial horizontal laser beams and detect the distance to obstacles based on the time-of-flight that the returning beams (as being reflected by these obstacle) take until being received by the SLR. Within, the angular resolution of SLRs refers to the amount of samples taking per degree. The amount of reflected laser points determine the resolution of obstacles.

Table 3. Existing ambient gait detection systems, their considered parameters, sensitivities, and study population and orientation (F: frontal, B: backwards, S: lateral, n.d.: indicating no information, BGS: background subtraction, DR: Doppler radar, EDF: erosion-dilation filter, GNN: global nearest neighbor, HMM: hidden Markov model, IQR: interquartile range; KC: 3D motion recorder™Kissei Comtec, KF: Kalman filter, KM: K-means, LMS: least mean square, PF: particle filter, RMSE: root mean square error, SD: standard deviation, Scanning laser rangefinders (SLRs): 04-LX-UG01: SLR URG04-LX-UG01, 04LX-F01: SLR UBG-04LX-F01, 30LX: SLR UTM-30LX.

	Sensor System			Resulting Sensitivity				Study Design	
Year	Sensor	Algorithm	Orient/Height	Detection Rate of Steps/Walks (in %)	Gait Velocity/Speed Error (cm/s)	Stride Length Error (cm)	Swing Time Error (s)	Reference System	Subjects (m/f); Age
2015 [28]	04-LX-UG01, UTM-30LX	KF, GNN	F 27 cm	Leg tracking (97.1%) Foot contact (99.3%)	n.d.	3.5 cm	n.d.	Vicon	7 (4/3); 70.9 years ± 3.5
2017 [29]	04LX-F01	KF/PF	F 40 cm	KF: 18.4% (10.5–30.1%) PF: 0.6% (0–2.3%)	KF: 7.9 (4.5–11.3) cm/s PF: 6.4 cm/s (4.2–9.9) RMSE	n.d.	n.d.	Vicon	4; 65 + years
2016 [30]	04LX-F01	HMM, KM, KF	F 40 cm walker	n.d.	n.d.	HMM: 8.9% ± 5.2% RB: 10.1% ± 6.8%	HMM: 10.9% ± 6.2% RB: 16.9% ± 5.7%	GAITRite	5; 65 + years
2014 [31,32]	SLR, 4 force sensors	BGS, DIET [13]	F/B 35 cm	n.d.	n.d.	3 cm	0.08 s	SIMI Motion	7 (5/2); 23–31 years
2009 [33]	UTM-30LX	LMS fitting [34]	F 10 cm	n.d.	n.d.	1.1 SD 0.8 cm	n.d.	n.d.	6 (3/3); n.d.
2017 [35]	UTM-30LX	n.d.	F 25 cm	n.d.	n.d.	25.9 cm (3.37%) ± 23.8 cm (3.53%)	0.091 s (22.9%) ± 0.051 s (12.1%)	KC	34 (21/13); 22–30 years
2015 [36]	UTM-30LX	KF, Catmull–Rom spline [37]	F/B	96.4% (tracking success rate)	n.d.	3–5 cm RMSE	n.d.	Vicon	7 (6/1); 23.0 ± 1.9 years
2017 [38]	Kinect	BGS [39] LSM, EDF, HMM	F	n.d.	0.3; SD 0.12 cm/s	0.6; SD 8.31 cm	n.d.	GAITRite	11 (7/4); 22–53 years
2017 [40]	DR, Precision Line RCR-50	Zero-crossing in time domain IQR filter	F 15 cm	n.d.	1.08 RMSE	n.d.	n.d.	Vicon, Kinect	8; seniors

As summarized in Table 3, most systems for automated detection of gait parameters apply SLRs, followed by systems that use red-green-blue (RGB) (D) cameras. Most approaches use a Kalman filter in combination with a background subtraction procedure and hidden Markov models for classification. In most cases, the SLR are aligned parallel to the walking direction of the subject and at a height of 20–40 cm, which corresponds approximately to the height of the knee or shin. No publication was found that placed the SLR orthogonally to the walking direction. In most publications, only subsets of the relevant gait parameters are described or evaluated, and the given parameters are usually also very specifically adapted to the respective scenario, which makes comparison difficult in many places. The number of subjects in most studies is in the single-digit range, rarely in the low to medium double-digit range. The age of the test persons also varies greatly from young adults (22–30 years) to seniors (67–92 years).

However, to the authors' best knowledge, so far only the application with a frontal placement of the SLR towards the walking patients has been investigated. While the frontal placement is suitable in a supervised clinical setting, it has limited practicability within everyday home scenarios, where movements have to be characterisable from the side. In addition, the sensitivity of both SLR types, the Hokuyo URG-04LX (herein referred to as SLR-04) and the Hokuyo UST-10LX (herein referred to as SLR-10) in regard to sensing gait parameters have yet to be compared.

Thus, this article introduces an SLR-based autonomous in-home sensor-system for unobtrusive long-term and privacy-preserving in gait monitoring that overcomes the requirement of frontal sensor placements. The system's sensitivity and both SLRs' sensitivity is evaluated in comparison to GAITRite measures (as reference system) with 86 subjects.

2. Materials and Methods

In this Section, we initially introduce unobtrusive gait monitoring (UGMO), which is followed by the description of the study design and the evaluation methodology.

2.1. Unobtrusive Gait Monitoring (UGMO)

The developed UGMO system (shown in Figure 2) has been designed for unsupervised sensitive monitoring (and assessment) of common gait-parameters within domestic environments. In order to affect the proband as little as possible, the device has a reasonably small size, and does not require any user interaction. Furthermore, UGMO can automatically detect time-series with gait activity and will only record these movements. The UGMO system consists of a measuring platform and a software based signal-processing chain, as described subsequently.

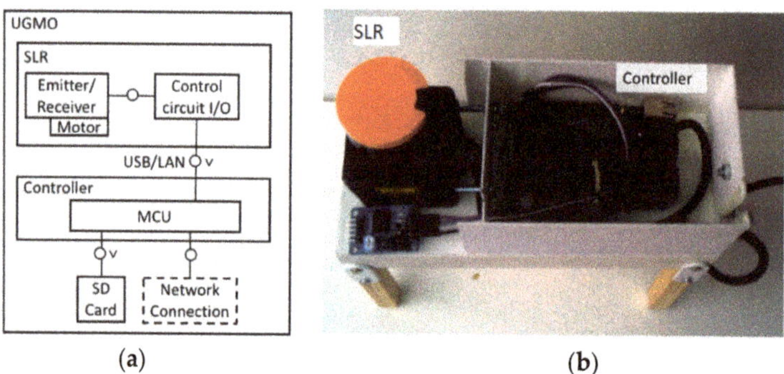

(a)   (b)

Figure 2. The resulting unobtrusive gait monitoring (UGMO) system: (**a**) the system components, (**b**) the device.

2.1.1. UGMO Hardware

The UGMO hardware combines a Hokuyo SLR with an ambient light sensor and a processing unit (based on a Raspberry Pi 3) within a handy form factor (L × H × W: 20 cm × 20 cm × 8 cm). By utilizing these sensors, the users' privacy is assured since only gait-related distance measures of feet and intensity of ambient lights are monitored.

The SLR is placed at a height of approximately 15 cm above ground, since being suitable for gait measurements. Two popular versions of the Hokuyo sensors—the SLR-04 and the SLR-10 have been evaluated for comparison. While the cheaper SLR-04 has been successfully applied for gait recognition [28–30], the SLR-10 could be expected to achieve higher sensitivity due to its four-fold scanning rate and coverage of an increased measuring area (as summarized in Table 4)—which becomes especially relevant in the case of scanning the gait of bypassing persons. However, it comes with a 40% increased price and thus might be considered only if achieving significantly higher results.

Table 4. Characteristics of the considered SLR.

SLR Scanner-Type	Hokuyo URG-04LX (SLR-04) [41]	Hokuyo UST-10LX (SLR-10) [42]
Scanning rate	10 Hz	40 Hz
Measuring area	2–560 cm	6–1000 cm
	240°	270°
Measuring Accuracy	±10 mm (0.20–1 m), ±3% (1–5.6 m)	±40 mm
Angular resolution	approx. 0.36°	approx. 0.25°
I/O	Universal series bus (USB)	Local-area network (LAN)
Power Supply	5V DC, 500 mA (800 mA during start up)	12VDC/24VDC, 150 mA (450 mA during start up)

Intended as a monitoring device, UGMO can either operate as standalone (by recording to a memory card) or can transmit recordings directly to the Internet. The UGMO's data recordings support sufficiently long recording durations: with each measure holding approx. 13 KB (resulting in 52 KB/s for SLR04 and 130 KB/s for the SLR10) and each walk (over a distance of approx. 5 m) approx. 3 MB, the UGMO could record approx. 355 days on a 32 GB memory card when assuming 30 walks per day and compression adding further power of 10, the data size is unproblematic. UGMOs power connection consists of a 5V DC, 700–1000 mA power supply for the Raspberry Pi 3 and a power supply for the SLR (see Table 4). With UGMO's hardware design being straightforward the following description focuses on the algorithmic approaches.

2.1.2. Signal-Processing

UGMO integrates the following signal-processing workflow (shown in Figure 3).

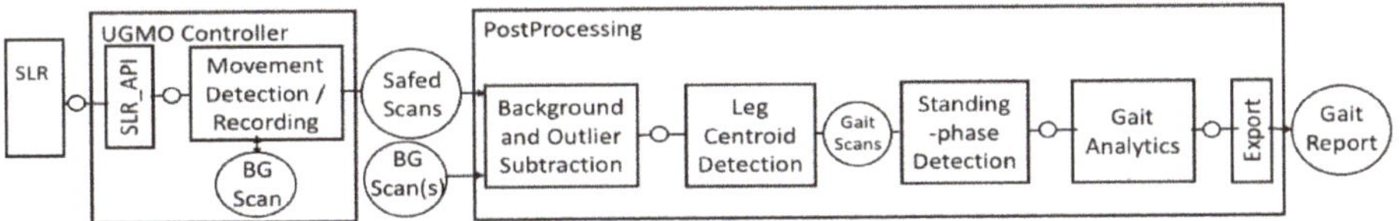

Figure 3. UGMO's signal processing workflow; ranged laser scanner; BG scan: background scan; rectangles indicate processing steps and circles indicate data storages.

The software has been developed via Python 3.

The **movement detection/recording** module handles the communication with the SLR, detects when a walk has been performed in front on the UGMO and records the SLR data of movement sequences. Therefore, the module initially (and regularly) collects a background scan (BG scan) against which subsequent scans are substituted. Movement is detected if scans significantly differ from the background. In these cases, the scans are recorded for later processing or could be transferred to a server for direct analysis via an available network connection. It has two parameters (the sensitivity parameter and delay parameter) to calibrate the accuracy of the movement-detection: The sensitivity parameter defines how many measured points (see angular resolution in Table 4 for each SLR) have to be different from the background laser scan. For the SLR-10 the sensitivity parameter has been set to 3 and for the SLR-04 4, respectively. The delay parameter describes how many consecutive laser scans have to pass the sensitivity (3 for SLR-04 and 27 for SLR-10) in order to start (and end) a walk. These settings have been chosen experimentally.

Background and outlier subtraction: for points that differ significantly from the background image, the presence of a movement is assumed and thus these points are further considered. Thus, the stored background image is subtracted from the current recorded (scan-) image by the following algorithm: angular points are compared among both images and if differentiating by less than a threshold (of 20 cm for the SLR-10 and 3 cm for the SLR-04), the resulting angular point-specific distant-measure is excluded from further investigations (by setting it to 0). An examplary resulting scan is shown in Figure 4b.

Next, in order to exclude temporal noise from the resulting subtracted image, only the remaining points that contain min. (5 for SLR-10, 2 for SLR-04) neighbouring points (that are not 0) are further on considered. Also, the neighboring points have to have a value difference of less than (10 cm SLR-10, 3 cm SLR-04).

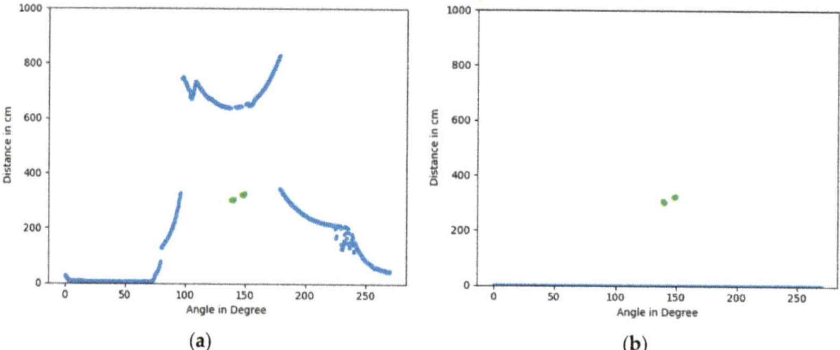

Figure 4. Examplary results of the background and outlier subtraction: (**a**) original image: steps (in green) and background (in blue) (**b**) results of background and outlier subtraction.

Leg centroid detection: In order to detect legs in the remaining distance points per scan, the k-nearest neighbour (knn) clustering with an intended cluster amount of 2 is applied. Subsequently, the cluster centers are calculated from the corresponding points per cluster. These two cluster centers represent the desired ankle (talus and tibia) positions of the distant and the frontal leg. Since considering the detected leg positions of all scans, the brief loss of the back leg is unproblematic and the algorithm is as well suited to cover the particular case of covert legs, where the distant leg (from sensor point of view) is briefly covert by the frontal leg (for a few milliseconds during the swing phase of the frontal leg) meanwhile no points are collected for the distant leg. For the leg centroid detection, SLR-specific parameter-settings have not to be differentiated.

Standing phase detection: In order to identify the standing phases (temporal and spatial), the ankle-positions within all scans of a detected walk are condensed into a single 2D image (see Figure 5a). The previously detected ankle positions are subsequently transformed from angular-

and distance-encoded vectors to concrete 2D positions via the following trigonometric functions (where α is the angle in degrees for the current SLR sample as shown in Figure 5a):

$$x = \text{distance} \times \cos(\alpha)$$

$$y = \text{distance} \times \sin(\alpha)$$

The resulting converted (geographically correct) visualization is shown in Figure 5b.

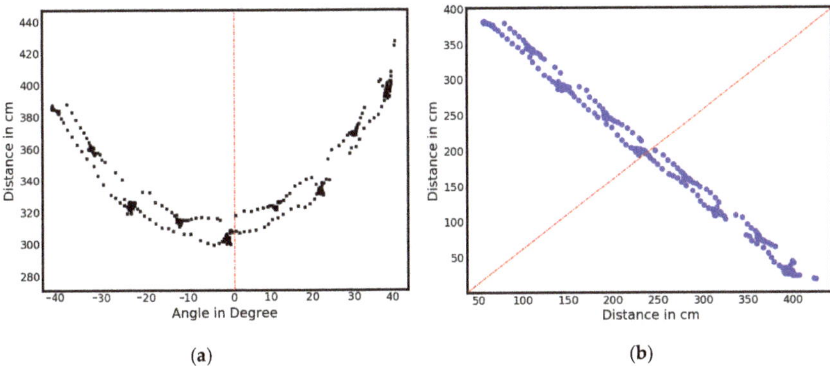

(a)

(b)

Figure 5. (a) Summary of all leg positions into a single image (b) after switch of coordinate system (Figure 5b: the SLR is placed at coordinate 0/0 with the center point of view facing along the $f(x) = x$ line).

Since in standing positions the ankles are positioned at the same coordinates for multiple (consecutive) scans, the corresponding regions can be calculated correspondingly via these concentrations (as shown for example in Figure 6). In order to identify these concentration points, the clustering algorithm DBSCAN has been used with the following parameter settings: Its maximal distance between intra cluster-points being generally set to 50 mm and the minimal number of points per cluster being set to 2 for the SLR-04 and to 7 for the SLR-10. Exemplary results of this standing phase detection are shown in Figure 6a for the SLR-04 and Figure 6b for the SLR-10 and indicate the higher amount of ankle measures to be considered for the SLR-10 in comparison to the SLR-04.

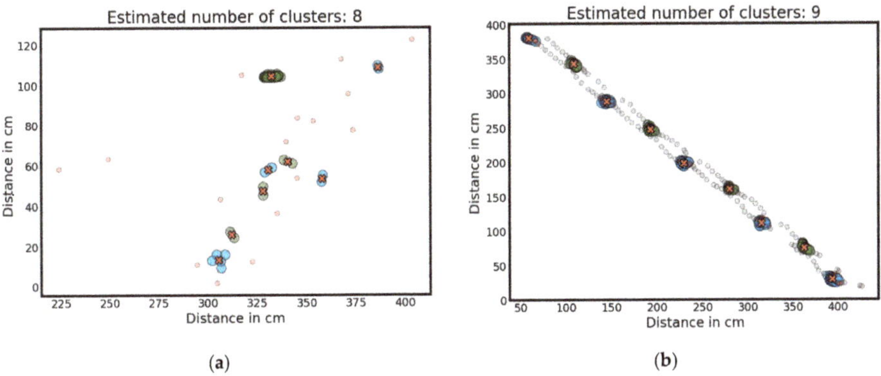

(a)

(b)

Figure 6. The results of the standing phase detection for an examplistical (better) identical walk representing the identified standing phases based on the DBSCAN clustering (with standing phases marked in color, general detected ankles as black dots, and corresponding standing positions marked via a red cross). (a) For the erroneous SLR-04 sensor and (b) for the SLR-10 sensor.

The centers of the identified clusters are calculated as the median of the timestamps of all ankle measures per cluster. Next to the median timestamp, the corresponding x and y coordinates of this ankle measure and the cluster's starting and ending time (representing first and last contact time) are considered of the are used for the static phase (see Figure 6). The use of the median was preferred over the first and last contact time, since it is expected to achieve more robust results.

The identified coordinates and timestamps are afterwards used within the gait analysis to extract the corresponding gait parameters.

In order to derive the common gait parameters velocity, cadence, walking distance, stance time, swing time and stride length, the contact times per standing phase (representing steps) and the associated step positions are further analysed within the **Gait Analytics** processing step. The analysis has been made using both, either the 'First Contact Time' or the 'Average Contact Time' to identify the sensitivity of both parameters. The steps for both parameters have then been matched to the GAITRite Analysis with a maximum time difference 'timedelta'.

While the calculation of the gait parameters itself is straightforward, the following three further pre-processing steps have to be conducted.

Initially, the steps are ordered ascendingly according to the time of recording. Consecutively, the orientation of the steps (left or right leg) is calculated for the initially step by detecting whether the walk is orientated from left to right or right to left and then whether the following step has an increased or decreased distance to the SLR. The orientations of subsequent steps are then altered.

Furthermore, each intermediate step (IM Steps, see Figure 7), being at the midpoint of one stride and orthogonally to the position of the standing leg (as shown in Figure 7), is calculated since being required for the calculation of the single-step parameter. Intermediate steps are calculated via 3 subsequent standing phases as follows. Among the first and the third standing phases (both of this leg) a line is assumed and the step position is assumed to be the junction, where an orthogonal line to these base line passes through the position of the second standing phase (of the other leg).

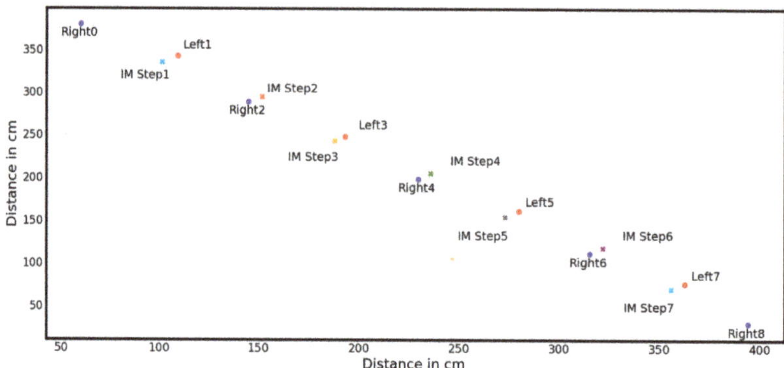

Figure 7. Calculation of steps as part of gait analysis (IM Steps representing calculated intermediate steps).

In the subsequent **Calculation of Gait Parameters**, the gait parameters are then calculated as described in Section 1 Table 2 based on the extracted spatio-temporal data (x,y coordinates and timestamps) of the detected steps.

The **export** format is based on the one of the GAITRite csv export (a tab-separated ASCII export file holding the field per step as summarized in Annex 1), with the difference of it being more easily readable for a human (and the common step count encoding of GAITRite has been excluded). Complete walks are saved in one row, with individual steps being saved in lists, instead of every single step having one row. The current export contains all described gait-parameters, namely:

- Per walk: subject ID, timestamp, distance, cadence, speed (speed and GAITRite's parameter of velocity are used synonymously);
- Per step: first contact time, last contact time, left/right stride length (cm), left/right stance phases (s), left/right swing phases.

2.2. Study Design

In order to evaluate UGMO's sensitivity regarding the detection of walks, steps and the corresponding gait parameters, the following study has been conducted: UGMO's sensitivity was compared to a 6 m GAITRite (with an active sensing area of 4.88 m) with GAITRite SW Version 4.8.7, acting as reference. To clarify the suitability of both SLRs, both have been used in parallel and have been placed on top of each other (the SLR-10 at a height of 9 cm and the SLR-04 at 18 cm, respectively) facing the GAITRite walkway at a distance of 3.6 m to the GAITRite center. The brief height alteration between both SLRs is unproblematic in regard to the systems' sensitivity, since both positions are centered around the ankle, which assures reasonable low variability regarding the measurement distances. Thereby, it is assured that all 3 sensors (the GAITRite, the SLR-04 and the SLR-10) record the same gaits. In order to achieve direct comparability among the systems, the SLR wider measurement angel (see Table 4) was restricted onto the GAITRite sensing area via visual covers as shown in Figure 8. To assure clock synchronization, all three devices were connected to the same measurement computer. The precision of the timestamps was recorded with 1000 Hz by all systems.

Within the study, the recording software was deployed on a standard PC (Windows 7 64bit 4 GB Ram, Python 3 and the GAITRite software).

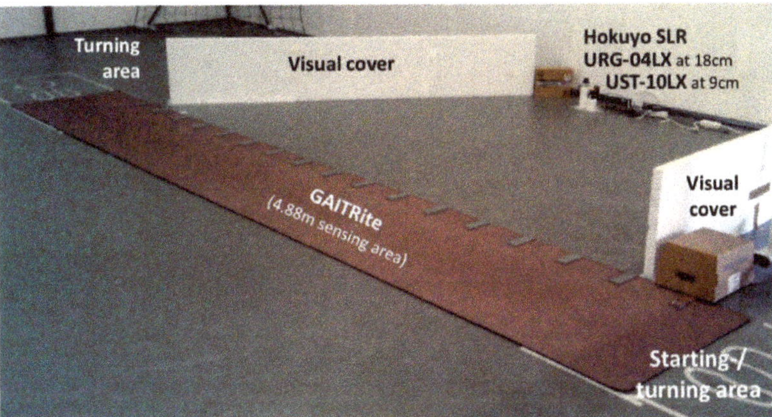

Figure 8. The measurement setup: Including the GAITRite and both SLRs with a visual shielding to limit their viewing angle on GAITRite's active sensing area and exclude other walks. Participants passed the GAITRite with turning in the marked turning areas 2 times for 6 min at various paces.

Within this setting, subjects were requested to walk continuously over the GAITRite to and fro for 6 min. In order to cover a wider spectrum of walking speeds, they were requested to pass this 6 min walk test twice—once at comfortable and once at quick pace. Since the systems' sensitivity is based on the number of scans per step, slower paces cause a higher number of scans per step than faster ones. Thus, a further investigation of slow paces was undertaken in order to overcome exhaustion of the participants as a result of the additional efforts.

We provided verbal, as well as written information for all potential participants and checked for inclusion and exclusion criteria (ability to walk with socks and without walkers and being able to pass the timed up and go (TUG) test within 10 s). The study received ethical approval by the ethical committee of the University of Oldenburg approval code number Drs. 33/2016.

2.3. Methodology

In order to study UGMO's sensitivity, the measurements of the SLRs and the GAITRite have been exported as csv files (covering all foot positions per subject in millisecond accuracy). Per subject, a list of all walks measured by GAITRite, SLR-04 and SLR-10 is extracted from the respective export files. When comparing the sensitivity of the automatic gait detection (separately per SLR), the first and last step (each as first contact time) from each walk were then extracted and compared to the GAITRite steps with a synchronization overlap time-delta. For this synchronization overlap, 3 s were determined initially as suitable when considering the amount of correctly associated steps among each UGMO version and the GAITRite (see Table 5).

Table 5. Suitability of synchronization overlap (bold indicating the selected optimum).

Synchronisation Overlap (s) between SLR and GAITRite	Number of Steps (% of Overall 56351 Considered Steps)	
	URG04LX	**UST-10LX**
4	43162 (75.6%)	55083 (97.7%)
3.5	43253 (76.8%)	55167 (97.9%)
3	**43260 (76.8%)**	**55181 (97.9%)**
2.5	43092 (76.5%)	55188 (97.9%)
2	42035 (74.6%)	55153 (97.9%)
1.5	37240 (66.1%)	54516 (96.7%)
1	25221 (44.8%)	46879 (83.2%)
0.5	11473 (20.4%)	23961 (42.5%)

If the steps of the GAITRite and SLR were within this time delta, the walk was treated as a correctly detected walk. For the evaluation of the detection accuracy of individual steps, each single step (of the sorted SLR step list) was compared and treated as correct if it had a matching counterpart within the sorted GAITRite list. This was the only step, in which the results of the different sensors were synchronized for evaluation purposes. Even though the clocks were only synchronised per subjects, the clock-drift remained uncritical, since every 5 m walk was synchronised separately among all systems. In addition, the gait parameters were calculated via UGMO's signal-processing chain per correctly detected walks. Afterwards, the parameters were averaged per walk separately for UGMO and GAITRite measures. In order to clarify the influence of gait speed on the systems sensitivity, the walks were separated into two groups according to the walking-past blocks: normal and fast walking speeds. Subsequently, the results per group were evaluated via Pearson correlation coefficient and the calculation of errors between both systems.

3. Results

3.1. Descriptive Statistics

Within the described evaluation setup, recordings of the gait of 92 subjects were recorded for evaluation purposes.

Among the recordings, six subjects were excluded due to the following errors: For two subjects the same ID has been used. Two additional subjects have not correctly executed the protocol, but have turned around already after 3 m instead of passing the full distance. For two additional subjects, no SLR measures were recorded during assessment. After initial exclusion of these six subjects the descriptive statistics (shown in Table 6) applies for the remaining 86 subjects.

Within the study overall 56,351 steps within an overall 7877 walks were recorded within approx. 8 h.

Table 6. The descriptive statistics of the considered cohort of 86 subjects (including 39 females). The leg-length was measured from the top of trochanter major till the bottom of the ankle and thus, represents the length of upper and lower limbs.

	Average	SD	Min	Max
Age (years)	59.6	22.8	21	82
Height (cm)	173.3	10.2	151	196
Weight (kg)	76.1	12.8	53	103
Left leg-length (cm)	80.8	5.59	67	94
Right leg-length (cm)	80.79	5.65	67	94

3.2. Influence of Scanning Laser Rangefinder (SLR) Frequencies and Resolution onto Step Detection Sensitivity

As summarized in Table 5, the SLR-10 has a significantly higher sensitivity (in terms of correctly detected steps) in comparison to the slower SLR-04. Since these variations in sensitivity might directly cover a specific type of walks, the systems' overall sensitivity to detect critical changes in gait might thereby exclude specific relevant walks (e.g., the slower one). In our perspective this is a relevant limitation that contradicts the applicability off the SLR-04 for this purpose. These results agree with the lower sensing quality of the SLR-04 and can be seen as a result from the lower measurement characteristics (namely the max. measurement distance, frequency and resolution). Thus, we further only considered the SLR-10 and excluded the SLR-04 from subsequent evaluations.

3.3. Sensitivity of Gait Parameters

For the subsequent separated grouped analysis for the walks with normal walking pace and the ones with fast walking pace, 254 walks could not be considered, since they were unrelated to the blocks of normal and fast walking, even though representing generally valid measures. This exclusion would not be required for normal use of the UGMO, but was only required for the subsequent evaluation.

Among the correctly detected 7623 walks, a further 144 walks (1.9%) had to be removed due to the following reasons:

- 75 walks (73 GAITRite and 2 SLR; 59 of them occurring in the fast pace group) had a distance of less than 3 m and thus were removed automatically (even though shorter distances can be expected to achieve reliable results either, we defined it as a min requirement to achieve comparability among the 4.88 m active GAITRite and the SLR).

- For 60 walks (0.8%; among them 48 of them occurred in the fast pace group) no gait parameters could be calculated due to an error in the SLR data representation.

- 9 walks (6 SLR and 3 GAITRite; all in the fast pace group) included stride-length of more than 2 m and thus were removed automatically

These filter steps are integrated in the UGMO platform, to exclude medically meaningless/ erroneous measures.

With the remaining correctly detected 7479 walks and 55,690 steps for UGMO and 48,011 for the GaitRite on a distance of approximately 34.8 km over approximately 7 h, UGMO's sensitivity to the gait parameters shown in Table 7 was evaluated in comparison to the GAITRite as reference. In order to classify UGMO's sensitivity regarding varying walking speeds the investigated walks were separated regarding the walking speeds into normal pace (3345 considered walks) and fast walking pace (4134 considered walks).

Table 7. UGMO's gait analysis sensitivity in comparison to GAITRite. The table shows the interquartile ranges and the 99 percentile over the median errors (SLR-GAITRite) over all walks per subject as error = abs(SLR value) = abs(GAITRite value) between SLR-10 and GAITRite; CC: Pearson correlation coefficient.

Parameter	Walking Speed	Min	1. IQR	Median	3. IQR	99%	Max	CC
Velocity [m/min]	normal	0	0.68	1.58	3.17	8.8	20.19	0.95
	fast	0	1.08	2.46	5.03	12.96	45.81	0.93
Left Stride Length Mean (cm)	normal	−68.66	−5.43	−2.49	−1.50	1.85	18.03	0.91
	fast	−53.59	−3.92	−2.33	−1.41	2.22	16.45	0.95
Right Stride Length Mean (cm)	normal	−56.46	−5.56	−3.30	−2.15	1.24	17.76	0.93
	fast	−42.75	−5.17	−3.44	−2.22	0.93	7.51	0.96
Cadence [1/min]	normal	−19.6	0.1	3.2	8.4	28.66	111.4	0.71
	fast	−23.4	−1.8	2.6	6.8	28.94	66.3	0.79
Left Stance Time Mean (s)	normal	−0.56	0	0.03	0.05	0.12	0.23	0.75
	fast	−0.47	−0.02	0	0.03	0.09	0.54	0.81
Right Stance Time Mean (s)	normal	−0.53	−0.10	−0.05	0	0.09	0.14	0.66
	fast	−0.43	−0.11	−0.058	−0.01	0.07	0.12	0.61
Left Swing Time Mean (s)	normal	−0.28	−0.04	−0.02	0	0.14	0.41	0.49
	fast	−0.17	−0.01	0.01	0.02	0.19	0.45	0.56
Right Swing Time Mean (s)	normal	−0.18	−0.04	−0.02	0	0.15	0.41	0.51
	fast	−0.23	−0.01	0.01	0.02	0.13	0.40	0.65
Walks' Distance [m]	normal	0	0.43	0.63	1.03	1,64	1.95	n.a.
	fast	0	0.39	0.63	1.04	1.58	2.08	n.a.

4. Discussion

Due to the study's population size and the wide distribution of subjects ages—ranging from 21 to 82 years with a mean age of 59.6 years and a standard deviation of 22.8 years—the results can be expected to be representative for the intended purpose to detect functional decline in aging adults.

In regard to the influence of the SLR type (as associated to varying data rates, measuring areas and angular resolutions), the SLR-10 achieves a much higher sensitivity in terms of the correct detection of steps (98% compared to 77%) and walks (97% compared to 66%) than the cheaper SLR-04, whose lower performance might have been affected by the sensors range, frequency and angular resolution characteristics. Thus, the SLR-10 should be applied instead of the SLR-04 to ensure the correct detection of most walks. With the rate of correct positive detected walks by the SLR-10—as compared to the GAITRite acting as reference measure—the UGMO is well suited to act as monitoring device. Thus, we could confirm UGMO's high sensitivity to detect bypassing walks automatically.

Considering UGMO's (with SLR-10) sensitivity regarding the common gait parameters velocity and stride length, the results are similarly promising. With UGMO's corresponding sensitivity being sufficient to detect typical age- and disease-related variations for velocity (as summarized in Table 8), UMGO's applicability to detect these meaningful variations for functional decline, since its 99 percentile error is well below the critical measurement range. Furthermore, the Pearson correlation coefficient is with 0.95 and 0.93 excellent for both considered walking paces [43]. As shown in Figure 9 all errors reside below the age- and disease-related variations and 95% and 81% of the measurement for normal and fast walking pace groups hold errors below a fourth of the minimal age- and disease-related variations. Since the remaining measures with higher errors were well distributed among the subjects, UGMO's velocity is sufficiently sensitive, especially if applied for repeated measures—an approach that is practical for both supervised and unsupervised settings.

Similarly, the stride length correlated with 0.91 to 0.96 excellent [43] and all errors at 99 percentile are well within the margin of age- and disease-related variations in stride length for both speeds and legs (compare Table 8). Thus, the sensitivity of UGMO's stride-length calculation could be confirmed as well.

Table 8. The sensitivity of UGMO's gait parameters with the SLR-10 in comparison to the expected variations as associated with common age- and disease-related variations (calculated as the difference between the normal gender-independent value and the corresponding disease-specific value, as discussed in Table 2).

Parameter	Common Age- and Disease-Related Variations		Error of SLR as 99 Percentile (Normal/Fast Walking Pace)
	Min [16]	Max [22]	
Velocity Diff [m/min]	23.8	42.4	8.8/12.96
Stride Length [cm]	30	58	1.85/2.22
Cadence Diff [1/min]	7.3	19.6	28.66/28.94

The sensitivity of UGMO's cadence measure is rather ambiguous (see Figure 10). With a correlation of 0.71 and 0.79 for the normal and fast walking paces, its sensitivity is rather modest [43]. Furthermore, only 71% and 87% of the measures in the normal and respectively fast walking pace groups fall below the minimal age- and disease-related variations. Consequently, the cadence parameter might only be sensitive if applied via repeated measures.

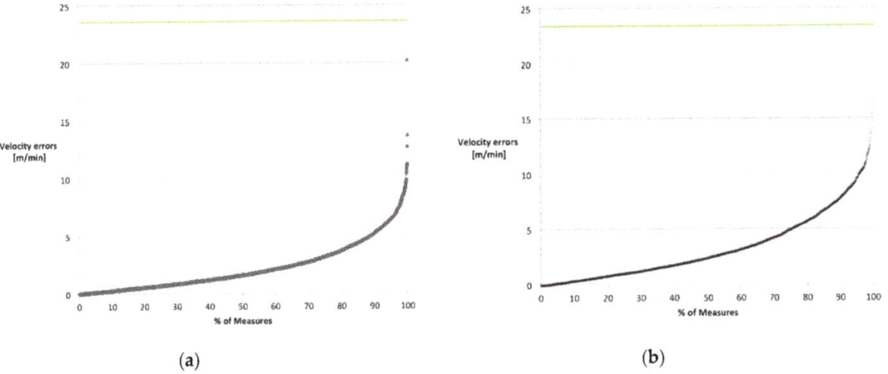

(a)

(b)

Figure 9. Error distribution of velocity measures separated by groups for (a) normal walking pace and (b) fast walking pace; green lines (at 23.8 m/min) identifies the minimal expected variance for common age- and disease-related variations.

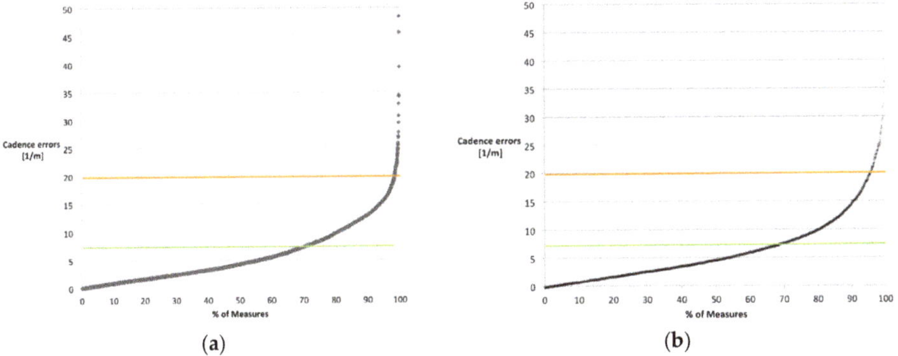

(a)

(b)

Figure 10. Error distribution of cadence measures separated by groups for (a) normal walking pace and (b) fast walking pace; green and orange lines (at 7.3 and 19.6. steps/min) identifies the minimal expected variance for common age- and disease-related variations and maximal ones respectively.

Comparing the UGMO's sensitivity to the reported ones of both existing systems, the velocity and stride-length are representative of existing SLRs (as summarized in Table 3) and corresponding depth-sensor based systems as summarized in [44]. For the velocity, the error is comparable to the reported errors of 3.84 m/min of other SLR systems. The achieved correlation of 0.95 to 0.93 is slightly below those of Kinect-sensor based systems, which regularly achieve correlations of up to 0.99. With the correlation of 0.95 and 0.93 UGMO's stride length is with median errors around 2.3 to 3.4 cm on par with the reported mean and root mean square errors of approximately 3 cm for other SLRs (see Table 3), despite the different viewing angles. The correlations of the stride lengths are slightly below Kinect-based systems, which correlated up to 0.99 compared to UGMO's 0.91 to 0.96. However, most of the Kinect-based systems have been evaluated for use with a frontal view on the movement.

The stance- and swing-time parameters correlate modestly with the once of the GAITRite. This might be related to the variation in the measurement setup—due to the UGMO's extended sensing area compared to the GAITRite. This might result in only UGMO detecting the potential variations in swing-time at beginning and ending of the walkway as transitioning to/from turning.

In general, the results indicate that some outliers occurred among all considered parameters (consider the large margin between the 99 and 100 percentile in Table 7), which intentionally have not been trimmed. These outliers might be related to the additional steps that have been recorded only by the UGMO and not by the GAITRite (as a consequence of UGMO's wider viewing angle, see walk distance in Table 7) and might include suddenly altered movements during transitioning to turning and, thereby, might rarely occur in realistic settings.

Furthermore, such rare outliers can be even filtered within UGMO by considering only consistent variations over multiple subsequent walks as relevant indicators for functional decline.

Since the variations of UGMO's sensitivity among the gait parameters for the normal and fast walking speed groups (see Table 7) were rather low, the variations of the sensitivity for slower walking speeds could be expected to be comparable as well, especially since the SLR will have more samples per step to be considered in the calculations. For velocity, the error decreases and the correlation becomes stronger with lower walking speeds, while for stride length the correlation decreases slightly with decreasing walking speeds.

Additional validations of the UGMO system are intended to confirm the system's sensitivity for slower walking speeds, different viewing angles, minimal and maximal distances and non-rectilinear walks among other influences expected for unsupervised applications. The current system is also not able to detect walks covering subjects in-between stop and or turn around, during which pets walk through the measuring area, or other conditions that might occur in a real-world setting. Thus, further developments in that regard are intended.

5. Conclusions

The article introduces the hardware and signal-processing tool chain of the unobtrusive gait monitoring (UGMO) system that detects variations in common gait parameters (such as velocity and stride length) of elderly people that have been shown to be a reliable indicator for functional and cognitive decline. Functional and cognitive decline has been shown to be strongly correlated to fall risks and being a leading cause of fatal injury and the most common cause of non-fatal trauma-related hospital admissions among older adults causing over $50 billion total medical costs in 2015. The novelty of UGMO in comparison to other SLR-based systems is that it supports the lateral supervision of walks (in contrast to the commonly used frontal recording), which is especially challenging due to the hidden leg problem, to be considered. Thereby, UGMO is expected to be highly applicable for unsupervised home assessment. By evaluating the UGMO system in comparison to the GAITRite, as a reference system, via 86 study participant with ages ranging from 21 to 82 years, with a mean age of 59.6 years and a standard deviation of 22.8 years, covering each passing twice the 6 min walk test under supervision, the following findings have been gained: comparing two SLR types, it has been shown, that the SLR-10 achieves a much higher sensitivity than the cheaper SLR-04 in terms of the correct detection of steps (98% compared to 77%) and walks (97% compared to 66%).

By using the SLR-10, the UGMO sensitivity in measuring gait parameters such as gait velocity and stride length is sufficient to detect reported age- and disease-related variations. Consequently, UGMO has been shown in a standardised supervised setting to be suitable to detect functional decline as associated with an increased fall risk. With the UGMO's applicability being confirmed within standardised settings (requiring lateral and continuous walks) we are looking forward to enhancing the system for more general scenarios and confirm its applicability to unsupervised unstandardised settings via additional studies.

Aside from their use for continuous monitoring within predestined groups, these sensors can also be expected to enhance knowledge about the reasons for falls and the impact of environmental factors' such as lighting conditions, daytime, flooring materials, obstacles, tiredness and activity levels on the quality and stability of gait. The associated causes and conditions of falling as a consequence of unstable gaits, being a fundamental requirement to implement safer environments, are not yet fully understood. Consequently, in order to gain insights on the genuine characteristics of gait and the related influences of environmental factors (such as lighting conditions or flooring), the UGMO represents a suitable sensor to generate new insights in this regard.

Author Contributions: S.F. and C.S. conceived and designed the experiments; C.S. developed the initial prototype and performed the experiments; S.F. and C.S. analyzed the data; N.V. contributed materials; all authors wrote and revised the paper.

Funding: This work was supported by the funding initiative Niedersächsisches Vorab of the Volkswagen Foundation and the Ministry of Science and Culture of Lower Saxony as a part of the Interdisciplinary Research Centre on Critical Systems Engineering for Socio-Technical Systems.

Acknowledgments: The authors like to thank Linda Büker for her support by conducting the experiments.

Conflicts of Interest: The authors declare no conflict of interest.

References

1. Florence, C.S.; Bergen, G.; Atherly, A.; Burns, E.; Stevens, J.; Drake, C. Medical Costs of Fatal and Nonfatal Falls in Older Adults. *J. Am. Geriatr. Soc.* **2018**, *66*, 693–698. [CrossRef] [PubMed]
2. Jager, T.E.; Weiss, H.B.; Coben, J.H.; Pepe, P.E. Traumatic brain injuries evaluated in U.S. emergency departments, 1992–1994. *Acad. Emerg. Med.* **2000**, *7*, 134–140. [CrossRef] [PubMed]
3. Jefferis, B.J.; Iliffe, S.; Kendrick, D.; Kerse, N.; Trost, S.; Lennon, L.T.; Ash, S.; Sartini, C.; Morris, R.W.; Wannamethee, S.G.; et al. How are falls and fear of falling associated with objectively measured physical activity in a cohort of community-dwelling older men? *BMC Geriatr.* **2014**, *14*, 114. [CrossRef] [PubMed]
4. Scheffer, A.C.; Schuurmans, M.J.; van Dijk, N.; van der Hooft, T.; de Rooij, S.E. Fear of falling: Measurement strategy, prevalence, risk factors and consequences among older persons. *Age Ageing* **2008**, *37*, 19–24. [CrossRef] [PubMed]
5. Schepens, S.; Sen, A.; Painter, J.A.; Murphy, S.L. Relationship Between Fall-Related Efficacy and Activity Engagement in Community-Dwelling Older Adults: A Meta-Analytic Review. *Am. J. Occup. Ther.* **2012**, *66*, 137–148. [CrossRef] [PubMed]
6. Zijlstra, G.A.R.; Van Haastregt, J.C.M.; Van Rossum, E.; Van Eijk, J.T.M.; Yardley, L.; Kempen, G.I.J.M. Interventions to Reduce Fear of Falling in Community-Living Older People: A Systematic Review. *J. Am. Geriatr. Soc.* **2007**, *55*, 603–615. [CrossRef] [PubMed]
7. Al-Aama, T. Falls in the elderly: Spectrum and prevention. *Can. Fam. Physician* **2011**, *57*, 771–776. [PubMed]
8. Grobe, S.; Kakar, R.S.; Smith, M.L.; Mehta, R.; Baghurst, T.; Boolani, A. Impact of cognitive fatigue on gait and sway among older adults: A literature review. *Prev. Med. Rep.* **2017**, *6*, 88–93. [CrossRef] [PubMed]
9. Mielke, M.M.; Roberts, R.O.; Savica, R.; Cha, R.; Drubach, D.I.; Christianson, T.; Pankratz, V.S.; Geda, Y.E.; Machulda, M.M.; Ivnik, R.J.; et al. Assessing the Temporal Relationship Between Cognition and Gait: Slow Gait Predicts Cognitive Decline in the Mayo Clinic Study of Aging. *J. Gerontol. Ser. A Biol. Sci. Med. Sci.* **2013**, *68*, 929–937. [CrossRef] [PubMed]

10. Savica, R.; Wennberg, A.M.V.; Hagen, C.; Edwards, K.; Roberts, R.O.; Hollman, J.H.; Knopman, D.S.; Boeve, B.F.; Machulda, M.M.; Petersen, R.C.; et al. Comparison of Gait Parameters for Predicting Cognitive Decline: The Mayo Clinic Study of Aging. *J. Alzheimers Dis.* **2016**, *55*, 559–567. [CrossRef] [PubMed]

11. Alzheimer's Association. 2012 Alzheimer's disease facts and figures. *Alzheimers Dement.* **2012**, *8*, 131–168. [CrossRef] [PubMed]

12. Murray, M.P.; Drought, A.B.; Kory, R.C. Walking Patterns of Normal Men. *J. Bone Joint Surg. Am.* **1964**, *46*, 335–360. [CrossRef] [PubMed]

13. Murray, M.P.; Kory, R.C.; Sepic, S.B. Walking patterns of normal women. *Arch. Phys. Med. Rehabil.* **1970**, *51*, 637–650. [PubMed]

14. Finley, F.R.; Cody, K.A.; Finizie, R. V Locomotion patterns in elderly women. *Arch. Phys. Med. Rehabil.* **1969**, *50*, 140–146. [PubMed]

15. Ostrosky, K.M.; VanSwearingen, J.M.; Burdett, R.G.; Gee, Z. A comparison of gait characteristics in young and old subjects. *Phys. Ther.* **1994**, *74*, 637–644. [CrossRef] [PubMed]

16. Kressig, R.W.; Gregor, R.J.; Oliver, A.; Waddell, D.; Smith, W.; O'Grady, M.; Curns, A.T.; Kutner, M.; Wolf, S.L. Temporal and spatial features of gait in older adults transitioning to frailty. *Gait Posture* **2004**, *20*, 30–35. [CrossRef]

17. Wang, F.; Stone, E.; Skubic, M.; Keller, J.M.; Abbott, C.; Rantz, M. Toward a passive low-cost in-home gait assessment system for older adults. *IEEE J. Biomed. Heal. Inform.* **2013**, *17*, 346–355. [CrossRef] [PubMed]

18. Hellmers, S.; Steen, E.-E.; Dasenbrock, L.; Heinks, A.; Bauer, J.M.; Fudickar, S.; Hein, A. Towards a minimized unsupervised technical assessment of physical performance in domestic environments. In Proceedings of the 11th EAI International Conference on Pervasive Computing Technologies for Healthcare (PervasiveHealth '17), Barcelona, Spain, 23–26 May 2017; ACM Press: New York, NY, USA, 2017; pp. 207–216.

19. Liu, L.; Stroulia, E.; Nikolaidis, I.; Miguel-Cruz, A.; Rios Rincon, A. Smart homes and home health monitoring technologies for older adults: A systematic review. *Int. J. Med. Inform.* **2016**, *91*, 44–59. [CrossRef] [PubMed]

20. Perry, J.; Burnfield, J.M.; Cabico, L.M. *Gait Analysis: Normal and Pathological Function*; SLACK Inc.: Thorofare, NJ, USA, 2010; ISBN 9781556427664.

21. Wick, J.Y.; Zanni, G.R. Tiptoeing Around Gait Disorders: Multiple Presentations, Many Causes. *Consult. Pharm.* **2010**, *25*, 724–737. [CrossRef] [PubMed]

22. Maki, B.E. Gait changes in older adults: Predictors of falls or indicators of fear. *J. Am. Geriatr. Soc.* **1997**, *45*, 313–320. [CrossRef] [PubMed]

23. Menz, H.B.; Latt, M.D.; Tiedemann, A.; Mun San Kwan, M.; Lord, S.R. Reliability of the GAITRite walkway system for the quantification of temporo-spatial parameters of gait in young and older people. *Gait Posture* **2004**, *20*, 20–25. [CrossRef]

24. Merriaux, P.; Dupuis, Y.; Boutteau, R.; Vasseur, P.; Savatier, X. A Study of Vicon System Positioning Performance. *Sensors* **2017**, *17*, 1591. [CrossRef] [PubMed]

25. Hellmers, S.; Fudickar, S.; Büse, C.; Dasenbrock, L.; Heinks, A.; Bauer, J.M.; Hein, A. Technology Supported Geriatric Assessment. In *Ambient Assisted Living*; Springer: Cham, Switzerland, 2017; pp. 85–100.

26. Byun, S.; Han, J.W.; Kim, T.H.; Kim, K.W. Test-Retest Reliability and Concurrent Validity of a Single Tri-Axial Accelerometer-Based Gait Analysis in Older Adults with Normal Cognition. *PLoS ONE* **2016**, *11*, e0158956. [CrossRef] [PubMed]

27. Dehzangi, O.; Taherisadr, M.; ChangalVala, R. IMU-Based Gait Recognition Using Convolutional Neural Networks and Multi-Sensor Fusion. *Sensors* **2017**, *17*, 2735. [CrossRef] [PubMed]

28. Yorozu, A.; Takahashi, M. Development of gait measurement robot using laser range sensor for evaluating long-distance walking ability in the elderly. In Proceedings of the 2015 IEEE/RSJ International Conference on Intelligent Robots and Systems (IROS), Hamburg, Germany, 28 September–2 October 2015; pp. 4888–4893.

29. Chalvatzaki, G.; Papageorgiou, X.S.; Tzafestas, C.S.; Maragos, P. Comparative experimental validation of human gait tracking algorithms for an intelligent robotic rollator. In Proceedings of the 2017 IEEE International Conference on Robotics and Automation (ICRA), Singapore, 29 May–3 June 2017; pp. 6026–6031.

30. Papageorgiou, X.S.; Chalvatzaki, G.; Lianos, K.-N.; Werner, C.; Hauer, K.; Tzafestas, C.S.; Maragos, P. Experimental validation of human pathological gait analysis for an assisted living intelligent robotic walker. In Proceedings of the 2016 6th IEEE International Conference on Biomedical Robotics and Biomechatronics (BioRob), Singapore, 26–29 June 2016; pp. 1086–1091.

31. Frenken, T.; Lohmann, O.; Frenken, M.; Steen, E.-E.; Hein, A. Performing gait analysis within the timed up & go assessment test: Comparison of aTUG to a marker-based tracking system. *Inform. Health Soc. Care* **2014**, *39*, 232–248. [CrossRef] [PubMed]

32. Fudickar, S.; Kiselev, J.; Frenken, T.; Wegel, S.; Dimitrowska, S.; Steinhagen-Thiessen, E.; Hein, A. Validation of the ambient TUG chair with light barriers and force sensors in a clinical trial. *Assist. Technol.* **2018**, 1–8. [CrossRef] [PubMed]

33. Pallejà, T.; Teixidó, M.; Tresanchez, M.; Palacín, J. Measuring Gait Using a Ground Laser Range Sensor. *Sensors* **2009**, *9*, 9133–9146. [CrossRef] [PubMed]

34. Ahn, S.J.; Rauh, W.; Warnecke, H.-J. Least-squares orthogonal distances fitting of circle, sphere, ellipse, hyperbola, and parabola. *Pattern Recognit.* **2001**, *34*, 2283–2303. [CrossRef]

35. Tanabe, S.; Ii, T.; Koyama, S.; Saitoh, E.; Itoh, N.; Ohtsuka, K.; Katoh, Y.; Shimizu, A.; Tomita, Y. Spatiotemporal treadmill gait measurements using a laser range scanner: Feasibility study of the healthy young adults. *Physiol. Meas.* **2017**, *38*, N81–N92. [CrossRef] [PubMed]

36. Yorozu, A.; Moriguchi, T.; Takahashi, M. Improved Leg Tracking Considering Gait Phase and Spline-Based Interpolation during Turning Motion in Walk Tests. *Sensors* **2015**, *15*, 22451–22472. [CrossRef] [PubMed]

37. Catmull, E.; Rom, R. A Class of Local Interpolating Splines. *Comput. Aided Geom. Des.* **1974**, 317–326. [CrossRef]

38. Dubois, A.; Charpillet, F. Measuring frailty and detecting falls for elderly home care using depth camera. *J. Ambient Intell. Smart Environ.* **2017**, *9*, 469–481. [CrossRef]

39. Dubois, A.; Charpillet, F. Human activities recognition with RGB-Depth camera using HMM. In Proceedings of the 2013 35th Annual International Conference of the IEEE Engineering in Medicine and Biology Society (EMBC), Osaka, Japan, 3–7 July 2013; pp. 4666–4669.

40. Rui, L.; Chen, S.; Ho, K.C.; Rantz, M.; Skubic, M. Estimation of human walking speed by Doppler radar for elderly care. *J. Ambient Intell. Smart Environ.* **2017**, *9*, 181–191. [CrossRef]

41. Hokuyo Automatic Co. Ltd. Scanning Laser Range Finder URG-04LX-UG01 Specifications. Available online: https://www.robotshop.com/media/files/pdf/hokuyo-urg-04lx-ug01-specifications.pdf (accessed on 26 September 2018).

42. Hokuyo Scanning Laser Range Finder UST-10LX Specifications. Available online: https://www.generationrobots.com/media/HokuyoUST-10LX/UST-10LX_Specification.pdf#page=1&zoom=auto,-107,848 (accessed on 26 September 2018).

43. Fleiss, J. *The Design and Analysis of Clinical Experiments*; John Wiley & Sons: New York, NY, USA, 1986. [CrossRef]

44. Springer, S.; Seligmann, G.Y. Validity of the Kinect for Gait Assessment: A Focused Review. *Sensors* **2016**, *16*, 194. [CrossRef] [PubMed]

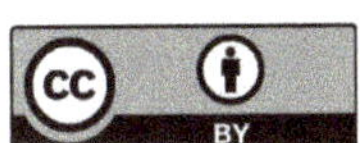 © 2018 by the authors. Licensee MDPI, Basel, Switzerland. This article is an open access article distributed under the terms and conditions of the Creative Commons Attribution (CC BY) license (http://creativecommons.org/licenses/by/4.0/).

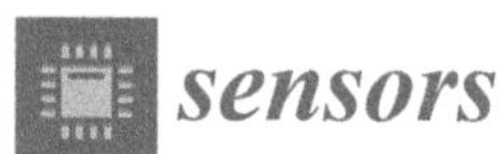 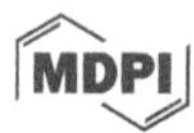

Article

Inertial Sensor Angular Velocities Reflect Dynamic Knee Loading during Single Limb Loading in Individuals Following Anterior Cruciate Ligament Reconstruction

Kristamarie A. Pratt [1,2,*] and Susan M. Sigward [1]

[1] Human Performance Laboratory, Division of Biokinesiology and Physical Therapy, University of Southern California, 1540 E Alcazar St., CHP-155, Los Angeles, CA 90089-9006, USA; sigward@pt.usc.edu

[2] Department of Rehabilitation Sciences, University of Hartford, 200 Bloomfield Ave, West Hartford, CT 06117, USA

* Correspondence: kristamarie.pratt@gmail.com; Tel.: +1-860-768-5266

Received: 6 September 2018; Accepted: 3 October 2018; Published: 15 October 2018

Abstract: Difficulty quantifying knee loading deficits clinically in individuals following anterior cruciate ligament reconstruction (ACLr) may underlie their persistence. Expense associated with quantifying knee moments (KMom) and power (KPow) with gold standard techniques precludes their use in the clinic. As segment and joint kinematics are used to calculate moments and power, it is possible that more accessible inertial sensor technology can be used to identify knee loading deficits. However, it is unknown if angular velocities measured with inertial sensors provide meaningful information regarding KMom/KPow during dynamic tasks post-ACLr. Twenty-one individuals 5.1 ± 1.5 months post-ACLr performed a single limb loading task, bilaterally. Data collected concurrently using a marker-based motion system and gyroscopes positioned lateral thighs/shanks. Intraclass correlation coefficients (ICC)(2,k) determined concurrent validity. To determine predictive ability of angular velocities for KMom/KPow, separate stepwise linear regressions performed using peak thigh, shank, and knee angular velocities extracted from gyroscopes. ICCs were greater than 0.947 (p < 0.001) for all variables. Thigh (r = 0.812 and r = 0.585; p < 0.001) and knee (r = 0.806 and r = 0.536; p < 0.001) angular velocities were strongly and moderately correlated to KPow and KMom, respectively. High ICCs indicated strong agreement between measurement systems. Thigh angular velocity (R^2 = 0.66; p < 0.001) explained 66% of variance in KPow suggesting gyroscopes provide meaningful information regarding KPow. Less expensive inertial sensors may be helpful in identifying deficits clinically.

Keywords: inertial sensors; anterior cruciate ligament; rehabilitation; knee; gyroscope; power; angular velocity

---

1. Introduction

Marker-based three-dimensional motion analysis is the current gold standard for quantification of movement deficits during dynamic tasks following knee injury or surgery. This technology uses three-dimensional marker positions (recorded at 250–340 Hz), and ground reaction force data (1360–1500 Hz) to calculate knee moments, angular velocities, and power. However, these analyses are complex, expensive, and time-consuming; thus, impractical in clinical settings. Two-dimensional video assessment using traditional video cameras or tablets (recording at 24–32 Hz) are becoming popular among clinicians for detection of movement impairments, but are limited to quantification of kinematics during tasks performed at slower speeds. Unfortunately, relevant knee loading deficits often coincide with much smaller differences in joint angle often making them difficult to observe clinically [1,2]. Differences in angles may be particularly difficult to detect during more dynamic tasks as individuals go through nearly 30–50 degrees of flexion in less than 200 milliseconds. Recent advances in wireless capabilities and data storage in wearable technology make inertial sensors more affordable and practical for movement assessments outside a motion analysis laboratory [3–7].

Individuals following anterior cruciate ligament (ACL) reconstructive surgery present with altered sagittal plane knee loading patterns that persist 6 to 24 months post-surgery. This coincides with the time when they are performing more demanding functional tasks and returning to participation in higher levels of physical activities and sports [8–11]. The presence of altered loading at this time is of particular concern as it is related to an increased risk for re-injury. A recent prospective study found that the odds of suffering a second ACL injury were 3.3 times greater in those who exhibited asymmetrical knee loading during a drop land at the time they returned to sports [12]. Biomechanically altered sagittal plane knee loading patterns following ACL reconstruction (ACLr) are characterized by decreased knee power absorption, angular velocities, and extensor moments in the reconstructed knee when compared to nonsurgical knee and healthy controls. They are commonly observed during portions of dynamic tasks that require eccentric control or deceleration (e.g., running, landing, hopping) [2,11,13,14]. Clinicians often rely on measures of function (i.e., how far an individual can hop) to assess knee function [15,16]; however, these assessments are not sensitive to altered knee mechanics identified with gold standard motion capture technology [1]. Marker-based three-dimensional motion analysis revealed that individuals who were able to pass clinical hop tests, determined by comparing the distance hopped between reconstructed and healthy limbs, continued to exhibit a 6% decrease in knee extensor moment and 43% decrease in knee power absorption in the reconstructed limb [1]. The inability to identify specific mechanical loading deficits with clinical assessments may underlie their persistence. Given the potential long-term consequences of persistent deficits, it is critical to develop clinically useful methods for identification and improvement of altered loading patterns beyond functional measures of performance.

Inertial sensors (accelerometer, gyroscope, and magnetometer) are commonly used to detect events or to calculate spatial-temporal variables; however, they can be affixed to body segments to measure segment angular velocities and accelerations. Despite the fact that kinematics are not the only variables considered in the calculation of power and joint moments, kinematic variables, specifically joint and segment angular velocities, may adequately reflect knee power absorption and knee extensor moments during dynamics tasks. Knee as well as thigh and shank angular velocities not only quantify how fast a segment rotates, but also provide a preliminary understanding of neuromuscular control of dynamic tasks. Individuals may employ subtle changes in joint kinematics and concurrently, segment kinematics, to alter forces and decrease knee loading during these dynamic tasks [17,18]. While calculations may be performed to quantify segment/joint angles using multiple sensors, recent studies have highlighted the ability of raw outputs of a single sensor to detect between limb differences in knee loading during gait [19,20] and a single limb loading task [17,21]. In individuals following ACLr between limb ratios in shank [19] and thigh [21] angular velocities have been related to knee moment and power deficits during gait and a single limb loading task, respectively. The strength of the relationship with knee power ratios during single limb loading resulted in strong diagnostic accuracy of between limb deficits in knee joint power using thigh angular velocity measured with inertial units [21].

These data suggest that inertial sensors may be able to provide a more accessible alternative to marker-based three-dimensional motion analysis for detection of loading impairments in a clinical setting, particularly during a single limb loading task. This is important as a recent study found that individuals progressing to running after ACLr exhibit deficits in not only knee power but also in knee angular velocity and knee extensor moments during this less demanding single limb loading task [22]. Quantification of these deficits outside of laboratory setting will allow rehabilitation specialist to ensure they are being addressed. This study aims to advance the previous work relating between limb ratios in inertial sensor outputs of segment angular velocity to knee power deficits during a single limb loading task [21]. Using the same subjects, the current manuscript's purpose is threefold: (1) to establish concurrent validity for measures of segment and joint angular between inertial sensors and the gold standard motion analysis system velocities, (2) to provide detailed methods for identifying inertial sensor outputs specific to knee power during the single limb loading task, and (3) to investigate the predictive value of between thigh and shank angular velocities and sagittal plane knee power and knee extensor moments in healthy and impaired limbs of individuals status-post ACLR during this task.

2. Materials and Methods

2.1. Participants

Twenty-one individuals (12 females; 28.8 ± 11.2 years) who had primary unilateral ACLr (11 right) using a bone-patellar-tendon-bone autograft, allograft, or hamstring autograft approximately 5.1 ± 1.5 months prior to testing participated. All participants reported that they were recreationally active prior to their injury (evaluated using Cincinnati Sports Activity questionnaire) [23]. Recreational athlete was defined as Level I or II on the Cincinnati Sports Activity scale. At the time of participation, individuals were actively attending physical therapy and had initiated a running progression within 2 months of testing.

Individuals were excluded from the study if they: (1) were not cleared by physical therapist to perform the functional activities, (2) had prior ACL injury and knee surgery on the contralateral limb, (3) had concurrent pathology or morphology that could cause pain or discomfort during physical activity, and (4) had any physical, cognitive, or other condition that may impair the individual's ability to perform the tasks proposed in this study. An a priori power analysis performed using pilot data from six individuals determined that 14 subjects would provide more than 80% power at the alpha level of 0.05.

2.2. Instrumentation

Kinematic data and ground reaction force data were collected using either a marker-based, 11-camera motion capturing system (Qualysis Inc., Gothenberg, Sweden) at a 250 Hz and force platforms at 1500Hz (Advanced Mechanical Technologies, Inc., Newton, MA, USA) or a 14-camera motion capturing system (BTS Bioengineering Corp., Milan, Italy) at 340 Hz and force platforms at 1360 Hz (BTS Bioengineering Corp., Milan, Italy). Two motion capture systems were used due to a transition to a new motion capture system during the study. Concurrently, inertial data was collected using four inertial sensors equipped with a triaxial accelerometers, gyroscopes, and magnetometers (Opal, APDM Inc., Portland, OR, USA). The primary variable of interest from the inertial sensors, angular velocity, was measured using the gyroscope. While direct measurements from the accelerometer and magnetometer were not used for analysis in this study, they remained active throughout data collection to increase accuracy of gyroscope measurements using APDM's proprietary algorithm. The range for the gyroscope in X and Yaxes was ±34.9 rad/s and Zaxis is ±26.8 rad/s. The gyroscope's noise density in X and Yaxes was 0.81 mrad/s/$\sqrt{Hz}$ and 2.2 mrad/s/$\sqrt{Hz}$ for Zaxis. Inertial data was recorded at 128Hz using Motion Studio software (APDM Inc., Portland, OR, USA). Data was synchronized and wirelessly streamed from all four sensors directly to the computer using "Robust Synchronized Streaming" mode. Data was buffered on the sensors to prevent data loss in the case of wireless interruptions.

2.3. Procedures

Testing took place in the University of Southern California's Human Performance Laboratory located at Completive Athletic Training Zone, Pasadena, CA, USA. All procedures were explained to each participant and informed consent was obtained as approved by the Investigational Review Board at University of Southern California Health Sciences Campus. Parental consent was obtained for all individuals under the age of 18 years. After consenting to participate, participant's age, height, weight, tibia length, knee medical history, and physical activity prior to injury were recorded.

Prior to testing, participants were asked to warmup on a stationary bike for five minutes. Reflective markers were placed on first and fifth metatarsals, distal end of second toes, medial and lateral malleoli, medial and lateral epicondyles of femurs, greater trochanters, posterior superior iliac spines, iliac crests, and L5S1 junction. In addition, tracking clusters, reflective markers attached to rigid plates, were secured bilaterally on participants' thighs, lower legs and heels of their shoes by the same examiner. After the static calibration trial all markers were removed, except tracking clusters, pelvis, and distal toe markers which remained on during testing.

Inertial sensors were placed on the mid-lateral thighs and shanks with the Xaxis aligned superior–inferior, bilaterally. Care was taken to align the Xaxis of thigh sensors with greater trochanters and lateral epicondyles of the femur, and Xaxis of shank sensors with lateral epicondyles and lateral malleoli (Figure 1). For testing the position of inertial sensors coincided with the position of the tracking marker clusters; therefore, they were affixed to the rigid plates firmly using elastic straps and tape.

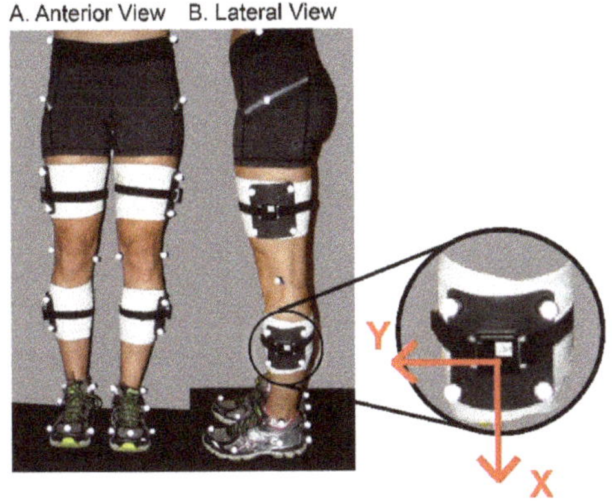

Figure 1. Orientation and location of inertial sensors and markers on thigh and shank during testing; Orientation of axes depicted on right.

2.4. Single Limb Loading Test

During testing, wearing their own athletic shoes, participants performed a dynamic single limb loading (SLL) task on each limb as described previously [21,22] (Figure 2). For this task, participants were instructed to stand on both feet on a single platform behind a tape line facing a target positioned on an adjacent force platform. The target was positioned a distance that was normalized to the length of each individual's tibia. Participants were instructed to leap forward onto the target on a single limb, to lower as far they can and then return to the start on two limbs. Participants were asked to complete the task in one fluid movement without pausing. To encourage fluid and continuous movement they performed three consecutive repetitions at their own self-selected pace for each trial. Participants performed SLL trials alternating between limbs beginning with the nonsurgical limb. A trial was considered acceptable when it contained presence of a distinct flight phase, maintenance of balance throughout the task and complete foot placement on the target force platform. The presence of a flight phase was considered as criteria for a successful trial to avoid instances of double limb support. It was determined by the absence of forces on either force plate prior to foot contact on the target force platform. Practice trials were allowed for individuals to become familiar with the task. Participants performed three trials on each limb.

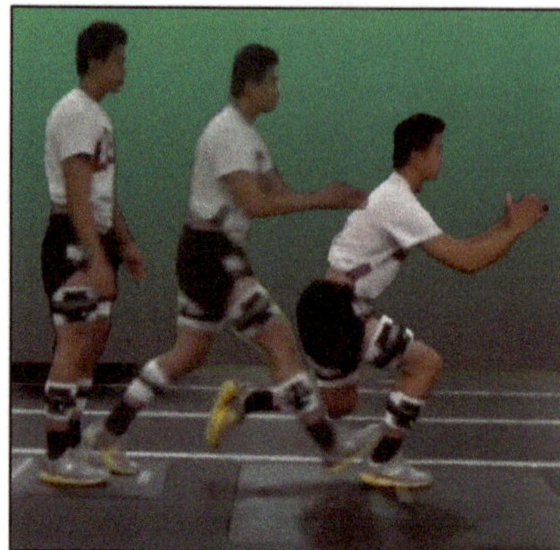

Figure 2. Single Limb Loading Test.

2.5. Data Analysis

Reconstructed three-dimensional marker coordinates (Qualysis Inc. Tracking Manager, Gothenberg, Sweden or BTS Bioengineering Corp SMARTtracker, Milan, Italy) were used in combination with force platform and anthropometric data to calculate joint kinematics, kinetics and energetics (Visual3DTM, Version 4.8, C-Motion, Inc., Rockville, MD, USA). Coordinate data was filtered using a fourth order, low pass, zero-lag Butterworth filter with frequency cut-off of 12 Hz. Data from the standing calibration trial was used to derive the local coordinate systems of body segments. Lower extremity segments were modeled as a frusta of cones, while the pelvis was modeled as a cylinder. Six degrees of freedom of each segment were calculated by transforming the triad of markers to the position and orientation of each segment during the standing calibration trial. Euler angles were used to calculate joint kinematics in the subsequent order: flexion/extension, abduction/adduction, and internal/external rotation. Joint angles were expressed as movement of the distal segment relative to the proximal segment. Standard inverse dynamic equations used kinematics, anthropometrics, and ground reaction forces to calculate internal net joint moments. Net joint power was calculated as the product of joint moment and joint angular velocity and normalized to body mass. Segment angular velocities measured with the marker-based motion analysis system were calculated with respect to the global coordinate system. Data obtained from Visual3D^{TM} were exported and analyzed using a customized MATLAB$^{®}$ program (Version R2014b, The MathWorks, Matick, MA, USA).

Signals from the inertial sensors placed on thighs and shanks were used to measure thigh and shank angular velocity, respectively. Angular velocity, a direct output of the gyroscope, in the Z-plane of the sensor were chosen to represent sagittal plane movement (Figure 1). Thigh and shank angular velocity measurements were negated on the right limb to coincide with the global coordinate system where knee flexion involved positive rotation from vertical of the proximal thigh and negative rotation of the proximal shank segment from vertical. Segment angular velocity data was low-pass filtered using a fourth order zero-lag Butterworth filter with a 15 Hz cutoff frequency. Knee joint angular velocity was calculated as the sum of thigh and shank angular velocities at each time point throughout the movement with positive rotation representing knee flexion. Thigh angles in the sagittal plane were calculated as the integral of the thigh angular velocity with respect to time. A thigh segment angle of 0 degrees corresponds to a vertical position of the thigh with and an angle of 90 degrees to a horizontal position. Segment angles were used for the purposes of event identification in the inertial sensor data. For the single limb loading task, individuals began the task with the knee in more extension and the thigh segment more vertical. During execution of the task, individuals flexed their knee on a planted foot moving the thigh to a more horizontal position and then extended the knee returning the thigh to a more vertical position (Figure 3A)

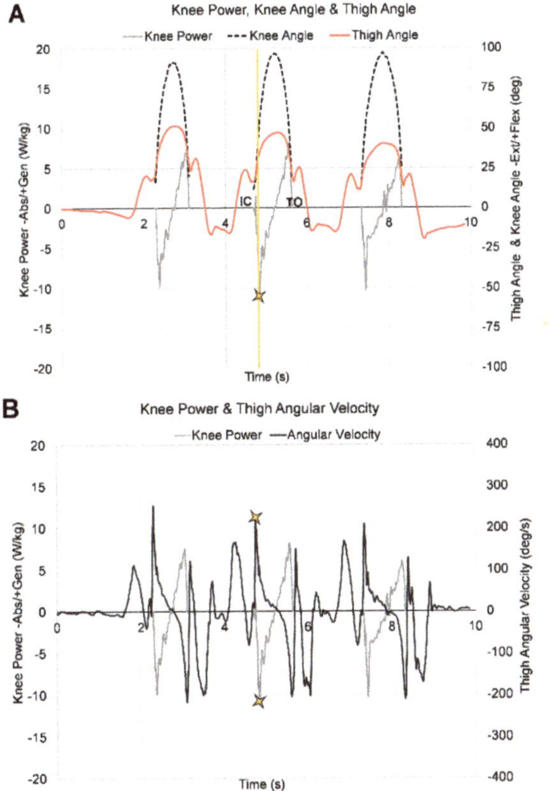

Figure 3. Three cycles of single limb loading task performed by one representative subject. (**A**) Marker-based knee angle (dashed black line), knee power (gray line), and inertial sensor thigh angle (red line); (**B**) Marker-based knee power (gray line) and inertial sensor thigh angular velocity (black line). Stars indicate the peak knee power absorption (**A**) and peak thigh angular velocity (**B**) identified after initial contact and before maximum knee flexion during the middle repetition of one trial.

All dependent variables were identified during the deceleration portion of stance phase of a single limb loading task. Stance phase was identified in the marker-based system using ground reaction forces, and in the inertial sensors using thigh angle measurements. For the marker-based motion capture system initial contact and toe-off were identified when the vertical ground reaction force was greater than 30 N and less than 30 N, respectively. For the inertial sensors, stance phase occurred between two local minimums of the thing angle, prior to and following a maximum thigh angle (Figure 3A, continuous red line). The local minimum thigh angle prior to the maximum thigh angle was initial contact and the local minimum thigh angle following was toe-off. Deceleration in the marker-based system was defined as the time between initial contact and peak knee flexion, and deceleration in the inertial sensors was defined as the time between the first local minimum thigh angle (initial contact) to the maximum thigh angle. Customized MATLAB® programs were used to identify variables of interest extracted from inertial sensors.

During deceleration, peak knee power absorption (Figure 3A) and peak knee extensor moments were identified using the marker-based motion capture system. Peak knee, thigh (Figure 3B), and shank angular velocities in sagittal plane were identified using both the marker based system and inertial sensors during the deceleration phase. The average of three trials (middle repetition of each trial) of each limb (ACL reconstructed (ACLr), nonsurgical (NonSx)) were used for analysis in both systems.

2.6. Statistical Analysis

To quantify the level of agreement between measurement systems, concurrent validity of shank, thigh, and knee angular velocity were determined using 2-way random intraclass correlation coefficients (ICC)(2,k). For clinical measurements agreement between measurement systems should exceed 0.90 to ensure reasonable validity.

To determine the best predictor of knee power absorption and knee extensor moment, two separate step-wise linear regressions were performed using shank, thigh, and knee angular velocities measured with inertial sensors. Peak knee power absorption (KPow) was the dependent variable for the first regression model and peak knee extensor moment (KMom) was the dependent variable for the second regression model. Peak shank (SAV), thigh (TAV), and knee (KAV) angular velocities from inertial sensors were independent variables. For both regression models, data from ACLr and Non-Sx limbs were considered together as initial multiple linear regression analysis that included limb as an independent variable determined that limb had no significant effect on the relationships (p = 0.072). Therefore, data presented below represents combined data from both limbs. One-tailed Pearson product–moment correlations were used to quantify the strength of the relationship between KPow and angular velocities and between KMom and angular velocities. A strong correlation was defined as a correlation greater than 0.75, a moderate correlation was defined as a correlation 0.50–0.75, and a weak correlation was defined as a correlation less than 0.5. Statistical analyses were performed using PASW software (version 18, SPSS, Inc., Chicago, IL, USA) with a significance level of $\alpha < 0.05$.

3. Results

Descriptive statistics for 21 participants can be found in Table 1. High intraclass correlation coefficients (ICC > 0.90) indicated strong agreement between measurement systems for KAV, TAV, SAV during SLL (Table 2).

Table 1. Descriptive statistics for the reconstructed (ACLr) and nonsurgical (Non-Sx) limb for joint and segment variables measured with marker-based motion capture and inertial sensor measurement systems; Data represents mean ± standard deviation and (range).

	ACLr Limb		Non-Sx Limb	
	Marker-Based	Inertial Sensor	Marker-Based	Inertial Sensor
Knee Power Absorption (W/kg)	5.8 ± 3.5 (1.3–15.4)	NA	9.2 ± 2.4 (5.6–14.7)	NA
Knee Extensor Moment (Nm/kg)	1.4 ± 0.4 (0.7–2.3)	NA	1.9 ± 0.2 (1.6–2.3)	NA
Knee Angular Velocity (deg/s)	328.0 ± 97.5 (154.4–521.2)	326.5 ± 100.6 (154.0–508.7)	420.1 ± 81.7 (249.6–543.3)	410.5 ± 84.55 (197.1–532.5)
Thigh Angular Velocity (deg/s)	156.0 ± 62.9 (48.7–276.0)	152.0 ± 67.2 (39.7–264.0)	210.0 ± 52.53 (108.0–308.0)	207.0 ± 54.0 (75.3–291.0)
Shank Angular Velocity (deg/s)	205.2 ± 53.8 (124.0–327.0)	195.1 ± 53.2 (119.8–301.3)	224.9 ± 33.79 (147.8–284.6)	221.5 ± 34.8 (125.7–270.7)

Table 2. Intraclass correlation coefficients (2,k) between marker-based motion capture and inertial sensor measurements for peak knee angular velocity, and peak thigh and shank angular velocities measured in all limbs, the reconstructed (ACLr) and nonsurgical (Non-Sx) limb.

	ALL Limbs	ACLr Limb	Non-Sx Limb
Knee Angular Velocity	0.978 **	0.989 **	0.950 **
Thigh Angular Velocity	0.967 **	0.947 **	0.973 **
Shank Angular Velocity	0.962 **	0.95 **	0.978 **

** Indicates significance; p < 0.001.

When considering joint and segment variables extracted from inertial sensors in a step-wise regression model predicting KPow, TAV(R^2 = 0.660, p < 0.001) was the only variable to enter the model; it explained 66% of variance in KPow during SLL. Peak KAV(r = 0.806, p < 0.001; Figure 4A) and TAV(r = 0.812, p < 0.001; Figure 4B; Equation (1)) were strongly correlated and SAV(r = 0.596, p < 0.001) was moderately correlated with KPow.

$$\text{Knee Power} = 0.042(\text{TAV}) - 0.087 \tag{1}$$

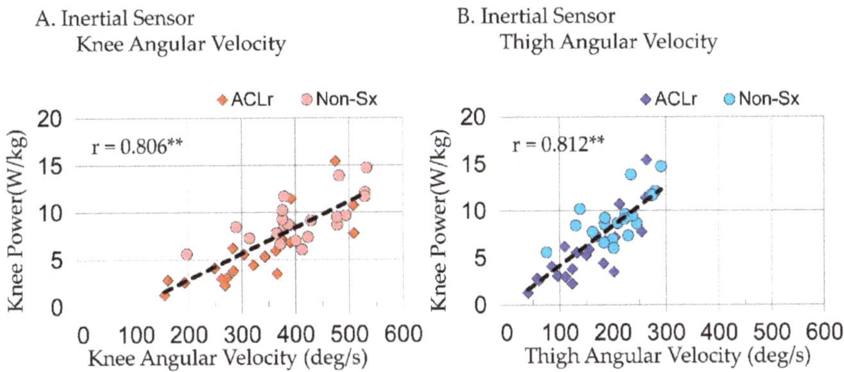

Figure 4. The relationship between peak knee power absorption and (**A**) peak knee angular velocities and (**B**) peak thigh angular velocities measured with inertial sensors in the reconstructed (ACLr) and nonsurgical (Non-Sx) limb; ** p < 0.001.

TAV (R^2 = 0.342, p < 0.001) was also the only variable to enter the KMom step-wise regression model when considering joint and segment variables extracted from inertial sensors. TAV explaining 34% of variance in KMom during SLL. Peak KAV(r = 0.536, p < 0.001; Figure 5A) and TAV(r = 0.585, p < 0.001; Figure 5B: Equation (2)) were moderately correlated with KMom and SAV(r = 0.345, p = 0.013) was poorly correlated.

$$\text{Knee Moment} = 0.004(\text{TAV}) + 0.585 \tag{2}$$

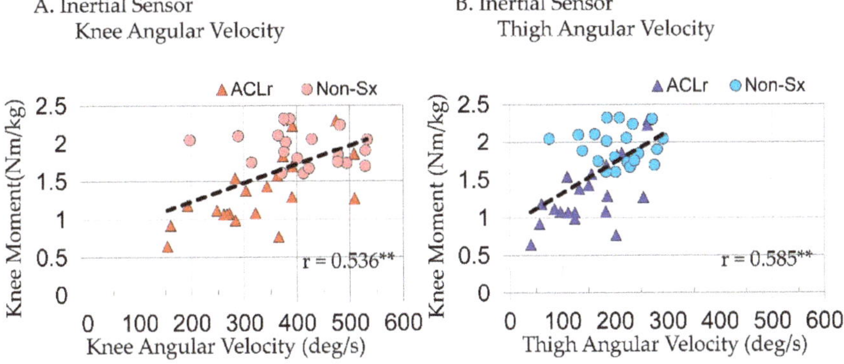

Figure 5. The relationship between peak knee extensor moments and (**A**) peak knee angular velocities and (**B**) peak thigh angular velocities measured with inertial sensors in the reconstructed (ACLr) and nonsurgical (Non-Sx) limb; ** p < 0.001.

Joint and segment angular velocities were positively correlated with peak KPow and peak KMom indicating faster velocities were related to larger peak knee power absorption and peak knee extensor moments.

4. Discussion

Findings from this study provide a foundation for using inertial sensors to detect altered knee loading without presence of force plates or marker-based motion system during this SLL task. Previous studies demonstrated that individuals post-ACLr exhibit deficits in dynamic knee loading that are challenging to detect in the clinic [1,14,22,24]. The inability to quantify common knee loading deficits in the clinic in individuals following ACLr is concerning as post-surgery these individuals aim to return to high level dynamic tasks, where the knee plays an essential role in force attenuation [25–27].

The results of this study suggest that segment angular velocities measured with inertial sensors and marker-based motion analysis systems provide similar information supporting use of inertial sensors in the clinic. The agreement between the marker-based system and inertial sensors was high, with ICCs ranging between 0.94 and 0.989, when measuring knee and segment angular velocities. While inertial sensors are a direct measurement of segment angular velocities and marker-based measurements involve calculations from marker positions, strong intraclass correlation coefficients confirm that both methods may be used to quantify thigh and shank angular velocities during this task. In addition, knee angular velocities that involve calculations in both measurement systems, also had strong intraclass correlation coefficients. Together, these data confirm that direct measurements from the gyroscope of inertial measurement devices and calculated joint measurements provide a feasible alternative for marker-based motion analysis systems. Future work is needed to determine if the strength of this relationship is consistent across other functional tasks.

Peak angular velocities coincided with peak knee power absorption just after initial contact (Figure 3B) as the knee is going into flexion (Figure 3A). When inertial sensor variables were considered together, sagittal plane peak thigh angular velocity was the best predictor of knee power absorption explaining 66% of the variance during single limb loading. After accounting for effects of thigh angular velocity, knee, and shank angular velocities did not add any additional information. The strength of the relationships suggests that angular velocity alone can provide meaningful information regarding knee power without marker-derived kinematics and ground reaction forces. This is not surprising as a between limb (surgical and non-surgical) ratio of thigh angular velocity in these same subjects was strong enough to identify knee power deficits with high sensitivity and specificity [21]. The correlation was slightly higher for thigh angular velocity; as a result, it was determined to be the stronger predictor of knee power when measured with inertial sensors.

Similarly, sagittal plane peak thigh angular velocity was the best predictor of peak knee extensor moments; however, it only explained 34% of the variance during single limb loading. Knee and shank angular velocities did not add any addition information. The moderate relationship between knee moment, and thigh ($r = 0.585$) and knee ($r = 0.536$) angular velocities suggests angular velocity measurements alone may provide some useful information regarding knee moment in the absence of ground reaction forces. However, it is not expected that these relationships are strong enough to add value to clinical decision making regarding knee moment deficits.

Using direct output of a single sensor on the thigh may be more practical for clinical use as it requires the purchase and application of fewer sensors. The use of a single sensor would provide clinicians with a simple tool that can be used to objectively quantify movement in the clinic and provide treatment rationales to third party payors. The strength of these relationships for knee power exceeded previously reported relationships between coronal plane thigh and shank angular velocities and knee adductor moments during single and double limb drop lands [18]. It is not surprising that segment angular velocity is more strongly related to joint power than moments given how they are calculated. Moreover, this SLL task required significant sagittal plane motion at the knee whereas frontal plane motion was limited. The testing procedures described in the current study allow for exploration of sagittal plane loading deficits commonly observed in individuals post-ACLr.

Shank angular velocity had a moderate relationship to knee power and poor relationship to knee moment. The range of angular velocities at the shank was smaller than those observed at the thigh and knee, but of similar magnitudes. When considered along with thigh angular velocity, shank did not add any additional information regarding knee power or moment. This suggests that motion at the thigh is more directly related to knee flexion during this single limb loading task. The instructions to perform the task encouraged individuals to lower themselves as far as they could. This may have resulted in large hip flexion angles increasing the contribution of thigh movement to knee flexion. However, future work is needed to determine if thigh and shank kinematics are reflective of hip and ankle kinematics, respectively.

Angular velocity measurements with inertial sensors provide meaningful information about an individual's ability to accommodate forces through their knee following ACL reconstructive surgery during phases of tasks that are too quick for our eyes and traditional video recorders to capture. It is likely that thigh angular velocity measured with inertial sensors is highly sensitive to difference in power observed between limbs or changes over time as the regression equation indicated that a 0.042 deg/s change in thigh angular velocity coincides with a 1 W/kg change in knee power absorption (Equation (1)). Interestingly, limb did not influence the relationship between sagittal plane angular velocities and knee power or knee moment during this task despite the presence of between limb differences in angular velocities and knee power at this time point in rehabilitation. This supports the use of the nonsurgical limb for comparison to assess knee loading asymmetries in the clinic, as seen commonly in assessment of rehabilitation progression [21,28–30]. While these findings set the foundation for quantifying knee power and moments with angular velocity measurements extracted from inertial sensors, they are limited to the single limb task assessed in this study. It is not clear if similar relationships exist during other dynamic tasks such running or hopping. For application of these data to the clinic, further work is needed to determine the sensitivity and specificity of these measures for quantifying altered knee loading.

5. Conclusions

Segment angular velocities measured with inertial sensor provide similar information to segment angular velocities measured with marker-based motion analysis systems. Furthermore, sagittal plane peak thigh angular velocity was the best predictor of peak knee power absorption and peak knee extensor moments. These findings suggest that in the absence of force platforms and a marker-based motion capture system, inertial sensors, more specifically a sensor placed on the thigh, may be useful in the clinic to quantify altered knee loading during a single limb loading task individuals following ACL reconstruction.

Author Contributions: Conceptualization, K.A.P. and S.M.S.; Methodology, K.A.P. and S.M.S.; Validation, K.A.P. and S.M.S.; Formal Analysis, K.A.P. and S.M.S.; Investigation, K.A.P.; Resources, S.M.S.; Data Curation, K.A.P. and S.M.S.; Writing-Original Draft Preparation, K.A.P. and S.M.S.; Writing-Review & Editing, K.A.P. and S.S.; Visualization, K.A.P.; Supervision, S.M.S.; Project Administration, K.A.P.

Funding: This research was supported in part by grant K12 HD0055929 from the National Center Medical Rehabilitation Research (NICHD) and the National Institute Neurological Disorders and 5R24HD065688-05 from the Eunice Kennedy Shriver National Institute of Child Health and Human Development, as part of the Medical Rehabilitation Research Infrastructure Network of the National Institutes of Health (NIH). Its contents are solely the responsibility of the authors and do not necessarily represent the official views of the NIH.

Acknowledgments: The authors would like to acknowledge CATZ Physical Therapy and Sports Performance Center for their support and assistance with this study.

Conflicts of Interest: The authors declare no conflict of interest.

References

1. Orishimo, K.F.; Kremenic, I.J.; Mullaney, M.J.; McHugh, M.P.; Nicholas, S.J. Adaptations in single-leg hop biomechanics following anterior cruciate ligament reconstruction. *Knee Surg. Sports Traumatol. Arthrosc.* **2010**, *18*, 1587–1593. [CrossRef] [PubMed]

2. Salem, G.J.; Salinas, R.; Harding, F.V. Bilateral kinematic and kinetic analysis of the squat exercise after anterior cruciate ligament reconstruction. *Arch. Phys. Med. Rehabil.* **2003**, *84*, 1211–1216. [CrossRef]

3. Fong, D.T.; Chan, Y.Y. The use of wearable inertial motion sensors in human lower limb biomechanics studies: A systematic review. *Sensors* **2010**, *10*, 11556–11565. [CrossRef] [PubMed]

4. Delahunt, E.; Sweeney, L.; Chawke, M.; Kelleher, J.; Murphy, K.; Patterson, M.; Prendiville, A. Lower limb kinematic alterations during drop vertical jumps in female athletes who have undergone anterior cruciate ligament reconstruction. *J. Orthopaedic Res.* **2012**, *30*, 72–78. [CrossRef] [PubMed]

5. Favre, J.; Jolles, B.M.; Aissaoui, R.; Aminian, K. Ambulatory measurement of 3d knee joint angle. *J. Biomech.* **2008**, *41*, 1029–1035. [CrossRef] [PubMed]

6. Dowling, A.V.; Favre, J.; Andriacchi, T.P. Inertial sensor-based feedback can reduce key risk metrics for anterior cruciate ligament injury during jump landings. *Am. J. Sports Med.* **2012**, *40*, 1075–1083. [CrossRef] [PubMed]

7. Havens, K.L.; Cohen, S.C.; Pratt, K.A.; Sigward, S.M. Accelerations from wearable accelerometers reflect knee loading during running after anterior cruciate ligament reconstruction. *Clin. Biomech.* **2018**, *58*, 57–61. [CrossRef] [PubMed]

8. Noehren, B.; Wilson, H.; Miller, C.; Lattermann, C. Long-term gait deviations in anterior cruciate ligament-reconstructed females. *Med. Sci. Sports Exerc.* **2013**, *45*, 1340–1347. [CrossRef] [PubMed]

9. Oberlander, K.D.; Bruggemann, G.P.; Hoher, J.; Karamanidis, K. Knee mechanics during landing in anterior cruciate ligament patients: A longitudinal study from pre- to 12 months post-reconstruction. *Clin. Biomech.* **2014**, *29*, 512–517. [CrossRef] [PubMed]

10. Roewer, B.D.; Di Stasi, S.L.; Snyder-Mackler, L. Quadriceps strength and weight acceptance strategies continue to improve two years after anterior cruciate ligament reconstruction. *J. Biomech.* **2011**, *44*, 1948–1953. [CrossRef] [PubMed]

11. Webster, K.E.; Gonzalez-Adrio, R.; Feller, J.A. Dynamic joint loading following hamstring and patellar tendon anterior cruciate ligament reconstruction. *Knee Surg. Sports Traumatol. Arthrosc.* **2004**, *12*, 15–21. [CrossRef] [PubMed]

12. Paterno, M.V.; Schmitt, L.C.; Ford, K.R.; Rauh, M.J.; Myer, G.D.; Huang, B.; Hewett, T.E. Biomechanical measures during landing and postural stability predict second anterior cruciate ligament injury after anterior cruciate ligament reconstruction and return to sport. *Am. J. Sports Med.* **2010**, *38*, 1968–1978. [CrossRef] [PubMed]

13. Oberlander, K.D.; Bruggemann, G.P.; Hoher, J.; Karamanidis, K. Altered landing mechanics in acl-reconstructed patients. *Med. Sci. Sports Exerc.* **2013**, *45*, 506–513. [CrossRef] [PubMed]

14. Ernst, G.P.; Saliba, E.; Diduch, D.R.; Hurwitz, S.R.; Ball, D.W. Lower extremity compensations following anterior cruciate ligament reconstruction. *Phys. Ther.* **2000**, *80*, 251–260. [PubMed]

15. Logerstedt, D.S.; Snyder-Mackler, L.; Ritter, R.C.; Axe, M.J.; Godges, J.J. Knee stability and movement coordination impairments: Knee ligament sprain. *J. Orthopaedic Sports Phys. Ther.* **2010**, *40*, A1–A37. [CrossRef] [PubMed]

16. Abrams, G.D.; Harris, J.D.; Gupta, A.K.; McCormick, F.M.; Bush-Joseph, C.A.; Verma, N.N.; Cole, B.J.; Bach, B.R., Jr. Functional performance testing after anterior cruciate ligament reconstruction: A systematic review. *J. Orthopaedic Sports Med.* **2014**, *2*. [CrossRef] [PubMed]

17. Yu, B.; Lin, C.F.; Garrett, W.E. Lower extremity biomechanics during the landing of a stop-jump task. *Clin. Biomech.* **2006**, *21*, 297–305. [CrossRef] [PubMed]

18. Dowling, A.V.; Favre, J.; Andriacchi, T.P. Characterization of thigh and shank segment angular velocity during jump landing tasks commonly used to evaluate risk for acl injury. *J. Biomech. Eng.* **2012**, *134*, 091006. [CrossRef] [PubMed]

19. Sigward, S.M.; Chan, M.S.M.; Lin, P.E. Characterizing knee loading asymmetry in individuals following anterior cruciate ligament reconstruction using inertial sensors. *Gait Posture* **2016**, *49*, 114–119. [CrossRef] [PubMed]

20. Patterson, M.R.; Delahunt, E.; Sweeney, K.T.; Caulfield, B. An ambulatory method of identifying anterior cruciate ligament reconstructed gait patterns. *Sensors* **2014**, *14*, 887–899. [CrossRef] [PubMed]

21. Pratt, K.A.; Sigward, S.M. Detection of knee power deficits following acl reconstruction using wearable sensors. *J. Orthopaedic Sports Phys. Ther.* **2018**, 1–24. [CrossRef] [PubMed]

22. Pratt, K.A.; Sigward, S.M. Knee loading deficits during dynamic tasks in individuals following anterior cruciate ligament reconstruction. *J. Orthopaedic Sports Phys. Ther.* **2017**, *47*, 411–419. [CrossRef] [PubMed]

23. Barber-Westin, S.D.; Noyes, F.R.; McCloskey, J.W. Rigorous statistical reliability, validity, and responsiveness testing of the cincinnati knee rating system in 350 subjects with uninjured, injured, or anterior cruciate ligament-reconstructed knees. *Am. J. Sports Med.* **1999**, *27*, 402–416. [CrossRef] [PubMed]

24. Sigward, S.M.; Lin, P.; Pratt, K. Knee loading asymmetries during gait and running in early rehabilitation following anterior cruciate ligament reconstruction: A longitudinal study. *Clin. Biomech.* **2016**, *32*, 249–254. [CrossRef] [PubMed]

25. Buczek, F.L.; Cavanagh, P.R. Stance phase knee and ankle kinematics and kinetics during level and downhill running. *Med. Sci. Sports Exerc.* **1990**, *22*, 669–677. [CrossRef] [PubMed]

26. Dai, B.; Butler, R.J.; Garrett, W.E.; Queen, R.M. Anterior cruciate ligament reconstruction in adolescent patients: Limb asymmetry and functional knee bracing. *Am. J. Sports Med.* **2012**, *40*, 2756–2763. [CrossRef] [PubMed]

27. Moolyk, A.N.; Carey, J.P.; Chiu, L.Z. Characteristics of lower extremity work during the impact phase of jumping and weightlifting. *J. Strength Conditioning Res.* **2013**, *27*, 3225–3232. [CrossRef] [PubMed]

28. Kvist, J. Rehabilitation following anterior cruciate ligament injury: Current recommendations for sports participation. *Sports Med.* **2004**, *34*, 269–280. [CrossRef] [PubMed]

29. Thomee, R.; Kaplan, Y.; Kvist, J.; Myklebust, G.; Risberg, M.A.; Theisen, D.; Tsepis, E.; Werner, S.; Wondrasch, B.; Witvrouw, E. Muscle strength and hop performance criteria prior to return to sports after acl reconstruction. *Knee Surg. Sports Traumatol. Arthrosc.* **2011**, *19*, 1798–1805. [CrossRef] [PubMed]

30. Myer, G.D.; Schmitt, L.C.; Brent, J.L.; Ford, K.R.; Barber Foss, K.D.; Scherer, B.J.; Heidt, R.S., Jr.; Divine, J.G.; Hewett, T.E. Utilization of modified nfl combine testing to identify functional deficits in athletes following acl reconstruction. *J. Orthopaedic Sports Phys. Ther.* **2011**, *41*, 377–387. [CrossRef] [PubMed]

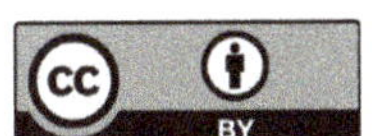

© 2018 by the authors. Licensee MDPI, Basel, Switzerland. This article is an open access article distributed under the terms and conditions of the Creative Commons Attribution (CC BY) license (http://creativecommons.org/licenses/by/4.0/).

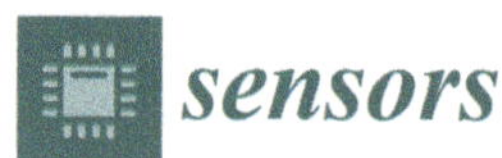 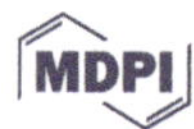

Article

A Fuzzy Tuned and Second Estimator of the Optimal Quaternion Complementary Filter for Human Motion Measurement with Inertial and Magnetic Sensors

Xiaoyue Zhang * and Wan Xiao

School of Instrumentation and Optoelectronic Engineering, Beihang University, Beijing 100191, China; xw7586@buaa.edu.cn
* Correspondence: zhangxiaoyue@buaa.edu.cn; Tel.: +86-10-8231-6547

Received: 4 September 2018; Accepted: 16 October 2018; Published: 18 October 2018

Abstract: To accurately measure human motion at high-speed, we proposed a simple structure complementary filter, named the Fuzzy Tuned and Second EStimator of the Optimal Quaternion Complementary Filter (FTECF). The FTECF is applicable to inertial and magnetic sensors, which include tri-axis gyroscopes, tri-axis accelerometers, and tri-axis magnetometers. More specifically, the proposed method incorporates three parts, the input quaternion, the reference quaternion, and the fuzzy logic algorithm. At first, the input quaternion was calculated with gyroscopes. Then, the reference quaternion was calculated by applying the Second EStimator of the Optimal Quaternion (ESOQ-2) algorithm on accelerometers and magnetometers. In addition, we added compensation for accelerometers in the ESOQ-2 algorithm so as to eliminate the effects of limb motion acceleration in high-speed human motion measurements. Finally, the fuzzy logic was utilized to calculate the fusion factor for a complementary filter, so as to adaptively fuse the input quaternion with the reference quaternion. Additionally, the overall algorithm design is more simplified than traditional methods. Confirmed by the experiments, using a commercial inertial and magnetic sensors unit and an optical motion capture system, the efficiency of the proposed method was more improved than two well-known methods. The root mean square error (RMSE) of the FTECF was less than 2.2° and the maximum error was less than 5.4°.

Keywords: human motion measurement; sensor fusion; complementary filter; fuzzy logic; inertial and magnetic sensors; ESOQ-2

---

1. Introduction

Human motion measurement is a key technology in rehabilitation, gait analysis, man–machine interaction, virtual reality, and other fields [1–4]. There are numerous kinds of human motion measurement techniques such as mechanical, magnetic, optical, acoustic, and inertial/magnetic. Most of these techniques require emissions from a source so as to track objects [5]. The magnetic measurement technique requires a self-excited stable magnetic field. The ultrasonic measurement technique needs to transmit ultrasonic waves. The optical measurement technique requires light to illuminate objects. However, no self-emission source is required for the inertial/magnetic measurement technique.

Motion measurement using inertial and magnetic sensors is a relatively new technique, which has received wide attention in recent years [4]. The inertial/magnetic measurement technique often uses a combination of micro-electromechanical system (MEMS) gyroscopes, accelerometers, and magnetometers, called magnetic, angular rate, and gravity (MARG) sensors [6]. MEMS sensors are usually low-cost, small in size, and can be manufactured into a wrist watch size [4], which is suitablefor the data collection of wearable devices. There are two advantages in the inertial/magnetic measurement technique, namely: one, is that the measurement technique itself has no inherent latency, and all delays are attributed to the data transmission, which is conducive to real-time measurement; and the other, is its lack of a necessary self-emission source [5]. This makes inertial/magnetic measurement systems easy to carry and use; moreover, the scope of use is not limited to a certain area.

We can obtain the motion of a human body by measuring the posture of the main limbs. In general, human motion can be seen as the movement of a kinematic chain composed of multiple independent limbs, and the members are bound by the connections between them. After the MARG sensors module has been fixed onto the main limbs of a human, the posture of the entire human body can be obtained by measuring the posture of each limb relative to the reference coordinate frame fixed with the earth [4]. According to the different data characteristics of the gyroscope, accelerometer, and magnetometer, a corresponding data fusion method is needed.

There are two principal methods of data fusion: the Kalman filter algorithm and the complementary filtering algorithm. The Kalman filter algorithm focuses on how to solve the effects of linear acceleration, environmental magnetic field abruption [7], and accelerometer and magnetometer data preprocessing algorithms [4]. There are also variations of the Kalman filter algorithm such as extended Kalman filtering [7,8] and the particle Kalman filter algorithm [9]. Time delay is one of the main downsides of the Kalman filter algorithm methods. The complementary filter algorithm is a method of data fusion for the MARG sensors in the frequency domain. The complementary filter algorithm mainly focuses on how to mix the accelerometer and magnetometer data so as to generate corrections, which can modify the quaternion calculated with the gyroscope data [5,10]. In addition, there is the gradient descent method that calculates attitudes by using an analytically derived and optimized gradient descent algorithm [11].

The purpose of this paper was to propose a simple structure complementary filtering algorithm that was suitable for measuring high dynamic human motion. In the current research, the complementary filter algorithm usually adopts a fixed conversion frequency, which is often difficult to adapt to high dynamic human motion. To address this problem, we proposed a complementary filter algorithm based on fuzzy logic and the Second EStimator of the Optimal Quaternion (ESOQ-2) algorithm. The fuzzy tuned algorithm was used to adjust the conversion frequency adaptively, which improved the adaptability of the algorithm for high dynamic human motion. The compensation of the accelerator for the ESOQ-2 algorithm can improve the adaptability of the proposed algorithm for high dynamic human motion. The MARG sensors' data were then input into the Fuzzy Tuned and Second EStimator of the Optimal Quaternion Complementary Filter (FTECF) to calculate the body posture. Then, the result was compared with the optical reference attitudes. The experimental results verified the performance of the proposed algorithm.

In Section 2, the basic definitions and details of the proposed algorithm are provided. Section 3 explains the measurement experiments with MARG sensors, and is devoted to the interpretation of the results. The final section provides some conclusions and future work.

2. Materials and Methods

This section is divided into two parts, the material used in the proposed algorithm (Sections 2.1–2.3) and the details of the proposed algorithm (Sections 2.4–2.6).

2.1. Coordinate System Definition

The inertial/magnetic measurement technique often refers to the body's limbs as rigid bodies [3]. The human body can be represented by 15 to 19 rigid body models that are connected to each other [12,13], so the overall body motion can be obtained by measuring the posture of each limb [9]. The human limbs are shown in Figure 1.

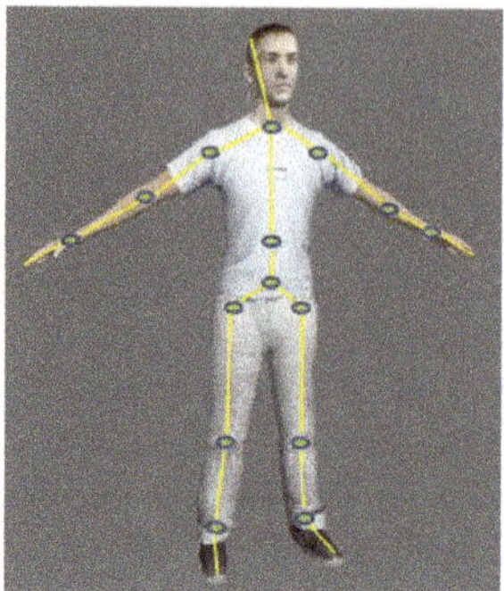

Figure 1. The segmentations of human limbs.

In this paper, we studied the generic limb posture measurement, which can be applied to all major limbs of the body. The upper limb movement is more agile and flexible than the other body limbs [9]. By convention, we chose the upper limb as the main research object [3,4,6,9,10]. In the upper limb, the more flexible upper arm movement was selected for detailed study.

The definition of the coordinate frames involved in the upper arm is illustrated in Figure 2. For the upper arm and MARG sensors, the coordinate frame was defined as B and S, respectively. In addition, the reference coordinate frame mounted on the earth was also defined as E.

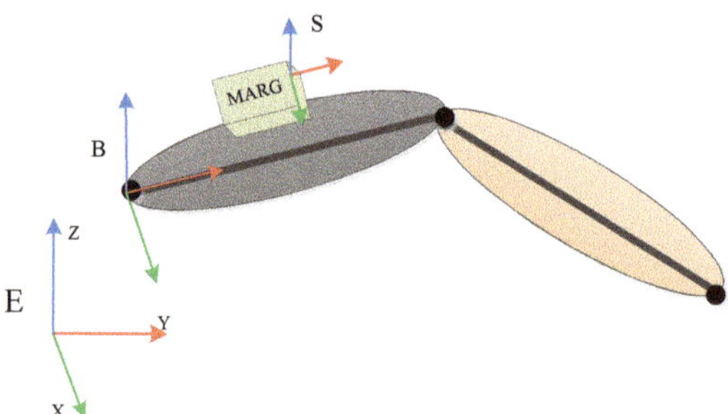

Figure 2. The definitions of the coordinate frames. E is the reference coordinate frame, which is mounted on the earth; B is the coordinate frame of the upper arm; S is the coordinate frame of the magnetic, angular rate, and gravity (MARG) sensor.

The reference coordinate for frame E is defined according to the orientation of the human body at the beginning of the measurement. The origin of the reference coordinate frame is in the vicinity of the human body in space. The directions of the three axes are defined as the Z-axis (upward in the direction of the gravity vector), the X-axis (pointing to the right of the body), and the Y-axis (pointing to the front of the body), which follow the right-handed coordinate system. Once the reference coordinate frame is defined, it is fixed in the space and does not change with the movement of the human body.

The coordinate of frame B is fixed to the human skeleton, and the origin can be set along the skeleton, usually at the rotation center of the limb. The T-pose is where the arms are straight forward, with the palms facing down and the thumb pointing straight ahead [14]. The upper arm coordinate frame and the reference coordinate frame maintain the same direction at the T-pose, and can be transformed into each other through a translation in space [10].

The origin of the coordinate of frame S is at the center of the three axes of the accelerometer, axially along the housing of the MARG sensors, and the directions of the three axes follow the right-handed coordinate system. The data output of each sensor is represented in the corresponding sensor coordinate frame.

For the sake of simplicity, we assumed that there was no relative displacement between the sensor and the upper arm, so the sensor coordinate frame and upper arm coordinate frame were considered to be identical. That is, the two frames had the same orientation, but with a different displacement.

2.2. Representation

The upper arm's movement information can be represented with Euler angles or quaternions [3]. This paper used the quaternion to calculate the rotational movement of the limb, and converted the quaternion into Euler angles for visual representation. The advantage of the Euler angles representation method is that it can intuitively represent a rotation. However, the Euler angles representation method is prone to the gimbal lock problem, resulting in the appearance of singularities. In contrast, the quaternion representation method can avoid the occurrence of singularities, and is more computationally efficient. In addition, the quaternion can be transformed with the attitude matrix and Euler angles [15].

In previous studies [4–6], the motion of the upper arm was usually described by the kinematics differential (Equation (1)).

$$\dot{q}_B^E = \frac{1}{2} q_B^E \otimes \overline{\omega}_B \tag{1}$$

where q_B^E denotes the quaternion from the upper arm coordinate frame, B, to the reference coordinate frame, E, which is calculated based on the gyroscope measurement. $\overline{\omega}_B = \begin{bmatrix} 0 & \omega_B^T \end{bmatrix}$ represents a four-element column vector, and $\omega_B = \begin{bmatrix} \omega_{B,x} & \omega_{B,y} & \omega_{B,z} \end{bmatrix}$ is the measured value of the triaxial gyro in the upper arm coordinate frame.

We can express a quaternion as follows:

$$q = q_0 + q_{vert} = q_0 + q_1 i + q_2 j + q_3 k \tag{2}$$

Then, Equation (1) can be written as a matrix as follows:

$$\begin{bmatrix} \dot{q}_{B,0}^E \\ \dot{q}_{B,1}^E \\ \dot{q}_{B,2}^E \\ \dot{q}_{B,3}^E \end{bmatrix} = \frac{1}{2} \begin{bmatrix} 0 & -\omega_{B,x} & -\omega_{B,y} & -\omega_{B,z} \\ \omega_{B,x} & 0 & \omega_{B,z} & -\omega_{B,y} \\ \omega_{B,y} & -\omega_{B,z} & 0 & \omega_{B,x} \\ \omega_{B,z} & \omega_{B,y} & -\omega_{B,x} & 0 \end{bmatrix} \begin{bmatrix} q_{B,0}^E \\ q_{B,1}^E \\ q_{B,2}^E \\ q_{B,3}^E \end{bmatrix} \tag{3}$$

If the gyroscope output, $\overline{\omega}_{B,t}$, and the fused quaternion, $q_{t-\Delta t}^E$, are known, then we can obtain the input quaternion as follows:

$$q_{gyr,t}^E = q_{t-\Delta t}^E + \dot{q}_{gyr,t}^E \Delta t \tag{4}$$

where Δt is the sampling time.

The motion of the upper arm can be represented by Euler angles (pitch–roll–yaw), as in Figure 3. The pitch angle is a rotation angle with respect to the X-axis of the coordinate frame, E. Similarly, we can define the roll angle and the yaw angle.

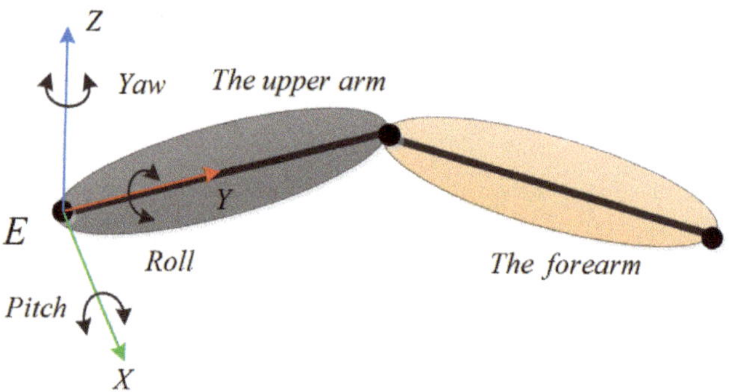

Figure 3. The definitions of the Euler angles.

2.3. Motion Speed

The maximum movement frequency of the upper arm of the human body is about 3.7 times per second [16], therefore, it is difficult for a person to maintain long-term high-speed movements. In this study, we choose two representative human motion speeds, namely: 0.5 movements per second (0.5 mov/s) and 2 movements per second (2 mov/s), representing human low-speed motion and human high-speed motion, respectively.

2.4. Description of the Proposed Algorithm

We proposed a complementary filter algorithm based on fuzzy logic and the ESOQ-2 algorithm. The block diagram of the algorithm is shown in Figure 4. The ESOQ-2 algorithm calculates the reference quaternion with accelerometers and magnetometers. The reference quaternion has a more precise dynamic response at a low frequency. In contrast, the input quaternion calculated by gyroscopes has a more precise dynamic response in high frequency. In this paper, a complementary filter fused the reference quaternion and input quaternion, and the conversion frequency was tuned by fuzzy logic.

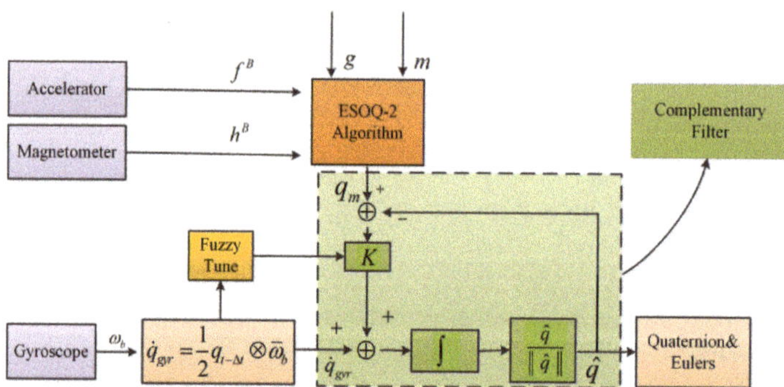

Figure 4. Block diagram of the proposed algorithm.

In order to analyze the complementary filter, we performed a Laplace transform (s is the Laplace operator) on q_m, $\dot{q}_{gyr}$, and $\hat{q}$. As shown in Figure 5, $q_m(s)$ is the Laplace transformation (LT) of q_m, and $sq_{gry}(s)$ denotes the LT of $\dot{q}_{gyr}$. $F_1(s)$ and $F_2(s)$ are two transfer functions and $F_1(s) + F_2(s) = 1$ [5].

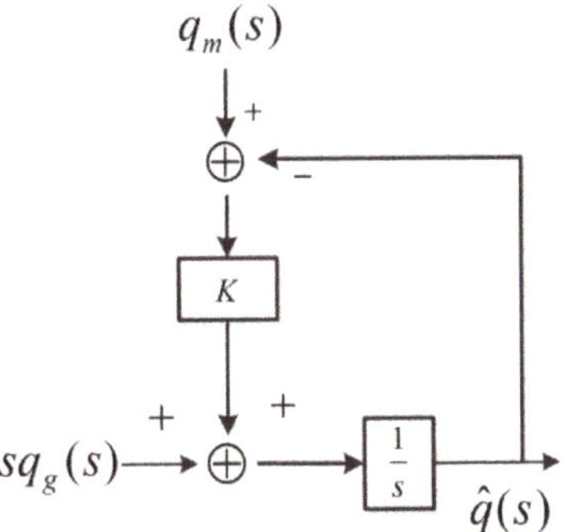

Figure 5. The frequency domain representation of the complementary filter.

$$F_1(s) = \frac{\hat{q}(s)}{q_m(s)} = \frac{K}{s+K} = \frac{1}{\tau s + 1} \tag{5}$$

$$F_2(s) = \frac{\hat{q}(s)}{q_{gry}(s)} = \frac{s}{s+K} = \frac{\tau s}{\tau s + 1} \tag{6}$$

$$\hat{q}(s) = F_1(s)q_m(s) + F_2(s)q_{gry}(s) = \frac{K}{s+K}q_m(s) + \frac{s}{s+K}q_{gry}(s) \tag{7}$$

$$f_c = \frac{1}{2\pi\tau} = \frac{K}{2\pi} \tag{8}$$

where $\tau = \frac{1}{K}$.

In Equation (7), $F_1(s)$ is equivalent to a low-pass filter and can filter out the high-frequency noise of the reference quaternion. $F_2(s)$ is equivalent to a high-pass filter, and can filter out the low frequency noise of the input quaternion. The conversion frequency of the complementary filter is f_c, in Equation (8), and can be adjusted by varying the filter gain, K [17].

The output of the complementary filter in the time domain in Figure 4 is as follows:

$$\hat{q}_t = [K(q_m - \hat{q}_t) + \dot{q}_{gyr}]\Delta t + q_{t-\Delta t} \tag{9}$$

By applying Equation (4) to Equation (9), we get the following [6]:

$$\hat{q}_t = (1 - \frac{K\Delta t}{1 + K\Delta t})q_{gry,t}^E + \frac{K\Delta t}{1 + K\Delta t}q_{m,t}^E \tag{10}$$

$$\hat{q}_t = (1 - \mu_t)q_{gry,t}^E + \mu_t q_{m,t}^E, 0 \leq \mu_t \leq 1. \tag{11}$$

where $\mu_t = \frac{K\Delta t}{1+K\Delta t} = 1 - \frac{1}{1+K\Delta t} = 1 - \frac{1}{1+2\pi f_c \Delta t}$, by using Equation (8) and $f_c \propto \mu_t$. Therefore, it can be seen from Equation (11) that tuning the fusion factor, μ_t, can change the conversion frequency, f_c, of the complementary filter. When μ_t increases, f_c correspondingly increases. At this time, the complementary filter output is more biased toward the reference quaternion, $q_{m,t}^E$. Similarly, when μ_t decreases, f_c decreases correspondingly, and the complementary filter is more biased to the input quaternion, $q_{gry,t}^E$.

To prevent the quaternion from being non-orthogonal, we performed orthogonalization on it.

$$\hat{q} = \frac{1}{\sqrt{\hat{q}_0^2 + \hat{q}_1^2 + \hat{q}_2^2 + \hat{q}_3^2}} \begin{bmatrix} \hat{q}_0 \\ \hat{q}_1 \\ \hat{q}_2 \\ \hat{q}_3 \end{bmatrix} \tag{12}$$

2.5. The ESOQ-2 Algorithm and Computation for the Accelerator

2.5.1. The ESOQ-2 Algorithm and Reference Quaternion

We calculated the reference quaternion by using the ESOQ-2 algorithm. The ESOQ-2 algorithm has been proposed for the Wahba problem [18]. The Wahba problem is used to estimate the attitudes of a body in the least-squares sense, by using the vector's reference values and the corresponding measurement values, as shown in Equation (13).

$$L_W(A) = \frac{1}{2}\sum_{i-1}^{n} \alpha_i \|Ar_i - b_i\|^2 = \min \tag{13}$$

where α_i represents the relative weight of the observation vector ($\sum_i \alpha_i = 1, i = 1 \sim n$). The weight is related to the data credibility of the ith observation vector.

In Equation (13), r is the n-dimensional vector defined in the reference coordinate frame, b is the corresponding vector definition in the body coordinate, and A is the attitude matrix from r to b. In this paper, n is 2, r represents the gravity vector and geomagnetic field vector defined in the reference coordinate frame, and b represents the accelerometer and magnetometer measurement vector. Assuming that in the quasi-static condition (limb motion acceleration is negligible when compared to gravitational acceleration) the magnetic field is not distorted, the attitude measurement in this paper was used to determine the body posture through the reference and measurement values of the gravity vector and the geomagnetic field vector.

The q-method demonstrates that the optimal quaternion, q_{opt}, is the eigenvector with the largest eigenvalue of the 4×4 symmetric matrix K [19],

$$Kq_{opt} = \lambda_{max}q_{opt} \tag{14}$$

Therefore, as long as the eigenvector with the largest eigenvalue of matrix K is obtained, the optimal attitude quaternion can be obtained.

The procedure for the ESOQ-2 algorithm is as follows:

(1) Calculate the structure matrix

$$K = \begin{bmatrix} B + B^T - tr[B]I_{3\times3} & z \\ z^T & tr[B] \end{bmatrix} \tag{15}$$

where $B = \sum_i \alpha_i b_i r_i^T$ is the attitude profile matrix, $I_{3\times3}$ is the 3×3 unit matrix, and z is the vector $z = \sum_i \alpha_i b_i \times r_i = \{B(2,3) - B(3,2), B(3,1) - B(1,3), B(1,2) - B(2,1)\}^T$.

(2) Calculate the maximum eigenvalue of the approximated matrix K

$$\lambda_{max} = \frac{1}{2}(\sqrt{2\sqrt{d} - b} + \sqrt{-2\sqrt{d} - b}) \tag{16}$$

where $b = -2(tr[B]) + tr[adj(B + B^T)] - z^T z, d = \det(K)$.

(3) Calculate the reference quaternion

From the formula $[(tr[B] - \lambda_{max})S - zz^T]e = Me = 0$, the best robustness vector can be obtained, so

$$q = \left\{ \begin{array}{c} (\lambda_{max} - tr[B])e_k \\ z^T e_k \end{array} \right\} \tag{17}$$

Thus, the direction of the optimal quaternion is obtained by normalizing q, that is, $q_{opt} = q/\sqrt{q^T q}$.

(4) Avoid singularity adjustment

For the singularity problem that this method may produce, the specific details of the solution are in the literature [19].

In this paper, the gravity vector is expressed as $g = \begin{bmatrix} 0 & 0 & 9.78 \end{bmatrix}^T$, assuming that the local geomagnetic vector modulus is h, and the declination angle of the local geomagnetic vector is ε. When the X-axis of the reference coordinate frame points to the east and the Y-axis points to the north, the geomagnetic vector can be expressed as $m = \begin{bmatrix} 0 & h\cos\varepsilon & h\sin\varepsilon \end{bmatrix}^T$.

2.5.2. Compensation for the Accelerator

The quasi-static condition in the ESOQ-2 algorithm is rare in human motion. Therefore, we needed to compensate the accelerator in order to handle a high dynamic movement. Because of the acceleration of the limb movement, the accelerometer output is the combination of the gravity acceleration and the motion acceleration. In this case, the input quaternion is more reliable, so we replaced the accelerometer's output with the gravitational acceleration vector calculated with the input quaternion. Based on the aforementioned concept, the input vectors, f, (gravity-related) for the ESOQ-2 algorithm were calculated using the following equations:

$$f^B = \begin{cases} \dfrac{f_{m,t}}{\|f_{m,t}\|}, & if \ \left|\|f_{m,t}\| - \|g\|\right| \leq \delta_a \ and \ \|\omega_{b,t}\| \leq \delta_w, \\[2ex] C_E^B \dfrac{g}{\|g\|}, & otherwise. \end{cases} \tag{18}$$

$$\begin{cases} \|f_{m,t}\| = \sqrt{f_{mx,t}^2 + f_{my,t}^2 + f_{mz,t}^2} \\[2ex] \|\omega_{b,t}\| = \sqrt{\omega_{bx,t}^2 + \omega_{by,t}^2 + \omega_{bz,t}^2} \end{cases} \tag{19}$$

$$C_E^B = \begin{bmatrix} q_{gyr,0}^2 + q_{gyr,1}^2 - q_{gyr,2}^2 - q_{gyr,3}^2 & 2(q_{gyr,1}q_{gyr,2} + q_{gyr,0}q_{gyr,3}) & 2(q_{gyr,1}q_{gyr,3} - q_{gyr,0}q_{gyr,2}) \\[1ex] 2(q_{gyr,1}q_{gyr,2} - q_{gyr,0}q_{gyr,3}) & q_{gyr,0}^2 - q_{gyr,1}^2 + q_{gyr,2}^2 - q_{gyr,3}^2 & 2(q_{gyr,2}q_{gyr,3} + q_{gyr,0}q_{gyr,1}) \\[1ex] 2(q_{gyr,1}q_{gyr,3} + q_{gyr,0}q_{gyr,2}) & 2(q_{gyr,2}q_{gyr,3} - q_{gyr,0}q_{gyr,1}) & q_{gyr,0}^2 - q_{gyr,1}^2 - q_{gyr,2}^2 + q_{gyr,3}^2 \end{bmatrix} \tag{20}$$

where $f_{m,t} = \begin{bmatrix} f_{mx,t} & f_{mx,t} & f_{mx,t} \end{bmatrix}$ is the accelerometer triaxial output data, and $\omega_{b,t}$ is the gyroscope triaxial output data. C_E^B represents the attitude transformation matrix from the reference coordinate frame (E) to the sensor coordinate frame (S) and the upper arm coordinate frame (B), assuming that the latter two coordinate frames are consistent in direction. $q_{gyr} = \begin{bmatrix} q_{gyr,0} & q_{gyr,1} & q_{gyr,2} & q_{gyr,3} \end{bmatrix}$ is the input quaternion. δ_a and δ_w are the corresponding thresholds for acceleration and angular velocity, respectively.

2.6. Quaternion Fusion Factor

In this paper, fuzzy logic was used to generate the fusion factor for the reference quaternion and the input quaternion. As a fuzzy input, $e1$ can be calculated as Equation (21), as follows:

$$e1 = \frac{\varsigma}{\varsigma + \|\dot{q}_{gyr}^E\|} \tag{21}$$

where the quaternion differential value, $\dot{q}_{gyr}$, is calculated from the gyroscope output. In addition, ς represents the minimum value of the angular velocity differential mode value $\|\dot{q}_{gyr}^E\|$ under normal human motion, which can be obtained through simple experiments.

The specific steps for designing a fuzzy controller are as follows [20]:

(1) Fuzzification

That is, a fuzzy set is used to represent real-valued signals. This paper used a single-valued method.

(2) Establish fuzzy inference rules

In this part, $e1$ is the fuzzy input, and u is the fuzzy output. The fuzzy output, u, was μ_t in the paper. From Equation (21), we can see that when the acceleration of the line motion was large, $\dot{q}_{gyr}$ increased and $e1$ decreased. According to Equation (11), μ_t should be tuned to be smaller, as the quaternion calculated by the gyroscope is more reliable. On the contrary, when the linear motion acceleration is small, $\dot{q}_{gyr}$ decreased and $e1$ increased. Therefore, μ_t should be tuned to be larger.

The rules of the fuzzy inference are set according to the aforementioned principles in Table 1.

Table 1. Fuzzy rules.

$e1$	u
small	small
large	large

The inference rule language is expressed as follows: Rule 1—if $e1$ is small, then u is small; Rule 2—if $e1$ is large, then u is large.

(3) Determine the weights and rule reliability

In practice, it is important to establish the relationship between the weights of the fuzzy rules and the reliability of the fuzzy rules in the knowledge base. There is a reversible mapping between the weights and the corresponding fuzzy rule confidence vectors.

(4) Choose the appropriate relationship generation method and inference synthesis algorithm

The selection of appropriate relationship generation methods and inference synthesis algorithms is required when designing a fuzzy controller. This article used the Z-shaped membership function and the S-shaped membership function in the MATLAB fuzzy toolbox. The fuzzy membership functions designed based on the fuzzy inference rules and rule reliability are shown in Figure 6.

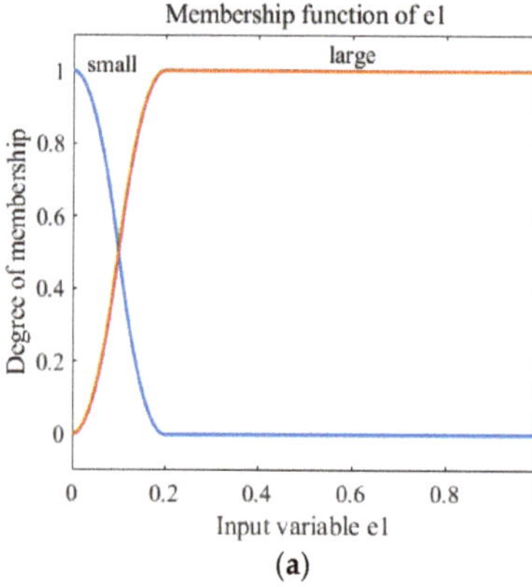

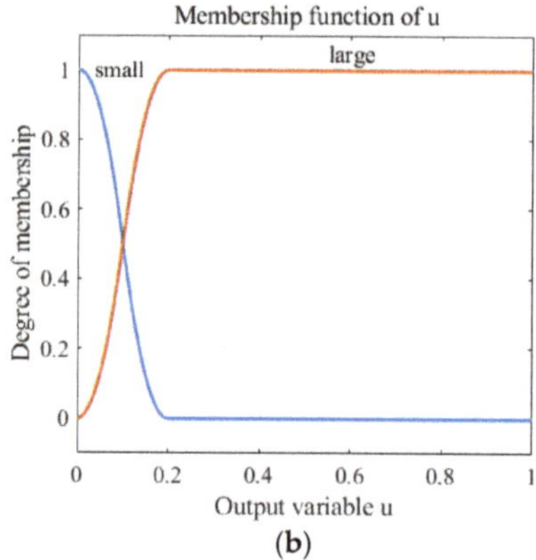

Figure 6. The fuzzy membership functions. (**a**) The input membership function. (**b**) The output membership function.

(5) Defuzzification

When the output of an inference process forms a fuzzy output set, it is necessary to compress its distribution in order to produce a single value that expresses the output of the fuzzy system, that is, anti-blurring. This study used the maximum membership degree average method.

3. Experimental Results and Discussion

In this section, we consider the experimental testbed and evaluate the performance of the proposed FTECF method at different test times and motion speeds. We also compare the FTECF with two other methods in terms of accuracy and structure, so as to further evaluate its performance.

To verify the proposed algorithm, we used the MARG sensors named MTi-3 [21]. MTi-3 is produced by Xsens Technologies (Enschede, The Netherlands). Figure 7a shows that we bound MTi-3 to the subject's right upper arm to measure its motion. All of the sensor signals were sampled at 100 Hz and were interfaced to a personal computer (PC) via a universal serial bus (USB) cable. The accompanying software MT manager provided the calibrated sensor measurements. An Oqus 7+ optical motion capture system (Qualisys, Göteborg, Sweden), shown in Figure 7b, provided the reference orientation, which captures motion by using passive reflective technology with three cameras [22]. The spatial positioning accuracy of Oqus 7+ is less than 1 mm, and the latency time is less than 4 ms.

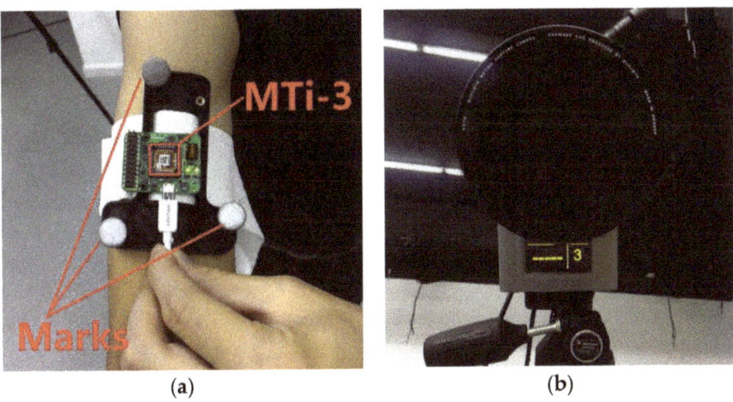

(a)   (b)

Figure 7. The experimental illustrations. (**a**) MTi-3 placed on the upper arm. (**b**) Oqus 7+.

In the experiment, the subject swung his upper arm according to the procedure of Figure 8. First, the subject stretched his upper arm and remained stationary at the T-pose for about 10 s, in order to calculate the initial position. Then, the subject swung his upper arm in the order of roll–pitch–yaw, and subsequently repeated the motion for about 55 s in the same order. As shown in Figure 8, we referred to the entire experiment as the 110 s test, and the approximately one-minute portion of the 110 s test as the 55 s test. By comparing the results of the two tests, we could conclude the influence of time on the algorithm. In addition, two motion speeds were mentioned in Section 2.3. In order to study the performance of the proposed algorithm at different motion speeds, we performed three trials for each speed.

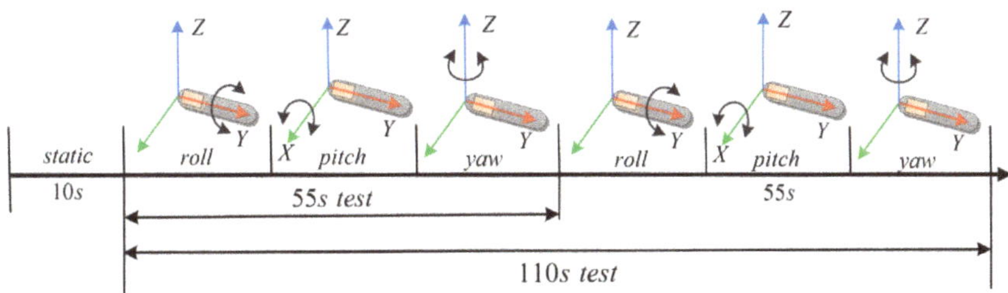

Figure 8. The experimental illustrations of motion.

Two other algorithms, Madgwick's method [11] and Yun's method [4], were used to compare the proposed FTECF method. In order to verify the orientation estimation accuracy, the root mean square error (RMSE) value of the Euler angles from the quaternion-based orientation was chosen as the criterion to evaluate the performance of the proposed FTECF method [4–6,10]. The calculation formula is as follows:

$$e_{RMSE} = \sqrt{\frac{\sum_{i=1}^{n} \left(\beta_{obs} - \beta_{tru} \right)^2}{n}} \tag{22}$$

where β_{obs} indicates the Euler angles calculated by the FTECF or other methods, the Euler angles, β_{tru}, are the reference attitudes, and n indicates the number of calculations.

Note that Yun's method was assumed in the quasi-static state, which means that the acceleration of motion is small relative to the acceleration of gravity. The experiment obviously did not meet this assumption. We performed Equations (18) and (19) on the QUEST algorithm in Yun's method (similar to the ESOQ-2 algorithm in this paper, which uses a gravitational acceleration vector and a geomagnetic vector to determine the attitudes).

The relevant parameter of the fuzzy tuned algorithm was selected as $\zeta = 0.0006325$. The corresponding thresholds for acceleration and angular velocity were $\delta_a = 0.1 \, \text{m/s}^2$ and $\delta_w = 10^{\circ}/s$, respectively. $\|g\|$ and $\|h\|$ were selected as $9.78 \, \text{m/s}^2$ and $0.6 \, \text{Gauss}$, respectively. The declination angle of the local geomagnetic vector ε was -58°.

3.1. The Effect of Motion Speed and Test Time on the Proposed FTECF

We plotted the typical measurements of the proposed FTECF at two motion speeds. Figures 9 and 10 are the typical measurement results of FTECF at 0.5 mov/s and 2 mov/s, respectively. In Figures 9a and 10a, the red solid lines indicate the Euler angles measured by the optical motion capture system, and the blue dotted lines indicate the Euler angles calculated by the FTECF. The blue lines in Figures 9b and 10b indicate the angle errors calculated by Equation (22). As can be seen from Figures 9b and 10b, in terms of the fluctuation of the error, yaw was the largest, pitch was second, and roll was the smallest. In addition, the results showed that the proposed FTECF maintained a RMSE within a certain range of accuracy.

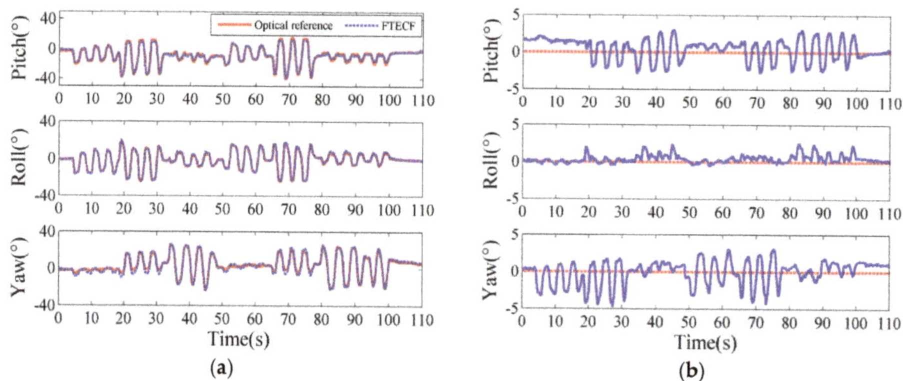

Figure 9. Typical results of the Fuzzy Tuned and Second EStimator of the Optimal Quaternion Complementary Filter (FTECF) at 0.5 mov/s. (**a**) The Euler angles of the optical and the proposed FTECF. (**b**) Euler angle errors.

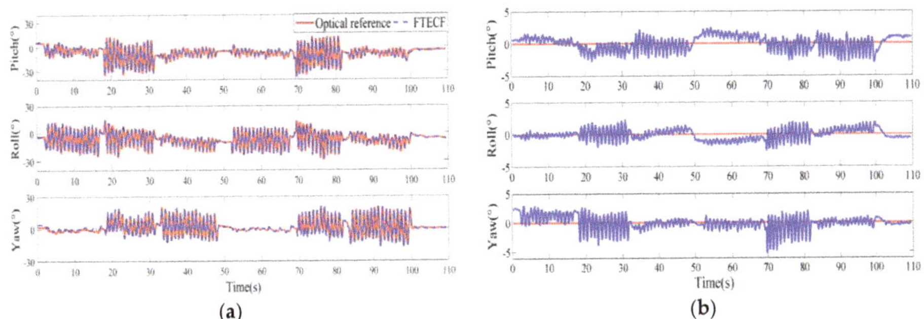

Figure 10. Typical results of FTECF at 2 mov/s. (**a**) The Euler angles of the optical and the proposed FTECF. (**b**) Euler angle errors.

Figure 11 shows the RMSE of the FTECF under four different test conditions. In Figure 11, the blue bars indicate the RMSE of the FTECF at the 0.5 mov/s, 55 s test condition. The meaning of the red, yellow, and purple bars can be inferred from the legend. In order to obtain the influence of the motion speed on the proposed algorithm, we compared the blue and yellow bars with a test time of 55 s, and the red and purple bars with a test time of 110 s. The results show that yaw had a smaller RMSE at higher motion speeds, while pitch and roll changed less at different motion speeds when compared with yaw. Similarly, in terms of the influence of test time on the proposed algorithm, we compared the blue and red bars with a motion speed of 0.5 mov/s, and the yellow and purple bars with a motion speed of 2 mov/s. From Figure 11, we can see that the three Euler angles showed a small change at different test times.

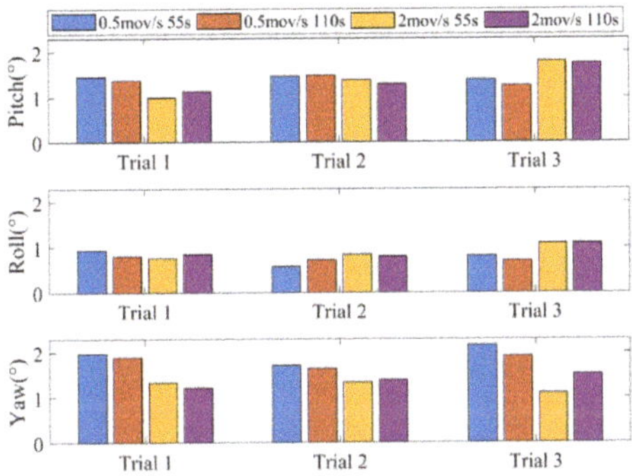

Figure 11. Root mean square error (RMSE) of the proposed FTECF method.

3.2. Compare the Proposed FTECF and the Other Two Methods

To compare the performances of the proposed FTECF and the other two methods, we listed each of the Euler angle's maximum RMSE from each method, as shown in Table 2. We also listed the maximum errors of each method. The maximum RMSE of each method and the smallest maximum error of the three methods are in bold.

Table 2 shows that the maximum RMSE of the FTECF was less than 2.2°, and the maximum error was less than 5.4°. In addition, the RMSE of the pitch and roll of the FTECF were also smaller than the other two methods, while the RMSE of the yaw was slightly larger than that in Madgwick's method.

The proposed FTECF found a balance between high precision and simple structure. Compared with the Kalman filter algorithm represented by Yun's method, the proposed method needed lower calculation costs and adapted well to high-speed human motion. The gradient descent algorithm represented by Madgwick's method was also simple in structure. However, the proposed method had a higher precision than Madgwick's method.

Table 2. Summary of errors. RMSE—root mean square error; FTECF—Fuzzy Tuned and Second EStimator of the Optimal Quaternion Complementary Filter.

Euler Angles (°)	FTECF	Madgwick's Method	Yun's Method
RMSE (pitch)	1.8024	**2.2313**	1.9024
RMSE (roll)	1.0884	1.2695	1.4793
RMSE (yaw)	**2.1605**	2.1393	**2.5881**
Maximum error	**5.376**	5.801	9.463

4. Conclusions

In this paper, we proposed a complementary filter, based on fuzzy logic and the ESOQ-2 algorithm, for human motion measurement. Firstly, the proposed method was effective at handling high dynamic movement with the fuzzy tuned algorithm and the compensation of the accelerator. The proposed algorithm did not accumulate errors under either 55 s and 110 s of measurement, indicating that it had the potential for long-term human motion measurement. Secondly, the RMSE of the proposed FTECF was less than 2.2°, which was comparable to the other two methods. In summary, this paper demonstrated the different speed motion measurements of the human upper arm by using the proposed method, and the results also illustrated its high accuracy.

Due to its high accuracy and computational efficiency, the proposed algorithm can be potentially implemented in a network of miniature MARG sensors for human body motion, forming a truly portable and ambulatory motion measurement system. The motion measurement system can be used in patient rehabilitation and behavioral monitoring. Future work will further study the influence of magnetic interference on the proposed algorithm. The complexity of the algorithm and the measurement effect for a longer time will also be studied. In addition, we will study the joint orientation assessment when the sensors are used in combination.

Author Contributions: X.Z. and W.X. conceived and designed the experiments; W.X. performed the experiments; X.Z. and W.X. wrote and approved the manuscript.

Funding: As part of the research project, this work was supported by the National Natural Science Foundation of China (61703024).

Acknowledgments: The authors are indebted to the NOKOV company for their cooperation in the previous experiments. Furthermore, we gratefully acknowledge the INFO.instrument company for letting us carry out the experiments of this paper in their optical motion capture lab.

Conflicts of Interest: The authors declare no conflict of interest.

References

1. Zhou, H.; Hu, H.; Harris, N.D.; Hammerton, J. Applications of wearable inertial sensors in estimation of upper limb movements. *Biomed. Signal Process. Control* **2006**, *1*, 22–32. [CrossRef]

2. Sabatini, A.M. Quaternion-based strap-down integration method for applications of inertial sensing to gait analysis. *Med. Boil. Eng. Comput.* **2005**, *43*, 94–101. [CrossRef]

3. Filippeschi, A.; Schmitz, N.; Miezal, M.; Bleser, G.; Ruffaldi, E.; Stricker, D. Survey of Motion Tracking Methods Based on Inertial Sensors: A Focus on Upper Limb Human Motion. *Sensors* **2017**, *17*, 1257. [CrossRef] [PubMed]

4. Yun, X.; Bachmann, E.R. Design, Implementation, and Experimental Results of a Quaternion-Based Kalman Filter for Human Body Motion Tracking. *IEEE Trans. Robot.* **2006**, *22*, 1216–1227. [CrossRef]

5. Fourati, H.; Manamanni, N.; Afilal, L.; Handrich, Y. Complementary Observer for Body Segments Motion Capturing by Inertial and Magnetic Sensors. *IEEE/ASME Trans. Mechatron.* **2014**, *19*, 149–157.

6. Tian, Y.; Wei, H.; Tan, J. An adaptive-gain complementary filter for real-time human motion tracking with MARG sensors in free-living environments. *IEEE Trans. Neural Syst. Rehabil. Eng.* **2013**, *21*, 254–264. [CrossRef] [PubMed]

7. Sabatini, A.M. Quaternion-based extended Kalman filter for determining orientation by inertial and magnetic sensing. *IEEE Trans. Biomed. Eng.* **2006**, *53*, 1346–1356. [CrossRef] [PubMed]

8. Brigante, C.M.N.; Abbate, N.; Basile, A.; Faulisi, A.C.; Sessa, S. Towards Miniaturization of a MEMS-Based Wearable Motion Capture System. *IEEE Trans. Ind. Electron.* **2011**, *58*, 3234–3241. [CrossRef]

9. Zhang, Z.Q.; Wu, J.K. A Novel Hierarchical Information Fusion Method for Three-Dimensional Upper Limb Motion Estimation. *IEEE Trans. Instrum. Meas.* **2011**, *60*, 3709–3719. [CrossRef]

10. Bachmann, E.R.; Mcghee, R.B.; Yun, X.; Zyda, M.J. Inertial and magnetic posture tracking for inserting humans into networked virtual environments. In Proceedings of the ACM Symposium on Virtual Reality Software and Technology, Baniff, AB, Canada, 15–17 November 2001; pp. 9–16.

11. Madgwick, S.O.; Harrison, A.J.; Vaidyanathan, A. Estimation of IMU and MARG orientation using a gradient descent algorithm. In Proceedings of the IEEE International Conference on Rehabilitation Robotics, Zurich, Switzerland, 29 June–1 July 2011; p. 5975346.

12. Baker, R. ISB recommendation on definition of joint coordinate systems for the reporting of human joint motion-part I: Ankle, hip and spine. *J. Biomech.* **2003**, *36*, 300–302. [CrossRef]

13. Yun, X.; Bachmann, E.R.; Mcghee, R.B. A Simplified Quaternion-Based Algorithm for Orientation Estimation from Earth Gravity and Magnetic Field Measurements. *IEEE Trans. Instrum. Meas.* **2008**, *57*, 638–650.

14. Roetenberg, D.; Luinge, H.; Slycke, P. Xsens MVN: Full 6DOF Human Motion Tracking Using Miniature Inertial Sensors. Xsens Motion Technol. BV. Available online: https://www.researchgate.net/publication/239920367_Xsens_MVN_Full_6DOF_human_motion_tracking_using_miniature_inertial_sensors (accessed on 17 October 2018).

15. Mortari, D. *ESOQ-2 Single-Point Algorithm for Fast Optimal Spacecraft Attitude Determination*; American Society of Mechanical Engineers: New York, NY, USA, 1997.

16. Chen, B. *Practical Ergonomics*; China Water Conservancy and Hydropower Press: Beijing, China, 2017; ISBN 978-7-5170-5668-3.

17. Bachmann, E.R. Inertial and Magnetic Angle Tracking of Limb Segments for Inserting Humans into Synthetic Environments. Ph.D. Thesis, Naval Postgraduate School, Monterey, CA, USA, 2000.

18. Wahba, G. A Least Squares Estimate of Satellite Attitude. *Siam Rev.* **2006**, *7*, 409. [CrossRef]

19. Mortari, D. Second Estimator of the Optimal Quaternion. *J. Guid. Control Dyn.* **2000**, *23*, 885–887. [CrossRef]

20. Zhang, G.L. *Fuzzy Control and MATLAB Applications*; Xi'an Jiaotong University Press: Xi'an, China, 2002; ISBN 7-5605-1067-1.

21. Data Sheet MTi 1-Series. Available online: https://www.xsens.com/download/pdf/documentation/mti-1/mti-1-series-datasheet-rev-d.pdf (accessed on 20 August 2018).

22. Oqus Cameras Products. Available online: https://www.qualisys.com/cameras/oqus/ (accessed on 20 August 2018).

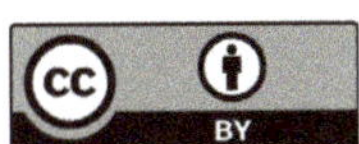

© 2018 by the authors. Licensee MDPI, Basel, Switzerland. This article is an open access article distributed under the terms and conditions of the Creative Commons Attribution (CC BY) license (http://creativecommons.org/licenses/by/4.0/).

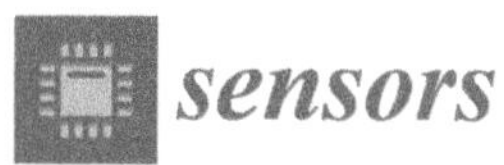 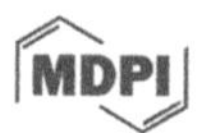

Article

A Self-Managed System for Automated Assessment of UPDRS Upper Limb Tasks in Parkinson's Disease

Claudia Ferraris [1,4,*], Roberto Nerino [1], Antonio Chimienti [1], Giuseppe Pettiti [1], Nicola Cau [2,3], Veronica Cimolin [2], Corrado Azzaro [3], Giovanni Albani [3], Lorenzo Priano [3,4] and Alessandro Mauro [3,4]

[1] Institute of Electronics, Computer and Telecommunication Engineering, National Research Council, 10129 Torino, Italy; roberto.nerino@ieiit.cnr.it (R.N.); antonio.chimienti@ieiit.cnr.it (A.C.); giuseppe.pettiti@ieiit.cnr.it (G.P.)
[2] Department of Electronics, Information and Bioengineering, Politecnico di Milano, 20133 Milano, Italy; nicola.cau@polimi.it (N.C.); veronica.cimolin@polimi.it (V.C.)
[3] Department of Neurology and NeuroRehabilitation, Istituto Auxologico Italiano, IRCCS, S. Giuseppe Hospital, 28824 Piancavallo, Italy; c.azzaro@auxologico.it (C.A.); g.albani@auxologico.it (G.A.); lorenzo.priano@unito.it (L.P.); alessandro.mauro@unito.it (A.M.)
[4] Department of Neurosciences, University of Turin, 10124 Torino, Italy
*   Correspondence: claudia.ferraris@ieiit.cnr.it; Tel.: +39-011-0905405

Received: 7 September 2018; Accepted: 15 October 2018; Published: 18 October 2018

Abstract: A home-based, reliable, objective and automated assessment of motor performance of patients affected by Parkinson's Disease (PD) is important in disease management, both to monitor therapy efficacy and to reduce costs and discomforts. In this context, we have developed a self-managed system for the automated assessment of the PD upper limb motor tasks as specified by the Unified Parkinson's Disease Rating Scale (UPDRS). The system is built around a Human Computer Interface (HCI) based on an optical RGB-Depth device and a replicable software. The HCI accuracy and reliability of the hand tracking compares favorably against consumer hand tracking devices as verified by an optoelectronic system as reference. The interface allows gestural interactions with visual feedback, providing a system management suitable for motor impaired users. The system software characterizes hand movements by kinematic parameters of their trajectories. The correlation between selected parameters and clinical UPDRS scores of patient performance is used to assess new task instances by a machine learning approach based on supervised classifiers. The classifiers have been trained by an experimental campaign on cohorts of PD patients. Experimental results show that automated assessments of the system replicate clinical ones, demonstrating its effectiveness in home monitoring of PD.

Keywords: Parkinson's disease; UPDRS; movement disorders; human computer interface; RGB-Depth; hand tracking; automated assessment; machine learning; at-home monitoring

---

1. Introduction

Parkinson's Disease (PD) is a chronic neurodegenerative disease characterized by a progressive impairment in motor functions with important impacts on quality of life [1]. Clinical assessment scales, such as Part III of the Unified Parkinson's Disease Rating Scale (UPDRS) [2], are employed by neurologists as a common basis to assess the motor impairment severity and its progression. In ambulatory assessments, the patient performs specifically defined UPDRS motor tasks that are subjectively scored by neurologists on a discrete scale of five classes of increasing severity. For upper limb motor function, the specific UPDRS tasks are Finger Tapping (FT), Opening-Closing (OC) and Pronation-Supination (PS) of the hand. During the assessment process, specific aspects of the movements (i.e., amplitude, speed, rhythm, and typical anomalies) are qualitatively and subjectively evaluated by neurologists to produce discrete assessment scores [3].

On the other hand, a quantitative, continuous and objective scoring of these tasks is desirable because the reliable detection of minimal longitudinal changes in motor performance allows for a better adjustment of the therapy, reducing the effects of motor fluctuations on daily activities and avoiding long term complications [4,5]. Currently, these goals are limited by costs, granularity of the UPDRS scale, intra and inter-rater variability of clinical scores [6].

Another desirable feature is the automation of the assessment, because it opens the possibility to monitor the motor status changes of PD patients more frequently and at home, reducing both the patient discomfort and the costs, so improving the quality of life and the disease management. Several proposed solutions, toward a more objective and automated PD assessment at home, mainly employ wearable and optical approaches [5,7], and make use of the correlation existing between the kinematic parameters of the movements and the severity of the impairment, as assessed by UPDRS [3,8–10].

Solutions for upper limb task assessment based on hand-worn wireless sensors (i.e., accelerometers, gyroscopes, resistive bands) [8–12] do not suffer from occlusion problems, but are more invasive for motor-impaired people with respect to optical approaches and, more importantly, with an invasiveness that can affect motor performance. Some optical-based approaches for hand tracking in the automated assessment of upper limb tasks of UPDRS have been recently proposed based on video processing [13], RGB-Depth cameras combined with colored markers [14], video with the aid of reflective markers [15], and bare hand tracking by consumer-grade depth-sensing devices [16–18].

In this context, tracking accuracy is an important requirement for a reliable characterization of motor performance based on kinematic features. The Microsoft Kinect® device [19,20] accuracy has been assessed in the PD context, resulting restricted to timing characterization of hand movement, due to the limitations of its hand model [21]. The Leap Motion Controller® (LMC) [22] and the Intel RealSense® device family [23] offer more complex hand models and better tracking accuracy. In particular, the LMC is imposing itself as a major technological leap and it is widely used in human computer interaction [24,25] and rehabilitation applications [26,27]. LMC tracking accuracy has been evaluated by a metrological approach mainly in quasi-static conditions [28,29], showing submillimeter accuracy, even if limited to a working volume. In healthcare applications, such as visually guided movements and pointing tasks, the accuracy in moderate dynamic condition is significantly lower, in comparison with the gold-standard motion capture systems [30–32]. The Intel RealSense® device family has been characterized for close-range applications [33], even if its hand tracking accuracy has been evaluated only for specific applications [19,34,35]. Its tracking firmware shows similar limitations in tracking fast hand movements, as discussed in [19,31] and in this paper. Furthermore, the typical short product life span of these devices and of the related software support [36] warns against solutions too dependent on closed and proprietary hardware and software.

Along this line of research, we propose as an alternative a low-cost system for the automated assessment of the upper limb UPDRS tasks (FT, OC, PS) at home. The system hardware is based on light fabric gloves with color markers, a RGB-Depth sensor, and a monitor, while the software implements the three-dimensional (3D) tracking of the hand trajectories and characterizes them by kinematic features. In particular, the software performs the real-time tracking by the fusion of both color and depth information obtained from the RGB and depth streams of the sensor respectively, which makes hand tracking and assessment more robust and accurate, even for fast hand movements. Moreover, the system acts at the same time as a non-invasive Human Computer Interface (HCI), which allows PD patients the self-management of the test execution. The automated assessment of FT, OC, PS tasks is performed by a machine learning approach. Supervised classifiers have been trained by experiments on cohorts of PD patients assessed, at the same time, by neurologists and by the system, and are then used to assess new PD patient performance. An important feature of our solution is that it does not rely on any particular hardware or firmware; it only assumes the availability of RGB and depth streams at reasonable frame rate.

The rest of the paper is organized as follows: first, the hardware and software of the automated assessment system are described, along with the details of its HCI. Then, the experimental setup for the comparison of the tracking accuracy [37] of the HCI respect to consumer devices is detailed. The experiments on PD patients, the kinematic feature selection and the supervised classifier training for the automated assessment are described in the following section. Finally, the Results section presents the tracking accuracy of our HCI with respect to consumer hand tracking devices, the discriminatory power of the selected parameters for motor task classification, and the classification accuracy obtained by the trained classifiers for upper limb UPDRS task assessment.

The overall results for the user usability of the HCI and on the accuracies in the automated assessment of upper limb UPDRS tasks demonstrate the feasibility of the system in at-home monitoring of PD.

2. Hardware and Software of the PD Assessment System

2.1. System Setup

The system hardware is built around a low-cost RGB-Depth camera, the Intel RealSense SR300®, which provides, through its SDK [23], synchronized RGB color and DEPTH streams at 60 frame/sec with resolution of 1280 × 720 and 640 × 480, respectively. The range of depth is from 0.2 m to 1.5 m for use indoors. The SR300 is connected via an USB 3 port to a NUC i7 Intel® mini-PC running Windows® 10 (64×) and equipped with a monitor for the visual feedback of the hand movements of the user. The user equipment consists of black silk gloves with imprinted color markers, which are used both for the gestural control of the system and for task assessments (Figure 1).

The system software is made by custom scripts written in C++ which run on the NUC. The software implements different functionalities: a Human Computer Interface (HCI) based on hand tracking, through the SR300 data stream acquisition, real-time processing and visual feedback; a movement analysis and characterization, through the processing of the fingertip trajectories obtained by the HCI; an automated assessment of the hand movements, through the implementation of trained supervised classifiers.

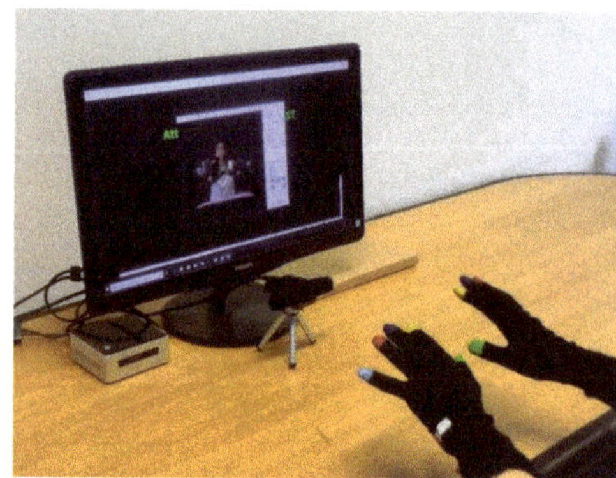

Figure 1. System for the upper limbs analysis: RGB-Depth camera (Intel RealSense® SR300); NUC i7 Intel® mini-PC; lightweight gloves with color markers.

2.2. System Software

2.2.1. Initial Setup for Hand Tracking

At startup of the management software, the system automatically performs an initial setup in which the user is prompted to stay with one hand up and open in front of the camera. During this phase, which lasts only a few seconds, global RGB image brightness adjustment, hand segmentation and color calibration are performed, with the SR300 in manual setting mode. The depth stream is acquired through access to the APIs of the SR300 SDK [23], and it is processed in the OpenCV environment to recover the centroid of the depth points closest to the camera, considered approximately coincident with the hand position [38]. The hand centroid is then used to segment the hand from the background and to define 2D and 3D hand image bounding boxes, both for color and depth images.

A brightness adjustment and a color constancy algorithm are performed to compensate for different ambient lighting conditions. First, the segmented hand RGB streams are converted into the HSV color space, which is more robust to brightness variations [38]. Afterwards, a color constancy algorithm is used to compensate for different ambient lighting conditions [39]. For this purpose, the white circular marker on the palm is detected and tracked by the Hough Transform [38] in the HSV stream. The average luminance is evaluated and used to classify the environmental lighting condition as low, normal or high intensity. The average levels of each HSV component are also evaluated to compensate for predominant color components, which can be due to different types of lighting, such as natural, incandescent lamps and fluorescent lamps: their values are used to scale each of the three HSV video sub-streams during the normal operation phase.

Depending on the measured lighting conditions on the glove (low, normal, high intensity), one triplet out of three of HSV threshold values is chosen for the marker segmentation process during the normal operation phase. These three triplets of thresholds were experimentally evaluated for every specific color of the markers in the three glove lighting conditions considered previously.

2.2.2. Continuous Hand and Finger Tracking

During the normal operation phase, the depth stream segmentation described in the setup phase is performed continuously and the 3D position of the hand centroid is used to update the 2D and 3D hand bounding boxes (Figure 2). The color thresholds, selected in the initial setup phase, are used to detect and track the color blobs of all the markers.

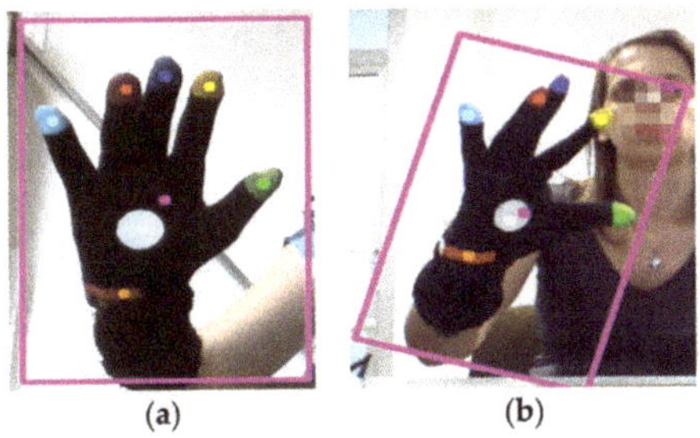

(a)   (b)

Figure 2. Result of the hand segmentation and the detection of color markers; bounding box of the hand with glove and centroids of the color blobs: (**a**) open hand in static and frontal pose; (**b**) semi-closed hand in dynamic and rotated pose.

To improve performance and robustness, the CamShift algorithm [38] was used for the tracking procedure. Cumulative histograms for glove and color markers are used to define the contours of the hand and each color marker more accurately. The 2D pixels of every color marker area are re-projected to their corresponding 3D points by standard re-projection [38], and their 3D centroids are then evaluated. Each 3D centroid is used as an estimation of the 3D position of the corresponding fingertip. The 3D marker trajectories are then used for movement analysis. The accuracy of the system in the 3D hand tracking of the movements, prescribed for upper limb UPDRS assessment, has been compared to other consumer hand trackers software (LMC and RealSense) and the comparison outcomes are shown in Results section.

2.2.3. Human Computer Interface and System Management

The hand tracking capability of the system and the graphical user interface (GUI) of the system management software are used to implement a HCI based on gestural interactions and visual feedback, which provides a natural interface suitable for subjects with limited computer skills and with motor impairments. During the assessment tasks session, the user is guided through the GUI menu by video and textual support and can make choices by simple gestures, such as pointing at the menu items to select and closing the hand or fingers to accept (Figure 3).

To remind the user of the possible choices, or when an incorrect sequence of actions takes place, suggestions are displayed as text output on the screen. At every point during the assessment session, the user can stop the session and quit, if tired, to avoid the onset of stress and/or anxiety. The data of the sessions (video of each task execution, user inputs, finger trajectories and assessment scores) are encrypted and recorded on the system hardware to provide remote supervising facilities to authorized clinicians.

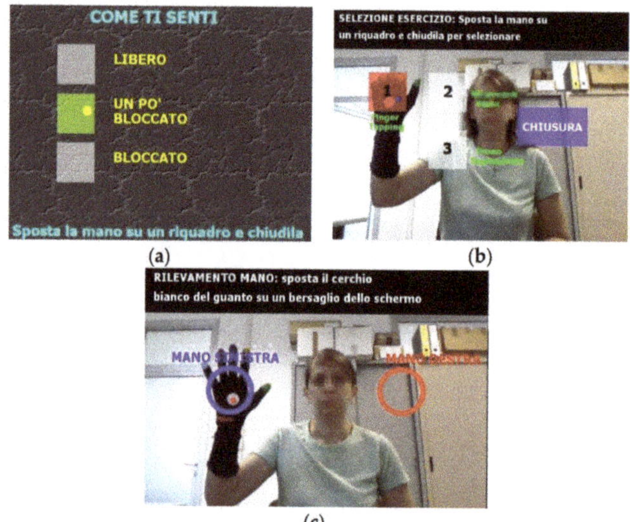

Figure 3. Human computer interface with natural gesture-based interaction: (**a**) patient's input of the perceived motor impairment condition (low, medium, high) by hand positioning and closing on the menu items; (**b**) selection of the motor test (1, FT; 2, OC; 3, PS) by hand positioning and closing on the menu items (**c**) selection of the hand (SX, DX) involved in the motor test by positioning of the hand inside one of the circular targets.

3. Performance Comparison of the HCI Hand Tracker with Consumer Devices

3.1. Experimental Setup

An experimental setup was built to evaluate and compare the accuracy of the HCI, the LMC® and the Intel RealSense® SR300 (Intel Corporation, Santa Clara, CA, USA) [40] in the hand tracking of the FT, OC and PS movements. The comparisons were made by using a DX400 optoelectronic system (BTSBioengineering, Milan, Italy) as gold reference (BTS SMART DX400©, 8 TVC, 100–300 fps) [41].

The LMC hand-tracking device [22] is built around two monochromatic IR cameras and three infrared LEDs, which project patternless IR light in a hemispherical working volume. The IR cameras reliably acquire images of the objects (hands) from 2 cm to 60 cm distance in the working volume, at a frame rate of up to 200 fps. To reduce possible interference among the several Infrared Radiation (IR) light sources of the different devices, the comparison was split into two experiments (Sections 3.1.1

and 3.1.2): in the first one, the HCI, the LMC and the DX400 were involved; in the second one, the HCI, the RealSense SR300 and the DX400 were involved. In both the experiments, the devices' accuracies were evaluated by comparison of the movements captured at the same time by the two devices with the DX400 reference system. It should be noted that we compared two SR300 devices; one is a component of the HCI of our system, and the other is an external device whose proprietary hand tracking firmware was to be assessed. In this case, we compared the performance of our tracking software, based on the processing of color and depth map of the SR300 implementing the HCI, with the proprietary one of the external SR300.

The movements were performed in the smallest working volume common to all the devices. Specifically, both the LMC and the SR300 used in the HCI have a working volume delimited by a truncated pyramid boundary, whose apex is centered on the device and whose top and base distances are defined by the reliable operating range. This range is established according to the device specifications [22,40] and the results of other experimental works [29,35], also taking into account a minimum clearance during movements, to avoid collisions. Consequently, we assume a reliable operating range for the LMC controller from 5 to 50 cm, while that of SR300 of the HCI can be safely reduced respect to the device specifications (20 to 120 cm) from 20 to 100 cm, considering the minimum spatial resolution necessary to track the colored marker at the maximum range. Therefore, the reliable working volume for the LMC is about 0.08 m^3, while that of the HCI is about 0.45 m^3, which is about six times bigger. Then, the smallest working volume common to all the devices is constrained by the LMC one, and therefore the accuracy evaluations and comparisons are limited to this volume.

In the two experiments, five healthy subjects (3 men/2 women) of different heights (from 1.50 to 1.90 m), aged between 25 and 65, were recruited to assess the accuracy of the devices in hand tracking of FT, OC and PS movements. The subjects had no history of neurological, motor and cognitive disorders. The rationale of this choice is to provide a data set of finger trajectories approximately filling the working volume, which are representative both of the specific movements and of the population variability. Moreover, we chose healthy subjects because their movements are faster and of greater amplitude with respect to motor-impaired PD subjects, and therefore they are more challenging for accuracy evaluations. During the experiments, the subjects were seated on a chair facing the HCI and the LMC (or the SR300, in the second experiment), with the chest just beyond the upper range of the working volume. A set of hemispherical retroreflective markers, with diameter of 6 mm, were attached on the fingertips of the subject wearing the HCI glove (Figure 4).

The subjects were told to perform the FT, OC and PS movements as fast and fully as prescribed in UPDRS guidelines [2], with the hand in front of the devices. The movements were performed in different positions, approximately corresponding to the corners and the center of the bounding box of the working volume, with the aid and the supervision of a technician. A total of nine hand positions were sampled in the working volume. The movements were first performed by the right hand in its working volume, then by the left one, after adjusting the chair and subject position to fit its corresponding working volume. The 3D trajectories of the fingers were tracked simultaneously by the HCI and by one of the other two devices, and were then compared with those captured by the DX400 optoelectronic system.

The different 3D positions of the reflective and colored fingertip markers correspond to a 3D displacement vector with constant norm of about 9 mm between their respective 3D centers. This vector was added to the 3D centers of the colored fingertip markers to estimate the "offset free" colored marker trajectory, which was used for the HCI accuracy estimation. To evaluate the influence of the gloves respect to the bare hand on the commercial system accuracy, we performed two preliminary tests. First, we compared the luminance of the IR images of both the bare hand and gloved one, as obtained from the SDKs of the two devices. Please note that, IR images are used as input for the proprietary hand tracking firmware of the LMC. We found no substantial differences between the IR images of the hand in the two cases; neither in the spatial distribution, nor in the intensity of the luminance. Second, as in [29], we compared the fingertip position of a plastic-arm model, fixed on a stand, in different static locations inside the working volume. In every location, we first put on and then removed the glove from the hand, looking at the differences in the 3D fingertip positions for the two conditions. Since we found position differences below 5 mm, we assumed the glove influence to be approximately negligible.

In both the experiments, we checked for possible IR interference among different devices by switching them on and off in all possible combinations, while keeping the hand steady in various positions around the working volume and looking at possible data missing or variations of tracked positions. A safe working zone of approximately $2 \times 2 \times 2$ m in size was found, where the different devices were not influenced by one another. The devices could almost frontally track the hand movement, without line of sight occlusions. In the safe working volume, the claimed accuracy of the DX400 is 0.3 mm, and all markers were seen, at all times, by at least six of the eight cameras placed in a circular layout and few meters around the working zone. Two calibration procedures were used in the two experiments to estimate the coordinate transformation matrices for the alignment of the local coordinate systems of the different devices to the reference coordinate system of the DX400 (Sections 3.1.1 and 3.1.2).

The devices have different sampling frequencies: a fixed sampling rate of 100 sample per second for the DX400, an almost stable sampling rate of 60 sample per second for the SR300, and a variable sampling rate, which cannot be set by the user, for the LMC, ranging from 50 to 115 samples per second in our experiments. Consequently, the 3D trajectory data were recorded and resampled by cubic spline interpolation at 100 samples per second to compare the different 3D measures at the same time. To compare the accuracy of the different tracking devices, we used the simple metrics developed in [37], which provides a framework for the comparison of different computer vision tracking systems (such as the devices under assessment) on benchmark data sets. With respect to [31], where the standard Bland-Altman analysis was conducted to assess the validity and limits of agreement for measures of specific kinematic parameters, we prefer to adopt the following more general approach and not to define, at this point, which kinematic parameters will be used to characterize the movements.

Consider two trajectories X and Y composed of 3D positions at a sequence of time steps i. According to [37], we use the Euclidean distance d_i between two samples positions x_i and y_i at time step i as a measure of the agreement between the two trajectories at time i. The mean D_{mean} of these distances d_i provides quantitative information about the overall difference between X and Y. Here we identify X trajectory as measured by the DX400 reference system, and the distances d_i can be interpreted as positional errors. Then, as in [37], we adopt the mean D_{MEAN}, the standard deviation SD, and the maximum absolute difference MAD $= |d_i|_{max}$ of the d_i sequence as useful statistics for describing the tracking accuracy. Furthermore, we note that, for the tracking accuracy evaluation of the FT, OC and PS movements, the absolute positional error in the working volume is not important; the correctly performed hand movements are necessarily circumscribed to a small bounding box positioned at the discretion of the subject in the working space.

On the other hand, we know the device measurements are subject to depth offsets increasing with the distance from the device [33]. For this reason, some pairs of trajectories may be very similar, except for a constant difference in some spatial direction; that is, an average offset vector $\bar{d}$ (translation) could be present between the trajectories. Since this offset vector is not relevant for characterizing the movements, we subtract it from the d_i sequence before evaluating the accuracy measures [37], (p. 4). The accuracies were evaluated comparing the finger trajectories measured at the same time by one device and the corresponding one measured by the DX400. Only the trajectory parts falling in the working volume were considered in the comparison. The final measure of the device accuracy is obtained by the average values of the D_{MEAN} and the SD evaluated for all the trajectories captured by the device in the working volume, while for the MAD value the maximum over all the trajectories in working volume is considered.

Custom C++ scripts were developed for both the experiments to collect the data through the SDK APIs of the devices, and custom Matlab® scripts (Mathworks Inc, Natick, MA, USA) were developed to perform the alignment of the finger trajectory data from different devices into the common reference frame of the DX400, and to evaluate accuracy measures (see Tables 1 and 2).

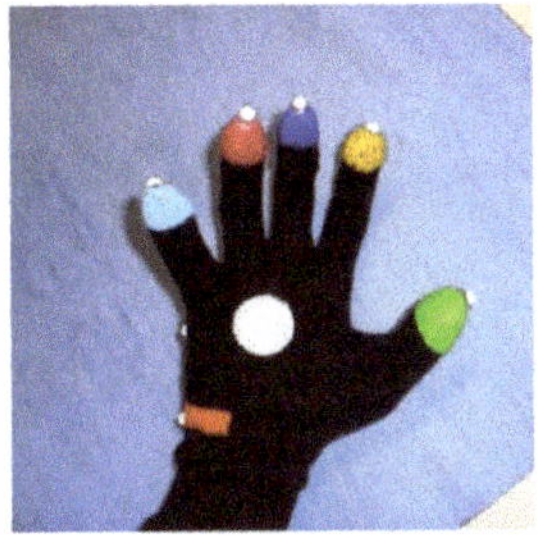

Figure 4. HCI glove with reflective markers on the finger tips.

Table 1. Accuracy of the HCI for FT, OC and PS movements.

Accuracy Parameters	FT	OC	PS
D_{MEAN} (mm)	2.5	3.1	4.1
SD (mm)	3	3.5	4
MAD (mm)	5.2	6.0	7

Table 2. Accuracy of the LMC for FT, OC and PS movements.

Accuracy Parameters	FT	OC	PS
D_{MEAN} (mm)	11.7	13.8	20.1
SD (mm)	13.3	22.8	26.6
MAD (mm)	32.1	35.2	45.1

3.1.1. Leap Motion and HCI Setup

The LMC was positioned facing the subject (the Y axis of the LMC reference system was pointing to the subject's hand) at about 10 cm away from the closest distance of the hand in the working volume, and it was firmly attached on a support to avoid undesired movements of the device. The RGB-Depth sensor of the HCI was placed 10 cm beyond and above the LMC, to avoid direct interferences with the LMC and to allow the maximum overlapping of the working volumes of the two sensors.

An external processing unit (Asus laptop Intel Core i7-8550U, 8 MB Cache) was used to run the scripts accessing the LMC proprietary software (LMC Motion SDK, Core Asset 4.1.1) for real-time data acquisition and logging. The final information provided by the scripts was the positions over time of 22 three-dimensional joints of a complex hand model, which includes fingertips. The LMC Visualizer software was used to monitor, in real time, the reliability of the acquisitions.

The calibration procedure, used to estimate the alignment transformation between the LMC controller and the DX400 coordinate frames, makes use of the same special V-shaped tool (Figure 5a) as in [29], which consists of two wooden sticks fixed on a support and two reflective markers fixed on the stick tips. The tool was moved around the working space and tracked both by the LMC and the DX400. The alignment transformation was estimated as the transformation (roto-translation) which best aligns the two set of tracking data by the two devices.

A different approach was used to estimate the alignment transformation between the coordinate frames of the SR300 device of the HCI and the DX400. A dihedral target, made of three planes orthogonal to each other, was built (Figure 5b). Seven reflective markers were attached at its center and along the axis at a fixed distance from the origin. The depth maps of the SR300 device of the HCI were processed to extract the planes, and to estimate the dihedral plane intersections and their origin in the local coordinate system [42]. The positions of the reflective marker on the plane intersections were measured by the DX400, in the global coordinate system. The alignment transformation was then estimated as the transformation which best aligns the two sets of data tracked by the two devices.

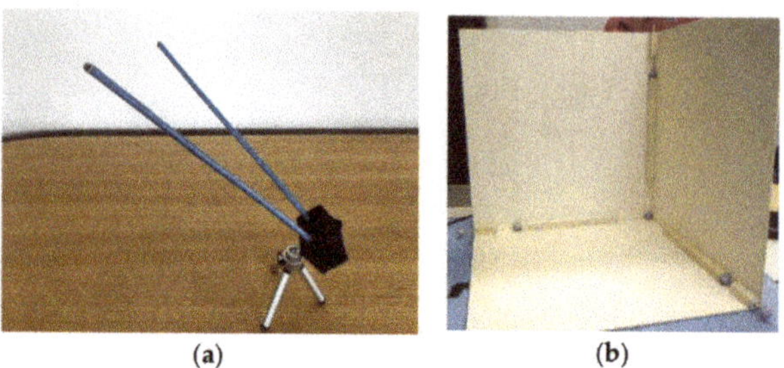

(a)   (b)

Figure 5. Calibration tools: (**a**) V-shaped tool; (**b**) Dihedral tool.

3.1.2. Intel SR300 and HCI Setup

We refer to Section 2.1 for a brief description of the RealSense SR300 features. In this experiment, the Intel SR300 was positioned facing the subject at about 20 cm away from the closest distance of the hand in the working volume, and it was firmly attached on a support to avoid undesired movements. The device transmitted 3D position data of hand and fingertips to the Asus laptop PC (Section 3.1.1) running specifically developed C++ scripts interfacing the SR300 SDK APIs [23] for real-time data acquisition and logging. The same approach described in Section 3.1.1 was used to estimate the alignment transformation between the coordinate frames of the SR300 device respect to the DX400. We note, as in Section 3.1, that we compared two SR300 devices; one is a component of the HCI of our system, and the other is an external device whose proprietary hand tracking firmware was to be assessed.

4. Automated Assessment of Upper Limb UPDRS Tasks

4.1. Clinical Data Acquisition

A cohort of 57 PD patients (37 men/20 women) was recruited to perform the FT, OC and PS tasks (UPDRS Part III, items 3.4, 3.5, 3.6) under the supervision of a neurologist expert in movement disorders and PD. The patients were chosen according the UK Parkinson's Disease Society Brain Bank Clinical Diagnostic standards and met the following criteria: Hoehn and Yahr score (average 2.1, min 1, max 4); age 45–80 years; disease duration 2–29 years. Patients were excluded if they had had previous neurosurgical procedures, tremor severity >1 (UPDRS-III severity score), or cognitive impairment (Mini–Mental State Examination score <27/30). All the patients were allowed to take their routine PD medications. Another cohort of 25 healthy controls (10 men/15 women), aged between 55 and 75, was recruited. Healthy Controls (HC) had no history of neurological, motor and cognitive disorders. Informed consent was obtained in accordance with the Declaration of Helsinki (2008). The study's protocol was approved by the Ethics Committee of the Istituto Auxologico Italiano (Protocol n. 2011_09_27_05).

The PD subjects were seated in front of the system, wearing the gloves of the HCI: their hand movements were acquired during UPDRS tasks execution and then analyzed by the system and scored by the neurologist at the same time. Some of the visual features of interest for the neurologist are rate, rhythm, amplitude, hesitations, halts, decrements in amplitude and speed, as indicated by the UPDRS. The neurologist classified the performances of the PD cohort in four UPDRS levels, i.e., 0 (normal), 1 (slightly impaired), 2 (mildly impaired), 3 (moderately impaired). No patient of the PD cohort was assessed as UPDRS 4 (i.e., severely impaired). The HC subjects performed FT, OC and PS tasks in the same environmental conditions and with the same setup of PD subjects. The system recorded the videos and the 3D trajectories of the PD and HC cohort performances, along with the assigned UPDRS scores of the PD cohort for each single task.

4.2. Movement Characterization by Kinematic Features

As mentioned in the Introduction, the automatic assessment of UPDRS tasks makes use of the well-established correlation existing between kinematic features of the movements and clinical UPDRS scores. An initial set of kinematic parameters, estimated from the 3D trajectories, were used to characterize the hand movements; these parameters are closely related to those features of the movement that are implicitly used by neurologists to score the motor performance of the patient.

The initial sets of kinematic parameters, considered to characterize the hand movements during the FT, OC and PS tasks, consisted of about twenty parameters per task. These parameters are closely related to those features of the movement that are implicitly used by neurologists to score the motor performance of the patient, as described in the Introduction. These initial sets could potentially include irrelevant and redundant parameters which can hide the effects of clinically relevant parameters and reduce the predictive power of the classifiers. Among the most used feature selection (FS) algorithms in machine learning, the Elastic Net (EN) [43] was chosen to reduce the initial parameter sets to the most discriminative subsets. EN is a hybrid of Ridge regression and LASSO regularization. EN encourages a grouping effect on correlated parameters which tends to be in or out of the model together. In contrast, the LASSO tends to select only one variable from the group, removing from the model the other ones. This behavior can generate incorrect models with our set of parameters, that address similar kinematic features and tend to be moderately correlated. In fact, we found this by inspection of the cross-correlation matrices of the parameters evaluated from the FT, OC and PS datasets. The EN selection procedure we used is based on the Matlab$^{®}$ implementation (lasso function with α parameter). The parameter α $(0 \leq \alpha \leq 1)$ controls the function behavior between a Ridge or a LASSO regression.

A dimensionality reduction of the parameter space was performed on the data sets by Principal Component Analysis (PCA), retaining the 98% of the data information content. The sets of parameters which contribute more to the eigenvectors of the PCA representation are compared with those selected by the EN, to check for possible inconsistencies. Depending on the value of α, the number of elements in the selected sets can change, even if the most important parameters remain the same. To stress the parameter correlation with UPDRS scores, the final set of selected parameters are chosen starting from the best ones among those of the EN sets, and taking those having absolute values of the Spearman's correlation coefficient ρ greater than 0.3, at a significance level $p < 0.01$. The selected parameters for FT, OC and PS are shown, respectively, in Tables 3–5 of the Results section. To avoid biasing the results by the different scaling of the parameters not related to clinical aspects, the PD parameters $p_{i\,PD}$ were normalized by the corresponding average parameter values of the HC subjects $p_{i\,HC}$ (Equation (1)); as expected, the average values for healthy subjects are always better than the $p_{i\,PD}$ ones.

$$p_{i\,PD\,Norm} = p_{i\,PD}/p_{i\,HC}, \tag{1}$$

The normalized parameters of Tables 3–5 are able to discriminate the different UPDRS classes for the FT, OC and PS tasks, highlighting the increasing severity of motor impairment by the corresponding increasing of their values. This is confirmed by the radar graphs of the mean values of the kinematic parameters versus UPDRS severity class, as shown in the Results section.

Table 3. List of significant parameters for Finger Tapping task.

Name	Meaning	Spearman Correlation Coefficient ρ
MOm	Mean of Maximum Opening	−0.45
MOv	Variability [1] of Maximum Opening	0.32
MOSm	Mean of Maximum Speed (opening phase)	−0.57
MOSv	Variability [1] of Maximum Speed (opening phase)	0.36
MCSm	Mean of Maximum Speed (closing phase)	−0.58
MCSv	Variability [1] of Maximum Speed (closing phase)	0.40
MAm	Mean of Movement Amplitude	−0.44
MAv	Variability [1] of Movement Amplitude	0.38
Freq	Principal Frequency of voluntary movement	−0.46
Dv	Variability [1] of Movement Duration	0.44

[1] Variability is equivalent to the coefficient of variation CV, defined as the ratio of the standard deviation σ to the mean μ, CV = σ/μ.

Table 4. List of significant parameters for Opening Closing task.

Name	Meaning	Spearman Correlation Coefficient ρ
MOSm	Mean of Maximum Speed (opening phase)	−0.61
MOSv	Variability [1] of Maximum Speed (opening phase)	0.42
MCSm	Mean of Maximum Speed (closing phase)	−0.58
MCSv	Variability [1] of Maximum Speed (closing phase)	0.56
MAm	Mean of Movement Amplitude	−0.57
MAv	Variability [1] of Movement Amplitude	0.34
Dv	Variability [1] of Movement Duration	0.55

[1] Variability is equivalent to the coefficient of variation CV, defined as the ratio of the standard deviation σ to the mean μ, CV = σ/μ.

Table 5. List of significant parameters for Pronation Supination task.

Name	Meaning	Spearman Correlation Coefficient ρ
MRm	Mean of Movement Rotation	−0.30
MRv	Variability [1] of Movement Rotation	0.31
MSSm	Mean of Maximum Speed (supination phase)	−0.48
MSSv	Variability [1] of Maximum Speed (supination phase)	0.36
MPSm	Mean of Maximum Speed (pronation phase)	−0.44
MPSv	Variability [1] of Maximum Speed (pronation phase)	0.43
Freq	Principal Frequency of voluntary movement	−0.43
DSv	Variability [1] of Supination Duration	0.34
DPv	Variability [1] of Pronation Duration	0.35

[1] Variability is equivalent to the coefficient of variation CV, defined as the ratio of the standard deviation σ to the mean μ, CV = σ/μ.

4.3. Automated UPDRS Task Assessment by Supervised Classifiers

Different supervised learning methods were evaluated for the automatic assessment of the FT, OC and PS tasks: Naïve-Bayes (NB) classification, Linear Discriminant Analysis (LDA) [44], Multinomial Logistic Regression (MNR), K-Nearest Neighbors (KNN) [45] and Support Vector Machine (SVM) with polynomial kernel [46]. The NB, LDA, MNR and KNN classifier evaluations were performed in the Matlab® environment using specific toolboxes. The SVM classifiers were implemented with the support of the LIBSVM library package [47], and the SVM kernel parameters optimized using a grid search of possible values. Three specific classifiers, one for each task, were trained for every method using the sets of "selected kinematic parameters vector–neurologist UPDRS score" pairs as input. The leave-one-out and the ten-fold cross validation have been used to evaluate the performance in terms of both accuracy and generalization ability. The accuracies of all the methods were compared both for binary classification (healthy subjects, Parkinsonians) and for multiclass classification (five classes: healthy and four UPDRS classes).

5. Results

5.1. Hand Tracking Accuracy of the HCI Compared to Consumer Devices

5.1.1. HCI—Leap Motion Tracking Accuracy Comparison

The comparison between the accuracy of the HCI tracker respect to the LMC was made for the FT, OC and PS task movements using the DX400 optoelectronic system as reference. The accuracy of HCI in FT, OC, and PS movement tracking, expressed as average values of the mean D_{MEAN}, the standard deviation SD, and the maximum absolute difference MAD (Section 3.1) over the whole set of trajectories are shown in Table 1, while in Table 2, the corresponding values for the LMC are shown.

Furthermore, examples of typical trajectories of the FT, OC and PS task movements are shown in Figure 6. Only the trajectories of representative fingers are considered here, to avoid overcrowded graphs. A reference system, whose X and Y axes are co-planar with the Z and X axes of the LMC, was chosen as the more convenient to represent at best the differences of the trajectories tracked by the different devices. The reference systems for the X and Y components of the OC and PS movements are indicated in Figure 7b,c, respectively. In Figure 6a, the distance between the index and thumb fingertips during the FT task movements is plotted, as estimated by the three devices. In Figure 6b, the Y component of the index finger movements during the OC task movements is plotted, positive when fingers move down and the hand closes (Figure 7b). In Figure 6c, the X component of the pinky finger for the PS task movements is plotted, positive when pinky finger moves left while rotating around the Y axis (Figure 7c). As can be seen in Figure 6a, the LMC shows good responsiveness to very quick FT movements (up to 7 FT cycles/sec), but the finger distance shows overshoots for medium-speed FT cycles and attenuations respect to the reference and the HCI values for high-speed FT cycles. Overall, many incomplete finger closures are present in the lower part of Figure 6a, along with unexpected offsets in slow-speed FT cycles. In contrast with LMC, the HCI response follows much better the reference system. Similar problems can be seen in Figure 6b for the OC task, where a good LMC response is obtained for medium-speed OC cycles, while unexpected offsets and attenuations are present for low and high-speed cycles. Again, the HCI response follows much better the reference system measurements.

The PS task is the most challenging one for the hand trackers, because finger velocity could reach more than 2 m/s. In this task the accuracy of HCI tracker is quite satisfactory as compared to the reference. In Figure 6c, the LMC results for the PS task seem better than those for FT and OC tasks, even if offsets and attenuations are still present. However, if we look at Figure 8, in which the three components of the position of the pinky fingertip during PS movements are shown, some instabilities in the LMC tracker become evident.

We remark that, during PS, the hand faces the LMC and performs PS rotating around its main axis Y (Figure 7c), while the pinky position moves almost along the X axis (Figure 7c). In Figure 8, the first 20 s corresponds to a correct estimation of the hand pose; during rotation, the fingers always point upward along the -Y axis (Figure 7c). Some occasional event of swapping of the X and Z components occurs in the period from 20 to 30 s, as confirmed also from the other finger position values output by the LMC tracker. These events correspond to an inversion of the rotation axis of the PS, from upward to downward, followed by a quick recovering of the correct orientation. Concerning the period from 30 to 45 s, we see that the inversion of the rotation axis of the hand is persistent and evident in the swap of the X, Y and Z components, causing a wrong estimation of the hand movement. In addition, in the final part of the PS period, this behavior leads to a misinterpretation of the performing hand: the task is executed with the right hand but LMC tracker assumes it is performed by the left hand.

Overall, these problems with the LMC tracker limit the feasibility and the accuracy of the kinematic characterization of the hand movements and, consequently, the motor performance assessment based on it.

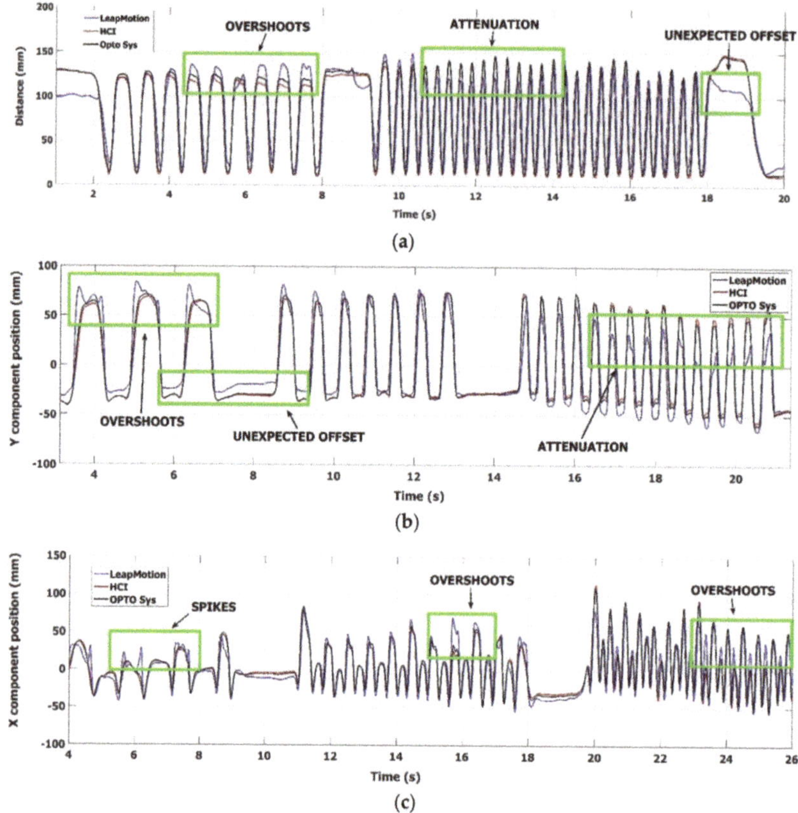

Figure 6. Comparison of the Leap Motion® tracker (blue solid line), the HCI tracker (red solid line) and the optoelectronic system (black solid line) during the execution of the FT, OC and PS motor tasks. The figures show the trajectories simultaneously measured by the three devices: (**a**) distance between thumb and index trajectories during the FT task; (**b**) Y component of the index trajectory during the OC task; (**c**) X component of the pinky trajectory during the PS task.

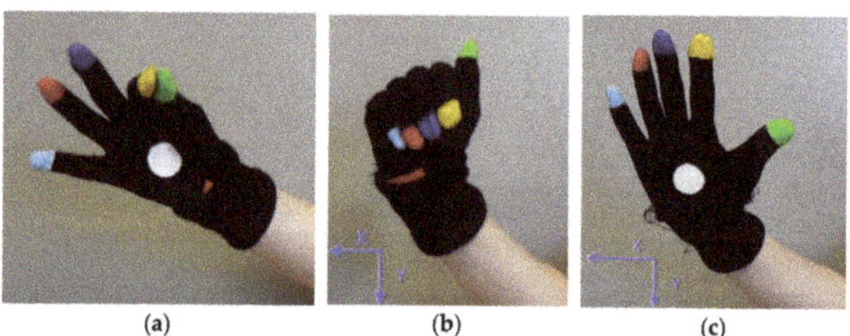

Figure 7. Hand pose without reflective markers during (**a**) FT, (**b**) OC, and (**c**) PS. For OC and PS the reference directions for the components of the movements are shown.

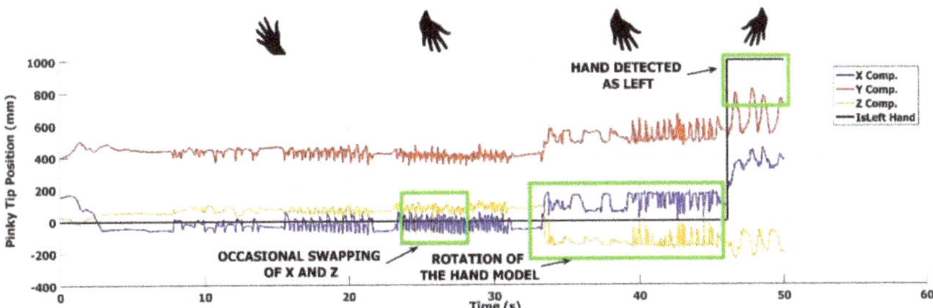

Figure 8. Example of Leap Motion® tracker failures in the pinky tip tracking during a pronation-supination task. The figure shows the three components of the 3D position of the pinky finger during the execution of the movement. After a 20 s period, where the hand pose is correctly estimated, a period of 10 s follows where occasional swapping of the X and Z components occurs. A persistent incorrect estimation of the hand pose occurs in the following 10 s, ending in the final part of the plot with a misinterpretation of the right-hand movements as performed by the left one.

5.1.2. HCI—RealSense SR300 Tracking Accuracy Comparison

The comparison between the accuracy of the HCI and the SR300 trackers was limited to FT task movements, both because the results provide significant indication on the accuracy and because of Intel's intention to discontinue the development of the hand tracking part of the camera firmware [40]. The accuracy of HCI in FT movement tracking, expressed as the average values of the mean D_{MEAN}, the standard deviation SD, and the maximum absolute difference MAD (Section 3.1) over the whole set of trajectories were: D_{MEAN} = 21.1 mm; SD = 32.5 mm; MAD = 56.3 mm.

A typical result of the FT task performance execution is shown in Figure 9, where the distance between the index and thumb fingertips is plotted. The accuracy of the SR300 tracking firmware as compared to the HCI and to the optoelectronic reference system is clearly limited, especially in the period from 14 to 20 s, where the SR300 tracked distance shows large errors as compared to the distance measured by the HCI and the reference system. This period corresponds to high-speed FT movements, where in many cases the closing distance in the FT cycle does not correspond to a true fingers closure (P1 in Figure 9), or the true maximum amplitude is missed (P2 in Figure 9).

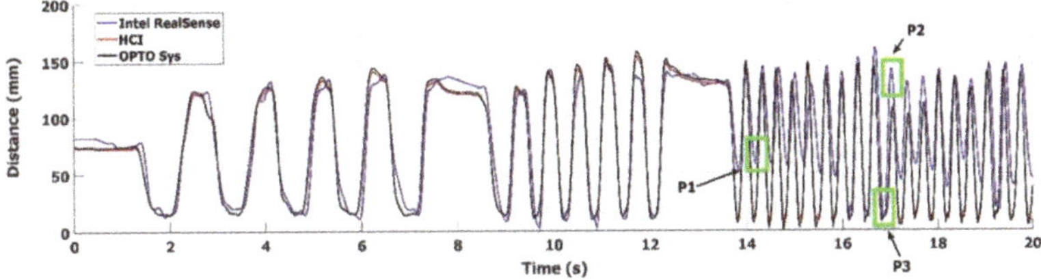

Figure 9. Comparison of the Intel RealSense® and the HCI trackers during the execution of FT task movements. The figure shows the estimated distance between the thumb and the index fingers measured by the Intel RealSense® tracker (blue solid line), the HCI tracking algorithm (red solid line) and the optoelectronic reference system (black solid line).

These problems are emphasized in Figure 10, where the 3D fingertip positions are re-projected on the SR300 RGB images. The incorrectly estimated closure of the peak P1 in Figure 9 is highlighted in Figure 10a, where the re-projected position of the index fingertip is incorrectly assigned to the middle fingertip (upper green filled circle). Some instability in the tracking of the hand model is apparent by comparison of Figure 10a,b, where two quite similar hand poses, corresponding to the peak P1 and P3 in Figure 9, gives a wrong distance estimation in Figure 10a and a correct one in Figure 10b.

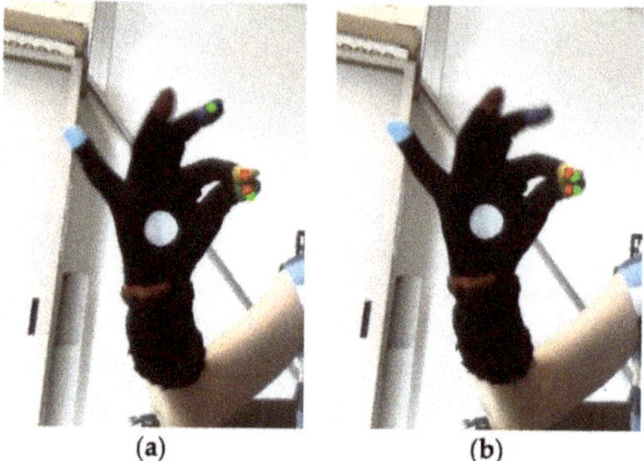

(a)   (b)

Figure 10. 2D re-projections on RGB images of the 3D fingertip positions. Thumb and index from Intel RealSense® tracker (green filled circles) versus thumb and index positions as estimated by the HCI tracker (red filled rectangles): (**a**) Incorrectly evaluated position of index finger by the Intel RealSense® tracker (joint on middle finger, P1 in Figure 9); (**b**) Correctly evaluated position of the index finger for Intel RealSense® tracker (P3 in Figure 9).

5.2. Selection of Discriminant Kinematic Parameters

The parameter selection procedure retains those kinematic parameters which best correlate with neurologist UPDRS scores of the FT, OC and PS tasks. The results of the selection are shown in Tables 3–5 for the FT, OC and PS tasks, respectively. The parameter labels, the parameter meaning and the Spearman's ρ values and sign of the correlation are shown in columns 1, 2 and 3, respectively. The good correlation of the selected parameters with the UPDRS scores is an important requirement for the automated assessment.

The mean values of the kinematic parameters versus the UPDRS severity class are shown in the radar graphs of Figure 11. The parameters were chosen such that increasing values indicate a worsening of the performance, which is visualized as a corresponding expansion of the related graph. As can be seen, almost all the selected parameters discriminate between different UPDRS severity classes. The different graphs are encapsulated and do not overlap, which means that, on the average, a monotonic increasing of the parameter value correspond to an increasing (i.e., worsening) of the UPDRS score.

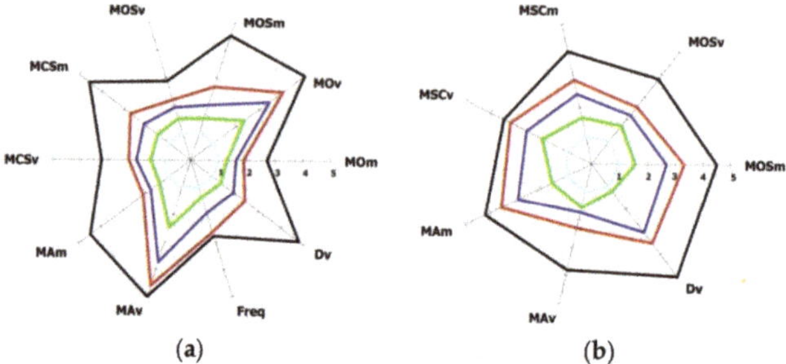

(a)   (b)

Figure 11. *Cont.*

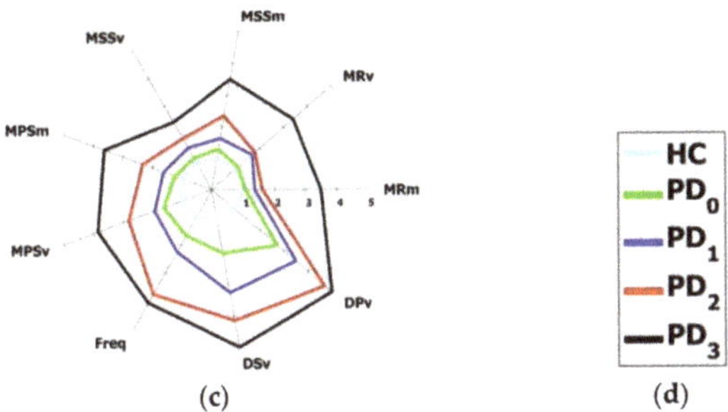

Figure 11. Radar plots of the mean values of the normalized kinematic parameters vs. the UPDRS severity class for the three upper limbs tasks: (**a**) Finger Tapping; (**b**) Opening-Closing; (**c**) Pronation-Supination. (**d**) Radar plots legend with HC and PD severity classes.

5.3. Accuracies of the Supervised Classifiers in UPDRS Task Assessment

The results of the preliminary comparison among different supervised learning methods are shown in Table 6, in which classification accuracies, resulting from the leave-one-out and 10-fold cross validation methods for binary and multiclass classification problems, are reported. The "HEALTHY vs. PD" columns refer to the binary classification problem (healthy versus parkinsonian subjects), while "HEALTHY vs. UPDRS" columns refer to the five-classes classification problem (healthy subjects versus UPDRS scores of parkinsonian subjects). The obtained results suggested the use of SVM, not only for an overall greater mean accuracy, but also for the ability to limit the classification errors to one UPDRS score, unlike the other methods that sometimes generated classification errors greater than one UPDRS score. This is also an important requirement for obtaining the best agreement with the standard neurological assessment.

Table 6. Accuracies of classifiers for cross validation method and classification test.

Task	Classifier	HEALTHY vs. PD		HEALTHY vs. UPDRS	
		Leave-One-Out	10-Fold [1]	Leave-One-Out	10-Fold [1]
FT	NB	91.19	91.70	59.94	59.45
	LDA	93.71	93.71	66.31	66.63
	MNR	95.60	95.60	73.35	73.06
	SVM	98.23	98.44	76.06	76.71
	KNN	93.71	94.10	69.69	69.22
OC	NB	86.67	86.16	58.19	58.84
	LDA	88.57	88.57	61.05	61.56
	MNR	90.48	91.44	65.95	66.21
	SVM	90.48	90.06	65.14	65.24
	KNN	89.52	90.34	59.14	59.17
PS	NB	98.97	98.97	56.67	56.79
	LDA	91.75	91.75	55.67	57.10
	MNR	98.97	98.70	56.79	56.51
	SVM	98.97	98.97	58.73	58.87
	KNN	98.97	97.94	57.82	58.25

[1] mean accuracy on 500 classification trials.

As a consequence of the preliminary comparison activity and focusing on the automated assessment of the UPDRS tasks, after the training by experimental data, the SVM supervised classifiers for the FT, OC and PS tasks have been validated by the leave-one-out cross validation method only on the PD cohort (four classes). The absolute classification error $e_c = |C_i - C'_i|$, defined as the difference between the UPDRS class C assigned by the neurologist and the estimated UPDRS class C', was never greater than 1 UPDRS class for all the tasks. Furthermore, the mean value of the error over the patients' cohort for FT, OC and PS task was 0.12, 0.27 and 0.60, respectively. The classification performance of the classifiers has been evaluated by their confusion matrices and expressed concisely in terms of accuracy, defined as the number of true positives plus the number of true negatives, divided by the total number of instances. In our experiment, we used multi-class classifiers trained on almost balanced classes. In this case, the per-class accuracy, where the class classification accuracies are averaged over the classes, is more appropriate [48]. The resulting accuracies values obtained by the cross-validation methods for the FT, OC and PS classifiers are 76%, 65% and 58%, respectively.

6. Discussion

In this paper, a self-managed system for the automated assessment of Parkinson's disease at home is presented. The core of the system is a low-cost non-invasive human computer interface which provides both a gesture-based interaction for the self-management of the task executions and, at the same time, the characterization of the patient movements by an accurate hand tracking.

Tracking accuracy is important because the automated assessment makes use of the correlation existing between kinematic parameters of the hand movements and the severity of the impairment.

6.1. Accuracy Comparison of the HCI Tracker Respect to Commercial Devices

We compared the accuracy of our HCI tracker with possible alternatives of widely used consumer hand tracking devices such as LMC and the Intel RealSense SR300.

The results of the comparison highlight some problems with these tracking devices. The accuracy of LMC in hand movement tracking is about ten times worse with respect to the HCI in the working volume, as shown in Tables 1 and 2 also in the trajectory example of Figures 7 and 8. In particular, the maximum absolute difference MAD has a considerably large value; this is probably due to some inconsistency in the tracking, which occurs randomly, as shown in Figure 8.

These results are consistent with those reported in [31,32] and in contrast to previous studies [28,29]. The fingertip speed is expected to increase from FT to OC movements and to reach maximum values for PS. A decrease in accuracy with speed is expected, and confirmed by the accuracy values of Tables 1 and 2 for both the HCI and the LMC, which become worse as movement speed increases. The accuracy of proprietary hand tracker of the SR300 in the working volume for FT movement is even worse respect to the HCI; amplitude attenuations and missed closures of the fingertips are present, as shown in Figure 9. For conciseness reasons, we averaged the accuracy values for all the hand trajectories in the working volume, but considering the not aggregated values, we noted a worsening of the accuracy for the performances whose hand position is far from the device, as expected.

Between the two devices, LMC is, at the moment, the only device able to track high-speed movements, but unexpected offsets and attenuations in the tracked trajectories are present and, for the most challenging high-speed movements of the PS task, severe inconsistencies on the fingertip and hand pose estimation occur. This is not unexpected, since the device is intended for general purpose applications, mainly in VR environments, while our tracking application is specialized on specific high-speed hand movements. On the other hand, the trajectories tracked by our HCI are satisfyingly close to those of the optoelectronic reference.

Another problem with LMC is the working volume, which is very limited (0.08 m^3) respect to the HCI one (0.45 m^3); the user is forced to perform the motor tasks in a constrained environment, and this is an important limitation for the usability of the device by motor impaired people.

Nevertheless, care must be taken in extrapolating these accuracy results to more general tracking applications; effects on accuracy due to the several infrared sources present in the experiment have been experimentally evaluated, but more systematic work is necessary to exclude any interference. Furthermore, the typical short product life span of these consumer tracking devices and of the related software support rise concerns on their widespread use. Intel's recent decision to discontinue the hand tracking firmware development for RealSense camera family is an example. Even if this decision has no impact on our PD assessment system, this is one more reason not to rely on solutions too dependent on closed and proprietary hand tracking firmware.

6.2. Kinematic Parameter Selection

A second goal of this work was the selection of the kinematic parameters of the hand movements which best correlate with clinical UPDRS scores. The Spearman non-parametric rank correlation was adopted to make the selection more robust to possible non-linear relationship between scores and parameters. The choice for this preliminary experiment to employ only one rater was dictated by the reason to not introduce, in the training datasets, different biases and noise due both to inter-rater disagreement and to the different sensitivity of the raters to specific motor aspects. The final choice for the best parameters was effective, as the radar plots of Figure 11 show, but heuristic, being based on the threshold on the Spearman correlation value combined with the visual evidence of discriminant power of the parameters on the radar plots. This discriminative power is different for each parameter; Freq for FT, or MRv and MRm for PS seem less discriminant than others when differentiating among the UPDRS classes (Figure 11), but only the last two have low correlation values. This indicates that the radar graphs catch only a part of the interdependence between UPDRS scores and parameters. Among the aspects not yet explored in this work, there is the integration of the assessments from more than one neurologist in the training set, and the pruning of some parameters of the selected set that are highly correlated each other.

6.3. Automated Assessments by Supervised Classifiers

The third goal of this work was the automation of the assessment by means of supervised classifiers trained on the selected parameters and the related UPDRS scores. SVM classifiers were chosen for their better performance on our training dataset with respect to the other types of classifiers we tested. We compared our results for classification accuracy with the results of some recent studies, even if many of them reported results only for the FT task and for binary classification (Healthy vs. Parkinsonian, HvsP). In particular, in [11], the UPDRS classes of the PD cohort were grouped, reducing the classification from multi-classes to a binary classification and declaring an accuracy for FT from 87.2% to 96.5%, depending on the grouping strategy. In [13], the HvsP binary classification was addressed, reporting a lower classification accuracy for FT (95.8%) with respect to our results, but on a wider cohort. In the same study, the results for the multi-classes classification are not directly comparable, since the classification was reduced to a 3-classes problem, resulting in a greater average classification accuracy for the FT task (around 82%). The classification results in [16] are limited to the HvsP binary classification for all the upper limbs UPDRS tasks. However, only the maximum accuracy for each classifier was included, ranging from 71.4% to 85.7%. Finally, the HvsP binary classification was also addressed in [18], and the results were reported for each UPDRS task; in this case, the classification accuracies ranged from 87.5% for PS to 100% for FT, but on a very limited number of HC and PD subjects. In conclusion, our results concerning the HvsP binary classification accuracy are overall better than the results of the previous studies mentioned [13,16,18] (see Table 6). Moreover, our results also seem good for the multi-classification case (e.g., [13]), considering that our classifiers addressed more classes than other studies. The classification accuracies obtained for the FT, OC and PS assessment tasks indicate that the classification errors were limited to 1 UPDRS class at most, and well below, on average. This result is compatible with the inter-rater agreement values usually found among neurologists for these tasks. A limitation of the present approach is that the subjectivity of the neurology judgment influences the machine learning process and, as a matter of fact, the classifiers mimic a particular neurologist. By using one neurologist, we reduce the inter-rater disagreement "noise" generally present in the training data of two or more neurologists but, of course, we reduce also the generalizing capabilities and the robustness of the automated assessment. Further work is required both to increase the training data set with the contribution of other neurologists and to harmonize their assessments. An important difference between the assessments of the system and those of the neurologists is that the system assesses the same motor performance with the same score, and do not show intra-rater disagreements. Summarizing, the results indicate that automated assessments of the upper limb tasks replicates the clinical ones, demonstrating its effectiveness in monitoring of PD at home. The present work is part of a project aimed at bringing the automated assessment of many UPDRS items into the home, for a more comprehensive assessment of the neuro-motor status of PD patients.

7. Conclusions

In this paper, a self-managed system for the automated assessment of Parkinson's disease at home is presented. The automated assessment is focused on upper limb motor tasks as specified by standard assessment scales. The core of the system is a low-cost human computer interface which provides gesture-based interaction for the self-management of the task executions and an accurate characterization of the patient movements by selected kinematic parameters. The hand tracking accuracy of the system has been compared favorably with popular consumer alternatives.

The correlation between selected kinematic parameters and clinical UPDRS scores of patient performance has been used for the automated assessment by a machine learning approach based on supervised classifiers. The classifiers were trained by the assessments collected by the system and by a neurologist on cohorts of PD patients in an experimental campaign. The results on trained classifier performance show that automated assessments of the system replicate clinical ones, demonstrating its effectiveness. Furthermore, the system interface allows gestural interactions with visual feedback, providing a system management suitable for motor impaired users in home monitoring of Parkinson's disease.

Author Contributions: C.F. and R.N. designed and developed the system, analyzed the PD data and wrote the paper; A.C. and G.P. gave technical support on the development and contributed to review the paper; N.C. and V.C. provided the optoelectronic facilities and data; C.A., G.A., L.P. and A.M. designed and supervised the clinical experiment on PD subjects and assessed the patients' performance.

Funding: This work was partially supported by VREHAB project, funded by the Italian Ministry of Health (RF-2009-1472190).

Conflicts of Interest: The authors declare no conflict of interest.

References

1.   Pal, G.; Goetz, C.G. Assessing bradykinesia in Parkinsonian Disorders. *Front. Neurol.* **2013**, *4*, 54. [CrossRef] [PubMed]

2.   Goetz, C.G.; Tilley, B.C.; Shaftman, S.R.; Stebbins, G.T.; Fahn, S.; Martinez-Martin, P.; Poewe, W.; Sampaio, C.; Stern, M.B.; Dodel, R. Movement Disorder Society-sponsored revision of the Unified Parkinson's Disease Rating Scale (MDS-UPDRS): Scale presentation and clinimetric testing results. *Mov. Disord.* **2008**, *23*, 2129–2170. [CrossRef] [PubMed]

3.   Espay, A.J.; Giuffrida, J.P.; Chen, R.; Payne, M.; Mazzella, F.; Dunn, E.; Vaughan, J.E.; Duker, A.P.; Sahay, A.; Kim, S.J.; et al. Differential Response of Speed, Amplitude and Rhythm to Dopaminergic Medications in Parkinson's Disease. *Mov. Disord.* **2011**, *26*, 2504–2508. [CrossRef] [PubMed]

4.   Espay, A.J.; Bonato, P.; Nahab, F.B.; Maetzler, W.; Dean, J.M.; Klucken, J.; Eskofier, B.M.; Merola, A.; Horak, F.; Lang, A.E.; et al. Movement Disorders Society Task Force on Technology. Technology in Parkinson's disease: Challenges and opportunities. *Mov. Disord.* **2016**, *31*, 1272–1282. [CrossRef] [PubMed]

5.   Patel, S.; Lorincz, K.; Hughes, R.; Huggins, N.; Growdon, J.; Standaert, D.; Akay, M.; Dy, J.; Welsh, M.; Bonato, P. Monitoring Motor Fluctuations in Patients with Parkinson's Disease Using Wearable Sensors. *IEEE Trans. Inf. Technol. Biomed.* **2009**, *13*, 864–873. [CrossRef] [PubMed]

6.   Richards, M.; Marder, K.; Cote, L.; Mayeux, R. Interrater reliability of the Unified Parkinson's Disease Rating Scale motor examination. *Mov. Disord.* **1994**, *9*, 89–91. [CrossRef] [PubMed]

7. Mera, T.O.; Heldman, D.A.; Espay, A.J.; Payne, M.; Giuffrida, J.P. Feasibility of home-based automated Parkinson's disease motor assessment. *J. Neurosci. Methods* **2012**, *203*, 152–156. [CrossRef] [PubMed]

8. Heldman, D.A.; Giuffrida, J.P.; Chen, R.; Payne, M.; Mazzella, F.; Duker, A.P.; Sahay, A.; Kim, S.J.; Revilla, F.J.; Espay, A.J. The modified bradykinesia rating scale for Parkinson's disease: Reliability and comparison with kinematic measures. *Mov. Disord.* **2011**, *26*, 1859–1863. [CrossRef] [PubMed]

9. Taylor Tavares, A.L.; Jefferis, G.S.; Koop, M.; Hill, B.C.; Hastie, T.; Heit, G.; Bronte-Stewart, H.M. Quantitative measurements of alternating finger tapping in Parkinson's disease correlate with UPDRS motor disability and reveal the improvement in fine motor control from medication and deep brain stimulation. *Mov. Disord.* **2005**, *20*, 1286–1298. [CrossRef] [PubMed]

10. Espay, A.J.; Beaton, D.E.; Morgante, F.; Gunraj, C.A.; Lang, A.E.; Chen, R. Impairments of speed and amplitude of movement in Parkinson's disease: A pilot study. *Mov. Disord.* **2009**, *24*, 1001–1008. [CrossRef] [PubMed]

11. Stamatakis, J.; Ambroise, J.; Cremers, J.; Sharei, H.; Delvaux, V.; Macq, B.; Garraux, G. Finger Tapping Clinimetric Score Prediction in Parkinson's Disease Using Low-Cost Accelerometers. *Comput. Intell. Neurosci.* **2013**, *2013*. [CrossRef] [PubMed]

12. Oess, N.P.; Wanek, J.; Curt, A. Design and evaluation of a low-cost instrumented glove for hand function assessment. *J. Neuroeng. Rehabil.* **2012**, *9*, 2. [CrossRef] [PubMed]

13. Khan, T.; Nyholm, D.; Westin, J.; Dougherty, M. A computer vision framework for finger-tapping evaluation in Parkinson's disease. *Artif. Intell. Med.* **2014**, *60*, 27–40. [CrossRef] [PubMed]

14. Ferraris, C.; Nerino, R.; Chimienti, A.; Pettiti, G.; Pianu, D.; Albani, G.; Azzaro, C.; Contin, L.; Cimolin, V.; Mauro, A. Remote monitoring and rehabilitation for patients with neurological diseases. In Proceedings of the 10th International Conference on Body Area Networks (BODYNETS 2014), London, UK, 29 September–1 October 2014; pp. 76–82.

15. Jobbagy, A.; Harcos, P.; Karoly, R.; Fazekas, G. Analysis of finger-tapping movement. *J. Neurosci. Methods* **2005**, *141*, 29–39. [CrossRef] [PubMed]

16. Butt, A.H.; Rovini, E.; Dolciotti, C.; Bongioanni, P.; De Petris, G.; Cavallo, F. Leap motion evaluation for assessment of upper limb motor skills in Parkinson's disease. In Proceedings of the 2017 International Conference on Rehabilitation Robotics (ICORR), London, UK, 17–20 July 2017; pp. 116–121. [CrossRef]

17. Bank, J.M.P.; Marinus, J.; Meskers, C.G.M.; De Groot, J.H.; Van Hilten, J.J. Optical Hand Tracking: A Novel Technique for the Assessment of Bradykinesia in Parkinson's Disease. *Mov. Disord. Clin. Pract.* **2017**, *4*, 875–883. [CrossRef]

18. Dror, B.; Yanai, E.; Frid, A.; Peleg, N.; Goldenthal, N.; Schlesinger, I.; Hel-Or, H.; Raz, S. Automatic assessment of Parkinson's Disease from natural hands movements using 3D depth sensor. In Proceedings of the IEEE 28th Convention of Electrical & Electronics Engineers in Israel (IEEEI 2014), Eliat, Israel, 3–5 December 2014.

19. Ferraris, C.; Pianu, D.; Chimienti, A.; Pettiti, G.; Cimolin, V.; Cau, N.; Nerino, R. Evaluation of Finger Tapping Test Accuracy using the LeapMotion and the Intel RealSense Sensors. In Proceedings of the 37th International Conference of the IEEE Engineering in Medicine and Biology Society (EMBC 2015), Milan, Italy, 25–29 August 2015.

20. Han, J.; Shao, L.; Shotton, J. Enhanced computer vision with Microsoft Kinect sensor: A review. *IEEE Trans. Cybern.* **2013**, *43*, 1318–1334. [CrossRef] [PubMed]

21. Galna, B.; Jackson, D.; Mhiripiri, D.; Olivier, P.; Rochester, L. Accuracy of the Microsoft Kinect sensor for measuring movement in people with Parkinson's disease. *Gait Posture* **2014**, *39*, 1062–1068. [CrossRef] [PubMed]

22. Leap Motion Controller. Available online: https://www.leapmotion.com (accessed on 3 August 2018).

23. Intel Developer Zone. Available online: https://software.intel.com/en-us/realsense/previous (accessed on 3 August 2018).

24. Lu, W.; Tong, Z.; Chu, J. Dynamic Hand Gesture Recognition with Leap Motion Controller. *IEEE Signal Process. Lett.* **2016**, *23*, 1188–1192. [CrossRef]

25. Bassily, D.; Georgoulas, C.; Guetler, J.; Linner, T.; Bock, T. Intuitive and Adaptive Robotic Arm Manipulation using the Leap Motion Controller. In Proceedings of the 41st International Symposium on Robotics (ISR/Robotik 2014), Munich, Germany, 2–3 June 2014.

26. Iosa, M.; Morone, G.; Fusco, A.; Castagnoli, M.; Fusco, F.R.; Pratesi, L.; Paolucci, S. Leap motion controlled videogame-based therapy for rehabilitation of elderly patients with subacute stroke: A feasibility pilot study. *Top. Stroke Rehabil.* **2015**, *22*, 306–313. [CrossRef] [PubMed]

27. Marin, G.; Dominio, F.; Zanuttigh, P. Hand gesture recognition with jointly calibrated Leap Motion and depth sensor. *Multimed. Tools Appl.* **2016**, *75*, 14991–15015. [CrossRef]

28. Weichert, F.; Bachmann, D.; Rudak, B.; Fisseler, D. Analysis of the Accuracy and Robustness of the Leap Motion. *Sensors* **2013**, *13*, 6380–6393. [CrossRef] [PubMed]

29. Guna, J.; Jakus, G.; Pogacnik, M.; Tomazic, S.; Sodnik, J. An analysis of the precision and reliability of the leap motion sensor and its suitability for static and dynamic tracking. *Sensors* **2014**, *14*, 3702–3720. [CrossRef] [PubMed]

30. Smeragliuolo, A.H.; Hill, N.J.; Disla, L.; Putrino, D. Validation of the Leap Motion Controller using markered motion capture technology. *J. Biomech.* **2016**, *49*, 1742–1750. [CrossRef] [PubMed]

31. Niechwiej-Szwedo, E.; Gongalez, D.; Nouredanesh, M.; Tung, J. Evaluation of the Leap Motion Controller during the performance of visually-guided upper limb movements. *PLoS ONE* **2018**, *13*, e0193639. [CrossRef] [PubMed]

32. Tung, J.Y.; Lulic, T.; Gonzalez, D.A.; Tran, J.; Dickerson, C.R.; Roy, E.A. Evaluation of a portable markerless finger position capture device: Accuracy of the Leap Motion controller in healthy adults. *Physiol. Meas.* **2015**, *36*, 1025–1035. [CrossRef] [PubMed]

33. Carfagni, M.; Furferi, R.; Governi, L.; Servi, M.; Uccheddu, F.; Volpe, Y. On the performance of the Intel SR300 depth camera: Metrological and critical characterization. *IEEE Sens. J.* **2017**, *17*, 4508–4519. [CrossRef]

34. Asselin, M.; Lasso, A.; Ungi, T.; Fichtinger, G. Towards webcam-based tracking for interventional navigation. In Proceedings of the Medical Imaging 2018: Image-Guided Procedures, Robotic Interventions, and Modeling, Huston, TX, USA, 10–15 February 2018; Volume 10576. [CrossRef]

35. House, R.; Lasso, A.; Harish, V.; Baum, Z.; Fichtinger, G. Evaluation of the Intel RealSense SR300 camera for image-guided interventions and application in vertebral level localization. In Proceedings of the Medical Imaging 2017: Image-Guided Procedures, Robotic Interventions, and Modeling, Orlando, FL, USA, 11–16 February 2017; Volume 10135. [CrossRef]

36. Intel RealSense SDK. Available online: https://software.intel.com/en-us/realsense-sdk-windows-eol (accessed on 6 August 2018).

37. Needham, C.J.; Boyle, R.D. Performance evaluation metrics and statistics for positional tracker evaluation. In Proceedings of the International Conference on Computer Vision Systems, Graz, Austria, 1–3 April 2003; Springer: Berlin/Heidelberg, Germany, 2003; pp. 278–289.

38. Bradski, G.; Kaehler, A. *Learning OpenCV: Computer Vision with the OpenCV Library*; O'Reilly Media: Sebastopol, CA, USA, 2008; 580p.

39. Lee, D.; Plataniotis, K.N. A Taxonomy of Color Constancy and Invariance Algorithms. In *Advances in Low-Level Color Image Processing*; Springer: Dordrecht, The Netherlands, 2014; pp. 55–94.

40. Intel RealSense Archived. Available online: https://software.intel.com/en-us/articles/introducing-the-intel-realsense-camera-sr300 (accessed on 11 August 2018).

41. BTS S.p.A. Products. Available online: http://www.btsbioengineering.com/it/prodotti/smart-dx (accessed on 11 August 2018).

42. Point Cloud Library. Available online: http://pointclouds.org (accessed on 3 August 2018).

43. Zou, H.; Hastie, T. Regularization and variable selection via the elastic net. *J. R. Stat. Soc. Ser. B* **2005**, *67*, 301–320. [CrossRef]

44. Fisher, A. The Use of Multiple Measurements in Taxonomic Problems. *Annu. Hum. Genet.* **1936**, *7*, 179–188. [CrossRef]

45. Data Mining: Practice Machine Learning Tools and Techniques. Available online: https://www.cs.waikato.ac.nz/ml/weka/book.html (accessed on 28 September 2018).

46. Vapnik, V.N. An overview of statistical learning theory. *IEEE Trans. Neural Netw.* **1999**, *10*, 988–999. [CrossRef] [PubMed]

47. Chang, C.C.; Lin, C.J. LIBSVM: A library for support vector machines. *ACM Trans. Intell. Syst. Technol.* **2011**, *2*, 27. [CrossRef]

48. Sokolova, M.; Lapalme, G. A systematic analysis of performance measures for classification tasks. *Inf. Process. Manag.* **2009**, *45*, 427–437. [CrossRef]

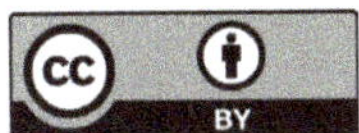

© 2018 by the authors. Licensee MDPI, Basel, Switzerland. This article is an open access article distributed under the terms and conditions of the Creative Commons Attribution (CC BY) license (http://creativecommons.org/licenses/by/4.0/).

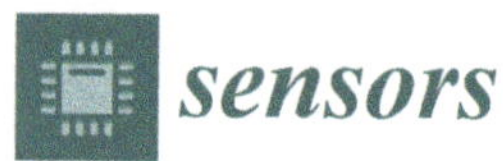 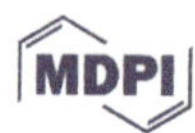

Article

Gait Study of Parkinson's Disease Subjects Using Haptic Cues with A Motorized Walker

Minhua Zhang [1], N. Sertac Artan [1], Huanying Gu [1], Ziqian Dong [1,*], Lyudmila Burina Ganatra [2], Suzanna Shermon [2] and Ely Rabin [2]

[1] College of Engineering and Computing Sciences, New York Institute of Technology, New York, NY 10023, USA; mzhang16@nyit.edu (M.Z.); nartan@nyit.edu (N.S.A.); hgu03@nyit.edu (H.G.)

[2] College of Osteopathic Medicine, New York Institute of Technology, 101 Northern Blvd, Glen Head, NY 11545, USA; lburina@nyit.edu (L.B.G.); sshermon@nyit.edu (S.S.); ely_rabin@sciarc.edu (E.R.)

* Correspondence: ziqian.dong@nyit.edu; Tel.: +1-646-273-6129

Received: 11 September 2018; Accepted: 17 October 2018; Published: 19 October 2018

Abstract: Gait abnormalities are one of the distinguishing symptoms of patients with Parkinson's disease (PD) that contribute to fall risk. Our study compares the gait parameters of people with PD when they walk through a predefined course under different haptic speed cue conditions (1) without assistance, (2) pushing a conventional rolling walker, and (3) holding onto a self-navigating motorized walker under different speed cues. Six people with PD were recruited at the New York Institute of Technology College of Osteopathic Medicine to participate in this study. Spatial posture and gait data of the test subjects were collected via a VICON motion capture system. We developed a framework to process and extract gait features and applied statistical analysis on these features to examine the significance of the findings. The results showed that the motorized walker providing a robust haptic cue significantly improved gait symmetry of PD subjects. Specifically, the asymmetry index of the gait cycle time was reduced from 6.7% when walking without assistance to 0.56% and below when using a walker. Furthermore, the double support time of a gait cycle was reduced by 4.88% compared to walking without assistance.

Keywords: Parkinson's Diseases; motorized walker; haptic cue; gait pattern; statistics study

---

1. Introduction

Individuals with Parkinson's disease (PD) may suffer from movement disorders [1]. The initial symptoms include involuntary tremors of hands, arms, or legs, slow movement, rigidity, and postural instability. These symptoms lead to different gait disturbances [2]. Stolze et al. found that people with PD had a significant spatiotemporal parameters reduction in step length and walking velocity compared with healthy individuals [3]. Individuals with PD may also experience difficulties in step initiation and in postural changes [4]. Although dopaminergic medications, which increase the levels of dopamine in the brain, may help improve gait, their effectiveness decreases as the disease progresses [5].

A growing body of research has demonstrated that individuals with PD can benefit from various cueing devices [6–8]. Individuals with PD increased their pedaling rate under auditory cueing (provided by a metronome) and visual cueing (presented as central road markers) conditions [9,10]. Individuals with PD can benefit from haptic (touch and proprioception) feedback to improve balance. Haptic cues from the use of a walking stick [11], and visual cues from a laser cane reduce forward/backward and side to side movements [6]. Gait patterns of PD patients walking straight on a level ground without assistance were well investigated [2,4,12,13].

The aim of this study is to investigate the immediate gait modifications of individuals with PD when they switch from walking without assistance to walking with a conventional and a motorized walker. We attempt to answer two questions: (1) Can haptic cues help improve the motor performance of patients? and (2) how effectively do PD subjects adapt to various speed cues?

Our analysis showed that test subjects walking with a conventional walker and a motorized walker showed better gait symmetry performance than walking without assistance. Subjects also walked faster with an increasing haptic speed cue and increased stride height and stride length while using the motorized walker with a speed cue above the medium speed range. We also observed that test subjects walking with a conventional walker and a motorized walker exhibited less double support time out of the gait cycle time. When walking with the motorized walker on a medium speed cue, subjects had on average 4.88% less double support time, which indicated a faster gait initiation under this condition.

2. Related Work

Human gait is the periodic movement of limbs, trunk, and arms during locomotion. The bipedal gait cycle consists of right-side and left-side steps. De Rossi et al. introduced a six-phase gait model, where each side has an initial, a swing, and a stance phase [14]. An eight-phase gait model was introduced that expands the initial phase into two additional sub phases: Initial contact and loading response phases [15]. Gait cycle time, stride length, stride height, gait initiation, and other gait parameters are of interest to clinicians in understanding the disease progression of patients with PD [13,16]. The stance phase for the control subjects occupies approximately 60% of the gait cycle, and the swing phase occupies the remaining 40% [17]. Individuals with PD have difficulty controlling balance and gait, which can lead to falling, injury, dependence, and loss of quality of life. Individuals with PD have shorter steps, reduced stride height, and extended stance phase compared to the healthy controls [18]. Impaired balance and gait, including freezing of gait, in PD has been attributed in part to changes in attention. Freezing of gait often occurs during situations requiring gait changes or divided attention such as turning or narrow passages [19]. PD subjects who experience freezing of gait have distinctive impairments in the bilateral coordination of locomotion [20].

External spatial and temporal cues help people with PD to overcome slowing of their gate. Auditory timing cues can have positive rehabilitative effects on various gait characteristics of PD [21], stroke [22], and hemiparesis [23] patients. For patients with PD, visual cues have shown to improve stride length, while auditory cues have shown to improve cadence [21]. However, the beneficial effects on gait can disappear when the visual and attentional cues are removed [24] . Thus, the cues should always be present to maintain their rehabilitative effects. Haptic cues from non-supportive manual contact with an external surface provides somatosensory information that individuals with poor balance improve the control of upright standing during intervention programs [25,26]. Such cues from assistive ambulatory devices such as walking canes and walkers might also improve stability and orientation during gait, but at the cost of reducing walking speed. People with PD walked with slower gait speed and reduced stride length when using a cane and a wheeled walker compared to walking without any device [27]. However, PD subjects produced natural gait pattern when using a wheeled walker, by not slowing velocity or increasing variability as other devices do [28]. In our present study, we tested whether gait of people with PD would improve when following haptic speed cues from a self-propelled walker, self-navigating walker.

3. Methods

In this study, we collected spatiotemporal postural and gait data from six PD subjects walking in a predesigned course via the VICON motion capture system (Vicon, Denver, CO, USA) under three conditions of manual gait aids: none (without assistance), with a conventional rolling walker, and with a motorized walker, where the motorized walker can be configured to operate at three different speed ranges: Low (32–52 cm/s), medium (52–72 cm/s), and high (72–96 cm/s). The speed is measured without any payload, where the walker's movement is propelled by its motors without users holding on to it to move around. We applied statistical analysis on the extracted gait features to determine the significance of the gait modifications and used asymmetry index [29] to analyze the bilateral coordination of the locomotion.

3.1. Subjects and Protocols

Six PD patients (five males and one female) between the ages of 44 and 77 (median: 66) and at Hoehn and Yahr stages 2–3, were recruited at the New York Institute of Technology College of Osteopathic Medicine to participate in this study. This study was reviewed and approved by New York Institute of Technology (NYIT) Institutional Review Board.The Unified Parkinson's Disease Rating Scale (UPDRS) scores for the subjects ranged from 18 to 33, and Mini-Mental State Examination (MMSE) scores ranged from 26 to 30. Years diagnosed was between 1 and 27 years (median: 24). Each patient was instructed to walk in a preset course for 5 meters including a 90-degree turn under the following haptic cue conditions: (1) Without assistance, (2) with a conventional walker, and (3) with a motorized walker with various speed cues.

Task: With each of the three experimental conditions, patients walked alongside a 25-foot board, then proceeded to make a 90 degree turn, and continued walking alongside another 25-foot board. The two boards were at a right angle to each other, and the patients walked on the left side of each board.

For each patient, two to three trials of walking without assistance, two to three trials of walking with a conventional walker, and six to ten trials of walking with a motorized walker were recorded. Incomplete trials were excluded from the study. Notations representing each trial are listed in Table 1. The speed configurations of the walker in this table are measured at zero load, which indicates that the walker is moving untethered, i.e., without having a patient holding on to it.

Table 1. Trial notations.

Notation	Definition
c	walking without assistance
mxx	walking with motorized walker, trial number XX
ml	walking with motorized walker, low speed cue: $[32, 52)$ cm/s
mm	walking with motorized walker, medium speed cue: $[52, 72)$ cm/s
mh	walking with motorized walker, high speed cue: $[72, 96)$ cm/s
w	walking with conventional walker

3.2. Apparatus

A nine-camera VICON motion capture system (Vicon, Denver CO) with a sampling rate of 100 Hz was used for recording the gait and postural parameters of the subjects by measuring ongoing position of reflective markers attached to the following body landmarks: Bilateral metatarsals, achilles tendons, lateral collateral ligaments of the knees, iliac crests, wrists, and acromions as shown in Figure 1. Two additional markers were placed on each walker.

A motorized walker as shown in Figure 2 was designed to provide speed control and navigation in a preset course [30] by instrumenting a conventional walker with two 64 mm, 12 V gear head motors (Am Equipment, Jefferson, OR) on the rear wheels, a URG-04LX-UG01 laser range sensor (Hokuyo Osaka, Japan, 2015), and a micro-controller board (stored inside the compartment under the walker seat).

The motorized walker was configured to move forward and turn at various pre-set speeds. When using the walker, the user holds the handles of the walker where a haptic cue is provided with the automatic movement of the walker that leads the user to move and turn at a pre-set speed. Table 2 shows the various speed configurations for the motorized walker. As an example, let us consider the *m*01 trial, i.e., the first trial with the motorized walker. The motorized walker accelerates up to the maximum speed of 32 cm/s. The average acceleration is 24 cm/s^2 and the acceleration time is 0.06 s to reach the maximum speed. The configuration parameters can be changed depending on the movement ability of PD patients. In this study, some patients had trials with up to the 80 cm/s maximum haptic speed cue. Upon sensing an obstacle in its path, as a safety measure, the motorized walker proportionally decreases its speed and comes to a full stop.

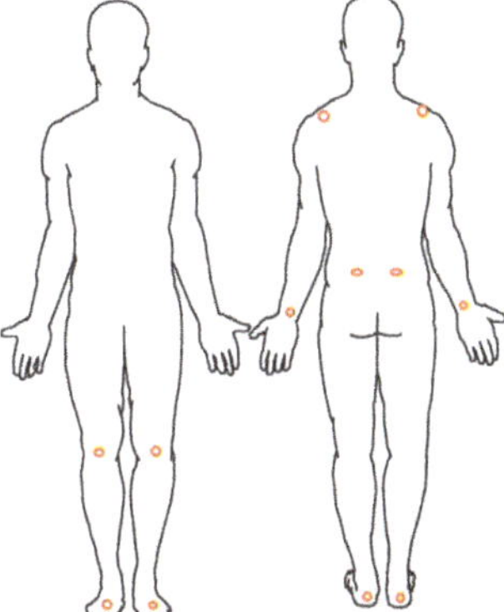

Figure 1. Red circles show the location of the retroreflective markers.

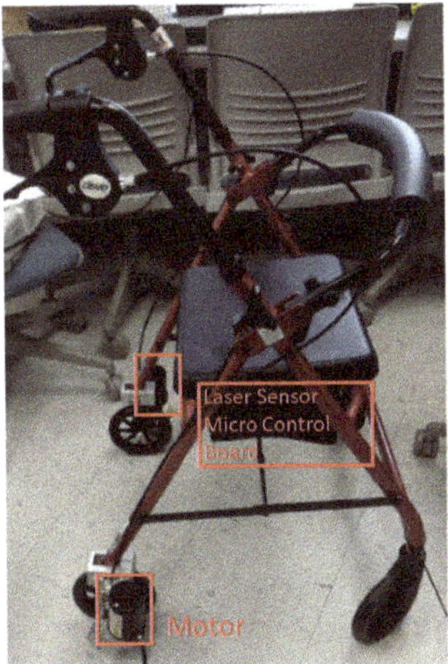

Figure 2. The motorized walker with speed control, preset course navigation, and obstacle avoidance.

Table 2. Speed settings for trials with the motorized walker.

Trial No.	Speed Range	Max Speed [cm/s]	Acceleration [cm/s^2]	Accel. Time [s]
m01	ml	32	24	0.06
m02	ml	44	24	0.06
m03	mm	52	24	0.06
m04	mm	60	20	0.1
m05	mm	64	20	0.1
m06	mh	72	12	0.2
m07	mh	80	12	0.2

3.3. Data Analysis

Gait is a complex sensorimotor activity that involves spatiotemporal coordination of the legs, trunk, arms, and dynamic equilibrium, all of which are affected by PD. Table 3 outlines the terminology used in the description of the gait model. The duration of a complete gait cycle is defined as the *gait cycle time* (GCT) [14,31] and shown in Figure 3a. GCT is divided into two phases: *Stance time* (ST) and *swing time* (SW). ST denotes the duration when the foot is on the floor, while SW denotes the duration when the foot is in the air. *Double support* (DS) denotes the period when both feet are on the floor. DS can be divided into *initial double support* (IDS), which denotes the duration between the initial foot's heel contact and the other foot's toe off, and *terminal double support* (TDS), which denotes the duration of the subsequent opposite-side heel contact and toe off [32].

Table 3. Terminology.

Terminology	Definition
GCT	Gait Cycle Time
SW	Swing Time
ST	Stance Time
DS	Double Support
IDS	Initial Double Support
TDS	Terminal Double Support
SH	Step Height
SL	Step Length

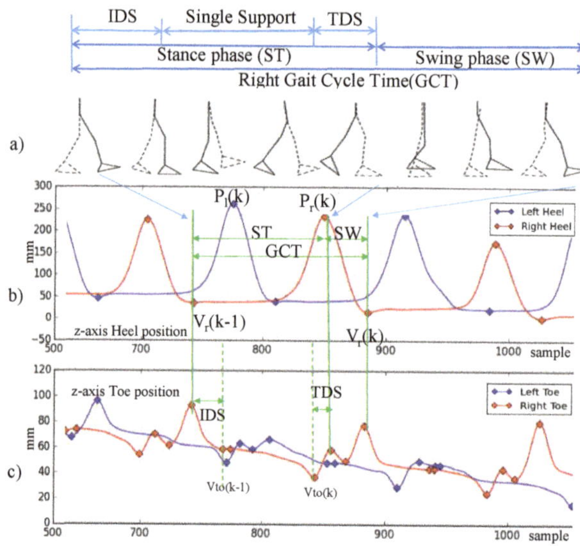

Figure 3. Gait cycle model. (**a**) Gait cycle model (**b**) z-axis heel position (**c**) z-axis toe position.

The gait parameters are calculated based on the spatiotemporal measurement of the marker locations attached on the subject's body. As shown in Figure 3b,c, we use the vertical heel and toe positions to identify the gait phases. We use the following spatial location measurements in identifying gait events and calculating gait parameters: $V(k)$ denotes the kth valley of the heel position in z-axis, $P(k)$ denotes the kth peak of the heel position in z-axis, and V_{to} denotes the nearest valley of the toe position in z-axis.

Gait Cycle Time (GCT) is calculated as the duration between two consecutive valleys of the heel position as:

$$GCT(k) = V(k) - V(k - 1) \tag{1}$$

Swing Time (SW) is calculated as the duration between two consecutive valley and peak of the heel position:

$$SW(k) = V(k) - P(k) \tag{2}$$

Stance Time (ST) is the remaining period of a GCT minus swing time:

$$ST(k) = GCT(k) - SW(k) \tag{3}$$

Initial Double Support (IDS) time is the duration between the valley of the heel position and its nearest valley of the toe position:

$$IDS(k) = V_{to} - V(k) \tag{4}$$

Terminal Double Support (TDS) time is the duration between the peak of the heel position and its nearest valley of the toe position:

$$TDS(k) = P(k) - V_{to} \tag{5}$$

Step height is the difference between the peak of the heel position and its nearest valley position:

$$SH(k) = P(k) - V(k - 1) \tag{6}$$

Step length is defined as the difference between the x coordinate of the heel position between two consecutive peaks:

$$SL(k) = P_x(k) - P_x(k - 1) \tag{7}$$

where the subscript x indicates the x coordinate. Finally, velocity is defined as the ratio of step length over gait cycle time:

$$Vel = \frac{SL}{GCT} \tag{8}$$

Previous studies showed that the ratio of stance/swing of healthy subjects is about 3:2 [33,34]. IDS warrants the upright stability during walking [35]. It reduces to zero when a subject is running, which means both feet are airborne twice during the gait cycle [36]. Sofuwa et al. [37] also showed that PD patients have decreased gait speed and stride length and increased double support time.

Morris et al. [38] reported that patients in the earlier stages of PD may have extended stance time which allows PD subjects maintain their gait stability. The IDS may increase in the the late stage of PD. This long IDS can give the impression that the PD subjects *glue* their feet on the ground.

4. Signal Processing for Gait Analysis

In this Section, we introduce the signal processing procedure for gait signal analysis. A block diagram of the procedure is outlined in Figure 4.

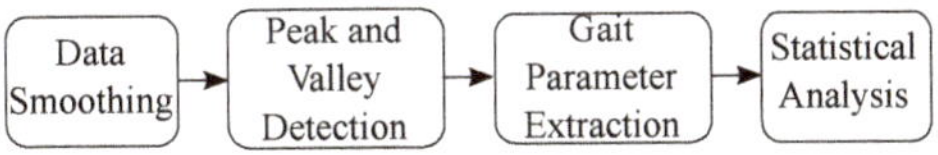

Figure 4. Signal processing procedure for gait analysis.

First, we smoothed raw data to remove noise and identify gait cycle based on [39] through peak and valley detections. Then, we extracted the gait parameters following the definition in Section 3.

Finally we studied the statistical significance of the observations. We explain each procedure in detail in the following section.

4.1. Data Smoothing

To remove noise in the measured signal to find peaks and valleys, two types of filters were evaluated for data smoothing: (1) Convolution [40], and (2) Savitzky-Golay low-pass filter [41]. Convolution did not decrease the amplitude of the signal and retained more of the gait details, and in general performed better than Savitzky-Golay low-pass filter in this context. Thus, we chose convolution for smoothing. A 40-sample Hanning window is used for convolution, so that the window size is less than half of the gait cycle time (0.5 s).

4.2. Peak and Valley Detection and Principle Gait Parameters Extraction

We implemented the peak and valley detection algorithm in Python based on the algorithm presented by Ferrari et al. [42]. We used the *argrelextrema* function from the SciPy Python library's signal processing toolbox [43] to identify the peak and valley candidates. Portions of the data that correspond to the turning phase might still be mistaken as peaks and valleys. To remove the turning phase peaks and valleys detection errors, only one peak between two valleys and only one valley between two peaks were selected. Figure 5 shows the peaks and valleys identified after the smoothing operation is completed and turning phase peaks and valleys are removed. Once the peaks and valleys are identified SW, ST, IDS, SL, and SH are calculated using (2)–(7).

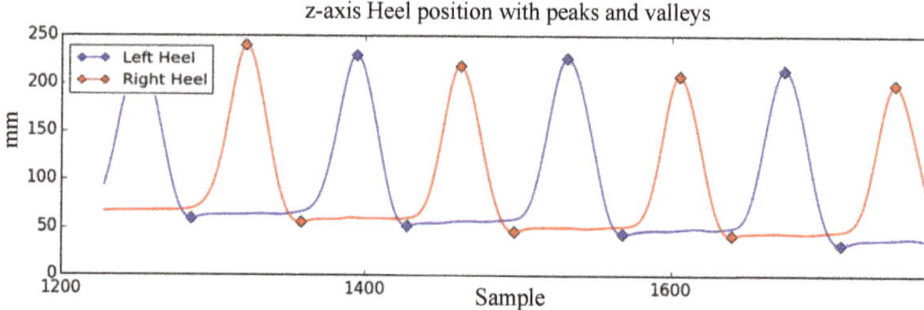

Figure 5. Peaks and valleys of z-axis heel position.

4.3. Statistical Analysis

In this study, we are interested in the variability among different sets of trials when subjects walk without assistance, with a conventional walker, and with a motorized walker providing haptic speed cues. Towards that goal, we evaluated the mean and standard deviation from the five sets of trials (c, ml, mm, mh, w) and applied statistical hypothesis testing. First, we apply Shapiro-Wilk test to verify that the data follow normal distribution ($p > 0.05$), then we applied t-test (alpha = 0.05) to test the null hypothesis that the gait parameters do not vary whether the patient is walking without assistance, or using a conventional walker or a motorized walker.

5. Results

In this Section, we present the results comparing the gait parameters observed at different trials and analyze gait symmetry and individual gait performance.

5.1. Gait Parameters

Table 4 shows the spatiotemporal gait parameters for all subjects measured (mean ± SD) for different trials, i.e., walking without assistance (c), walking with a conventional walker (w), and walking with the motorized walker (m) with low (ml), medium (mm), and high (mh) speed cues.

The subjects' walking speed follows the cueing speed of the motorized walker. More specifically, PD subjects walking velocity is 29.24 ± 7.94 cm/s on low speed cues; 52.80 ± 10.56 cm/s on medium speed cues; and 67.33 ± 11.67 cm/s on high speed cues.

We observed that the stride height and stride length also increase as the cueing speed increases. At the lowest cueing speed, the subjects have the lowest stride height (SH: 14.52 ± 4.09 cm) and shortest stride length (SL: 49.72 ± 12.58 cm). At the highest cueing speed, the subjects have the highest stride height (SH: 21.08 ± 2.97 cm) and length (SL: 74.76 ± 12.11 cm).

In Table 5, we show that there was a significant difference in walking patterns for subjects walking with the motorized walker with medium speed cue (mm) and walking without any assistance (c) in all gait parameters ($p < 0.05$) with the exception of IDS ($p = 0.059$). Conversely, the difference is insignificant between walking without assistance and motorized walker with high speed cue (mh), and conventional walker (w) in all gait parameters with the following exceptions for both cases: SW, SL, and Vel, where the differences are significant ($p < 0.05$). These results suggest that motorized walker at medium speed cues has the largest gait modification in PD subjects.

Table 6 summarizes the ratio of ST, IDS, and TDS periods in a gait cycle. Accordingly, the motorized walker reduces the PD subjects' ST over GCT when the speed cues increase (74.40%, 73.10%, 71.53% respectively in ml, mm, mh). This suggests that PD subjects use less time on the ground when the speed cue increases. PD subjects walking without assistance present higher IDS and TDS to GCT ratios ($IDS/GCT = 18.75\%$, $TDS/GCT = 16.88\%$), while PD subjects walking with motorized walker on medium speed cues (mm) have lower ratios ($IDS/GCT = 15.66\%$, $TDS/GCT = 15.09\%$). This corresponds to 3.09% and 1.79% lower IDS/GCT, and TDS/GCT ratios, respectively. These observations may indicate PD subjects have less hesitation in initiating a step when walking with motorized walker on medium speed cues.

Table 4. Mean and standard deviation of gait parameters for Parkinson's disease (PD) subjects walking without assistance (c), with conventional walker (w), and with motorized walker (m) at low (ml), medium (mm), and high (mh) speed cues.

Gait Parameters			m		
(unit)	c	w	ml	mm	mh
GCT (s)	1.29 ± 0.25	1.34 ± 0.21	1.68 ± 0.28	1.4 ± 0.2	1.31 ± 0.13
SW (s)	0.35 ± 0.05	0.39 ± 0.06	0.43 ± 0.10	0.38 ± 0.06	0.38 ± 0.06
ST (s)	0.94 ± 0.22	0.95 ± 0.2	1.25 ± 0.28	1.02 ± 0.17	0.94 ± 0.1
IDS (s)	0.24 ± 0.69	0.24 ± 0.11	0.28 ± 0.14	0.22 ± 0.01	0.21 ± 0.06
TDS (s)	0.22 ± 0.03	0.22 ± 0.12	0.25 ± 0.13	0.21 ± 0.13	0.21 ± 0.05
SL (cm)	92.98 ± 1.24	70.61 ± 27.70	49.72 ± 12.58	68.59 ± 11.86	74.76 ± 12.11
SH (cm)	21.19 ± 3.14	20.78 ± 3.40	14.52 ± 4.09	19.02 ± 3.31	21.08 ± 2.97
Vel (cm/s)	75.28 ± 12.99	65.89 ± 17.36	29.24 ± 7.94	52.80 ± 10.56	67.33 ± 11.67

Table 5. *p*-values for the pairwise comparison of gait parameters for PD subjects walking without and with motorized walker.

Gait Parameters	Pairwise Comparison of *p*-Value		
(unit)	c vs. mm	c vs. mh	c vs. w
GCT (s)	0.006	0.459	0.245
SW (s)	0.014	0.025	0.002
ST (s)	0.016	0.959	0.686
IDS (s)	0.059	0.754	0.216
TDS (s)	0.004	0.142	0.154
SL (cm)	$\ll 0.01$	0.001	$\ll 0.01$
SH (cm)	0.001	0.866	0.583
Vel (cm/s)	$\ll 0.01$	0.002	0.07

Table 6. The ratio of stance time (*ST*), initial double support (*IDS*), and terminal double support (*TDS*) in a gait cycle.

Gait Parameters		m			
	c	ml	mm	mh	w
ST/GCT	72.76%	74.40%	73.10%	71.53%	70.98%
IDS/GCT	18.75%	16.78%	15.66%	15.72%	17.48%
TDS/GCT	16.88%	14.94%	15.09%	16.18%	16.59%
IDS/ST	25.77%	22.56%	21.43%	21.98%	24.63%
TDS/ST	22.45%	20.08%	20.65%	22.62%	23.37%

5.2. Gait Symmetry

Gait symmetry is defined as the perfect agreement between the actions of the lower limbs [44]. *Asymmetry index*, denoted as I_a can be used to quantify gait symmetry or asymmetry [29]:

$$I_a = \frac{X_L - X_R}{\max(X_L, X_R)} \times 100 \tag{9}$$

where, $X \in [GCT, SH, SL, \text{Vel}]$, and subscripts L and R represent left side and right side, respectively. $I_a \in [-1, 0)$ represents right asymmetry (i.e., the value of the gait parameter is higher on the right side), and $I_a \in (0, 1]$ represents left asymmetry. $I_a = 0$ when there is no asymmetry.

Table 7 shows the asymmetry indices of gait parameters. Our results indicate that PD subjects exhibit better overall gait symmetry when they use a motorized or conventional walker compared to walking without assistance. The GCT asymmetry indices ($I_{a,GCT}$) of motorized walker (below 0.1 to 0.56%) or conventional walker (0.53%) are much lower than walking without assistance (6.7%).

Table 7. Asymmetry indices for straight walking.

Gait Parameters		m			
	c	ml	mm	mh	w
$I_{a,GCT}$	6.7%	0.56%	<0.1%	<0.1%	0.53%
$I_{a,SH}$	5.7%	−3.99%	3.46%	2.12%	1.48%
$I_{a,SL}$	−1.8%	−2.10%	1.44%	1.33%	−3.25%
$I_{a,\text{Vel}}$	3.4%	−9.50%	1.48%	2.03%	−2.75%

For the stride height asymmetry index ($I_{a,SH}$), similarly, the subjects have more symmetric foot-raising posture with either of the walkers compared to walking without assistance (5.7%). Subjects using the conventional walker (1.48%) show better stride height symmetry compared to using the motorized walker (between −3.99 and 2.12%). For the stride length and velocity asymmetry index ($I_{a,SL}$, $I_{a,\text{Vel}}$), subjects using the motorized walker with medium and high speed cues show better symmetry with regards to stride length ($I_{a,SL}$) at 1.41% and 1.33%, respectively compared to walking without assistance and walking with the conventional walker.

5.3. Individual Gait Performance

In this Section, we study the individual PD subject's (P1–P6) trials and compare the results of gait performance for each individual. To determine whether cue speed affects (1) the quality of gait performance matching the cue speed and/or (2) amelioration of PD gait symptoms, we organize the trials such that, for each subject, the speed cue starts at a low speed, and gradually increases to higher speeds.

Figure 6a–f show the GCT for each subject for different trials (based on the notation introduced in Table 1). Each bar corresponds to the mean GCT value for a different trial in seconds. The blue bars represent the mean values for the left side, orange bars represent the mean values for the right side, and the error bars indicate the variance of GCT for each case. Trials with noisy or corrupted data due to the data acquisition issues are excluded. The individual GCT bar chart indicates PD subjects need time to adapt to the motorized walker. We observe that PD subjects have high GCT and GCT variance when they start to use the motorized walker. However, after the first one to three trials, GCT drops to a relatively lower level and fluctuates in a smaller range. For instance, for subject P1, GCT $\in [1.5, 1.7]$ during the first three trials using the motorized walker, but drops to $[1.3, 1.4]$ after that.

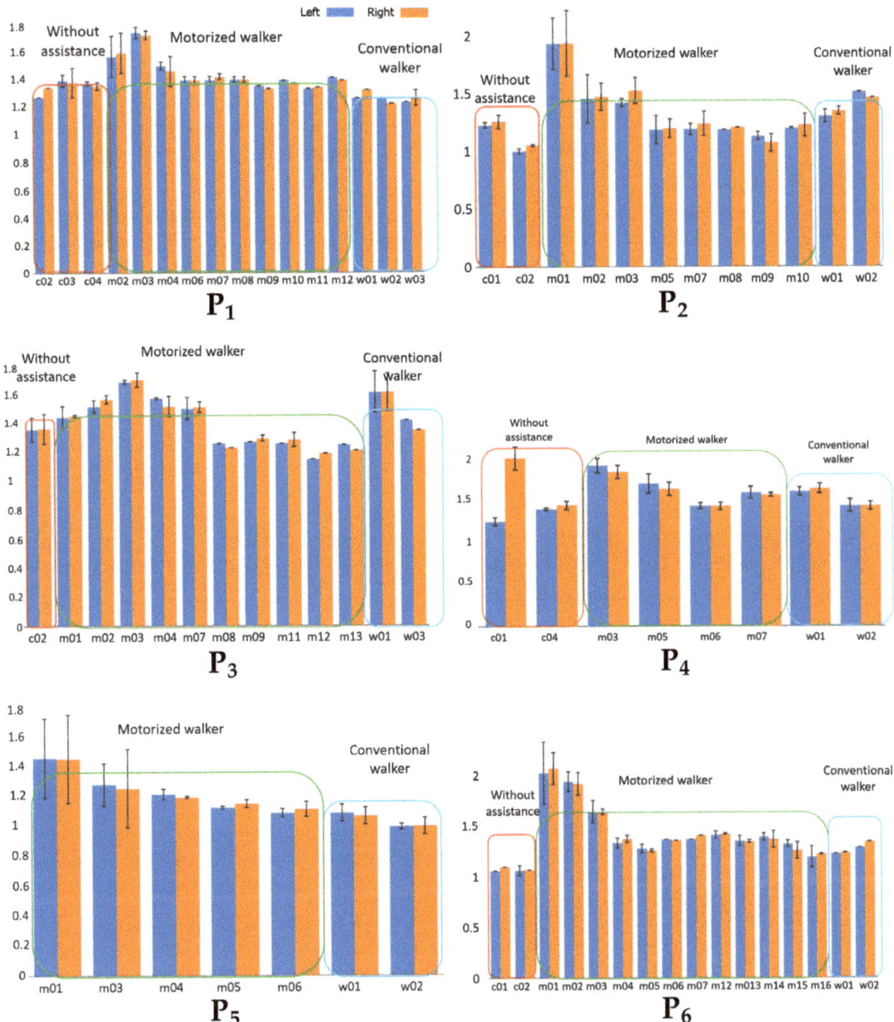

Figure 6. Gait cycle time (GCT) for each of the 6 subjects (P_1–P_6) without assistance, with motorized walker, and with conventional walker.

6. Discussion

In this study, we observed that the study subjects using a motorized walker exhibit a walking pattern with more symmetric performance on both sides. The study subjects' walking velocity increased as the speed cue increased. We also observed that study subjects required a few trials to get used to the motorized walker. While initial trial shows large variabilities, as the number of trials increases, GCT variability decreases. Our study provides further evidence that PD subjects exhibit a natural gait pattern, when using a wheeled walker without slowing down [28]. The subjects' gait performance under different haptic speed cues also provide insights on immediate gait modification under these speed cues conditions.

Although, with six subjects, the current study can provide some insights, a wider perspective can be achieved if the sample size is increased in a future study. In particular, more subjects at each PD stage, and more subjects based on years from diagnosis and age can help evaluate the efficacy of the motorized walker at different stages of the disease.

The availability of a large group of subjects can also enable protocols that can evaluate parameters at higher granularity. Another possible extension to this work is to reverse the order of the speed cues, starting from higher speed cues to lower speeds to see the impact on the adaptation of using the motorized walker. Conversely, speed cues can also be randomized to investigate the impact of initial cues to the overall adaptation.

Hausdorff et al. [20,45] have proposed that gait control impairments (gait asymmetry, and bilateral dyscoordination), even during periods in which freezing is not present, set the stage for the occurrence of a freezing of gait (FOG) episode. Our study shows that the walker can immediately modify the gait regulation of PD subjects, demonstrating more bilateral gait symmetry. In this case, it can be hypothesized that the motorized walker providing haptic cues can possibly improve the bilateral coordination of locomotion and can potentially reduce the FOG occurrence in PD subjects. Future work with a long-term use of the motorized walker will allow enough FOG episodes to be observed. In parallel, new analytic models should be developed to provide quantitative analysis of gait performance to evaluate the efficacy of the intervention.

7. Conclusions

We studied the immediate gait modifications of individuals with Parkinson's disease, comparing between walking without assistance to walking with a conventional and a self-navigating motorized walker that provides haptic speed cues. We observed that the subjects' gait exhibited more symmetry with reduced initial double support time when walking with a walker compared to walking without assistance. When using a motorized walker with medium speed cues, subjects' IDS and TDS ratios to GCT were reduced by 3.09%, and 1.78% compared to walking without assistance, respectively, with an overall 4.88% reduction in double support time. During the individual analysis, we observed a learning curve for the subjects to get used to the motorized walker. This usually took one to three trials, after which GCT variability was reduced. The test subjects' walking velocity was strongly related to the speed cues. When the cueing speed increased, we observed a decrease in the GCT, SW, ST, and IDS, while SL, SH, and velocity increased. Reduced step initiation time and increased stride length and height indicated improvement in gait for the test subjects. The gait improvements indicate the test subjects exhibit a gait pattern closer to healthy controls with better gait symmetry and balance. More symmetry in bilateral locomotion is promising for improved balance of the subjects in reducing potential fall risks. The motorized walker can be adopted as a rehabilitation device in gait training. The use of a customized motorized walker also has potential to mitigate the freezing of gait episodes by providing continuous haptic cues for subjects to follow without divided attention.

Author Contributions: E.R. and Z.D. conceived and designed the study; L.G., S.S. and E.R. conducted subject recruitment and data collection; M.Z., N.S.A., H.G., and Z.D. conducted data processing and statistical analysis; M.Z. and N.S.A. prepared the manuscript; all authors contributed to the editing and proofreading of the manuscript.

Funding: This research is partially funded by a New York Institute of Technology Institutional Support for Research and Creativity (ISRC) grant.

Conflicts of Interest: The authors declare no conflict of interest.

Ethics Statement: All subjects gave their informed consent for inclusion before they participated in the study. The study was conducted in accordance with the Declaration of Helsinki, and the protocol was approved by the Ethics Committee, the Institution Review Board (IRB) of New York Institute of Technology (Protocol BHS-892).

References

1. Morris, M.E. Movement disorders in people with Parkinson disease: A model for physical therapy. *Phys. Therapy* **2000**, *80*, 578.
2. Jankovic, J. Parkinson's disease: Clinical features and diagnosis. *J. Neurol. Neurosurg. Psychiatry* **2008**, *79*, 368–376. [CrossRef] [PubMed]
3. Stolze, H.; Kuhtz-Buschbeck, J.P.; Drücke, H.; Jöhnk, K.; Illert, M.; Deuschl, G. Comparative analysis of the gait disorder of normal pressure hydrocephalus and Parkinson's disease. *J. Neurol. Neurosurg. Psychiatry* **2001**, *70*, 289–297. [CrossRef] [PubMed]
4. Jöbges, M.; Heuschkel, G.; Pretzel, C.; Illhardt, C.; Renner, C.; Hummelsheim, H. Repetitive training of compensatory steps: A therapeutic approach for postural instability in Parkinson's disease. *J. Neurol. Neurosurg. Psychiatry* **2004**, *75*, 1682–1687. [CrossRef] [PubMed]
5. Protas, E.J.; Mitchell, K.; Williams, A.; Qureshy, H.; Caroline, K.; Lai, E.C. Gait and step training to reduce falls in Parkinson's disease. *Neuro Rehabil.* **2005**, *20*, 183–190.
6. McCandless, P.J.; Evans, B.J.; Janssen, J.; Selfe, J.; Churchill, A.; Richards, J. Effect of three cueing devices for people with Parkinson's disease with gait initiation difficulties. *Gait Posture* **2016**, *44*, 7–11. [CrossRef] [PubMed]
7. Rabin, E.; Chen, J.; Muratori, L.; DiFrancisco-Donoghue, J.; Werner, W.G. Haptic feedback from manual contact improves balance control in people with Parkinson's disease. *Gait Posture* **2013**, *38*, 373–379. [CrossRef] [PubMed]
8. Franzén, E.; Gurfinkel, V.S.; Wright, W.G.; Cordo, P.J.; Horak, F.B. Haptic touch reduces sway by increasing axial tone. *Neuroscience* **2011**, *174*, 216–223. [CrossRef] [PubMed]
9. Gallagher, R.; Damodaran, H.; Werner, W.G.; Powell, W.; Deutsch, J.E. Auditory and visual cueing modulate cycling speed of older adults and persons with Parkinson's disease in a Virtual Cycling (V-Cycle) system. *J. Neuro Eng. Rehabil.* **2016**, *13*, 77. [CrossRef] [PubMed]
10. McIntosh, G.C.; Brown, S.H.; Rice, R.R.; Thaut, M.H. Rhythmic auditory-motor facilitation of gait patterns in patients with Parkinson's disease. *J. Neurol. Neurosurg. Psychiatry* **1997**, *62*, 22–26. [CrossRef] [PubMed]
11. Boonsinsukh, R.; Saengsirisuwan, V.; Carlson-Kuhta, P.; Horak, F.B. A cane improves postural recovery from an unpracticed slip during walking in people with Parkinson disease. *Phys. Therapy* **2012**, *92*, 1117. [CrossRef] [PubMed]
12. Pun, U.K.; Gu, H.; Dong, Z.; Artan, N.S. Classification and visualization tool for gait analysis of Parkinson's disease. In Proceedings of 38th Annual International Conference of the IEEE Engineering in Medicine and Biology Society (EMBC), Orlando, FL, USA, 16–20 Augest, 2016; pp. 2407–2410.
13. Hausdorff, J.M. Gait dynamics in Parkinson's disease: common and distinct behavior among stride length, gait variability, and fractal-like scaling. *Chaos Interdisciplin. J. Nonlinear Sci.* **2009**, *19*, 026113. [CrossRef] [PubMed]
14. De Rossi, S.; Crea, S.; Donati, M.; Reberšek, P.; Novak, D.; Vitiello, N.; Lenzi, T.; Podobnik, J.; Munih, M.; Carrozza, M. Gait segmentation using bipedal foot pressure patterns. In Proceedings of The Fourth IEEE RAS/EMBS International Conference on Biomedical Robotics and Biomechatronics, Roma, Italy, 24–27 June, 2012; pp. 361–366.
15. Kong, K.; Tomizuka, M. Smooth and continuous human gait phase detection based on foot pressure patterns. In Proceedings of 2008 IEEE International Conference on Robotics and Automation, Pasadena, CA, USA, 19–23 May 2008; pp. 3678–3683.
16. König, N.; Singh, N.B.; Baumann, C.R.; Taylor, W.R. Can Gait Signatures Provide Quantitative Measures for Aiding Clinical Decision-Making? A Systematic Meta-Analysis of Gait Variability Behavior in Patients with Parkinson's Disease. *Front. Human Neurosci.* **2016**, *10*, 319. [CrossRef] [PubMed]
17. Alvarez-Alvarez, A.; Trivino, G. Linguistic description of the human gait quality. *Eng. Appl. Artif. Intell.* **2013**, *26*, 13–23. [CrossRef]
18. Frenkel-Toledo, S.; Giladi, N.; Peretz, C.; Herman, T.; Gruendlinger, L.; Hausdorff, J.M. Effect of gait speed on gait rhythmicity in Parkinson's disease: Variability of stride time and swing time respond differently. *J. Neuroeng. Rehabil.* **2005**, *2*, 23. [CrossRef] [PubMed]

19. Spildooren, J.; Vercruysse, S.; Desloovere, K.; Vandenberghe, W.; Kerckhofs, E.; Nieuwboer, A. Freezing of gait in Parkinson's disease: The impact of dual-tasking and turning. *Mov. Disord.* **2010**, *25*, 2563–2570. [CrossRef] [PubMed]

20. Plotnik, M.; Giladi, N.; Hausdorff, J.M. Bilateral coordination of walking and freezing of gait in Parkinson's disease. *Eur. J. Neurosci.* **2008**, *27*, 1999–2006. [CrossRef] [PubMed]

21. Suteerawattananon, M.; Morris, G.; Etnyre, B.; Jankovic, J.; Protas, E. Effects of visual and auditory cues on gait in individuals with Parkinson's disease. *J. Neurol. Sci.* **2004**, *219*, 63–69. [CrossRef] [PubMed]

22. Roerdink, M.; Lamoth, C.J.; van Kordelaar, J.; Elich, P.; Konijnenbelt, M.; Kwakkel, G.; Beek, P.J. Rhythm perturbations in acoustically paced treadmill walking after stroke. *Neurorehabil. Neural Repair* **2009**, *23*, 668–678. [CrossRef] [PubMed]

23. Patton, J.L.; Kovic, M.; Mussa-Ivaldi, F.A. Custom-designed haptic training for restoring reaching ability to individuals with poststroke hemiparesis. *J. Rehabil. Res. Dev.* **2006**, *43*, 643. [CrossRef] [PubMed]

24. Morris, M.E.; Iansek, R.; Matyas, T.A.; Summers, J.J. Stride length regulation in Parkinson's disease. *Brain* **1996**, *119*, 551–568. [CrossRef] [PubMed]

25. Baldan, A.; Alouche, S.; Araujo, I.; Freitas, S. Effect of light touch on postural sway in individuals with balance problems: a systematic review. *Gait Posture* **2014**, *40*, 1–10. [CrossRef] [PubMed]

26. Shull, P.B.; Damian, D.D. Haptic wearables as sensory replacement, sensory augmentation and trainer–A review. *J. Rehabil. Res. Dev.* **2015**, *12*, 59. [CrossRef] [PubMed]

27. Bryant, M.S.; Pourmoghaddam, A.; Thrasher, A. Gait changes with walking devices in persons with Parkinson's disease. *Disabil. Rehabil. Assistive Technol.* **2012**, *7*, 149–152. [CrossRef] [PubMed]

28. Kegelmeyer, D.A.; Parthasarathy, S.; Kostyk, S.K.; White, S.E.; Kloos, A.D. Assistive devices alter gait patterns in Parkinson disease: Advantages of the four-wheeled walker. *Gait Posture* **2013**, *38*, 20–24. [CrossRef] [PubMed]

29. Vagenas, G.; Hoshizaki, B. A multivariable analysis of lower extremity kinematic asymmetry in running. *Inter. J. Sport Biomech.* **1992**, *8*, 11–29. [CrossRef]

30. Rabin, E.; Dong, Z. Motorized walker, 2018. US Patent 9,968,507, 15 May, 2018.

31. Salarian, A.; Russmann, H.; Vingerhoets, F.J.; Dehollain, C.; Blanc, Y.; Burkhard, P.R.; Aminian, K. Gait assessment in Parkinson's disease: Toward an ambulatory system for long-term monitoring. *Trans. Biomed. Eng.* **2004**, *51*, 1434–1443. [CrossRef] [PubMed]

32. Zijlstra, W.; Hof, A.L. Assessment of spatio-temporal gait parameters from trunk accelerations during human walking. *Gait Posture* **2003**, *18*, 1–10. [CrossRef]

33. Rahul, A.; Mohanty, R.; Tharion, G. Effectiveness of an Articulated Knee Hyperextension Orthosis in Genu Recurvatum. *Online J. Health Allied. Scs.* **2014**, *13*, 8.

34. Winter, D.A.; Patla, A.E.; Frank, J.S.; Walt, S.E. Biomechanical walking pattern changes in the fit and healthy elderly. *Phys. Therapy* **1990**, *70*, 340–347. [CrossRef]

35. Ounpuu, S. The biomechanics of walking and running. *Clinics Sports Med.* **1994**, *13*, 843–863.

36. Novacheck, T.F. The biomechanics of running. *Gait Posture* **1998**, *7*, 77–95. [CrossRef]

37. Sofuwa, O.; Nieuwboer, A.; Desloovere, K.; Willems, A.M.; Chavret, F.; Jonkers, I. Quantitative gait analysis in Parkinson's disease: Comparison with a healthy control group. *Arch. Phys. Med. Rehabil.* **2005**, *86*, 1007–1013. [CrossRef] [PubMed]

38. Morris, M.E.; Iansek, R.; Matyas, T.A.; Summers, J.J. Ability to modulate walking cadence remains intact in Parkinson's disease. *J. Neurol. Neurosurg. Psychiatry* **1994**, *57*, 1532–1534. [CrossRef] [PubMed]

39. Boulgouris, N.V.; Hatzinakos, D.; Plataniotis, K.N. Gait recognition: A challenging signal processing technology for biometric identification. *Signal Process. Mag.* **2005**, *22*, 78–90, doi:10.1109/MSP.2005.1550191. [CrossRef]

40. Styblinski, M.; Tang, T.S. Experiments in nonconvex optimization: stochastic approximation with function smoothing and simulated annealing. *Neural Networks* **1990**, *3*, 467–483. [CrossRef]

41. Press, W.H.; Teukolsky, S.A. Savitzky-Golay Smoothing Filters. *Comp. Phys.* **1990**, *4*, 669–672. [CrossRef]

42. Ferrari, A.; Ginis, P.; Hardegger, M.; Casamassima, F.; Rocchi, L.; Chiari, L. A Mobile Kalman-Filter Based Solution for the Real-Time Estimation of Spatio-Temporal Gait Parameters. *Trans. Neural Syst. Rehabil. Engineering* **2016**, *24*, 764–773. [CrossRef] [PubMed]

43. SciPy.org, scipy.signal.argrelextrema. 2017. Avaliable online: https://docs.scipy.org/doc/scipy/reference/generated/scipy.signal.argrelextrema.html (accessed on 18 October 2018)

44. Herzog, W.; Nigg, B.M.; Read, L.J.; Olsson, E. Asymmetries in ground reaction force patterns in normal human gait. *Med. Sci. Sports Exerc.* **1989**, *21*, 110–114. [CrossRef] [PubMed]
45. Plotnik, M.; Hausdorff, J.M. The role of gait rhythmicity and bilateral coordination of stepping in the pathophysiology of freezing of gait in Parkinson's disease. *Mov. Disord.* **2008**, *23*. [CrossRef] [PubMed]

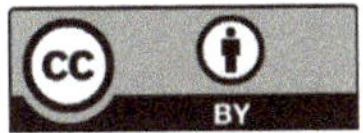

© 2018 by the authors. Licensee MDPI, Basel, Switzerland. This article is an open access article distributed under the terms and conditions of the Creative Commons Attribution (CC BY) license (http://creativecommons.org/licenses/by/4.0/).

MDPI
St. Alban-Anlage 66
4052 Basel
Switzerland
Tel. +41 61 683 77 34
Fax +41 61 302 89 18
www.mdpi.com

Sensors Editorial Office
E-mail: sensors@mdpi.com
www.mdpi.com/journal/sensors

www.ingramcontent.com/pod-product-compliance
Lightning Source LLC
LaVergne TN
LVHW071608170726

843515LV00008B/2347